PEDIATRIC INTENSIVE CARE

edited by

ELIEZER NUSSBAUM, M.D.
Associate Professor
Department of Pediatrics
University of California, Irvine
Director, Pediatric Pulmonary Center
and Intensive Care Unit
Miller Children's Hospital Medical Center
Long Beach, California

FUTURA PUBLISHING COMPANY
Mount Kisco, New York
1984

Published by
Futura Publishing Company, Inc.
295 Main Street, P.O. Box 330
Mount Kisco, New York 10549

L.C. #: 83-80676
ISBN #: 0-87993-199-X

Dedication

To Sara

Contributors

Stephen C. Aronoff, M.D., Assistant Professor of Pediatrics, Case Western Reserve University, School of Medicine, and Attending Physician, Rainbow Babies and Children's Hospital, Cleveland, Ohio

Morris J. Asch, M.D., Associate Clinical Professor of Surgery and Pediatrics, University of California, Los Angeles, Center for the Health Sciences, Los Angeles, California

James A. Baker, M.D., Associate Clinical Professor of Pathology, University of California Medical Center, Irvine, and Associate Pathologist, Memorial Hospital Medical Center, Long Beach, California

George Bisset, III, M.D., Assistant Professor of Pediatrics, Tulane University, School of Medicine, New Orleans, Louisiana

Laurence Carnay, M.D., Assistant Clinical Professor of Neurology, University of California Medical Center, Irvine, California

Barry B. Ceverha, M.D., Clinical Instructor of Neurological Surgery, University of Southern California, School of Medicine, and Director, Intensive Surgical and Trauma Unit, Memorial Hospital Medical Center, Long Beach, California

Seymour R. Cohen, M.D., F.A.A.P., Chief, Division of Otolaryngology, Children's Hospital of Los Angeles, and Clinical Professor of Surgery, University of Southern California, School of Medicine, Los Angeles, California

William Dean Davies, M.D., F.A.C.S., Clinical Assistant Professor of Surgery, University of Southern California, School of Medicine, Los Angeles, California

Martha I. Ellington, R.R.T., Respiratory Therapy Supervisor, Pediatric Intensive Care, Memorial Hospital Medical Center, Long Beach, California

Jerry Z. Finklestein, M.D., Adjunct Professor of Pediatrics, University of California, Los Angeles, School of Medicine, and Director, Pediatric Hematology and Oncology, Memorial Hospital Medical Center, and Chief, Division of Pediatric Hematology and Oncology, Harbor/UCLA Medical Center, Torrance, California

Barry Fisher, M.D., Associate Director, Pediatric Pulmonary Center, Good Samaritan Hospital, Phoenix, Arizona

Stanley P. Galant, M.D., Clinical Professor of Pediatrics, University of California Medical Center, Irvine, California

Hugo L. Folli, Pharm.D., Coordinator, Children's Pharmacy, Memorial Hospital Medical Center, Long Beach, California

Gerald R. Greene, M.D., M.P.H., Associate Adjunct Professor of Pediatrics, and Director, Division of Pediatric Infectious Diseases, and Director, Pediatric Inpatient Service and Intensive Care Unit, University of California Medical Center, Irvine, California

Stephen Hirschfeld, M.D., Associate Professor of Pediatrics, Tulane University, School of Medicine, New Orleans, Louisiana

Hector E. James, M.D., Associate Professor of Neurosurgery and Pediatrics, University of California Medical Center, San Diego, California

Emily J. Kahlstrom, M.D., Assistant Professor of Pediatrics, Director, Pediatric Pulmonary Division, LAC-University of Southern California Medical Center, Los Angeles, California

Beverly Morgan, M.D., Professor and Chairman, Department of Pediatrics, University of California, Medical Center, Irvine, California

Stuart C. Morrison, M.B., Ch.B., M.R.C.P., Assistant Professor of Radiology, Case Western Reserve University, School of Medicine, and Radiologist, University Hospitals of Cleveland, Cleveland, Ohio

Christopher J.L. Newth, M.B., Ch.B., F.R.C.P.(C)., F.R.A.C.P., Associate Professor of Pediatrics and Anesthesia, and Director, Pediatric Intensive Care and Respirology, University of California Medical Center, San Francisco, California

Eliezer Nussbaum, M.D., Associate Professor, Department of Pediatrics, University of California, Irvine, and Director, Pediatric Pulmonary Center and Intensive Care Unit, Miller Children's Hospital Medical Center, Long Beach, California

Neil J. Sherman, M.D., Assistant Clinical Professor of Pediatrics and Surgery, University of Southern California Medical Center, Los Angeles, California

William T. Speck, M.D., Professor and Chairman, Department of Pediatrics, Case Western Reserve University, School of Medicine, and Director, Department of Pediatrics, and Chief, Division of Infectious Diseases, Rainbow Babies and Children's Hospital, Cleveland, Ohio

Robert Stern, M.D., Associate Professor of Pediatrics, Case Western Reserve University, School of Medicine, Rainbow Babies and Children's Hospital, and Director of Pediatric Pulmonary Clinic and Pulmonary Function Laboratory, Cleveland, Ohio

Kathleen Tripp, R.N., M.S., Pediatric Pulmonary Center, Good Samaritan Hospital, Phoenix, Arizona

Barry S. Yulish, M.D., Assistant Professor of Radiology, Case Western Reserve University, and Radiologist, University Hospitals of Cleveland, Cleveland, Ohio

Foreword

Since the end of World War II, spectacular progress has occurred in the field of pediatrics. One of the more recent developments, pediatric intensive care, introduced the concept of multidisciplinary management of critically ill children in a specialized area by full time nursing and medical personnel.

This approach to delivery of critical care for children was a natural consequence by pediatricians and hospitals when faced with the need to improve medical care but minimize costs. Previously, in the 1950s, the development of complex surgical procedures led to the introduction of recovery rooms. In the 1960s, the admission of newborns of increasing prematurity led to neonatal intensive care units. In the 1970s, increasing numbers of critically ill infants and children led to the formation of pediatric intensive care units in most North American hospitals.

The rapid and continuous growth of this specialized field of critical care has revealed an extreme shortage of trained personnel and an acute lack of readily available information. *Pediatric Intensive Care* helps to meet this educational need by presenting the combined knowledge and clinical experience of 26 authors who review a wide range of relevant topics. The result is a text which provides an invaluable reference for managing the critically ill child.

A.W. Conn, M.D., B.Sc(Med), F.A.C.A., F.R.C.P(C), F.A.A.P.
Professor
Hospital for Sick Children and University of Toronto
Ontario, Canada

Contents

Contributors v
Foreword *A.W. Conn, M.D.* ix
Introduction *Eliezer Nussbaum, M.D.* 1

Part I Central Nervous System Failure and Resuscitation

Chapter 1 Intracranial Dynamics 5
Hector E. James, M.D.

2 Drowning and Near-Drowning in Children with Main Emphasis on Cerebral-Cardiopulmonary Resuscitation 25
Eliezer Nussbaum, M.D.

3 Coma in Infants, Children and Adolescents . 35
Hector E. James, M.D.

4 Head Injury in Infants, Children and Adolescents 55
Hector E. James, M.D.

5 Status Epilepticus 79
Laurence Carnay, M.D.

6 Management of Central Nervous System Infections in Infancy and Childhood 95
Stephen Aronoff, M.D., and William Speck, M.D.

Appendix 1 Guidelines for the Critical Care of Patients with Reye's Syndrome A.1
Eliezer Nussbaum, M.D.

Part II Management of Acute Cardiovascular Disorders

Chapter 7 Pediatric Cardiovascular Monitoring 123
George Bisset, III, M.D., and Stephen Hirschfeld, M.D.

8 Diagnosis and Management of Circulatory Insufficiency and Shock ... 137
Stephen Hirschfeld, M.D., and George Bisset, III, M.D.

9 Pediatric Cardiopulmonary Resuscitation (CPR) ... 149
Stephen Hirschfeld, M.D., and George Bisset, III, M.D.

10 Cor Pulmonale in Children ... 159
Beverly Morgan, M.D.

Part III Pulmonary Failure and Disorders of the Respiratory Tract

Chapter 11 Radiologic Evaluation of Emergencies of the Respiratory Tract in Infants and Children ... 173
Barry S. Yulish, M.D., and Stuart C. Morrison, M.D.

12 Respiratory Failure ... 269
Eliezer Nussbaum, M.D.

13 Acute Epiglottitis and Croup ... 277
Christopher Newth, M.D.

14 The Diagnosis and Therapy of Status Asthmaticus ... 299
Stanley P. Galant, M.D.

15 Adult Respiratory Distress Syndrome in Children ... 309
Emily Kahlstrom, M.D.

16 Pleural Effusion in Children ... 325
Robert Stern, M.D.

17 Respiratory Care of the Pediatric Patient ... 339
Martha Ellington, R.R.T.

Part IV Trauma, Acute Poisoning and Bleeding Disorders

Chapter 18 Trauma Injuries in Children ... 371
Morris Asch, M.D., and Neil Sherman, M.D.

19 Spinal Cord Injury in Infants and Children . 393
Barry Ceverha, M.D.

20 Burns in Children 409
Morris Asch, M.D., and William Dean Davies, M.D.

21 Pediatric Poisoning 427
Hugo Folli, Pharm.D.

22 Bleeding and Clotting Disorders 457
Jerry Finklestein, M.D., and James Baker, M.D.

Part V Infections

Chapter 23 Intensive Care of Children with Infections ... 481
Gerald R. Greene, M.D.

Part VI Foreign Bodies

Chapter 24 Foreign Bodies in Children 517
Seymour Cohen, M.D.

Part VII Sudden Infant Death Syndrome

Chapter 25 Near Miss Sudden Infant Death Syndrome and Physiology/Methodology of Sleep Apnea 545
Barry Fisher, M.D., and Kathleen Tripp, R.N.

Index 579

Introduction

The new field of critical care is a milestone in the evolution of pediatrics. This volume represents the first attempt in combining multiple disciplines related to the field of pediatric intensive care. The difficult task of presenting the "state of the art" in pediatric intensive care was accomplished with the help of 26 contributors, nationally and internationally known in their fields. The book comprises 26 chapters and is organized in such a fashion as to allow the reader to follow the text in a systematic and comprehensive manner.

The book is composed of seven major parts including:

- Central nervous system failure and resuscitation
- Management of acute cardiovascular disorders in children
- Pulmonary failure and disorders of the respiratory tract
- Miscellaneous—including trauma, acute poisoning, bleeding disorders in children and burns, etc.
- Acute infections in children
- Foreign bodies
- Near-miss sudden infant death syndrome in children

The book emphasizes recent advances in critical care medicine in the pediatric age group; new technology in organ-system monitoring; approaches to diagnosis and therapeutic modalities.

The material is geared to health personnel involved in the care of the critically ill child including pediatricians, intensive care specialists, anesthesiologists, cardiologists, pulmonologists and also nurses, respiratory therapists, residents and students.

The style of the book and its organization are suitable for those interested in pathophysiology or up-to-date technology, while for others, the clinical material may be of benefit from the practical aspect. A multisystem approach is emphasized in this volume and will undoubtedly benefit the reader who may be faced with a complex of disorders in the pediatric intensive care unit.

The first three parts cover a majority of problems encountered in the practice of pediatric intensive care. The first part deals with the central nervous system on a broad spectrum basis and introduces the reader to various aspects of intracranial dynamics, cerebral resuscitation, coma, new theories in status epilepticus and the management of central nervous system infections in infants and children. The second part deals with management of acute cardiovascular disorders, describing in a meticulous manner the new approaches to cardiovascular monitoring, diagnoses and management of cardiovascular insufficiency, cardiopulmonary resuscitation and cor pulmonale in children. Part III is devoted to the respiratory tract and is divided into upper and lower airways. This part covers first grade emergencies such as acute epiglottitis and croup, status asthmaticus, respiratory failure and adult respiratory distress syndrome. Pathophysiology of respiratory failure and adult respiratory distress syndrome are described in such detail allowing the reader to gain the basic concepts of pulmonary mechanics, oxygen transport and hemodynamics. Parts IV, V and VI cover the scope of common pediatric emergencies such as trauma, burns, acute poisoning and acute infections while the concluding section deals with the newly-popular topics of sudden infant death syndrome and the physiopathology of sleep apnea.

—Eliezer Nussbaum, M.D.
Associate Professor of Pediatrics
University of California, Irvine
Director, Pediatric Pulmonary Center
and Intensive Care Units
Miller Children's Hospital
Memorial Hospital Medical Center
Long Beach, California

Part I

Central Nervous System Failure and Resuscitation

One of the major concerns of pediatric critical care is the insult inflicted upon the central nervous system of a child. It has been recognized that severe hypoxic/anoxic encephalopathy may result in irreversible brain damage. For that reason, the importance of cerebral resuscitation is emphasized. During the past decade much information has been accumulated concerning cerebral physiology and the relative importance of intracranial pressure (ICP) and cerebral perfusion pressure (CPP) upon the outcome of children who suffer from cerebral hypoxia and subsequently cerebral edema.

This first section provides comprehensive approaches to issues dealing with: functional or pathological injury to the central nervous system; and diagnosis, monitoring, therapy and prognosis. This part is composed of six chapters which are organized in a systematic manner beginning with intracranial dynamics followed by specific disease entities such as near-drowning, coma, head injury in infants and children, Reye's syndrome, status epilepticus and meningoencephalitis. The reader will find this part useful because it covers common, as well as unusual, CNS problems encountered in the daily practice of pediatric critical care.

We all regard the brain as "the main computer" with other systems or organs secondary in importance. Because of the brain's vital importance to the rest of the volume, I have chosen to introduce this part first.

1

Intracranial Dynamics

Hector E. James, M.D.

Introduction

The unique situation of the brain and its coverings within the rigid skull create a propensity for intracranial hypertension to occur as a response to many disease processes that affect the brain, be they vascular, inflammatory, traumatic or neoplastic. The Monro-Kellie[32] hypothesis states that the sum of the volumes of brain blood, cerebrospinal fluid and other components remains constant. As a consequence, addition of further volume (i.e. a tumor) creates a rise in intracranial pressure. Intracranial pressure causes cerebral dysfunction by mechanical distorsion (shifts) and/or impairment of cerebral blood flow and consequently, cerebral ischemia. Problems relating to these changes, diagnosis, management and how they affect outcome, encompass much of the practice of pediatric intensive care.

Monitoring of vital physiological parameters in a pediatric intensive care unit allows better management of disorders of body homeostasis in the acutely ill child by identifying the alterations before an irreversible pathological state is reached. Thus, monitoring of intracranial pressure (ICP) is a way to follow changes in pressure and compliance in a child with a brain insult, permitting then correct decisions in reference to duration and cessation of therapy.

Anatomy

The brain is partially compartmentalized by the dural attachments: the falx cerebri incompletely separating the right hemisphere from the left, the tentorium cerebelli separating incompletely the supra- from the infratentorial structures. Communication exists between the right and left supratentorial compartments by the interhemispheric cisterns and inside the brain, by the third ventricle. Communication between the supra- and infratentorial compartments is accomplished via the aqueduct of Sylvius in the brain stem, and the subarachnoid cisterns (perimesencephalic and ambient) outside the brain stem at the tentorial incisura. The intracranial compartment communicates freely with the spinal compartment via the subarachnoid space at the level of the foramen magnum. All the sites of communication are normally patent; however under pathological conditions shifts of structures may seclude the spaces, and give rise to complete compartmentalization. The degree of displacement of structures from one compartment to the other will depend on rate of growth of an intracranial mass, the local anatomy, the physical properties of the shifted portion of the brain, and the pressure gradient between the involved compartments. Usually, the more rapid the change, the least tolerated it will be, and symptomatology with rapid deterioration will be evidenced.

The brain is composed of blood vessels, cerebrospinal fluid (CSF) containing cavities and white and grey matter. The brain parenchyma is formed by water and organic material. Brain water constitutes 90% of the newborn brain and steadily decreases with age to approximately 65%. The white matter consists of axons and myelin sheaths that increase rapidly in the first three years of life, with scattered astrogliao cells. The fibers tend to run in a uniform fashion and will respond to changes in pressure according to the vector of the force and direction of the fibers. Within the white matter lie the deep grey masses of basal ganglia that tend to buttress the region against distorting forces (i.e. ventricular expansion in hydrocephalus). The grey matter is quite different in architecture than the white; the extracellular space is smaller than the white matter and the matrix consists of interspersed cells, dendritic processes and axons. The arteries and veins run vertically through the brain giving off capillaries at right angles.

The intracranial volume increases rapidly in early life, the brain attaining 75% of its adult size by 18 months of age. The final intracranial volume will be approximately 1900 ml by adult life, eighty percent being brain, 10% blood and 10% CSF.[16] The blood volume of the brain appears to be in the range of 3 to 4 ml/100 gm of brain tissue.[16]

Physiology

Cerebrospinal Fluid (CSF)

The CSF is formed mostly in the choroid plexus (approximately 80%) and the remainder in the interstitial spaces of the brain; the production rate is 0.33 ± 2 ml/minute.[31,39] The production rate is not affected by ICP unless it is so high as to reduce cerebral blood flow.[3] From the choroid plexus the CSF circulates in the ventricular system by bulk flow to the exit point in the roof of the fourth ventricle (foramina of Luschka and Magendie) into the subarachnoid space of the basal cisterns and spinal canal, or up through the tentorial incisura, then to the cerebral subarachnoid spaces to the primary sites of reabsorption in the arachnoid villi. These are located at the level of the venous sinuses, primarily sagittal and the transverse ones. The arachnoid villi are microscopic valves which open at 5 torr and reabsorption does increase in the face of higher ICP.[10,48,49]

Vascular

The arterial supply to the brain under normal conditions is via the carotid and vertebral arteries; and the venous drainage through the sinuses at the base, primarily the transverse and then the jugular veins. The pterygoid venous plexii and facial venous drainage can account for part of the intracranial venous return. From area to area of the arterial supply of the anterior, medial and posterior cerebral arteries, the capillary density is extremely variable and seems to either correlate with local density of synapses or with areas where the blood brain barrier is absent, such as the area postrema or supraoptic hypothalamic nuclei. The majority of the capillaries are anatomically different from the rest of the body, since they are nonfenestrated and have tight junctions between cells. These junctions are felt to be the anatomical site of the blood brain barrier, and they make it difficult for non lipid-soluble substances to enter the interstitial space.

The intracranial blood volume increases during development so that it reaches 200 ml in adult humans. Most of it is in the venous sinuses and pial veins. Cerebral veins are thin walled and because of this they may be significantly compressed and may affect blood volume before giving resistance to flow. The cortical surface veins enter the sagittal sinuses in an S-shaped fashion, so that they will collapse if no blood is entering them, preventing backflow from the sinuses to the veins. Intracranial hypertension may compress the veins in their trajectory through the subarachnoid space thus interfering with venous return and raising ICP even further.[42]

The most important factors controlling intracranial blood volume are the partial tension of arterial carbon dioxide (Pa_{CO_2}) and the local metabolic requirements of the brain.[7,38] Increases in Pa_{CO_2} lead to vasodilatation and increasing cerebral blood flow (CBF); thus, increases between 20 and 100 torr of Pa_{CO_2} are accompanied by linear increments of CBF. Increasing the Pa_{CO_2} from 20 to 40 torr doubles CBF and, thus, intracranial blood volume.[36,38] Control of the small arterioles and capillaries within the brain is closely related to local metabolism, possibly by pH changes in the interstitial fluid as a consequence of metabolic products and vasoactive substances. Consequently, an increase in local metabolism is accompanied by an increase in local flow, without change in cerebral perfusion pressure. When the pressure of oxygen is below 50 torr, cerebral blood flow increases dramatically. Hyperbaric oxygenation will result in cerebrovascular vasoconstriction and a decrease in cerebral blood flow.[33]

Cerebral blood flow is 75 to 80 ml/100 gm/minute in the grey matter, and 25 ml/100 mg/minute in the white matter. It appears to follow the Poiseuille law. Under most conditions, the length of the blood vessels and the viscosity can be considered constant. Therefore, in order to maintain a constant blood flow only the radius of the arteries and the pressure gradient across the brain can be varied. CBF is maintained at a constant rate over a large range of perfusion pressures. The effective perfusion pressure for the cerebral circulation is approximated by measuring the difference between arterial and intracranial pressure. The ability of the vascular bed to maintain constant flow in the face of changing perfusion pressure is believed to be a myogenic response of the muscular arterial walls to changes in transmural pressure.[2,9] As pressure drops the transmural pressure is decreased, arterioles dilate, flow resistance drops and despite a dropping perfusion pressure, the CBF remains stable. This will lead to an increase in arteriolar blood volume and a change in intracranial blood volume from the venous to the arterial side of the circulation. The normal range of cerebral autoregulation appears to be between 45–170 torr.[20] At the lower limits of autoregulation (range of 40–50 torr), the CBF begins to decrease; when the perfusion pressure reaches 25–30 torr, CBF falls to 50% of control.[20] As the upper limit is passed, there can be disruption of the blood brain barrier with increasing CBF and subsequent cerebral edema.[11] Above and below the range of good autoregulation, the flow is passively dependent on the cerebral perfusion pressure.[20]

After cerebral trauma autoregulation may be impaired in one area and preserved in another or may be globally lost throughout the cerebral hemispheres.[5] Therefore, although in normal brain a close relationship exists between cerebral perfusion pressure and blood flow, this relationship is lost in a variable fashion in the presence of intracranial pathology. When this situation exists increased blood pressure will increase CBF and consequently total cerebral blood volume. In turn, increasing blood volume will increase ICP. Conversely, reduction of systemic blood pressure will reduce CBF, cerebral blood volume and ICP. Consequently, under these conditions a reduction of blood pressure can, by producing a reduction of perfusion pressure, reduce CBF sufficiently to create cerebral ischemia and metabolic impairment. Cerebral edema may follow ischemia.[49] In edematous tissue the relationship of perfusion pressure to CBF is disturbed, and CBF correlates well with tissue water content, whereas perfusion pressure plays a less significant role.[24,25]

If sufficient injury to the brain and/or repeated elevations of ICP have occurred, massive vasodilatation can occur—a phenomenon termed *vasoparalysis,* in which ICP rises to the levels of blood pressure.[19] This represents a final stage of decompensation.

Cerebral perfusion pressure (CPP) can maintain a normal CBF

when over 40 torr. Under this value CBF falls and cerebral-arteriovenous oxygen difference increases rapidly.[11] No EEG changes are noted until CBF falls to 60–40% of normal, time when there is slowing in the tracing. Under 40% of normal, the EEG trace becomes flat, anaerobic metabolism increases and cerebral levels of adenosine triphosphate fall.[34] Likewise, decreasing CBF produces a steady impairment of evoked somatosensory potential transmission, so that at a CBF of less than 20 ml/100 gm/minute, evoked responses are no longer recorded.[1]

Figures 1, 2, 3 and 4 summarize the effects of PaO_2, $PaCO_2$, and perfusion pressure on CBF.

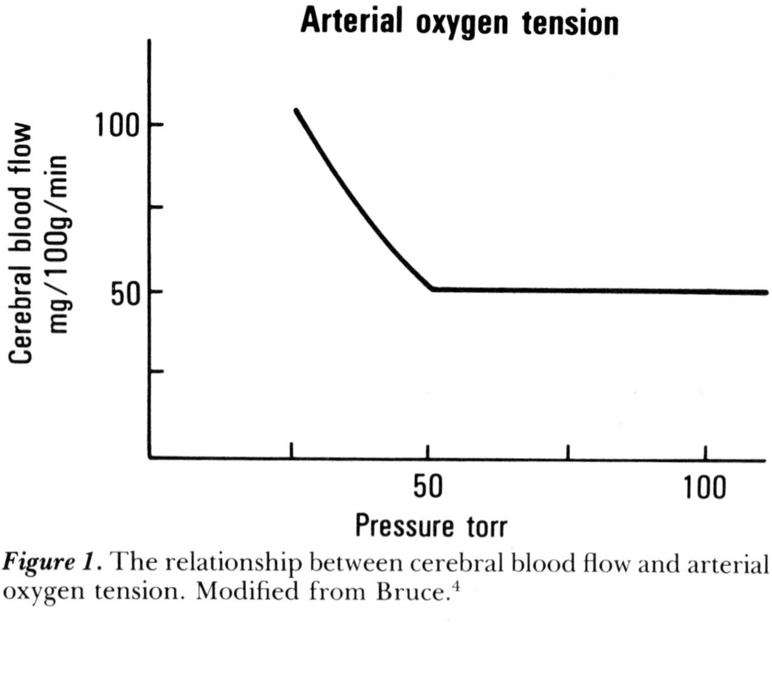

Figure 1. The relationship between cerebral blood flow and arterial oxygen tension. Modified from Bruce.[4]

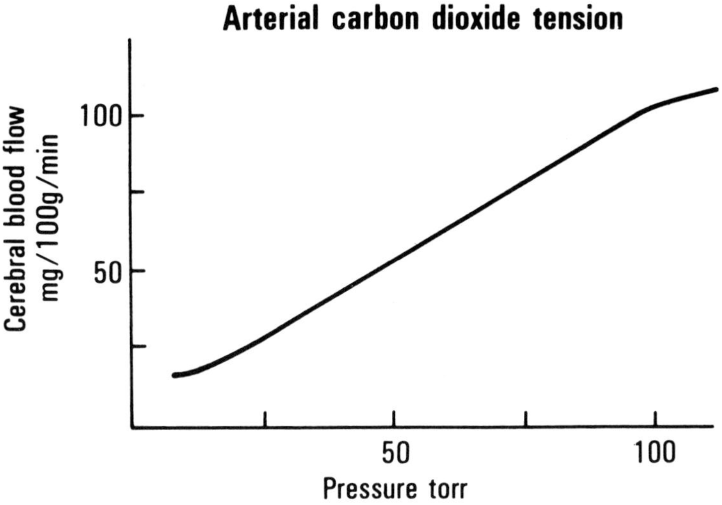

Figure 2. The relationship between cerebral blood flow and arterial carbon dioxide. Modified from Bruce.[4]

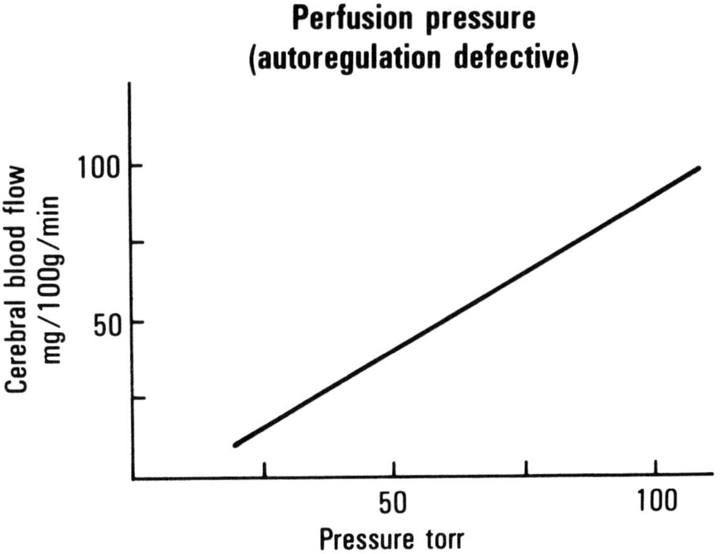

Figure 3. The relationship between cerebral blood flow and perfusion pressure in the presence of defective autoregulation. Modified from Bruce.[4]

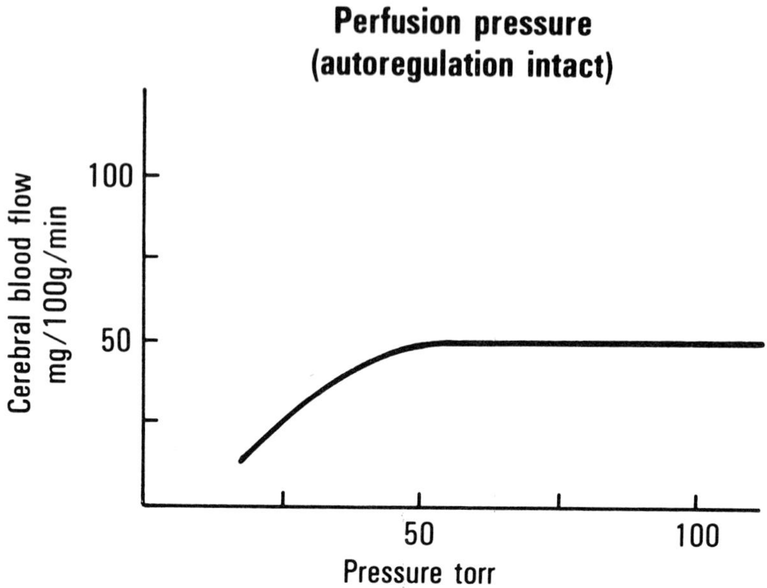

Figure 4. The relationship between cerebral blood flow and perfusion pressure in the presence of intact autoregulation. Modified from Bruce.[4]

Volume-Pressure Relationships

When an intracranial mass is progressively expanded, such as a balloon, there is little increase in ICP at first because an equivalent volume of CSF and venous blood can be expelled from the cranial cavity to accommodate the mass.[17] The addition of further volume, however, leads to a progressive rise in ICP when no further fluid can be expelled from the intracranial compartment. As discussed earlier, the Monro-Kellie[32] hypothesis states that the sum of the volumes of brain, blood, CSF and other components remains constant. In this case, a change in volume within one of these components is offset by an equal and opposite change in some other compartment. This accounts for the lack of change of ICP in the initial stages of enlargement of an intracranial mass. If the brain were completely incompressible and the cranium were non-

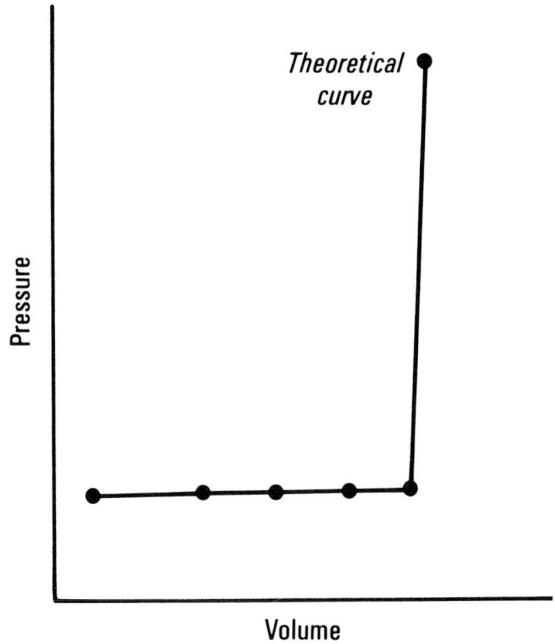

Figure 5. Theoretical volume-pressure curve that would be obtained assuming that the Monro-Kellie hypothesis was correct.

expandable the addition of volume to the intracranial space would lead to a theoretical pressure-volume curve (Fig. 5). However, the biological curve is not the same as the theoretical curve (Fig. 6).[19] At the inflection point of the volume-pressure curve, the residual displaceable volume is exhausted so that further relatively small changes in volume will lead to a large increase in pressure. (See Fig. 6.) This phenomenon has also been seen in children with hydrocephalus[43] and in patients with tumor, head injury and cerebrovascular disease.[27,28] The critical factor is the increase in pressure that results from a given increase in intracranial volume. This is a measure of a gradient in the volume-pressure curve at any point. Thus, the following formula may be employed:

$$\text{elastance} = \frac{\text{increase in pressure}}{\text{increase in volume}} = \frac{\Delta P}{\Delta V}$$

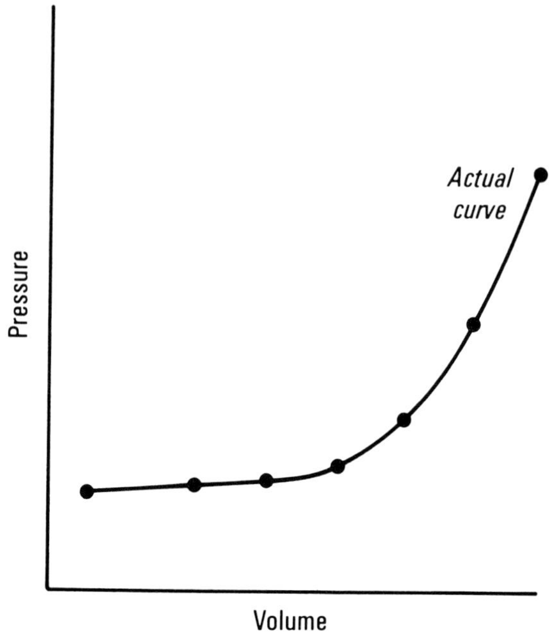

Figure 6. The biological volume-pressure curve obtained in animals with an expanding epidural balloon.[19]

The term *elastance* then is the reverse of the term *compliance,* thus:

$$\text{compliance} = \frac{1}{\text{elastance}}$$

The biphasic volume-pressure curve may best be understood by considering the initial, rather flat portion of the curve as related mainly to CSF buffering. As the volume changes continue, CSF buffering becomes exhausted and the elastic properties of the cerebral substance and blood vessels play the major buffering role as the volume-pressure rises steeply. If elastance is low the patient has volume reserve, but at high elastance small increases in volume may lead to fatal increases in pressure.[4]

A single pressure measurement is not sufficient to define the position of the patient on any given volume-pressure curve, and this reflects different reserve for residual displacement of volume.

To define the relative "tightness" of the intracranial space it is important to take into account not only ICP but also to estimate the compliance or the elastance. For that purpose the volume-pressure response[26] and the pressure-volume index[23] have been described. As defined by Miller[26] the *volume-pressure response* is expressed in torr, and it is the change in ICP seen immediately prior to and after the injection of 1 ml of saline in 1 second into the ventricular catheter employed for continuous ICP monitoring. This response is increased in parallel to the increase in ICP, and is correspondingly reduced following surgical decompression and reduced ICP.[26] The *pressure-volume index* (PVI) as defined by Marmarou et al.,[23] is the slope of a line obtained by plotting the logarithm of the CSF pressure against changes in CSF volume. This line is a straight one. The result is a number which when high indicates a soft compliant system, and when decreased it indicates a tight system. A PVI can be determined in practice by recording the ICP (Po), adding a fixed volume in a bolus injection (ΔV), then recording the peak pressure recorded (Pp) in a similar way to the volume-pressure response. But then, different from the volume-pressure response, the PVI is calculated by dividing the volume (ΔV) by the logarithm of the ratio Pp/Po. Once determined, the compliance at any given ICP can be easily calculated.[23] The normal PVI for an adult is 25 ml. It is important to realize that the PVI applies only to the CSF space, and consequently, if these spaces are distorted a change in the volume-pressure curve may develop. It follows that the measurement of compliance at any time gives information that is subject to rapid change.[44]

Intracranial Pressure

Normal Intracranial Pressure

Under normal conditions, recording pressures anywhere in the CSF-craniospinal axis yields the same values, because freely circulating CSF has a pressure-equalizing effect. The normal tracing of a continuous recording displays vascular and respiratory oscillations.[35] The vascular waves are due to arterial pulsations in larger vessels within the brain which produce an oscillation in the volume of the ventricular system. The respiratory wave is synchronous with alterations in the central venous pressure, reflecting intrathoracic pressure.

The normal ICP in the human adult and child is under 15 torr (204 mm H_2O). In the infant it is under 8–10 torr.[8,47] The ICP does not remain at a given value, but fluctuates constantly. Some procedures such as coughing or straining can produce short transient elevations of ICP to values of 80–100 torr, without apparent distress to the patient.

Raised Intracranial Pressure

A persistent elevation of ICP over 8–10 torr in the infant or over 15–20 torr in the child or adult is defined as *raised intracranial pressure.*[8,26,47] When ICP rises, obstruction of the CSF pathways can occur and consequently the ICP recording, to be reliable, has to be measured rostral to the obstruction.[19,45] In other words, pressure at the time of lumbar puncture may be much lower than intracranial pressure in the face of intracranial pathology, and therefore may not only confuse the clinician, but also may be dangerous due to continuous leakage of CSF at the puncture site.[26]

Although ICP may be increased artificially above the blood pressure in experimental preparations, this would rarely occur in clinical conditions. Accordingly, from the standpoint of pediatric practice, the arterial pressure should be regarded as the upper limit of ICP. As the ICP rises, the respiratory fluctuations become less prominent and the arterial component of the pressure wave increases.[50] In the practical setting, the visible widening of the pulse pressure in the continuous ICP monitor should alert the clinician to worsening elastance, and reciprocally decreased pulse pressure will indicate improving intracranial volume-pressure relationships. Rising intracranial pressure also becomes more passively related to changes in arterial pressure; simultaneous recording of ICP and blood pressure is therefore of great importance in a child with intracranial hypertension.

In the classical monographs on ICP recording in clinical practice, Lundberg[21,22] described three types of pressure waves. The most serious is the Type A or plateau wave, which consists of a sudden elevation of 50 torr or more, with durations of more than 5 minutes. These waves can recur frequently accompanied by neurological changes. The Type B wave is a rhythmic variation of ICP with a peaked increase in the range of 20–50 torr; it is related to changes in respiration and can accompany the Cheyne-Stokes pattern of breathing. At times, the presence of Type B waves serves as a prelude to plateau waves. Type C waves represent a rhythmic variation that is uncommonly seen, which run at 4–8 waves per minute and seem to correspond to changes in arterial pressure accompanying variations in activity of the vasomotor center, such as the Traube-Hering-Mayer phenomenon.

Increased ICP results from any addition to the volume of the intracranial constituents in excess of the compensatory capacity of the system (see volume-pressure relationships). The extent of the rise will depend upon the volume added, the rate at which it occurred, the state of the intracranial volume at the time of the additive, and the relative volumes of CSF and blood available for displacement.

Pathology

As lesions expand or the brain becomes larger due to swelling or edema, shifts occur with herniation of intracranial structures from one compartment to another. To a certain extent this may be viewed as another stage of compensatory mechanisms with expulsion of blood or CSF, produced by a differential pressure between intracranial areas. This may account for the presence of a normal ICP in the face of a significant brain shift that is sometimes seen.[26] In these cases ICP was elevated at one time prior to the shift. Compliance measurements should, even in the presence of normal ICP, give values that reflect brain tightness.[30]

When a supratentorial mass expands, the medial aspect of the temporal lobe is displaced into the tentorial hiatus and the cisterna ambiens becomes obliterated. This leads to an obliteration of the communication between the infra- and supratentorial subarachnoid spaces. This in turn leads to brain stem distortion and ischemia, causing its dysfunction[12] with subsequent impairment of the level of consciousness due to poor reticular formation activity. This is due to compression of the cerebral peduncles against the temporal lobe or the sharp dural edge of the tentorium. Corticospinal tract dysfunction follows, giving rise to ipsilateral or contralateral hemiparesis and since the third cranial nerve passes through the tentorial hiatus from the infratentorial compartment to the supratentorial, its compression at this point causes impairment of its function. This will lead to ipsilateral pupillary dilation since the third nerve produces myosis.[14] Therefore, the syndrome of *transtentorial herniation* is characterized by progressive impairment of consciousness, pupillary dilation ipsilateral to the expanding mass, and contralateral or ipsilateral hemiparesis. The ipsilateral pupillary dilation occurs in about 80% of the cases and the hemiparesis is ipsilateral in only about 50% of all cases.[6] It is the most frequently identified clinical syndrome of herniation. It can occur bilaterally, such as in the case of diffuse swelling secondary to trauma or diffuse encephalopathies. If the herniation continues untreated there is progressive caudal deterioration with Cheyne-Stokes respirations, central neurogenic hyperventilation, decerebration, apnea and death.[37] This could be due to downward axial shift with buckling of the brain stem, and the "fixed" basilar artery does not accompany the brain stem movement to the same degree, then the ventral perforating branches to the brain stem are elongated, stretched and therefore create ischemia of this structure.[12]

Tonsillar or *foramen magnum* herniation can be an end stage phenomenon due to caudal displacement of the brain stem and cerebellar tonsills, with or without the vermis, into the foramen magnum. This then results into progressive impairment of consciousness, bradycardia, hypertension, respiratory irregularity and apnea.

Upward tentorial herniation occurs when the infratentorial pressure is higher than the supratentorial pressure, leading to upward displacement of the cerebellar vermis into the incisura, compressing the brain stem, giving impairment of consciousness and respiratory irregularity. The posterior cerebral arteries may be kinked and their flow impaired from the posterior fossa to the supratentorial compartment. Ischemia of occipital lobe can then lead to the cortical blindness that is seen with this syndrome.

Cingulate or *subfalcine* herniation occurs due to supratentorial herniation from one compartment to the other, underneath the falx cerebri. This can create compression of an anterior cerebral artery which will lead to ischemia of the corresponding portion of the motor cortex. Consequently, loss of function of the contralateral leg as well as bladder control impairment may be seen.

In assessing a clinical or experimental setting the pediatrician must keep in mind the difference between *cerebral edema* and *cerebral swelling*. Throughout this text *cerebral edema* will be employed when there is (or suspected to be) an increase in brain tissue water. An example of this would be iatrogenic water overload. *Cerebral swelling* is defined as cerebral vascular engorgement, as a consequence of increased intracerebral blood volume. An example of this would be the early phases of pediatric head injury. This does not mean that in the clinical setting these two may not combine. Further clarification of these concepts will occur in the *Physiopathology* section of this chapter and in *Chapter Four.*

Physiopathology and Clinical Considerations

In its simplest interpretation the effect of a rise in ICP is to reduce cerebral perfusion pressure and, consequently, blood flow. Therefore, in its most severe form at the time of carotid angiography in a patient with very elevated ICP, the contrast material is seen to stop at the carotid siphon (pseudo-occlusion) because it cannot enter the intracranial compartment. This is the angiographic diagnosis of brain death.[18] The changes of cerebral blood flow and autoregulation with ICP have been discussed in the *Vascular* section of this chapter.

The pediatrician must not fall into the dangerous situation of placing too much emphasis on the level of ICP, as the relationship between ICP and the clinical state of the patient is not always direct. In certain situations high ICP has been seen in patients without neurological dysfunction.[15] On the one extreme, one may see a patient with a structural brain lesion and high ICP improve dramatically with reduction of the same, and on the other hand an unconscious patient with good compliance and low ICP, remain unconscious. Repeated episodes of a rise in ICP can have cumulative effects, and at times may be disastrous. As a general rule, ICP has a deleterious effect that becomes progressively worse with time.[26]

In considering the assessment and management of a child with intracranial hypertension one should mentally exercise the factors that increase elastance that may be shifting the volume-pressure curve to the left, or in other words, increasing brain "tightness."

Table I
Factors Increasing/Decreasing ICP

Factors Increasing ICP	*Factors Decreasing ICP*
Hypoventilation	Hyperventilation
Hypercarbia	Hypertonic diuretics:
Arterial hypertension	Mannitol
Seizures	Urea
Impaired venous return	DMSO
Intracranial mass	Arterial hypotension
Hydrocephalus	Corticosteroids
Certain anesthetic agents	Barbiturates
	CSF drainage
	Head elevation

These are: arterial hypertension (vasocongestion); intracranial mass; hydrocephalus brain herniation; and, some anesthetics.[41] Hypoventilation, hypercarbia, impaired venous return and water intoxication can increase intracranial pressure (Table I).

Decreasing intracranial elastance can be obtained by employing hypertonic diuretics (mannitol, urea, dimethyl sulfoxide),[13,16,29] arterial hypotension,[26] corticosteroids,[29] drainage of CSF, barbiturates and some anesthetics.[41]

Maintaining a normal ICP and compliance is often done just by correcting any of the above factors that can impair ICP regulation. Understanding the underlying physiopathology, volume-pressure relationships and cerebral hemodynamics is the single most important therapeutic tool that the pediatrician and intensivist have available. There is no single ideal therapy for ICP. The selection of the therapy must be directed to correcting the underlying physiopathology and this will be discussed in the subsequent chapters.

Acknowledgment: The preparation of this chapter and the following chapters 3 and 4 was kindly and efficiently executed with the secretarial assistance of Yvette Cabrera.

References

1. Astrup J, Symon L, Branstron NM, et al: Cortical evoked potential and extracellular potassium and hydrogen at critical levels of brain ischemia. *Stroke* 8:51–57, 1977.
2. Bayliss WM: On the local reaction of the arterial wall to changes of internal pressure. *J Physiol* 28:220–231, 1902.
3. Bering EA, Jr, Sato O: Hydrocephalus: Changes in the formation and absorption of cerebrospinal fluid within the cerebral ventricles. *J Neurosurg* 20:1050–1063, 1963.
4. Bruce DA: The pathophysiology of increased intracranial pressure. *Current Concepts,* Scope Publications, Upjohn Co., 1978.
5. Bruce DA, Langfitt TW, Miller JD, et al: Regional cerebral blood flow, intracranial pressure and brain metabolism in comatose patients. *J Neurosurg* 38:131–144, 1973.
6. Cabieses F, Jeri R: Transtentorial temporal lobe herniation. *Acta Neurol Lat Amer* 2:201–211, 1954.
7. Cohen PJ, Alexander SC, Smith TF, et al: Effects of hypoxia and normocarbia on cerebral blood flow in conscious man. *J Appl Physiol* 23:183–189, 1967.
8. Donn SM, Phillip AGS: Early increase in intracranial pressure in preterm infants. *Pediatrics* 61:904–907, 1978.
9. Folkow B: Descriptions of the myogenic hypothesis. *Circ Res* 15 (Suppl I):279–287, 1964.
10. Gomez DG, Potts DG, Deonarine V: Arachnoid granulations of the sheep: Structural and ultrastructural changes with varying pressure differences. *Arch Neurol* 30:169–175, 1974.
11. Haggendal E, Lofgren J, Nillson NJ: Effects of varied CSF pressure on cerebral blood flow in dogs. *Acta Physiol Scand* 79:262–271, 1970.
12. Hassler O: Arterial pattern of human brain stem. 'Normal' appearances and deformation in expanding supratentorial conditions. *Neurology* 17:368–375, 1967.
13. James HE, Langfitt TW, Kumar VS, et al: Treatment of intracranial hypertension. *Acta Neurochirurg* 36:189–200, 1977.
14. Jefferson G: The tentorial pressure cone. *Arch Neurol Psychiat* 40:857–876, 1938.
15. Johnston I, and Paterson A: Benign intracranial hypertension. II. CSF pressure and circulation. *Brain* 17:301–312, 1974.
16. Khul DE, Reivich M, Alavi A, et al: Local cerebral blood volume determined by three-dimensional reconstruction of radionuclide scan data. *Circ Res* 36:610–619, 1975.
17. Langfitt TW: Increased intracranial pressure. *Clin Neurosurg* 16:436–471, 1969.
18. Langfitt TW, and Kassel NF: Non-filling of cerebral vessels during angiography: Correlation with intracranial pressure. *Acta Neurochirurg* 14:96–104, 1966.
19. Langfitt TW, Weinstein JD, Kassell NF: Cerebral vasomotor paralysis produced by intracranial hypertension. *Neurology* 15:622–641, 1965.

20. Lassen NA: Control of cerebral circulation in health and disease. *Circ Res* 34:749–760, 1970.
21. Lundberg N: Continuous recording and control of ventricular fluid pressure in neurosurgical practice. *Acta Psychiatr Neurol Scand* 36:1–193 (suppl. 149), 1960.
22. Lundberg N: Monitoring of intracranial pressure. *In* Critchley M, O'Leary JL, Jennet B. (eds): *Scientific Foundations of Neurology*. London, Heinemann, 1972, pp. 356–371.
23. Marmarou A, Schulman K: Pressure-volume relationships—basic aspects. *In* Mclaurin R. (ed): *Head Injuries*. New York, Grune & Stratton, 1976, pp. 233–266.
24. Marshall LF, Bruce DA, Graham DI, et al: Alterations in behavior, brain electric activity, cerebral blood flow and intracranial pressure produced by triethyl tin sulfate-induced cerebral edema. *Stroke* 7(1):21–25, 1976.
25. Meinig G, Reulen HJ, Magavly C: Regional CBF and cerebral perfusion pressure in global brain edema induced by water intoxication. *Acta Neurochirurg* 29:1–13, 1973.
26. Miller JD: Volume and pressure in the craniospinal axis. *Clin Neurosurg* 22:76–105, 1975.
27. Miller JD, Garibi J: Intracranial volume/pressure relationships during continuous monitoring of ventricular fluid pressure. *In* Brock M, Dietz H (eds): *Intracranial pressure: Experimental and Clinical Aspects*. Berlin, Springer, 1972, pp. 270–274.
28. Miller JD, Garibi J, Pickard JD: Induced changes of cerebrospinal fluid volume. Effects of continuous monitoring of ventricular fluid pressure. *Arch Neurol* 28:265–269, 1973.
29. Miller JD, Leech PJ: Assessing the effects of mannitol and steroid therapy on intracranial volume-pressure relationships. *J Neurosurg* 42:274–281, 1975.
30. Miller JD, Pickard JD: Intracranial volume-pressure studies in patients with head injury. *Injury* 5:265–269, 1974.
31. Milhorat TH: *Hydrocephalus and the Cerebrospinal Fluid*. Baltimore, Williams & Wilkins Co., 1972.
32. Monro A: *Observations on the Structure and Function of the Nervous System*. Edinburgh, Creech & Johnson, 1783.
33. McDowell DG: Interrelationships between blood oxygen tension and cerebral blood flow. *In* Payne JP, Hill DW (eds): *Oxygen Measurements in Blood and Tissue*. London, Churchill, 1966, pp. 205–214.
34. McKenzie EI, McGeorge AP, Graham DI, et al: Breakthrough of cerebral autoregulation and the sympathetic nervous system. *In* Ingvar, DH, Lassen NA (eds): *Cerebral Function, Metabolism and Circulation*. Copenhagen, Munksgaard, 1977, pp. 48–49.
35. O'Connel JEA: The vascular factor in intracranial pressure and the maintenance of the cerebrospinal fluid circulation. *Brain* 66:204–228, 1943.
36. Phelps ME, Grubb RL, Ter Pogossian MM: Correlation between $PaCO_2$ and regional blood volume by X-ray fluorescence. *J Appl Physiol* 34:741–747, 1973.

37. Plum F, Posner JB: *Diagnosis of Stupor and Coma.* Philadelphia, Davis Co., 1980.
38. Reivich M: Arterial PCO_2 and cerebral hemodynamics. *Am J Physiol* 206:25–35, 1964.
39. Sato O, Bering EA: Extraventricular formation of cerebrospinal fluid. *Brain Nerv* 19:883–885, 1967.
40. Schuier FJ, Hossman KA: Experimental brain infarcts in cats. II. Ischemic brain edema. *Stroke* 11:593–600, 1980.
41. Shapiro HM: Intracranial hypertension. Therapeutic and anesthetic considerations. *Anesthesiology* 43:445–471, 1975.
42. Shapiro HM, Langfitt TW, Weinstein JD: Compression of cerebral vessels by intracranial hypertension: II. Morphological evidence for collapse of vessels. *Acta Neurochirurg* 12:223–233, 1966.
43. Shulman K, Marmarou A: Pressure-volume considerations in infantile hydrocephalus. *Dev Med Child Neurol* 13:90–95 (Suppl 25), 1971.
44. Sklar FH, Blashvilli I: The pressure-volume function of brain elasticity. *J Neurosurg* 47:670–679, 1977.
45. Smyth GE, Henderson WR: Observations on the cerebrospinal fluid pressure on simultaneous ventricular and lumbar punctures. *J Neurol Psychiatry* 1:226–237, 1938.
46. Tsuruda J, James HE, Camp PE, et al: Acute dimethyl sulfoxide therapy in experimental brain edema. Part 2: Effect of dose and concentration on intracranial pressure, blood pressure and central venous pressure. *Neurosurg* 10:355–359, 1982.
47. Vidyasagar D, Raju TNK: A simple noninvasive technique of measuring intracranial pressure in the newborn. *Pediatrics* 59: 957–961(suppl), 1977.
48. Welch, Friedman V: The cerebrospinal fluid valves. *Brain* 83: 454–469, 1961.
49. Welch K, Pollay M: Perfusion of particles through arachnoid villi of the monkey. *Amer J Physiol* 210:651–654, 1961.
50. Wright RD: Experimental observations on increased intracranial pressure. *Aust NZJ Surg* 7:215–235, 1938.

2

Drowning and Near-Drowning in Children with Main Emphasis on Cerebral-Cardiopulmonary Resuscitation

Eliezer Nussbaum, M.D.

Introduction

Brain injury following submersion is frequently observed in the pediatric age group.[1–4]

Only in recent years has the concept of cerebral resuscitation been emphasized[5–7] in comparison to previous years where therapy in near-drowned children focused on cardiopulmonary resuscitation alone. Therefore, a new concept was adopted, namely, cerebral-cardiopulmonary resuscitation. During the last decade more information has been accumulated regarding cerebral physiology and the importance of intracranial presure (ICP) and cerebral perfusion pressure (CPP) measurement in the management of children who incurred severe cerebral anoxic insult resulting in cerebral edema[8] and rise in ICP.[9] The near-drowned child who is severely comatose has, in general, a poor prognosis.[4–7,10–12] Since his outcome cannot be reliably predicted on the basis of clinical evaluation alone, it was apparent that continuous ICP measurements may be of paramount importance in directing therapy as well as helping to predict outcome. Our previous studies[9] have demonstrated the value of ICP and CPP monitoring as an objective prognostic tool in the near-drowned child who is severely comatose upon admission to the hospital.[9]

Incidence

Drowning and near-drowning remain among the leading causes of death in the pediatric age group, reaching epidemic proportions in areas which are heavily populated with swimming pools and beaches. A high percentage of brain damage was reported in those who survived.[2,5,9,11] It is estimated that in the United States alone 8,000 victims die each year as a result of drowning and that 40% are children under four years of age. It is also believed that boys are at higher risk than girls. Teen-aged boys (swimmers and nonswimmers) and unsupervised toddlers are included in the high risk category.

Definitions

- *Drowning:* A victim who dies within 24 hours.
- *Near-Drowning:* A victim who survives for more than 24 hours.
- *Secondary Drowning:* Recurrence of respiratory distress following apparent successful resuscitation.

Types of Near-Drowning (or Drowning)

Wet drowning or near-drowning is associated with aspiration in about 85% of the cases and dry drowning or near-drowning is associated with laryngospasm without aspiration in 15% of the cases resulting also in asphyxia. The onset of secondary drowning is within a few minutes to 24 hours following submersion. It is complicated by pulmonary edema, aspiration pneumonitis, fever, seizures and headaches.

It is agreed that all near-drowning victims, even if alert and breathing should be hospitalized at least 24–48 hours for observation.

Pathophysiology

Contrary to previous investigations, the clinical picture is not altered whether the victim aspirated fresh water or salt water.

Aspiration of salt water results in shift of fluids from the intravascular compartment into the alveolar space with concomitant basement membrane damage and leakage of albumin. In turn, patients may suffer from pulmonary edema with subsequent hypoxia, hypoxemia, acidosis and circulatory collapse. Initially, the near-drowned victim may be cyanotic, and distressed, associated with diffuse crepitant rales, rhonchi and wheezing.

The near-drowned victim who becomes comatose as a result of submersion will be discussed in detail later in the chapter.

Fresh water aspiration may result in wash-out of alveolar surfactant and damage to capillary and alveolar Type II cells. This may result in atelectasis, ventilation/perfusion ($\dot{V}_A\dot{Q}_C$) mismatching with subsequent hypoxia, intrapulmonary shunting and hypoxemia. Pulmonary hypertension, pulmonary edema and circulatory collapse may be inevitable. Despite the potential hemodynamic and pulmonary differences between fresh water and salt water drowning the therapeutic approach should be similar.[7–9] Following submersion the near-drowned victim may experience combined respiratory as well as metabolic acidosis secondary to severe hypoxia, respiratory failure and accumulation of lactic acid. It should be remembered that severe anoxic encephalopathy often results in cerebral edema, poor CPP and brain damage.

Therapy

We believe that successful resuscitation means an individual with intellectual integrity and an individual without brain damage. In order to achieve this goal aggressive management should be introduced with maximal attention to cerebral resuscitation.[5–7,9] It is recognized that severe cerebral anoxic insult may result in anaerobic metabolism and metabolic acidosis, reduction in adenosine-triphosphate (ATP) availability with subsequent impairment of sodium-potassium pump, cytotoxic cerebral edema, rise in ICP and decreased tissue perfusion (low CPP).[8,10] For these reasons rise in ICP should be prevented and the failing brain should be resuscitated.

Neurological Classification of Near-Drowned Children and their Therapy

We followed Conn's and Modell's classification of near-drowned children based on victim's neurological status.[5–7]

Category A (Awake)

Patients in this category were awake and alert upon admission or following pulmonary resuscitation (CPR). Baseline arterial blood gases and chest roentgenogram were obtained and the patients were observed in the pediatric intensive care unit (PICU) for 24–48 hours. Upon discharge home instructions were given to all patients regarding observation for possible neurological changes.

Category B (Blunted)

Patients in this group suffered from some degree of hypoxia and were partially comatose with blunted response to verbal stimuli. They responded to painful stimulation and maintained normal pupillary response. Although their levels of consciousness were somewhat depressed, all their peripheral reflexes were normal. These patients initially received diuretics and intravenous fluid restriction to about 30%–50% of maintenance to achieve a urine output of about 1 cc/kg/hr. They were provided with oxygen by mask and also dexamethasone sodium phosphate with antacids. Category B patients were closely monitored in the PICU for at least 48 hours.

Category C (Comatose)

Children in this group suffered severe hypoxic insult and were in coma. They were further divided into three subgroups:

C_1 (Decorticate): Flexor response to pain and irregular respirations with varying amplitudes;

C_2 (Decerebrate): Deeper stage of coma with extensor response to pain, hyperventilation, fixed and dilated pupils and minimal response to pain; and

C_3 (Flaccid): Still deeper stage of coma with no response to pain, fixed and dilated pupils, no spontaneous respirations or shallow and frequently ineffective breaths, hypotension and poor peripheral perfusion.

Therapy of Patients in Category C

Our detailed protocol followed the recommendations of other investigators who advocate full scale cerebral resuscitative measures in those near-drowned children who became comatose.[4–10]

Ventilation. Patients were hyperventilated and hyperoxygenated. Positive end expiratory pressure (PEEP) was kept between 2 and 6 cm H_2O. The level of inspired oxygen and PEEP were adjusted to maintain PaO_2 above 150 mm Hg. Tidal volume, minute ventilation and the ratio of inspiration to expiration were manipulated to keep $PaCO_2$ between 20 and 25 mm Hg. Serial arterial blood gases via an arterial line were obtained.

Hydration. Placement of central venous line (CVP) was helpful in assessment of fluid balance. In hypotensive patients a Swan-Ganz flow directed catheter was inserted in order to measure pulmonary capillary wedge pressure or cardiac output. Fluids were restricted to 30%–50% of normal maintenance. Furosemide 1 mg/kg was given intravenously to all children upon admission in order to minimize pulmonary and/or cerebral edema. Urine output was kept at approximately 1 cc/kg/hr and CVP at 3–8 mm Hg.

Temperature. Rectal temperature was kept at (30° ± 1° C) using a cooling mattress.

Muscular Paralysis. In order to prevent any movement, to minimize muscle rigidity and to control ventilation, pancuronium (Pavulon) 0.1 mg/kg intravenous was given every 2–4 hours as needed for continuous complete muscle paralysis. This measure was taken to minimize the risk of raised ICP.

ICP and CPP Measurements. From admission to our PICU, ICP was continuously monitored by means of a Richmond Screw.[9] ICP was kept below 15 mm Hg and CPP above 50 mm Hg. CPP was calculated as the difference between mean systemic blood pressure ($\overline{BP}$) and mean ICP ($\overline{ICP}$).[9] $CPP = \overline{BP} - \overline{ICP}$. $\overline{BP}$ was kept above 60 mm Hg.

Induction of Pentobarbital Coma. When ICP was sustained above 15 mm Hg for more than five minutes barbiturate coma was induced.[9] Subsequent doses of pentobarbital were guided by CPP and barbiturate levels. Mean arterial blood pressure ($\overline{BP}$) was kept between 60 and 90 mm Hg and CPP > 50 mm Hg. Intravenous drip with dopamine ranging from 5–15 mcg/kg/min was given when mean arterial blood pressure dropped below 60 mm Hg. Pentobarbital was administered intravenously first as a bolus 3–5 mg/kg followed by 1–2 mg/kg hourly to maintain serum level between 2.5 and 4.0 mg%. Pentobarbital was stopped if $\overline{BP}$ dropped below 60 mm Hg despite the use of dopamine or if serum level exceeded 4 mg%.

Other Measures. *Mannitol.* If ICP exceeded 20 mm Hg despite the above measures, manual hyperventilation was begun. When ICP did not fall below 20 mm Hg, mannitol 0.5 gm/kg was given intravenously followed by hourly 0.1 gm/kg until ICP fell below 20 mm Hg. Serum osmolality was kept below 320 mOsm/L and above this level mannitol was withheld.

Dexamathasone Sodium Phosphate. Loading dose was 0.5 mg/kg followed by maintenance of 0.25 mg/kg every six hours.

Other Physiological Parameters or Monitoring. Electroencephalogram (EEG), electrocardiogram, and cerebral perfusion scans for tissue viability were performed in patients with coma.

We applied the protocol to all patients in coma.

When category C patients responded to therapy or if ICP was maintained below 15 mm Hg for 48–72 hours, slow rewarming by 1° C per two hours was initiated and $PaCO_2$ was gradually brought to 35 mm Hg. If this was followed by normal ICP and CPP for at least 12 additional hours pancuronium and pentobarbital were discontinued and the surarachnoid bolt was removed within the following 12 hours. However, if after 48 hours of therapy EEG was isoelectric, cerebral perfusion was not demonstrated by nuclear scan and examination did not elicit any neurological activity, we concluded that it was likely that brain death or severe damage had occurred.

Discussion

In our experience,[9] hyperventilation was by far the most effective method in controlling a rise in ICP. Hyperventilation induces respiratory alkalosis and cerebrovascular constriction with subsequent modulation of cerebral blood flow and lowering ICP. Continuous ICP monitoring is therefore essential in assessing cerebral perfusion pressure and guiding appropriate therapy. Table I outlines the complications of ventilatory support.

Although hypothermia is recommended by various investigators who believe that this approach can decrease oxygen consumption and protect the brain which has suffered severe anoxic insult,[6] side effects of such therapy should not be ignored. (See Table V.)[6]

While previous studies have emphasized the difference between fresh water and salt water aspiration, the primary importance of hypoxia is recognized today. Since in our experience the clinical picture is not altered whether the victim aspirated fresh water or salt water, our protocol was applied equally to all cases of near-drowning. The author believes that victims should be fully resuscitated regardless of their condition because the brain may be severely insulted but still capable of recovery. This approach requires maximal attention to cerebral resuscitation with ICP monitoring since a rise in intracranial pressure may precede clinical deterioration. We again emphasize the importance of cerebral and cardiopulmonary resuscitation since it is currently recognized that cardiopulmonary resuscitation is a misleading concept and rather the concept of cardiopulmonary-cerebral resuscitation should be adopted.

Recent published studies concluded that near-drowning in fresh water does not cause permanent pulmonary dysfunction.[13]

Table I

Complications of Ventilatory Support

↓ Venous return
↓ Cardiac output
↑ Intracranial pressure
Pneumothorax
Cardiac tamponade
Subglottic stenosis
Airway plugging (inability to cough)
Arrhythmia

Table II

Role of Barbiturate Therapy in Cerebral Resuscitation

General
Protection against CNS damage induced by hypoxia
Reduction in brain metabolism

Specifics
Suppression of catecholamine synthesis
↙ ↘
- Decreasing membrane permeability
- Lowers cerebral oxygen demand by decreasing glycolysis lipolysis and protein synthesis

Vasoconstriction and shunting blood to areas with high O_2 demand (modulating cerebral blood flow)
Lowering ICP and improvement of cerebral perfusion
Minimizing damage from free O_2 radicals

It is therefore important to assure the parents that if a child survives submersion, acquiring permanent pulmonary disability is unlikely. Our recently published study had correlated outcome with ICP and CPP levels.[9] Children with ICP equal or less than 20 mm Hg and CPP equal or above 50 mm Hg had an excellent survival prognosis of 92% while 100% of those with ICP above 20 mm Hg and CPP of less than 50 mm Hg had expired. Although CPP is dependent on ICP, using both values provides better indication of prognosis than either parameter alone. Also arterial blood pH below 6.9 was associated with poor prognosis (either death or severe brain damage). Although the use of ICP and CPP could predict

Table III

Barbiturate Toxic Side Effects

- Arrhythmia
- May lower myocardial contractility and decrease cardiac output (myocardial depressant)

Table IV

The Effect of Hyperbaric Oxygenation on Cerebral Edema*

Cerebral Vasoconstriction Combined with *Increased Oxygen Availability*

↓	↓
Decreasing cerebral blood flow	Relieving cerebral anoxia
↓	
Minimizing cerebral edema	
↓	
Lowering ICP	
↓	
Improving CPP	
↓	
Minimizing cerebral ischemia	

*Research is currently being conducted in various centers studying the effect of hyperbaric oxygenation on cerebral edema.

either death or survival, these parameters were not useful in predicting those children who may recover neurologically intact or with severe brain damage.[9] Core temperature did not seem to be of value in predicting outcome.

Contrary to previous investigators who base their prognosis on clinical parameters alone, the author stresses the importance of objective assessment by utilizing continuous ICP and CPP moni-

Table V

Effects of Hypothermia (Advantages and Disadvantages)

- Hyperventilation → altered consciousness → respiratory depression → respiratory acidosis
- Reduced coronary perfusion
- Cardiac arrhythmia
- Decreased cardiac output
- Left shift of oxyhemoglobin curve
- Anaerobic metabolism and lactic acidosis
- Decreased O_2 consumption → protection of tissues and vital organs

toring.[9] The author favors the use of the subarachnoid bolt for continuous ICP monitorings since it is accepted as a safe modality. This technique should not be applied to all near-drowning victims but rather only to those who are comatose or manifest neurological deterioration.

References

1. Fandel I, Bancalari E: Near-Drowning in children: Clinical aspects. *Pediatrics* 58:573, 1976.
2. Pearn JH, Bart RD, Yamaoka R: Neurologic sequelae after childhood near-drowning: A total population study from Hawaii. *Pediatrics* 64:187, 1979.
3. Pearn J: Survival rates after serious immersion accidents in childhood. *Resuscitation* 6:271, 1978.
4. Dean JM, Kaufman ND: Prognostic indicators in pediatric near-drowning: The Glasgow coma scale. *Crit Care Med* 9:536, 1981.
5. Conn AW, Edmonds JF, Barker GA: Cerebral resuscitation in near-drowning. *Pediatr Clin of North Am* 26:691, 1979.
6. Conn AW: Near-drowning and hypothermia. CMA J 120:397, 1979.
7. Conn AW, Montes JE, Barker GA, et al: Cerebral salvage in near-drowning following neurological classification by triage. *Canad Anaesth Soc J* 27:201, 1980.
8. Ignelzi R: Cerebral edema: Present perspectives. *Neurosurgery* 4:338, 1979.
9. Nussbaum E, Galant S: Intracranial pressure monitoring as a guide to prognosis in the near-drowned, severely comatose child. *J Pediatr* 102:215, 1983.
10. Hoff BH: Multisystem failure: A review with special reference to drowning. *Crit Care Med* 7:310, 1979.
11. Orlowski JP: Prognostic factors in pediatric cases of drowning and near-drowning. *JACEP* 8:176, 1979.
12. Frates RC: Analysis of predictive factors in the assessment of warm-water near-drowning in children. *Am J Dis Child* 135:1006, 1981.
13. Jenkinson SG, George RB: Serial pulmonary function studies in survivors of near drowning. *Chest* 77:777, 1980.

3

Coma in Infants, Children and Adolescents

Hector E. James, M.D.

Introduction

We will consider *coma* as a disturbance of consciousness in which the child cannot respond to the environmental stimuli, and therefore cannot give an arousal response. We will employ for this purpose the constellation of inability to open eyes, give a verbal response and follow commands.

In this section we will not consider coma following head injury, and the reader is referred, for that information, to *Chapter Four.*

Coma differs from normal sleep state in that in sleep there is voice arousal and in coma there is not.

Stupor is a state in which the child may appear in light sleep, will have an arousal response to voice or touch, but the response will be slow and incomplete. Speech will be limited and the voice will trail off. The stimuli being withdrawn will permit the patient to return to the previous state.

Obtundation carries a similar meaning to stupor and cannot be differentiated from it in a precise way. A similar concept applies for *semi-coma. Lethargy* is meant to reflect a mild impairment of consciousness.

Impairment of consciousness without coma is a practical term used to cover the previous statements. One can infer that the normal waking state is absent, but the patient is not at the worst depth of impairment—that of coma.

Coma signifies a preterminal state of brain function in many disease entities and should therefore be considered as a life-threatening state by the people initially in contact with the child. The therapeutic attempts of the first few minutes often determine whether the child will survive, whether he will have irreversible brain damage, whether he will have a severe or mild intellectual impairment or whether he will be normal.

Physiopathology

There are multiple etiologies, other than trauma, for coma in an infant, child or adolescent. The causes may be of a congenital nature (i.e. intracranial hypertension due to hydrocephalus); due to infection (i.e. meningitis in infants); metabolic (i.e. diabetic coma); vascular (i.e. hypertensive encephalopathy); due to disorders of water and electrolyte balance (i.e. iatrogenic water intoxication and hyponatremia); and intoxications (i.e. tricyclic antidepressants). An attempt to classify these is seen in Table I.

Infection of the nervous system as a cause of coma is not uncommon. Bacterial infections in infants may cause meningitis and be complicated by coma and hypothermia. Inhabitants of the maternal gastrointestinal tract are the most common culprits, particularly E. coli, Klebsiella, Aerobacter and pseudomonas. Prema-

Table I

Causes of Coma in Children

Trauma
Infection
Intoxication
Developmental anomalies
Metabolic
Neoplastic
Vascular
Seizures

ture rupture of the amniotic membranes increases the risk. Haemophilus influenzae type B is a common bacterial cause of meningitis between two months and three years; meningococcus and pneumococcus is seen in older children. If the invasion of the nervous system occurs in the evening, no obvious prodromus is present and the child may be found comatose next morning. Pneumoccocal meningitis may occur because of a communication of the sinuses or airway with the subarachnoid space. Tuberculous meningitis may be very insidious but fulminant and devastating in many occasions.

Meningitis is a misnomer since the inflammation of the meninges does little to cause dysfunction. The pediatrician should realize that the disease is a meningocerebritis, with vascular occlusions of small and large arteries, brain swelling of varying degrees, and intracranial hypertension.[1,2]

Brain abscesses can present with coma with or without seizures. Patients with right to left cardiac shunts are at highest risk, because the "filtering" action of the lungs of bacteria has been removed. Brain abscesses cause coma by mass effect, displacements, intracranial hypertension, and cerebral ischemia. These patients are at high risk of death with transtentorial herniation. Most brain abscesses, but not all, are supratentorial in the middle and anterior cerebral artery distribution.

Viral encephalitis may cause acute profound coma with or without seizures. The disease is thought to be due to direct action of the agent on neurones and glia. Reactive hyperemia commonly presents with severe brain swelling and intracranial hypertension. If neuronal damage is severe, recovery will be associated with limited neurological recovery. Encephalitis caused by a specific virus tends to cluster geographically and seasonally. Thus the Arbo viruses tend to occur in warm weather (arthropod-borne viruses). Enteroviruses are associated with gastroenteritis and tend to occur in late summer. Some follow common childhood illnesses and have a seasonal incidence typical of each illness; examples are mumps, rubella, chickenpox and the like. Herpes virus encephalitis incidence is not truly known, and in its most clearly recognized form may be difficult to differentiate from a brain abscess.

Rickettsial infections have a geographical incidence and characteristic course, coma being associated with the most severe infections. They will most commonly have the manifestations of diseases in the form of fever, skin rash, headaches, which permit a prompt diagnosis.

Fungal meningitis is not uncommon in patients on oncological services or with debilitating diseases, all relatively immunosuppressed. In otherwise healthy children, fungal meningitis may cause infection because of geographical exposure. Impairment of consciousness may occur early in the disease, but frank coma is usually delayed.

A summary of coma due to infection is listed in Table II.

Postinfectious or parainfectious encephalomyelitis are diseases of the central and peripheral nervous systems which may follow common childhood disease. It is not known whether these are caused by direct invasion of the virus to the nervous system, or by an altered hypersensitivity or immune states, or a combination of both. Pathologically, one sees inflammatory cells around blood vessels, perivascular demyelination, varying degrees of axonal destruction, and these conditions can be duplicated in the experimental model by injection of brain extract with adjuvant. Clinically, they are characterized to follow a viral infection and develop fever, headache, and impairment of consciousness occurs rapidly. *Acute hemorrhagic leukoencephalopathy* has a course similar to those previously considered, but there is no history of previous viral illness. At times they

Table II

Coma Due to Infection

- *Active Infection*
  - Bacterial
    - meningitis—cerebritis
  - Fungal: Geographical or in the immunosuppressed
  - Protozoan
    - Amebic meningo-cerebritis
    - Cysticercosis
    - Malaria
  - Rickettsial
  - Viral encephalitis
- *Post-infectious or Parainfectious*
  - Acute hemorrhagic leukoencephalopathy
  - Encephalomyelitis
  - Reyes syndrome
- *Overwhelming Systemic Infection*

present without fever, there is a rapidly deteriorating level of consciousness, and the hallmark is that in the spinal fluid there is pleocytosis of mononuclear as well as red blood cells, with frequently elevated protein.

Reye's syndrome (acute encephalopathy and fatty degeneration of the liver) is characterized by a prodromal period with a viral illness, with subsequent vomiting, headaches, a rapidly deteriorating level of consciousness and seizures, and may be fatal within hours. Abnormal liver enzyme studies and clotting abnormalities confirm the diagnosis. Intracranial hypertension is usually present.[3]

Coma may follow overwhelming systemic infections (septic shock) due to systemic hypotension and toxic infection determined by bacterial toxins, and diminished host resistance or adrenal failure.

Coma due to *intracranial tumors* is not uncommon since tumors of the nervous system are second only to lymphomas in children. They may cause coma by the mass effect of the tumor and displacement of brain and/or posterior fossa structures with intracranial hypertension, or by creating obstructive hydrocephalus and thus leading to intracranial pressure. On occasions, tumors may hemorrhage into themselves and cause an acute rise in intracranial pressure, creating a rapid downhill course. Tumor infiltration in childhood is usually caused by perivascular and subarachnoid leukemic infiltrates in acute leukemia. The incidence of meningeal involvement at some time of the course of the illness has increased to more than 50% of cases due to longer survival. The impaired level of consciousness in these children is attributed to elevated intracranial pressure.

A summary of the causes of coma associated with intracranial tumors is listed in Table III.

Coma due to *intoxications* is not uncommon in children and adolescents. This can occur following voluntary intake of drugs or alcohol, or accidental ingestions. About 2,000 children die each year from poisoning.[4] The most common drugs ingested by children are usually combinations, analgesics, nonbarbiturate sedatives and psychopharmacologic agents.[5] Many cases are confused with encephalitis because they present with confusion, impairment of consciousness and seizures. All drugs that act as central nervous system depressants cause impairment of consciousness by acting

Table III
Neoplastic Causes of Coma

Intracranial Hypertension
Mass effect of tumor
Obstructive hydrocephalus due to tumor
Acute hemorrhage into tumor
Meningeal and subarachnoid tumor spread
Distortion and Infiltration of the Activating Reticular System
Diencephalic tumors
Hypothalamic tumors
Brain stem tumors

on the reticular activating system and related structures. Thus, depression of the activity of the reticular systems affects vasomotor center function, and the normal tonic vasoconstrictor peripheral activity is lost; consequently, heat loss follows as skin vessels dilate and hypotension ensues. Death from exposure will then occur. The heat loss is not counteracted by the normal central mechanisms of shivering because of central nervous system depression. Extreme overdosification by drugs and alcohol can also depress the respiratory center enough to cause respiratory arrest.

The most common intoxications and poisons are listed in Table IV.

Coma due to *metabolic causes* is not uncommon to the pediatric population. In the infant and young child, severe dehydration or significant electrolyte imbalance can occur rapidly, and progressively impair consciousness to a comatose state. This may be due to cellular dysfunction due to pH or ionic imbalance with cytotoxic failure, associated or not with seizures. Likewise, fluid overload is not unusual in the hospital setting, with water intoxication and hypoosmolality, cytotoxic failure, and convulsions are the consequences. Another iatrogenic cause of coma may be due to chronic parental nutrition and/or parenteral hyperalimentation. In liver or renal failure the alterations of metabolites, electrolytes and pH can progressively alter cerebral function and create a progressive encephalopathy due to a combination of these abnormalities. The coma will characteristically wax and wane with the disease process.

Table IV
Coma Due to Intoxications of Common Poisons

Heavy Metals
- lead
- mercury (organic)
- thallium

Pharmacological Agents
- phenobarbital and others
- phenytoin
- antidepressants
  - tricyclic
  - others
- phenothiazines
- opiates
- methadone
- glutethimide
- tranquilizers
- antihistamines

Alcohol

Drugs
- opiates and related

Venoms
- snake bites
- tick paralysis

Miscellaneous
- botulism
- carbon monoxide
- organic phosphates
- petroleum products

Vitamin deficiency states and malnutrition will lead to cytotoxic failure with progressive impairment of consciousness due to the ensuing encephalopathy and/or seizures. Alterations in ventilation and/or ventilation/perfusion in the lungs can create a severe encephalopathy proportional to the hypercarbia, hypoxemia and impaired venous return, with underlying intracranial hypertension.

Metabolic causes for coma are summarized in Table V.

Vascular causes of coma are listed in Table VI. They may be consequences of cardiac disease, central vasomotor reflexes or cardiac disease, central vasomotor reflexes or cardiac output that create a sudden or chronic reduction in cerebral perfusion and ischemia. Likewise, sudden hypotension due to systemic hemorrhage will have the same effect due to the lack of neuronal and glial metabolic substrate. Intracranial hemorrhage of nontraumatic origin may follow clotting plasma factor or platelet deficiencies or occur as a response to disseminated intravascular coagulation. In the premature newborn intracranial hemorrhage is commonly seen in the subependymal regions, at times extending into the deep

Table V

Coma Due to Metabolic Causes

Alterations of pH
- acidosis
- alkalosis

Organ or System Dysfunction
- hepatic failure
- renal failure
- diabetes mellitus
- hyper-hypoglycemia
- porphyria
- chronic lung disease
- hypercarbia
- hypoxemia
- pickwickian syndrome

Alterations of Water Balance
- injudicious intravenous therapy
- diabetes insipidus
- inappropriate ADH syndrome
- nephrogenic diabetes insipidus

Electrolyte Alterations
- hyper-hyponatremia
- hyper-hypocalcemia
- hyper-hypomagnesemia
- osmotic abnormalities
- chronic parenteral nutrition

Vitamin Deficiency and Dependency States
- nicotinic acid
- pantothenic acid
- pyridoxine
- thiamine (Leigh's disease)
- cyanocobalamine

Table VI
Vascular Causes of Coma

Cardio-Pulmonary Alterations
Asystole
Breath-holding spells
Syncope (vagal collapse)
Ventricular fibrillation
Vasomotor Alterations
Hypertensive encephalopathy
Hypotension—shock
Blood Vessel Alterations
Aortic stenosis
Embolizations
Thrombosis
Vasculitis
Polyarteritis nodosa
Lupus erythematosus
Granulomatous angiitis
Hemorrhagic Alterations
Deficiency of plasma clotting factors
Disseminated intravascular coagulation
Platelet dysfunction
Intracranial hemorrhage

white matter and causing mass effect. It is a more dramatic clinical condition when they occur in the cerebellum. Encephalopathy following vasculitis is a rare condition in children but may follow connective tissue disease such as lupus erythematosus. Microvascular occlusions can lead to tissue ischemia and progressive coma with or without seizures.

Impairment of consciousness of an insidious nature with respiratory irregularity and apnea may be seen in Arnold-Chiari malformations, the Dandy-Walker syndrome and other posterior fossa developmental anomalies due to brain stem distortion and ischemia.[6] A similar insidious problem may occur in bicompartmental hydrocephalus with an isolated fourth ventricle.[7] Untreated hydrocephalus can give rise to intracranial hypertension and coma.

A list of congenital anomalies that can cause coma is seen in Table VII.

Table VII

Coma Due to Developmental Anomalies

Hydrocephalus with intracranial pressure
Chiari malformation (without spina bifida)
Arnold-Chiari malformation
Arterio-venous malformations
Posterior fossa cysts
Dandy-Walker malformation
Arachnoid cysts
Bicompartmental hydrocephalus

Diagnosis

Therapy Directed Diagnosis

The most important aspect of the initial contact with a child with impairment of consciousness is assessing the severity of the impairment and determining airway control. A practical rule is if the patient is in coma, that is to say unable to open his eyes to stimuli, unable to follow commands and speak, artificial airway should be established and the patient intubated. This becomes even more important in the patient with seizures. (See Table VIII.)

Airway control will assure adequate ventilation, normoxia and normocapnia. These are important factors to ascertain adequate cerebral blood flow, metabolism and to reduce possibly elevated intracranial pressure. Seizures have a profoundly deleterious effect on the brain not only from the standpoints of brain metabolism and tissue acidosis, but also because of the dramatic increase in intracranial blood volume that they produce. Once the airway is assured the seizures can be medically controlled (i.e. diazepam intravenously 0.25–0.50 mg/kg/dose). For further explanation on the effects of ventilation and seizures on intracranial volume-pressure relationships, the reader should review *Chapter One.*

Following the previous steps ascertaining the state of the systemic blood pressure, pulse and placement of venous lines should already have been performed or should then be completed. Systemic hypotension should be corrected preferably with colloid, or

Table VIII
Therapy Directed Diagnosis in Non-Traumatic Coma

Airway assessment and control
  If in coma: intubate and ventilate
  If seizing: intubate and ventilate
    (Diazepam: 0.25–0.5 mg/kg/IV)

Blood pressure and pulse assessment
  Intravenous lines
  If hypotensive: correct (prefer colloid over cristalloid)

More through physical and neurological exam

If etiology unclear or suspected abuse: immediate computed tomography

Simultaneous to placement of intravenous lines
  Blood samples: CBC, glucose, BUN, creatinine,
    Electrolytes, calcium, magnesium, prothrombin time, SGOT, ammonia
  Immediately following administer G/W 50% (0.5–1.0 gm/kg)
  Toxic screen or blood ethanol level as indicated
  Arterial blood gas sample

Indwelling bladder catheter

Arterial line placement

If infant with open fontanelle and not bulging: lumbar puncture. If closed skull or obvious ICP: CT scan first.

judicious use of crystalloid. Liberalizing fluids will create a prompt shift of free water into an injured brain that can be deleterious if intracranial hypertension is present. An indwelling bladder catheter is a must in a comatose patient since marked distension due to urinary retention can account for combativeness, systemic hypertension and/or poor assessment of fluid balance.

The next step is a more thorough assessment of the patient's systemic and neurological exam as further history is obtained from the family, if available.

The absence of a history of trauma does not mean that silent trauma did not occur, such as in child abuse. The presence of bruises, old or new and/or the presence of preretinal hemorrhages should indicate to the physician that a significant brain injury is present and an immediate noncontrast CT scan is indicated. Thus, mass lesions due to intracranial hematomas may be detected and promptly treated.

Hypoglycemia should be suspected in any child in coma, and blood for glucose determination, together with a hemogram, electrolytes, prothrombin time, SGOT, blood ammonia, creatinine, calcium, magnesium, and toxic screen should be done when felt appropriate. This should be followed by 50% glucose (0.5–1.0 gm/kg) intravenously, as a therapeutic trial.

The patient's breath should be checked for ketosis, alcohol, uremia or hepatic fetor and aromatic intoxications.

Nuchal rigidity in the older child may indicate meningitis or subarachnoid hemorrhage. If intracranial hypertension is suspected, a CT scan should be performed immediately rather than a diagnostic lumbar puncture. This is done to determine that there is no intracranial mass that may follow the lumbar puncture with sudden deterioration due to herniation. *(See Chapter Four.)* In the infant, coma may follow meningitis abruptly and if the anterior fontanelle is patent and no obvious intracranial hypertension is evident, lumbar puncture should be done prior to CT scan, and immediate broad spectrum intravenous antibiotic therapy commenced.

If abdominal examination reveals no abdominal sounds, pursuit of a ruptured viscus should be the reason for an abdominal x–ray. Hyperactive bowel sounds may signify that the systemic hypotension is due to intra-abdominal hemorrhage.

The respiratory pattern and thoracic examination may indicate the presence of pneumonia, and in the infant this may be associated with significant impairment of consciousness.

Coma due to intoxication is often very difficult to diagnose or document. In the adolescent, ethanol intoxication should be considered and detected on breath. A blood alcohol level should be drawn and sodium bicarbonate should be added to the parenteral infusate to alkalinize and increase urine output, thus enhancing alcohol clearance. Anticonvulsant intoxication should always be suspected in a child on such medication when impairment of consciousness is seen. The pupillary examination may be of assistance in guiding the diagnosis as to the type of drug that caused the coma. (See Table IX). However, the physician should be aware that there is great variability in pupillary response. Combination

Table IX
Pupillary Examination and Coma

Mydriasis	*Miosis*
Amphetamines	Barbiturates
Antihistamines	Opiates
Atropine	Propoxyphen
Botulism	Meperidine
Cocaine	Methadone
Ephedrine	Carbon monoxide
Ethyl alcohol	Organophosphates
Glutethimide	Thallium
Snake venom	

of agents may manifest their effect on the pupil by varying its size; anoxia will cause the pupil to dilate. Pupillary inequality may be present in ingestions, as has been seen with barbiturate overdose.[8] With intoxications, fixed dilated pupils are not an indication to withdraw therapy. Amphetamines, antidepressants, antihistamines, glutethimide, phenothiazines and salicylates tend to cause seizures.

Definitive Diagnosis

Having performed the initial phases of management and not having encountered the final diagnosis for the coma state, definitive diagnostic testing should continue with the patient now in the intensive care setting. Improved toxicological analysis has allowed for identification of most poisons and intoxicants; however, there is commonly a delay of some hours. Awaiting these results should in no way indicate withholding therapy despite, what seems to be, a child in extremis. Mass lesions and congenital anomalies that can cause coma such as hydrocephalus should have been by now excluded with the computed tomogram. Hepatic and renal causes will be documented with the blood tests sent upon admission. An altered prothrombin time, an elevated SGOT and serum ammonia level will indicate Reyes syndrome, which can be confirmed by a percutaneous liver needle biopsy. Altered serum electrolytes, calcium or magnesium levels, will confirm the presence of coma due to iatrogenic imbalance, consequences of diarrhea and dehydration, diabetes insipidus, inappropriate ADH syndrome and related conditions.

Appropriate testing for porphyria will follow a history of discoloration of the urine and abdominal pains. Hypoglycemia from multiple causes is extremely common and will be documented by the admission blood measurement and by its response to the hypertonic parenteral glucose administration. Addison's disease and Cushing's disease usually present with other systemic signs prior to the onset of coma. Pheochromocytoma is rare, its history very vague, but the fluctuations in blood pressure together with a history of alterations of bowel habits may indicate the need for the catecholamine urine and serum determinations.

Hypercapnia may be a cause of coma and is usually associated with chronic lung disease and/or cystic fibrosis, the history usually being available for these due to their chronicity. Massive obesity should indicate to the physician that the hypercapnia is due to the Pickwick syndrome. The patients rarely lose consciousness early in the disease, but often become obtunded and are easily aroused.

Loss of consciousness due to seizures is a common occurrence in children, and accordingly should always be strongly considered in the diagnosis. Usually, but not always, the postictal depression follows a major motor seizure. Since the fall from a seizure may lead to head trauma, the differential diagnosis as to the cause of coma is not easy if signs of trauma are present. A CT scan is then mandatory. In most children there is a history of previous seizures, which then aids in the differential diagnosis. The pediatrician must be aware that seizures may have no motor evidence, and that electrical seizures may cause impairment of consciousness only documented as due to convulsions by an EEG.

The lumbar puncture will document the presence of meningitis in an infant in coma, and will also be suspicious for encephalitis. Definitive cultures for bacterial organisms will follow in meningitis. Viral cultures, for the most part, are not available except for tissue or secretion samples. Herpes encephalitis is strongly suspected when there is a history of maternal infection at delivery in newborns. Blisters, CSF changes indicative of possible encephalitis, an EEG with temporal lobe abnormalities, and a CT scan showing low density images in those areas, are indicative of possible encephalitis. Definitive diagnosis is obtained by retrieval of the organism from the brain culture or its presence in the electron microscopy examination. Bacterial brain abscesses are diagnosed by computed tomography and not by CSF changes *(vide supra)*.

Therapy

In the section on *Therapy Directed Diagnosis* the importance of urgent initial steps in the management of a child in coma was discussed with the objective of minimizing further brain insults by secondary complications such as hypoxia, hypercarbia, seizures, impaired cerebral autoregulation, hypothermia and hypotension.

Having identified the specific cause of coma, the appropriate specific therapeutic measures may be taken.

In the case of bacterial meningitis, initial broad spectrum antibiotic coverage may be adjusted to match the identified organism and antibiotic sensitivities. In meningitides and encephalitides underlying volume-pressure relationships may be so altered that intracranial hypertension may be a major determinant in outcome. It therefore follows that in the severe cases, intracranial pressure monitoring is an important adjuvant in the management of these patients.

Encephalopathies due to drowning, hypoxemia, hypercarbia, Reyes syndrome, are likewise managed with aggressive control of intracranial dynamics with intracranial pressure monitoring, ventilation support, maintenance of cerebral perfusion, and when available, cerebral blood flow measurements.[9,10]

In mass lesions such as brain tumors and brain abscesses, improving intracranial compliance can be promptly performed by ventilation and diuretic agents and steroids. *(See Chapter One.)* If obstructive hydrocephalus is present the only therapeutic measure that will relieve the problem is the insertion of ventricular drainage: brief relief will be obtained by medications that transiently reduce CSF production, such as furosemide or acetazolamide.[11]

Specific intoxicants will be best managed with the previously outlined initial steps and subsequent specific antidotes or therapies according to their availability. As a general rule, gastric lavage and enhancement of diuresis are good adjuvants to therapy in any intoxication that has been ingested.

Identification of an underlying metabolic disease, hormonal deficit or vitamin deficiency will guide the appropriate therapy.

Seizures are managed initially as previously outlined and then therapeutic blood levels of the chosen agent(s) should be determined to minimize the risk of recurrence of coma. There is no substitute for good airway management until the seizures are well controlled.

Prognosis

The outcome of a child in coma will be determined by the following parameters: etiological agent causing coma; time of detection of coma; rapidity and effectiveness of initial management; the subsequent management during the course of coma; and the availability of pediatric rehabilitation facilities and support systems.

The *type and the severity of causative agent* is definitely of utmost importance. Thus, in the situation of a severe carbon monoxide exposure, the neuronal destruction may be so extensive that a vegetative state may be the final outcome. On the other hand, a milder intoxicant can be associated with a total recovery. As a general rule, outside of intoxications nearly all causations of coma can be reversed to allow for a good recovery. Such a statement applies to those situations where prompt detection and effective therapy are instituted. This is due to the fact that the consequence of brain insult leads to secondary problems that can lead to brain ischemia and hypoxia.

The *time of detection* of coma is of utmost importance in reference to final outcome. A bacterial Gram-negative meningitis if detected early will naturally have a much better prognosis than if detected late. In the latter case, the occlusive disease involving the major and smaller arteries secondary to direct extension of the infection in the subarachnoid space is commonly associated with areas of brain ischemia that will lead to permanent damage.

The *rapidity and effectiveness of initial therapy* follow in importance to time of detection in reference to outcome. As an example, recurrent seizures can impair ventilation and if not properly treated can lead to hypoxia, hypercarbia, brain acidosis, intracranial hypertension and neuronal damage. Prompt effective airway control and anticonvulsive therapy will minimize those changes.

The *subsequent successful management during the course of the coma* not only will be the result of the physician's expertise and the strength of the host, but more often the result of a pediatric intensive care unit team. Infants and children in coma represent very brittle patients who need constant medical-nursing attention 24 hours a day. The often complicated therapy instituted to support these children mandates experienced pediatric nursing willing to withstand the grueling tension associated with such medicine. Prompt detection of such complications as a pneumothorax following mechanical ventilation can be not only life-saving, but also a strong factor in quality of outcome. As expectations rise in the often successful therapy of children in coma, so does the requirement for further sophistication in care. The unit that will render the best care to the pediatric patient is not only the one that effectively does the initial resuscitation and therapy, but continues an intensive care unit course with minimal complications.

The continued care of a child to fullest recovery is tantamount to follow-through to early pediatric rehabilitation support. This implies a *team* of therapists skilled in pediatric occupational, physical and speech therapies. This team in order to be effective, must also be able to follow-through into the appropriate school level and coordinate special resources as needed. The team must have a rehabilitation physician, psychologist, nurse coordinator and social worker.

Irreversible Coma

Coma depassé indicates a concept of dying as a process over time, rather than an event, occurring instantaneously. The patients are suffering from unresponsiveness and unreceptiveness from which they will never recover. The concept does not imply an understanding of underlying physiopathology, but it implies that recovery should not occur. *Cerebral death* and *brain death* have one more conclusive expression: There is evidence by physiological or radiological or histochemical studies that there is irrevocable brain damage. In making the statement of brain death one indicates that there will be a cardiovascular-respiratory collapse within hours or days despite heroic measures, which will fulfill the more traditional medico-legal criterion of death. One must tolerate only substantial

Table X

Definition of Irreversible Coma*

Unreceptivity and unresponsiveness to intense painful stimulation.
No movement or breathing—observed at least 1 hour by physicians. Respirator may be turned off for 3 minutes if Pa_{CO_2} is normal at beginning of trial and patient has been breathing room air for 10 minutes.
No reflexes—including pupillary, vestibular, other brain stem. Postural: also includes deep tendon reflexes and plantar response.
Flat EEG—increased gains for at least part of run: noncephalic and electrocardiogram obtained simultaneously.
All tests to be repeated at least 24 hours later with no change.
The etiology of the coma is not hypothermia (temperature below 32° C) or central nervous system depressants.

*Modified from the Ad Hoc Committee of the Harvard Medical School.[12]

error in deciding that the brain is alive when in fact it is dead, rather than an error in the opposite direction.

The *legal* concept of cerebral death varies among countries and even within individual states in the United States, and one must be informed of the often changing legislation. For the most part, the report of the Ad Hoc Committee of the Harvard Medical School is followed[12] with minor variations by most medical groups. The variations that are most commonly seen relate to the presence or absence of deep tendon reflexes, and whether a repeat set of studies are needed 24 hours later. (See Table X.)

Prevention

The best therapy for nontraumatic coma is to prevent its occurrence in day-to-day living. Restricting access to medications, intoxicants and poisons is a must. Appropriate lids for common indications will minimize the hazards of accidental ingestions. Appropriate instruction to school children and adolescents as to the problems with drugs and alcohol is needed, and should be encouraged. Instruction and supervision of children with platelet or clotting factor deficiencies should not only be directed to the child, but also to the family to minimize the exposure to head injuries.

Hydrocephalic children with or without Arnold-Chiari malformation, should be routinely checked on a periodic basis to determine that insidious shunt dysfunction or loculation of the ventricular system does not occur.[7,13] Instructions to the parents as to the potential for dysfunction of a shunt should be thorough, so that they may promptly identify and seek aid should an acute shunt obstruction occur. This will avoid the development of severe intracranial hypertension and brain ischemia.

Hospitalized patients on prolonged parenteral nutrition are always at risk of osmolality and electrolyte imbalance, or calcium, magnesium and zinc deficiencies. Accordingly, these should be routinely assessed to prevent brain dysfunction.

It is obvious that no therapy can take the place of common sense and education to prevent the frequent accidents, intentional and unintentional acquisition of poisons and diseases that may lead to coma. School education at all levels with parental involvement is society's best investment in that respect.

References

1. Blackwood W, Corsellis JAN (eds): *Greenfield's Neuropathology.* Third Edition, London, Arnold Co., 1976.
2. Baird DR, Whittle HC, Greenwood BM: Mortality from pneumococcal meningitis. *Lancet* 2:1344–1346, 1976.
3. Trauner DA: Reye's syndrome. *In Current Problems in Pediatrics,* Chicago-London, 1982, Year Book Medical Publishers, Inc., Volume 12, pp. 1–31.
4. Dreisbach RH: *Handbook of Poisoning.* Seventh Edition, Los Altos, Lange Medical Publications, 1971.
5. Pierce AW, Jr: Salicilate poisoning. Pediatrics 54:342–347, 1974.
6. Matson DD: *Neurosurgery of Infancy and Childhood.* Second Edition, Springfield, Illinois, Charles C. Thomas, 1969.
7. Foltz EL, DeFeo DR: Double compartment hydrocephalus—A new entity. *Neurosurgery* 7:551–559, 1980.
8. Mathew H: Acute poisoning: Some myths and misconceptions. *Br. Med. J* 1:519–522, 1971.
9. Bruce DA, Berman WA, Schut L: Cerebrospinal fluid pressure, monitoring in children: Physiology, pathology and clinical usefulness. In *Advances in Pediatrics,* New York, New York Medical Publishers, 1977. Volume 24, pp. 223–290.
10. James HE, Langfitt TW, et al: Treatment of intracranial hypertension. *Acta Neurochirurg* 36:189–200, 1977.

11. Harbaugh RD, James HE, Marshall LF, et al: Acute therapeutic modalities for experimental vasogenic edema. *Neurosurgery* 5:656–665, 1979.
12. Beecher HK: A definition of irreversible coma: Report of the Ad Hoc Committee of the Harvard Medical School to examine the definition of brain death. *JAMA* 205:85, 1968.
13. James HE, Schut L: Pitfalls in the diagnosis of arrested hydrocephalus. *Acta Neurochirurg* 43:13–17, 1978.

4

Head Injury in Infants, Children and Adolescents

Hector E. James, M.D.

Introduction

In children aged from one to five years, accidents are the most common cause of death and close to 30% of the deaths are due to head injuries. Twenty percent of deaths are a result of traffic accidents alone and almost 75% of all pediatric hospitalizations due to trauma are due to head trauma.[1–6] Over the past years the hospitalizations for head injury due to child abuse have increased.[7] Seventy-three percent of deaths that occur from head injury occur in the first 48 hours of hospitalization.[1] Of the children who are hospitalized and who subsequently die, 50% of them were not in coma upon admission.[8]

The mortality rate in children with head injury in the literature varies widely. Thus Bruce et al[9] report an overall mortality rate of 9% in severe head injury with modern aggressive management with a team consisting of pediatric neurosurgeons, pediatric intensivists and easy access to computed-tomography. Whereas, Carlsson et al[10] and Becker et al[11] report a mortality in patients, under 19 years of age, of 20–25%, and Jennet et al[12] reported 35%. If the children present to the hospital in decerebrate posturing the mortality has been reported at 44%, 50%, and 71%.[13–15]

The impression that the biological response to head injury in children differs from that of adults,[3,4,9] together with the fact that patients under 19 years of age have lower mortality when compared to similar adult patients due to a lower secondary mortality,[10,11] makes aggressive specialized management an absolute necessity if a good outcome is to be obtained. Our understanding of the effects of the initial traumatic injury on the brain is, at best, limited, and there are no means at present of treating the mechanical effects produced by the traumatic insult. Consequently, all therapy is directed to preventing a secondary brain insult from the consequences of head injury: hypoxia, hypercarbia, arterial hypotension, seizures and intracranial hypertension. All these parameters can be monitored, assessed and treated, and these should ideally start at the scene of the accident.

The ability to adequately manage the child with severe head injury should entail the combination of a series of resources, which at present consists of: a pediatric intensivist, pediatric neurosurgeon, pediatric intensive care unit and pediatric nursing, and ready access to computed tomography and operating room suite. If one analyzes the above referred outcome in the literature, one can start to dissect the reason behind the discrepancy in the numbers. Some series are reported prior to computed tomography availability, others are reported where there is no pediatric intensivist and/or pediatric neurosurgeon, and others where transportation from the scene of an accident as well as support at the scene, are inadequate or delayed. The author in a past experience[16] in 157 hospitalized pediatric head injuries noted that three patients transported over a great distance without adequate care at the scene and during transport, died within 72 hours of admission. Of the remaining 12 severe injuries (Glasgow Coma Scale eight or less), only one further mortality occurred. Thus, with the support system previously outlined, the data of Bruce et al[17] in our opinion, are realistic figures for the outcome of head injuries in children.

Pathology

Anatomical Pathology

As in the adult, there can be a wide array of pathology to the skull and brain in head injured children.[1,3,4,14,17] Bruises and abrasions, linear fractures and subgaleal masses, comminuted skull fractures, compound skull fractures and subsequent development of growing skull fractures (leptomeningeal cysts) weeks after the impact may be seen.[3] Intracranial hemorrhage may be a consequence of the injury, and this may lead to epidural, subdural or intracerebral hematomas. A combination of these may exist in the same patient.[18]

The elasticity of the young skull gives the child certain advantage over the adult, since it allows certain "plasticity" (deformation) to the system, neutralizing some of the forces on the brain on impact.[4] If the force of the blow is greater than the tensile strength of the bone, a fracture will occur. High velocity impacts create, on the other hand, severe acceleration—deceleration movements of the brain and skull that yield far more injury.

Skull fractures at the base can be accompanied by dural tears that then lead to CSF fistula. The more common locations are in the floor of the frontal fossa related to the cribriform plate, and in the petrous bone.[3,4] The former will manifest itself as obvious or silent CSF rhinorrhea, the latter as otorrhea. The presence of fistulae can create a pathway for bacteria into the subarachnoid space, and meningitis will follow.

The most common autopsy finding in pediatric head injuries is a swollen brain with congestion of the vessels and flattened gyri.[18] This is a consequence of the response of the brain to impacts that occur in angular acceleration movements of the cranium and the brain, against irregular bony surfaces at the anterior and middle fossas. In severe cases, contusions in the corresponding cortical surfaces are seen.[18] The brain swelling is probably magnified by the hypoxic–ischemic insult that can occur at the time of impact and impaired cerebrovascular autoregulation. (See Chapter One.)

The hemorrhages that follow head injury, be they mild or severe, may create an obstruction to CSF flow and lead to post-traumatic hydrocephalus. The obstruction to CSF flow occurs mostly in the subarachnoid space of the base and/or the arachnoid granulations, sites of CSF reabsorption.

Radiological Pathology

From what has been stated in the previous section one can infer that the most common computed tomogram finding in a child with significant head injury is the presence of subarachnoid blood. This is seen in 79% of the children and is noted as a sheet-like high density at the level of the falx cerebri and tentorium. In 49% of the cases, diffuse swelling is seen.[17] This is seen on CT as crowding of the lateral and third ventricles, without displacement from their normal position, with obliteration of the cisterns and subarachnoid spaces.[19] This is not accompanied by low density images, but, if anything, the white matter images might be more prominent than normal.[19] With the advent of high resolution CT equipment, cerebral contusions are not uncommonly seen (10% of cases). These are represented by areas on the surface of the brain of low density patches (cerebral edema) with spots of high density areas (the hemorrhages). These are thought to represent radiologically the cortical contusions described pathologically by Lindenberg et al.[18] Subdural hematomas are seen in 8% of children,[17] epidural hematomas in 6.5% and they are very uncommon under two years of age. This is thought to be due to the strong adherence under two years of age between the dura mater and the inner table of the skull, since bone growth is occurring primarily from the outer dural layers. Intracerebral hematomas are seen in 5% of cases.[17] With high velocity injuries, the acceleration–deceleration forces may produce sheer injuries in the white matter and brain stem. With high resolution scans these may be seen as small areas of patchy hemorrhages with or without low density lesions.

As the acute phase passes, changes may be seen in the CSF pathways represented by irregular accumulations of low density (CSF-like) areas over the convexities. These, characteristically, may change in shape and location when seen on sequential scans.[9] They do not have to be treated operatively.[9] In cases of severe head injuries, brain atrophy may become manifest a few weeks postimpact, seen by enlargement of the cisterns, ventricles and sulci, while retaining the acute angles of the ventricles.This must be differentiated from post-trauma hydrocephalus in which there is rounding of the ventricular angles, significant enlargement of the temporal horns, accompanied by a lack of clinical improvement. This may represent low or high pressure hydrocephalus and the differential diagnosis of atrophy versus normal pressure and/or arrested hydrocephalus is at times very difficult and usually based on clinical criteria.[20]

Physiopathology

The most common finding in head injury is the presence of subarachnoid blood and diffuse brain swelling.[9] Cerebral blood flow measurements in these patients show it to be increased and this is accompanied by an increase in blood brain volume.[19] Consequently, intracranial compliance will be altered and ICP elevations are common.[17,21] If ICP is not controlled, cerebral perfusion will falter and secondary repeated episodes of ischemic-hypoxia can ensue.[22] Seizures may complicate the course since post-traumatic epilepsy[23] seems more common in children than in the adult occurring in 6 to 14% of the cases.[1,14,17] Seizures can increase brain acidosis due to hypoventilation and thus affect cellular metabolism. They can lead to hypercarbia, consequent cerebral vasodilatation and further increase cerebral blood volume. By impairing ventilation, seizures can then lead to hypoxemia, impairment of cerebral metabolism and further cerebral vasodilatation. For further description of the effects of head injury on volume-pressure relationships, the reader should refer to *Chapter One.*

Intracranial hematomas can create cerebral dysfunction by mechanically distorting the brain and brain stem on one hand, and on the other, by raising ICP. Progressive mass effect will lead to herniations and impairment of cerebral perfusion. Therefore, they should be rapidly diagnosed and promptly removed.

In certain severe cases the acceleration–deceleration injury complicated by a rotational component, can lead to diffuse axonal injury of the white matter.[24] This has been seen in the clinical setting as well as the subhuman primate.[25] It is a distinctive clinicopathological injury and it is characterized by having no lucid interval after it, a low incidence of skull fractures, a low incidence of contusions, and intracranial hematoma.[24] In these cases the prognosis is extremely guarded.

Clinical Presentation and Diagnosis

The clinical presentation from the didactic standpoint may be divided into injuries of the skull and injuries of the brain.

Injuries of the Skull

These can be contusions and abrasions that will mandate the standard topical care and assessment of the child's tetanus prophylaxis. In infants, a subgaleal mass over the parietal convexity is a common occurrence following a fall and a striking of that region. It may not be noticeable until a day after the impact. There is not uncommonly an underlying *linear skull fracture.* The fracture *per se* requires no therapy and the hematoma will slowly resolve; however, follow-up anteroposterior and lateral plain roentgenograms are recommended 7–8 weeks following the injury to ascertain that a growing skull fracture (leptomeningeal cyst) is not occurring.[26,27] This is particularly important under two years of age, since the force of the rapidly growing brain can spread the fracture edges apart when a dural tear has occurred.

In more severe cases a child may present with a *comminuted depressed fracture* with or without an overlying interruption of skin (*compound fracture*). These are of importance since underlying dural tears can favor seizures, infection, meningitis and brain abscesses.[28] Therefore, prompt operative treatment is indicated. In cases of child abuse, a comatose child may present scalp bruise(s) and the etiology may be unclear. Funduscopic examination, not uncommonly, reveals pre-retinal hemorrhages that indicates a violent force being applied to the cranium.[7]

Periorbital ecchymosis immediately following impact will indicate a direct impact to the orbit. However, following a *fracture at the base* of the skull in the frontal region, retro-orbital bleeding will seep forward to the outer canthus, under the conjunctiva then to the conico-conjunctival junction, forming a sharp crescentic margin; because of gravity, it collects more in the lower half of the eye. This will classically take hours or a day to develop.[29] Bruises behind the ear are similar indications of fracture at the base in the posterior aspect of the middle fossa (Battle's sign),[29] and also develop gradually. Fractures at the base may lead to leakage of CSF such as can be seen in the region of the cribriform plate (rhinorrhea) or in the middle ear (otorrhea). The fluid is more often bloodstained than clear. The above physical findings are of importance since often skull roentgenograms do not reveal fractures because of their small size and the difficulty in visualization of structures of the base. Hemotympanum represents a fracture of the base with bleeding in the middle ear. Recognizing this is not only of value in ascertaining the magnitude of the injury, but will also mandate postdischarge otolaryngology follow-up. Hearing difficulty may ensue which, properly diagnosed and managed, will permit the child to have appropriate school performance.

Injuries of the Brain

There are multiple ways of classifying brain injuries and we will maintain certain flexibility in that respect.

The most common form of head injury is the *transient mild* "stunning" effect, in which the child stops activities for a matter of seconds and then resumes them. *Cerebral concussion* is a term commonly employed for a more significant impact to the skull. In this condition there is a transient loss of consciousness of a minute or more, and with return of consciousness the patient "is not well," is dazed, may or may not cry, and loses appetite. Vomiting is commonly present and resolves spontaneously.[30,31] The patient's lethargy may last hours or a few days. With return of function, the child may have residual headaches, short attention span and behavior problems, and in most cases these disappear within days or weeks of the injury.

In an attempt to define in mathematical terms the probability of various outcomes following head injury, studies have been made, derived from combinations of predicted features in an individual patient.This was done in an attempt to obtain a reliable prognosis as to the final outcome in a severely head injured patient within the first few days of injury.[12] These data come from a large volume data bank. In the study, the importance of deferring prognostic statements until six hours after injury has been emphasized by the authors and a 24-hour postinjury assessment is more reliable.[32] *Coma* in these studies is then defined by the best predictors of outcome, as an inability to open eyes spontaneously or with stimulation, to obey commands, or to speak.[32] Other factors of importance in outcome were pupil responsiveness and eye movement. Thus, in a large series of comatose patients from severe head injury who had no spontaneous eye opening within 24 hours of the injury, 64% were dead or vegetative at six months; of those with eye opening within 24 hours of injury only 30% were vegetative.[12] At six months the difference in recovery was evident: 54% of those able to open their eyes within 24 hours had a moderate to good recovery, while 26% of those did not.[12] From these studies and the head injury data bank, the Glasgow Coma Scale was created.[12,32] This scale relates, in mathematical terms, eye opening in response to any stimuli, verbal behavior and motor response by grading them (Table I). The lowest score is 3 (the worst), and the maximum is 15 (the best).

These studies and the Glasgow Coma Scale provide the opportunity for comparison of clinical trials, management and communication of patients with head injury and comparison of therapeutic trials. Obviously, because of speech and intellectual development, this scale does not apply to patients under two years of age. The mean age of the patients in the Jennet et al[12,32] studies was 33 years. It is obvious from the above that the scale was designed for head injury and therefore to employ it for other conditions is not valid, since it does not base itself on a data bank other than head injury. Likewise, the scale will be affected by intercurrent conditions such as drugs or alcohol ingested prior to the injury.

We will be describing therapy for head injuries on the basis of the Scale. We will define as a *mild* head injury those patients with scores of 13–15; *moderate* head injury, those with scores of 9–12; and a score of 8 and under as *severe* head injury.

Therapy

From the point of view of management we will divide therapy into skull therapy and brain therapy.

Therapy for Skull Injuries

Subgaleal hematomas require no therapy and needle drainage should be avoided to minimize the risk of infection.[3] They will spontaneously resolve in a matter of days. Scalp abrasions require thorough cleansing and an assessment of tetanus prophylaxis. Scalp lacerations should be cleaned and debrided thoroughly with prompt suture. The galea is extremely vascular and exsanguina-

Table I

Glasgow Coma or Responsiveness Scale

Eye Opening (E)		*Best Motor Response (M)*		*Verbal Response (V)*	
spontaneous	E4	obeys	M6	orientated	V5
to speech	3	localizes	5	confused conversation	4
to pain	2	withdraws	4	inappropriate words	3
nil	1	abnormal flexion	3	incomprehensible sounds	2
		extends	2		
		nil	1	nil	1

tion will occur if not sutured promptly. Following cleansing, a vertical mattress suture with a curved needle and number 3 or 4 "o" nylon is indicated. The vertical mattress suture is a hemostatic suture and if knotted tightly will stop galeal hemorrhage. An assessment of tetanus prophylaxis should then be performed.

For the depressed fractures with or without a compound component, the patient will be taken to the operating room by the neurosurgeon for exploration, repair of possible dural tears, debridement and elevation of fragments.[3,23] It would be appropriate to suture the laceration while awaiting the operating room, since exsanguination may occur. Forty-eight hour broad-spectrum intravenous antibiotic coverage is felt appropriate.

Basilar skull fractures should be admitted for bedrest and observation. Assessment of the clinical state should be accompanied by close monitoring of the rectal temperature. If a febrile spike should occur, then blood and CSF cultures (lumbar puncture) should be promptly taken and immediate broad-spectrum intravenous antibiotics initiated. When the organism and the appropriate antibacterial sensitivities are identified, the changes in the antibiotic regime can be made. There seems to be little grounds for placing a patient with basilar skull fracture on antibiotics upon admission since this may lead to resistant strains complicating the clinical course.[33] Twenty-four to forty-eight hours following cessation of symptomatic CSF fistula, progressive ambulation in the hospital may be initiated. Forty-eight hours later, if no leakage and no fever are noted, the patient may be discharged and followed closely, initially, as an outpatient.

A treatment diagram is seen in Table II.

Table II

Management of Skull Injuries

Subgaleal Hematoma
- No therapy.

Linear Skull Fracture
- Monitoring of neurological status.
- No therapy.
- In the child under two years, repeat anteroposterior and lateral skull film at two months (to exclude leptomeningeal cyst).

Depressed Skull Fracture
- Close monitoring of neurological status.
- Urgent elevation and exploration of fracture.

Compound Depressed or Linear Skull Fracture
- Close monitoring of neurological status.
- Emergency debridement and repair.
- Tetanus prophylaxis assessment.
- 48-hour broad spectrum intravenous antibiotic coverage.
- Follow-up skull anteroposterior and lateral skull x-ray (to exclude leptomeningeal cyst, determine bone healing).

Basilar Skull Fracture
- Close monitoring of neurological status.
- Absolute bedrest.
- No antibiotics.
- 24 hours after cessation of otorrhea or rhinorrhea, progressively ambulate for 24–48 hrs. If no recurrence, may discharge from hospital.
- If febrile spike, perform lumbar puncture and blood sample for cultures, commence broad spectrum antibiotic therapy, await sensitivities.
- If CSF cultures positive, treat for two weeks.
- If CSF fistula persists for more than one week of rest, operative repair indicated.

Scalp Laceration
- Debridement and repair with tight sutures promptly.
- Tetanus prophylaxis assessment.

Therapy for Brain Injury

The following discussion of therapy for brain injury will be divided into mild, moderate, and severe according to the Glasgow Coma Scale previously described.

Management of the Mild Head Injury. This applies to the patients with Glasgow Coma scores of 13 or more, or infants who fall, are "stunned," cry and then are seen fully alert and normal. If complicating factors such as skull injuries are not present and abuse is not suspected,[7] following observation in the emergency room as felt necessary, the patient may be discharged with appropriate instructions. If concern exists, the patient should be examined the next day. Skull radiographs are not necessary under these circumstances, if the physical examination is unremarkable. The presence of a subgaleal hematoma or a scalp laceration should mandate radiographs, for the reasons previously explained. Likewise, skull radiographs as well as a skeletal survey should be performed when abuse is suspected. Skull radiographs are most informative when clinically indicated.[34,35]

A category of its own is the child or adolescent who, following minor head injury, has recurrent vomiting. The hallmark of this patient is that although initially lethargic and with no evidence of a focal neurological finding, the child has a recuperating level of consciousness but continues with bouts of emesis that are exacerbated by changes in position or turning in bed. This may persist for several days. Positional vertigo in the child who is able to describe it, is often the only finding. The syndrome ceases on its own, and if the patient is quite alert, anti-emetics may be indicated when it is past 48 hours of the injury.

Patients, especially infants, with recurrent vomiting must be hospitalized and placed on maintenance intravenous fluid therapy consisting of dextrose 5% and 0.2 or 0.45 normal saline solution with potassium supplement, to avoid dehydration. Therapy can then be discontinued when oral tolerance of fluids is documented.

Management of Moderately Severe Brain Injuries. This applies to patients with a Glasgow Coma Score of 9–12, and to infants who, following a fall, remain irritable, lethargic and/or have recurrent emesis. It also applies to patients who have post-traumatic convulsions.

These patients should be thoroughly assessed and observed in the hospital. (See Table III). Skull radiographs and/or CT scan are not absolutely mandatory upon admission unless focal skull injury or complicating factors are present. To routinely attempt to perform these studies upon admission will yield a very poor study that may obscure the picture because of lack of cooperation and/or combativeness. Attempts to sedate these patients will lead to hypoventilation, furthering of brain swelling, and create intracranial

Table III

Outline of the Management of the Moderately Severe Brain Injury

G.C.S. 9 to 12
or
Lethargic, Irritable Infants with Emesis

↓

admit to PICU

↓

Observation
elevation of head or bed 10–15°
maintenance of intravenous fluids

↓

History of seizures:
phenytoin 5 mg/kg IV slowly,
repeat at 30–60 minutes
then maintenance

if no seizure history:
no prophylaxis

↓

If seizures occur

If level of consciousness deteriorates

If improvement → discharge

↓

Intubate—CT scan
For seizures: diazepam (0.25 mg/kg/dose)

↓

Management of severe brain injury *(Table IV)*

G.C.S. = Glasgow Coma Scale; PICU = Pediatric Intensive Care Unit

hypertension that will mandate intubation, mechanical ventilation, and aggressive support that could otherwise be avoided.

These patients should be admitted to the pediatric intensive care unit and closely observed. If deterioration of consciousness ensues and/or seizures occur, they should immediately be intubated, paralyzed, and a CT scan should immediately be performed in search of a progressive mass lesion.

Following admission, these patients should have elevation of the head of the bed by 10–15 degrees (*see Chapter One*), intravenous maintenance fluid therapy and no medication. If seizures occurred following the accident, seizure prophylaxis should be promptly instituted to avoid worsening of intracranial dynamics due to their deleterious effect. This may be done by slowly administering intravenous of phenytoin in saline solution, at 5 mg/kg with a repeat dose of 5 mg/kg 30–60 minutes later, and maintenance then of 5 mg/kg/day should follow the same day (divided into 12-hour doses). Nursing and in-house physician personnel should be instructed as to the significance and detection of seizures, since they may occur with minimal motor movement or none at all. If seizures should occur despite phenytoin therapy, no compromise should be made and the patient should be intubated, hyperventilated and administered a diazepam intravenously (0.25 mg/kg) bolus.

Most patients with moderate head injuries will recover without further ado or therapy. The majority of them, within 24–36 hours of the injury, are next to baseline status.

The pediatric patients who are not improving at 48 hours of injury and who have not had a CT scan, should be then promptly studied. This is due to the fact that in children it is common for epidural hematomas to become overtly manifest at 48 hours, whereas in the adult it does so at 24 hours.[36] For that reason a 24-hour hospitalization observation period is only valid for the child that has returned or nearly returned to baseline status. In children who have not, a 48-hour observation is mandatory.[36] In some cases the subdural hematomas do not enlarge enough to be symptomatic until after the hospitalization.[37] To rely on plain radiographs to state whether an intracranial hematoma is present or not is erroneous since no fractures were seen in 15%[36] and 19%[38] of patients with extradural hematomas, or in 23% of the subdural hematoma patients and 17% of intracerebral hematomas.[36]

A lucid interval was obtained by history in 68% of children with epidural hematomas, and 57% had no disturbance of consciousness at the time of injury.[38] It therefore follows that to rely on a history of post-traumatic loss of consciousness to attempt to define whether a hematoma is present or not, is unreliable.

Management of Severe Brain Injuries. Upon arrival or during transport, patients will be assessed as having Glasgow Coma scores of 8 or less, or they will be infants with severe obtundation, with or without seizures, and/or obtunded infants with multiple trauma. (See Table IV.)

Table IV

Outline of the Early Management of the Severe Brain Injury

G.C.S. 3 to 8
or
Infants with Unresponsiveness

↓

Emergency room:
intubation and ventilation
arterial gases
blood screening tests
dexamethasone 1 mg/kg/IV
phenytoin 5 mg/kg/IV
indwelling Foley catheter
nasogastric tube
cervical spine lateral film

↓

CT scan with scanogram

If operative lesion	If no operative lesion
O.R.	PICU
	arterial line
	central line
ICP monitor	ICP monitor

↓

PICU Management *(Table V)*

If not already intubated, these patients should be promptly intubated with minimal neck manipulation. Prompt intubation will not only allow for adequate oxygenation, but also lower the Pa_{CO_2} and improve pH. With this the ICP will be normalized and cerebral perfusion pressure (CPP) will improve. Simultaneously placing adequate venous lines, a lateral plain radiograph is obtained for signs of cervical injury or instability with the head maintained in the neutral position. The neurological and systems evaluation will be done while waiting for the cervical film to be processed.

Indwelling Foley catheter and nasogastric tube placement will follow and administration of 1 mg/kg/dose of dexamethasone intravenously. Following this, phenytoin will be given, 5 mg/kg/dose in a slow intravenous administration in normal saline, over 15–20 minutes. This should be repeated half an hour to an hour later (total of 10 mg/kg/loading dose). The patient should be promptly transported to the CT scan. A lateral scanogram of the skull will take the place of a lateral skull film for expediency, and a fast scan of the cranium will follow. If mass lesions in the form of subdural or epidural hematomas are present, the patient will be promptly taken to the operating room for their evacuation. If on the other hand no operative lesions are detected, then the patient is placed in the pediatric intensive care unit (PICU) where an arterial line, central venous or Swan-Ganz catheterization should be performed. A chest radiograph is then obtained to document the position of the endotracheal tube, state of the lungs and location of lines (Fig. 1).

Following evacuation of an intracranial hematoma or, if no operative lesion is present, upon arrival to the PICU an intracranial monitoring device is placed. This will permit assessments of ICP, intracranial elastance and CPP, and will give a course for appropriate therapy to be instituted in a timely fashion. There are multiple techniques for monitoring intracranial pressure and many devices are commercially available. The most commonly employed methods are intraventricular catheters or subdural devices. As a general rule, the author prefers to employ a ventricular catheter if the ventricles are clearly seen on CT scan, or the subdural screw when the ventricles are collapsed from swelling or edema. This will avoid unnecessary cannulations of the brain. The techniques for their placement and their advantages and disadvantages have been previously described by us.[39,40,41] The intraventricular catheter will for the most part give a slightly (2–4 torr) higher pressure and a wider pulse pressure than the subdural recordings. (See Fig. 1.) The ventricular catheter will permit for drainage of CSF intermittently as needed, as an adjuvant of ICP therapy.[41]

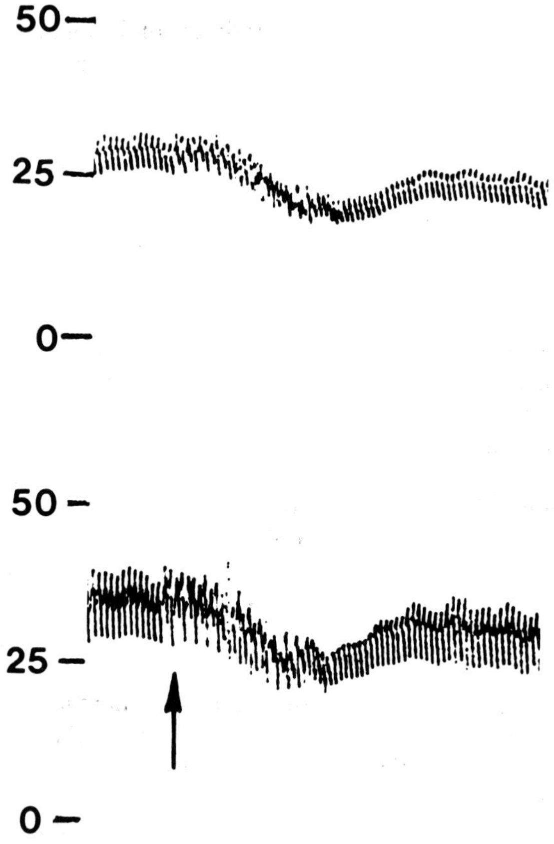

Figure 1. ICP recordings from an intraventricular catheter (lower tracing) and a subarachnoid screw (upper tracing). Continuous ICP recording demonstrating the respiratory and vascular variations. The superior tracing corresponds to a subarachnoid screw and the inferior tracing to an intraventricular catheter. Both recordings are simultaneously performed in the same patient for comparison. At the arrow, transient mechanical hyperventilation was instituted.

Most patients with head injury have elevated ICP upon admission[22] and this is significantly higher in patients with intracranial post-traumatic hematomas.[22] If properly managed initially, the first ICP readings are more commonly low due to intubation and early management therapy, but in the subsequent hours it will steadily or rapidly rise. In the majority of pediatric patients ICP will be controlled with hyperventilation and sedation (diazepam 0.25 mg/dose or thiopental 1.0–1.5 mg/kg/dose or meperidine 0.5–1.0 mg/kg/dose). If ICP is not maintained with this regime under 15 torr, additional therapy should be promptly instituted, since rapid bouts of ICP will be deleterious on the brain and lead to a poor outcome.[42] Fluid maintenance should be initially given and restriction of fluids may be indicated to maintain a serum osmolality in the 300–310 mOsm. If serum osmolality is below that and ICP is poorly controlled, a mannitol bolus of 0.5–1.0 gm/kg can be employed.[43] If serum sodium is high or if there is a contraindication to hypertonic diuretics, furosemide 0.5–1.0 mg/kg intravenously will have a similar effect on ICP.[44] If persistent fluctuations over 15 torr occur, a mannitol infusion parallel to the existing intravenous maintenance fluids may be given (1–2 gm/kg/ every 8 hours),[43] or alternating bolus administrations of mannitol (0.5–1.0 gm/kg) with furosemide (0.5–1.0 mg/kg).

If serum osmolality is over 310 mOsm/L alternative therapy to control ICP may be obtained by increasing ventilation and reducing the $Paco_2$ further to the low twenties. If on the other hand, hyperventilation is maximized, barbiturate therapy is needed. This can be done with intermittent bolus administration of pentobarbital 2.0 or 2.5 mg/kg or thiopental 1.0–1.5 mg/kg. If this regime fails, a continuous infusion of thiopental can be done.[17]

Failure to control ICP with this regime should lead to a barbiturate coma by monitoring blood levels frequently (3–5 mg%) and by EEG (isoelectric tracing). Hypothermia may be employed as an adjuvant therapy.[17,21]

At all times the systemic state of the child should be closely monitored and corrected where needed. Cerebral perfusion pressure should be over 40 torr at all times. Therefore, systemic arterial pressure (SAP) should always be maintained and normalized. One of the hazards of aggressive therapy for reducing ICP is that all the methods of treatment tend to reduce SAP. Medications should be administered slowly, especially the barbiturates, because of their strong hypotensive effects. Due to these concerns, volume and cardiac output measurements are extremely important in the pediatric patient undergoing aggressive therapy and they should have Swan-Ganz catheters in place for that purpose.

The effect of steroids on the course and outcome of head injuries is controversial. Several studies in the literature have given contradictory results. It is now clear that the pure anti-edema effect of steroids is limited, while the clinical efficiency in conditions other than head injury is considerable.[45–50] They seem to improve cell membrane function,[51,52] blood brain barrier integrity,[53,54] improve intracranial compliance[42] and normalize and stabilize cerebral blood flow.[50] Faupel et al[45] in a double-blind study on the effects of dexamethasone on severe closed head injuries in adult patients noted an improvement in the quality of survival and a reduction in mortality.

In that study, 100 mg of dexamethasone was given initially, and 100 mg was again given six hours later. The patients were then maintained on 16 mg a day for eight days and the therapy then abruptly stopped. A similar finding has been noted in a limited preliminary study in children with severe head injuries.[16] In this study children were given 1 mg/kg/dose upon arrival and then maintained on 1 mg/kg/day (divided into 8-hour dosages) for eight days. No deleterious effects were noted from this therapy. All patients received regularly antiacid suspensions through the nasogastric tube.[16]

A treatment diagram for severe head injury is seen in Table V.

Prognosis

The prognosis will be related to the magnitude of the injury, the presence or absence of associated injuries, the promptitude of management, the effectiveness and expertise of managing physicians and ancillary personnel, and finally the quality of rehabilitation services.

In a large present day therapy series of 85 children with severe head injury a useful recovery was seen in 87.5%.[17] A Glasgow Coma score higher than 5 was always associated with a good recovery. Overall persistent vegetative state was seen in 3.5% of pa-

Table V
Outline of the Treatment of the Severe Brain Injury

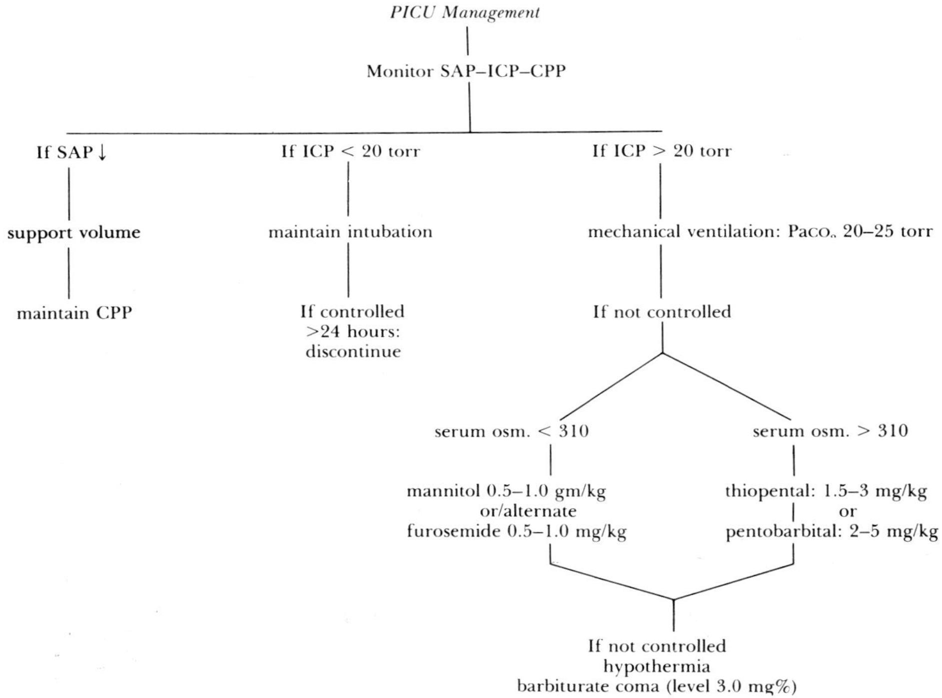

tients. Glasgow Coma scores of 3 or 4 were associated with poor outcome or death in 23% of patients. The overall mortality of the series was 9%. The worst prognostic findings were: flaccidity, fixed dilated pupils and absent oculovestibular responses.[17] Twenty-nine percent of patients who had fixed dilated pupils upon presentation had a poor outcome.[17]

On the other hand, nothing definitive in reference to outcome can be stated early in the disease due to unpredictable variables. Thus, children who initially seem severely diseased can have a good recovery.[16,17] Also, 90% of the total recovery a patient will have following a head injury will occur within six months of the insult.

Pediatric rehabilitation is a major component of the recovery phase of head injury. This should be instituted vigorously and early to permit the best results.

Prevention

Prevention is the most important facet of the care of infants, children, and adolescents, if we are to avoid the painful outcome of head injury.

Exposure of infants to high places, high chairs poorly constructed or without restraints, is to be condemned. The transportation of infants in the arms of an adult in a motor vehicle should not be permitted. Infants, children, and adolescents should always be restrained, since the mortality and severity of head injury is directly related to the lack of restraints. Motorcycle and bicycle riders, aside from appropriate indoctrination of common sense traffic behavior, should always wear protective helmets.

Identification of potential child abuse cases and assessment of other siblings in the family should always be a part of the practice of the pediatrician and ancillary personnel. This may prevent a child from suffering a severe brain injury at a later date.

References

1. Jamieson D, Kaye HH: Accidental head injury in childhood. *Arch Dis Child* 49:376–381, 1974.
2. Klonoff H: Head injuries in children: practice, accident conditions,

accident proneness and sequelae. *Am J Public Health* 62:2405–2417, 1971.

3. Matson DD: *Neurosurgery of Infancy and Childhood.* Second Edition, Springfield, Illinois, Ch. C. Thomas, 1969, pp. 217–359.
4. Mealey J: *Pediatric Head Injuries.* Springfield, Illinois, Ch. C. Thomas, 1968.
5. Partington NW: The importance of accident proneness in the etiology of head injuries in childhood. *Arch Surg* 35:215–223, 1960.
6. Proctor H: Head injuries. *Physiotherapy* 59:380–400, 1973.
7. James HE, Schut L: The neurosurgeon and the battered child. *Surg Neurol* 2:415–418, 1974.
8. Hendricks EB, Harwood-Nash DC, Hudson AR: Head injuries in children: A survey of 4,465 consecutive cases at the Hospital for Sick Children, Toronto, Canada. *Clin Neurosurg* 11:46–65, 1964.
9. Bruce DA, Schut L: Recent advances in the treatment of head injuries. *Pediatr Ann* 5:643–656, 1976.
10. Carlsson CA, Von Essen A, Lofgren A: Factors affecting the clinical course of patients with severe head injury. *J Neurosurg* 29:242–251, 1968.
11. Becker DP, Miller JD, Ward JD, et al: The outcome from severe head injury with intensive management. *J Neurosurg* 47:491–502, 1977.
12. Jennett B, Teasdale G, et al: Predicting outcome in individual patients after severe head injury. *Lancet* 1:1031–1034, 1976.
13. Hendrick EB: The use of hypothermia in severe head injury in childhood. *Arch Surg* 79:362–364, 1959.
14. Gruszkiewicz J, Doron Y, et al: Recovery from severe cranio-cerebral injury in brain stem lesions in childhood. *Surg Neurol* 1:197–201, 1973.
15. Bricolo A, Turazzi S, Alexandre A: Decerebrate rigidity in acute head injury. *J Neurosurg* 47:680–698, 1977.
16. James HE, Madauss WC, Tibbs PA, et al: The effect of high dose dexamethasone in children with severe head injury. *Acta Neurochirurg* 45:225–236, 1979.
17. Bruce DA, Raphaely RC, Goldberg AI, et al: Pathophysiology, treatment and outcome following severe head injury in children. *Child's Brain* 5:174–191, 1979.
18. Lindenberg R, Fisher RS, Durlacher S, et al: The pathology of the brain in blunt head injuries of infants and children. *International Congress Neuropathology Proceedings,* Excerpta Medica (Amsterdam) 1:477–479, 1955.
19. Zimmerman RA, Bilaniuk LT, Bruce DA, et al: Computed tomography of pediatric head trauma. Acute general cerebral swelling. *J Radiol* 126:403–408, 1978.
20. James HE, Schut L: Pitfalls in the diagnosis of arrested hydrocephalus. *Acta Neurochir* 43:13–17, 1978.
21. James HE, Langfitt TW, et al: Management of intracranial hypertension. *Acta Neurochir* 36:189–200, 1977.
22. Miller JD, Becker DP, Ward JD, et al: Significance of intracranial hypertension in severe head injury. *J Neurosurg* 47:503–516, 1977.

23. Jennett B: Early traumatic epilepsy, incidence and significance after non-missile injuries. *Arch Neurol* 30:394–398, 1974.
24. Graham DI, Adams JH, Gennarelli TA, et al: Diffuse axonal injury in non-missile head injury. *International Conference on Neurotraumatology*. Edinburgh, September 1982, pp. 22.
25. Adams JH, Gennarelli TA, Graham DI: Brain damage in non-missile head injury. *In* Smith WT, Cavanagh JB, (eds): *Recent Advances in Neuropathology*. Edinburgh, Churchill Livingstone, 1981.
26. Till K: *Pediatric Neurosurgery*. Blackwell Scientific Publications, 1975.
27. Sato O, Tsugane R, Kageyama N: Growing skull fractures of childhood. *Child's Brain* 1:148–157, 1975.
28. Jennett WB, Miller JD: Infection after depressed fracture of skull. *J Neurosurg* 36:333–339, 1972.
29. Lewin W: *The Management of Head Injuries*. Baltimore, Williams and Wilkins Co., 1966.
30. Rickham PP: Head injuries in childhood. *Helv Chir Acta* 28:560–575, 1961.
31. Schintker MT: A syndrome of cerebral concussion in children. *J Pediatr* 35:557–561, 1949.
32. Jennett B, Teasdale G: Aspects of coma after severe head injury. *Lancet* 1:878–881, 1977.
33. Ignelzi RJ, VanderArk GD: Analysis of treatment of basilar skull fractures with and without antibiotics. *J Neurosurg* 43:721–726, 1975.
34. Roberts F, Shopfner CE: Plain skull roentgenograms in children with head trauma. *Am J Roentgen* 14:230–240, 1963.
35. Vance BM: Fracture of the skull. *Arch Surg* 14:183–192, 1927.
36. Galbraith S, Smith J: Acute traumatic intracranial hematomas without skull fracture. *Lancet* 1:501–503, 1973.
37. Gutierrez FA, Raimondi AJ: Acute subdural hematoma in infancy and childhood. *Child's Brain* 1:269–290, 1975.
38. Choux M, Grisoli F, Peragut JC: Extradural hematomas in children. *Child's Brain* 1:337–347, 1975.
39. James HE, Bruno L, et al: Methodology for continuous recording of intraventricular and subarachnoid pressure in clinical practice. *Acta Neurochir* 33:45–51, 1976.
40. James HE, Bruno L, et al: Intracranial pressure monitoring with a subarachnoid bolt in children. *Surg Neurol* 3:313–315, 1975.
41. James HE, Langfitt TW, et al: Analysis of the response to therapeutic measures to reduce intracranial pressure in head injured patients. *J Trauma* 16:437–441, 1976.
42. Miller JD: Volume and pressure in the craniospinal axis. *Clin Neurosurg* 22:76–105, 1975.
43. James HE: Methodology for the control of intracranial pressure with hypertonic mannitol. *ICP IV*, Springer-Verlag, pp. 653–655, 1979.
44. Cottrell JE, Robustelli A, Post K, et al: Furosemide and mannitol induced changes in intracranial pressure and serum osmolality and electrolytes. *Anesthesiology* 47:28–30, 1977.
45. Faupel G, Reulen HJ, Muller D, et al: Double-blind study on the

effects of dexamethasone on severe closed head injuries. *In* Pappius H, Reulen H, (eds): *Dynamics of Brain Edema.* Berlin-Heidelberg-New York, Springer, 1976, pp. 337–343.

46. Gailicich JH, et al: Use of dexamethasone in the treatment of cerebral oedema associated with brain tumours. *Lancet* 81:46–53, 1961.
47. Gobiet W: The influence of various doses of dexamethasone on intracranial pressure in patients with severe head injuries. *In* Pappius H, Reulen H, (eds): *Dynamics of Brain Edema.* Berlin-Heidelberg-New York, Springer, 1976, pp. 351–335.
48. Long DM, et al: The response of human cerebral edema to glucosteroid administration. *Neurology* 16:521–528, 1966.
49. Meinig G, Aulich A, Wende S, et al: The effect of dexamethasone and diuretics on peritumoral brain edema: Comparitive study of tissue water content and computed tomography. *In* Pappius H, Reulen H, (eds): *Dynamics of Brain Edema.* Berlin-Heidelberg-New York, Springer, 1976, pp. 301–305.
50. Weinstein JD, Toy FJ, Jaff ME, et al: The effects of dexamethasone on brain edema in patients with metastatic brain tumors. *Neurology* 23:121–129, 1973.
51. Demopoulos HB, Milvy P, Kakari S, et al: Molecular aspects of membrane structure in cerebral edema. *In* Reulen HJ, Schurmann K, (eds): *Steroids and Brain Edema.* Berlin-Heidelberg-New York, Springer, 1972, pp. 29–39.
52. Pappius HM: Effects of steroids on cold injury edema. *In* Reulen HJ, Schurmann K, (eds): *Steroids and Brain Edema.* Berlin-Heidelberg-New York, Springer, 1972, pp. 57–63.
53. Hansebout RR, Lewin MG, Pappius HM: Evidence regarding the action of steroids in injured spinal cords. *In* Reulen HJ, Schumann K, (eds): *Steroids and Brain Edema.* Berlin-Heidelberg-New York, Springer, 1972, pp. 153–155.
54. Lewin MG, Pappius HM, Hansebout RR: Effects of steroids on edema associated with injury of the spinal cord. *In* Reulen HJ, Schumann K, (eds): *Steroids and Brain Edema.* Berlin-Heidelberg-New York, Springer, 1972, pp. 101–112.

5

Status Epilepticus

Laurence D. Carnay, M.D.

Introduction

Status epilepticus may be defined as a continuous seizure, lasting at least 30 minutes, and is classified into: *convulsive status epilepticus* in which the patient does not recover to a normal alert state between tonic-clonic attacks; *nonconvulsive status epilepticus* such as complex partial or absence in which the patient is in a "twilight state"; and *continuous partial status epilepticus* in which consciousness is preserved.

Convulsive tonic-clonic status epilepticus is a neurological emergency which requires immediate and effective treatment. It is estimated that 8000 persons are hospitalized each year for major motor status, and mortality is in the range of 6–30%.[1] Death and permanent neurological sequelae may result from the underlying disease process or is a consequence of the metabolic, cardiopulmonary or autonomic derangements which inevitably accompany major motor status.[2] (*See Table I.*)

Our concern for the swift treatment of status is supported by the clinical experience that status becomes self-sustaining, and by experimental data demonstrating neuronal necrosis in paralyzed, oxygen-ventilated and metabolically stabilized animals. In these studies, neuronal damage resembles that found in hypoglycemia

Table I
Complications of Status Epilepticus

Central Nervous System	
Excessive neuronal firing	
Increase in cerebral metabolic rate	
Depletion of neuronal ATP	
Increase levels of arachidonic acid and prostaglandins	
Change in membrane structure and ion transport	
Loss of vascular auto regulation	
Increase in cerebral venous pressure	
Inhibition of brainstem respiratory centers	
Cerebral edema (not common)	
Inhibition of protein synthesis	
Cell damage and death	
Metabolic	*Renal*
CO_2 narcosis	Acute tubular necrosis
Hyperkalemia	Myoglobinuria secondary to rhabdomyolysis
Lactic acidosis	
Hypertension	
Hypoglycemia	
Cardiopulmonary	*Autonomic*
Pneumonia, aspiration	Hyperpyrexia
Pulmonary edema—may be neurogenic	Hypersecretions—sweat, salivation, tracheal-bronchial
High output failure	Fluid and electrolyte imbalance
Cardiac arrhythmias	
Hypotension and shock	

which suggests depletion of substrate as a critical factor in neuronal necrosis even in nonconvulsive status epilepticus.[3,4] Thus, the goal of cessation of tonic-clonic motor activity in the presence of an EEG showing continuous seizure activity must now be questioned.

Pathophysiology

The development of cortical seizures may be a consequence of several parameters. Intrinsic neuronal membrane instability may lead to paroxysmal depolarization shifts (PDS) resulting in spontaneous depolarization. Recruitment of the surrounding neurons may lead to spreading of the epileptiform discharge. Such spreading is enhanced by dysfunction of usual inhibitory mechanisms and establishment of independent foci with subsequent spread of excitable activity to brain stem and spinal motor neurons with resultant clinical seizure activity.[5]

The development of status from an epileptiform disturbance is also based on the establishment of oscillatory epileptiform discharges between cortical and subcortical sectors with propagation of epileptiform activity via normal neuronal circuits. Such oscillatory discharges may result from a maintained elevation of extracellular potassium due to changes in neuromal-glial interaction. Univalent potassium is known to displace bivalent cations from fixed anionic sites in the resting membrane with resultant cooperative transformation of the resting neuronal membrane into its excited state.[6] Membrane instability is also enhanced during repeated seizures due to changes in phospholipid-protein arrangements in synaptic plasma membranes.

Oscillatory discharges are also initiated by recurrent excitatory synaptic drives resulting in neuronal hypersynchrony as well as backfiring antidromic spikes.

When the spread of spontaneous neuronal discharges is confined to the cortex and subcortical regions, the clinical expression of the paroxysm is *partial simple.* With spread through the corticothalamic pathways to the midbrain, paroxysms reascend bilaterally to both hemispheres and caudally to the brainstem giving rise to *secondary generalized* seizure activity. Finally, oscillatory disturbances may involve both hemispheres, the diencephalon, and brainstem simultaneously resulting in *primary generalized* seizure activity.

Cerebral blood flow increases at the onset of generalized seizures due to the loss of cerebral vascular autoregulation in the presence of systemic arterial hypertension.[7] Initially, the increased blood flow and enhanced delivery of glucose and oxygen are protective to the brain since cerebral metabolic rate (CMR) is increased during status epilepticus. This increase in CMR is also observed in paralyzed and ventilated animals and thus must be considered to be due to intrinsic neuronal activity.[8] As lactic acid accumulates during convulsive status epilepticus, progressive systemic hypotension occurs with a consequent reduction in cerebral blood flow. This may explain the neuropathological damage seen during prolonged status. Cerebral venous pressure increases during status and can result in petechial hemorrhages in the subpial cortex.[9]

Respiratory compromise in status epilepticus occurs as a result of aspiration, atelectasis and pulmonary shunting as well as inhibition of brainstem respiratory centers. Excessive bronchial secretions and neurogenic pulmonary edema related to autonomic discharges and bronchial constriction may result in hypoxia and hypercapnia. Cardiac instability and further reduction in cerebral blood flow occur and become the major cause of the morbidity and mortality in status.[10]

In the neonate, glycogen mobilization is slow due to decreased phosphorylase levels and to immaturity of the glial cells in which glycogen is stored. Thus, even though the cerebral metabolic rate in the neonate is lower compared with the adult, glucose metabolism is more critical in the immature brain.

Activation of phosphorylase is reduced in the neonate since glial cells have few beta adrenergic receptors which are required to produce cyclic AMP.[11] In addition, energy from ketone bodies which accounts for up to one-third of the energy consumed by newborn brains in many species, is reduced since regeneration of NAD from NADH is reduced in the status induced anoxic state.[12] Thus, there is an increased demand for already deficient glucose metabolism. Finally, the ability of glycolytic pathways to utilize glucose outstrips facilitated transport of glucose across the blood-brain barrier. A therapeutic consequence of these facts is the raising of blood glucose concentrations in the neonate results in an increase in the glucose carrying capacity of the blood-brain barrier.

Pathology

Ischemic neuronal changes in the hippocampus, layers 3, 5 and 6 of the cerebral cortex, with Purkinje cells of the cerebellum in the thalamic and basal ganglia have been documented after status epilepticus.[13] The distribution of these pathological changes is similar to those seen after cerebral hypoxia and hypoglycemia. Similar changes in the paralyzed–ventilated animal models suggest that excessive neuronal firing with increased cerebral metabolic rate and changes in membrane configuration contribute to the pathological changes. Children are more prone to permanent brain damage than adults after status epilepticus. Neuronal changes occur in one hour in children and after six hours in adults.[9] Wasterlain has demonstrated that seizure activity in young rodents slowed brain development by inhibition of cerebral protein synthesis and dissociation of brain polyribosomes.[14] A consequence of this inhibition is a reduced content of myelin lipid and synaptic proteins as well as a decreased rate of intercellular connections.

Clinical Presentation

Seizures may be classified on the bases of clinical manifestations, anatomical origin and electroencephalographic pattern. It was not until the 1960s that a standardized classification was established by the *International League Against Epilepsy*. An adaptation of this classification is seen in Table II.

It is apparent in Table II, that there are as many varieties of status epilepticus as there are types of seizures. The clinical presentation will depend on the place of origin within the brain and the degree of spread of the epileptiform discharge. Another help-

Table II

International Classification of Epileptic Seizures*

Partial Seizures (seizures beginning locally)
Partial seizures with elementary symptoms generally without impairment of consciousness, for example, focal motor seizures
Partial seizures with complex symptoms generally with impairment of consciousness, such as temporal lobe or psychomotor seizures
Partial seizures secondarily generalized
Generalized Seizures (bilateral symmetrical and without local onset)
Absences (petit mal)
Bilateral massive epileptic myoclonus
Infantile spasms
Clonic seizures
Tonic seizures
Tonic-clonic seizures (grand mal)
Atonic seizures
Akinetic seizures
Unilateral Seizures
Unclassified Epileptic Seizures

*Adapted from Gastaut H: Clinical and electroencephalographic classification of epileptic seizures. *Epilepsia,* 11:102–113, 1970.

ful classification as proposed by Treiman, Delgado-Escueta[5] considers status as falling into two types: (1) *convulsive status* which includes primary generalized major motor status, partial or focal status and generalized major motor status with partial onset, and (2) *nonconvulsive status* or prolonged epileptic fugue state which includes spike wave stupor and partial complex or psychomotor status. The awareness of nonconvulsive status of absence and partial complex status is most important since recent studies have demonstrated that partial complex status may produce chronic memory loss and symptoms similar to the Klüver-Bucy syndrome.

The most common form of status epilepticus is *generalized tonic-clonic status.* The true incidence is unknown but has been reported to be around 5% of all hospital admissions for epilepsy. It occurs in patients with known epilepsy as well as in individuals who have never had a previous seizure. The incidence of status is much greater in symptomatic rather than idiopathic epilepsy.

According to Aicardi,[16] in 21% of children with status epilepticus, the status was superimposed on a chronic static encephalopathy or seizure. In this group rapid discontinuation of antiepileptic drugs or fever secondary to a systemic noncentral nervous system infection were the two most common antecedents. Another 26% had an acute insult to the central nervous system such as trauma, infection, metabolic, toxins or tumors. In the remaining 53%, no cause of the status was defined, but this study was done prior to the advent of CAT scanning. In 75% of all cases of status epilepticus in children the occurrence is before the age of three. The younger the child at the age of status, the greater the likelihood that the status will be symptomatic.

When status occurs late in the course of idiopathic epilepsy it is presumed that prior neurological damage plays a critical role in the increased excitability and spread of the seizure focus.

Generalized tonic status is much less common than tonic-clonic status. It occurs in those patients with known seizure disorders and usually in those children with Lennox-Gastaut syndrome. This syndrome is characterized by tonic seizures, atypical absence seizures and mental retardation.

Generalized myoclonic status consists of rhythmic repetitive focal or generalized muscular contractions without alteration of consciousness. This disorder is associated with toxic, metabolic encephalopathic processes as well as anoxic brain damage and degenerative brain disease.

Simple partial (focal) status epilepticus occurs when the seizure focus is localized to one area of the brain. The clinical presentation of seizures (focal motor, focal sensory, focal autonomic) is determined by the seizure location within the brain and its spread. About 60–80% of convulsive status seizures have a partial onset which then progresses to generalized tonic-clonic seizures. It is reasonable to suspect a structural lesion in these patients although this is less valid in children than in adults. This group may not respond to treatment as easily as patients with primary generalized clonic-tonic status.

In *nonconvulsive status epilepticus,* absence status has been termed "petit mal" status, spike wave stupor and prolonged epileptic twilight state. It is characterized by nearly continuous aberrant behavior and responsiveness that ranges from mild confusion to stupor. Although tonic-clonic activity is usually not present, myoclonic twitching is seen in 50% of these patients. This disorder occurs most frequently in those patients who have preexisting epilepsy with 30% of this group experiencing absence only during the status episode.[17] After a period of unresponsiveness with improvement and worsening, the patient returns rapidly to an alert consciousness with minimal or no sequelae.

It is this abrupt termination in absence status which distinguishes it from the very rare *complex partial status epilepticus,* in which each of the repeated attacks is followed by a partial recovery ending in a prolonged recovery period. In addition to the clinical distinction between the two forms of nonconvulsive status, the EEG in absence status is characterized by generalized diffuse spike and polyspike wave complexes, while in the complex partial status there are focal spikes, sharp waves and slowing which secondarily generalize. The spikes and slow waves fluctuate with the clinical level of awareness.

Status Epilepticus in the Neonate

Four types of status epilepticus are observed during the first month of life.[18]

Clonic motor status can be circumscribed and confined to the hand, one side of the body or occur bilaterally but asynchronally. These seizures are associated with metabolic disorders and were formerly the most common seizure in the neonate accounting for

30–50% of neonatal seizures. As the etiologic spectrum has changed, metabolic disorders account for a much smaller percentage of neonatal seizures. Clonic status is also uncommon in hypoxia and meningitis but is present in approximately 30% of neonates in which the etiology is unknown.

Tonic postural status is commonly seen after hypoxia. It may occur without accompanying changes in the EEG as well as with a build-up of abnormal paroxysmal activity. It is possible that this seizure type which many consider the most common type of seizure in the newborn, is not truly epileptic but is a brainstem disinhibition phenomenon.

Slow myoclonus status is rare and is a consequence of perinatal hypoxia.

Electrical status in the newborn may occur without any clinical seizure activity and occurs in infants with severe forebrain dysfunction and usually implies a poor prognosis.

Finally, subtle seizures as described by Volpe,[19] characterized by brief eye movements, swimming movements, apnea or mouthing movements, and may represent serial seizure activity rather than status. The distinction is easily determined by continuous EEG monitoring.[20] However, at the present time, these seizures should be treated to prevent neuronal damage, inhibition of cerebral protein synthesis and dissociation of brain polyribosomes as described by Wasterlain.[21] Another rationale for vigorous treatment of the seizure types in the neonate is that brain glucose can decrease drastically because of increased glycolysis while blood glucose levels remain relatively unchanged.[22]

Treatment

Major motor status epilepticus is a life-threatening medical emergency which must be treated promptly and preferably by a well staffed Intensive Care Unit. Death during tonic-clonic status may be due to circulatory collapse, to the basic disease process, or to over-medication. Tonic-clonic status epilepticus causes one-third of all epilepsy related deaths.[5] Time is a critical factor in the treatment of status epilepticus, but the actual choice of anticonvulsant is less important than a thorough understanding of the pharmacokinetics of the drug used and an appreciation of the supportive measures necessary to prevent brain damage and death. Initial priorities are directed towards maintaining respiration and circulation and correcting metabolic disturbances. (See Table I).

Supportive Care

The child should be positioned to insure an adequate airway and to prevent injury against hard objects, as well as to prevent suffocation by pillows and blankets. Vital signs are taken and an oral airway is inserted while oral suctioning clears airway secretions. Oxygen should be given to alleviate hypoxia. If there is any doubt as to the adequacy of respiratory exchange, prompt endotracheal intubation is advised.

Initial Diagnostic Testing and Evaluation

Blood is drawn for glucose, BUN, electrolytes, calcium toxic screen and anticonvulsant blood levels. Arterial blood gases are also drawn. An intravenous line is secured and 2 cc per kilogram of 50% dextrose solution is infused. Severe metabolic acidosis (pH less than 7.1) is corrected by injection of bicarbonate. A brief history is obtained to determine if the child has a known seizure disorder, maintenance dosage of anticonvulsant and degree of compliance. In children with known seizures, the most common cause of status is the sudden decrease in anticonvulsant dosage or discontinuation of the medication. Further history is sought regarding recent head injury, systemic and CNS infections and ingestion of toxic substances. The general physical examination is used to establish or rule out site of infection or trauma as well as to ascertain the patient's general medical condition. The neurological examination is initially directed to the fundi, pupils and elicitation of focal motor deficit. The physician should also keep in mind other precipitating factors of status which may not be readily apparent on examination such as hypocalcemia, hyponatremia, hypoglycemia, hepatic or renal failure, withdrawal from sedatives, sleep deprivation, new CNS insult, drug intoxication and diagnostic procedures in hospital.

Anticonvulsant Therapy

Once supportive and diagnostic steps are performed, treatment with anticonvulsant medication is begun with the goal of cessation of convulsive activity within 30 minutes. The drugs employed must be able to cross the blood-brain barrier rapidly and should be administered intravenously to obtain effective serum and brain levels quickly. Intramuscular, oral and rectal administration are to be avoided due to slowness and variability of absorption.

Since there is no ideal drug for treating status, treatment regimes are varied. The ideal drug should stop seizures as well as remain long enough in the brain to prevent recurrence of seizures. The drug should also be free of undesirable side effects such as depression of consciousness, hypotension and respiratory depression. Unfortunately, such a drug has not been developed at this time. Some clinicians recommend a treatment regime beginning with diazepam followed by a loading dose of phenytoin.[5,15] Others advise the initial use of phenobarbital in loading doses with the avoidance of diazepam because of its known additive interaction with barbiturates and resultant respiratory depression.[23] Since the best regime is the one the physician knows best, both regimes and ancillary treatment programs will be discussed. (See Table III.)

Diazepam is often used as the initial drug to control seizures. It enters the brain within 10 seconds after administration and stops clinical seizures within three minutes in one-third of the patients with status and within five minutes in 80% of all cases.[15] The initial dose is 0.3 mg per kilogram given no faster than 2 mg per minute with 20 mg being the maximum loading dose. Side effects include respiratory depression or arrest, hypotension, sedation, laryngospasm and paradoxical tonic seizures.[24] Unfortunately, recurrence of seizures after intravenous diazepam is due to a rapid distribution out of the intravascular space with serum concentrations falling by more than 50% during the first 15 minutes after intravenous administration.[25] For this reason, a long-acting drug must be given immediately to insure long-term seizure control since use of a slow continuous intravenous diazepam drip in the pediatric age group is hazardous.

One of the most common errors in the management of status epilepticus is to treat status with repeated doses of intravenous

Table III

Outline Management of Status Epilepticus

Restore Homeostasis
Assure adequate respiratory exchange
Insert oral airway, administer oxygen and intubate prn
Protect child from physical harm
Draw blood for glucose, BUN, calcium, electrolytes, CBC, ABG and anticonvulsant level
Begin IV infusion of D5¼ saline and bolus of 50% D/W 2 cc/kg
Monitor BP, respirations, EKG and EEG
Brief History and Baseline Exam
Is there history of epilepsy, noncompliance, infection or trauma?
Treatment of Status
Choose phenobarbital-phenytoin, or diazepam-phenytoin-phenobarbital treatment plan
Phenobarbital 15–20 mg/kg and infuse at initial dosage of 5 mg/kg. Monitor respirations and intubate if the full loading dose is used. If after 30 minutes status not stopped, infuse phenytoin 18 mg/kg at a rate of 50 mg/min. Slow rate if hypotension occurs.
Diazepam 0.3 mg/kg up to 20 mg and infuse at a rate of 2 mg/min. Load with phenytoin as above. If seizures persist after 30 minutes, load with phenobarbital as above.
If treatment using methods of phenobarbital or diazepam fails consider paraldehyde infusion 200 mg/kg followed by continuous infusion of 20 mg/kg or employ short acting barbiturates.

diazepam, allowing toxic concentrations of diazepam and its metabolites to accumulate. Another benzodiazepine, lorazepam, may soon be available after studies of clinical effectiveness are complete. Lorazepam is much less extensively redistributed than diazepam. Thus, despite a shorter elimination half-life, the duration of action of lorazepam is greater than diazepam since diazepam's anticonvulsant activity is terminated by rapid and extensive tissue distribution rather than elimination.[26]

There is much discussion in the literature as to whether phenobarbital or phenytoin should be given simultaneously with diazepam in the treatment of status epilepticus. There are specific indications and contraindications for either drug. Phenytoin is preferred when intracranial hemorrhage or trauma is suspected since it does not depress respiration or alter the level of consciousness to the degree as does phenobarbital after an equivalent loading dose. Phenobarbital is certainly the drug of choice when status presents in a child with disorders of cardiac condition, allergy to phenytoin, or leukemia. Since the cardiorespiratory depressant effect of phenobarbital and diazepam may be additive, most reviews on status recommend phenytoin as the primary long-acting anticonvulsant in the treatment of status epilepticus.[5,15,27,28]

Although phenytoin can be detected in the cortex one minute after injection, it requires 15 minutes to reach peak brain levels. Since phenytoin, like diazepam, is rapidly distributed, a large loading dose must be given to maintain adequate blood and brain levels, but unlike diazepam, once this equilibrium is established brain/plasma ratios remain constant.

A loading intravenous phenytoin dose of 18 mg per kilogram provides an initial serum phenytoin level greater than 25 mcg per cc.[29] Phenytoin cannot be added to solutions containing glucose and may be diluted in normal saline at a concentration of 1 to 10 mg per cc. This solution may be infused at a rate not to exceed 50 mg per minute. Plasma levels above 10 mcg per cc are maintained for 12–24 hours following loading intravenous injection. Blood pressure, heart rate and EKG should be monitored during loading infusion. Hypotension is the most common complication seen during intravenous phenytoin but rarely occurs in the pediatric age group.

Intramuscular phenytoin should never be used in the treatment of status epilepticus. Peak serum concentrations occur 24 hours after a single intramuscular injection of phenytoin and are significantly lower than the same dose given intravenously. If treatment with diazepam and phenytoin is not successful in stopping status epilepticus, phenobarbital may then be infused.

Phenobarbital alone may be the initial drug used in the treatment of status. Certainly those pediatric intensive care units with extensive experience in using barbiturates during cerebral resuscitation may favor the use of phenobarbital as the initial treating anticonvulsant medication. The loading dose of phenobarbital is between 15–20 mg per kilogram. Phenobarbital is infused at an initial dosage of 5 mg per kilogram and at a rate of 30 mg per minute. Unlike diazepam, or shorter-acting barbiturates such as thiopental or amobarbital, at least 20 minutes is required for effective amounts of phenobarbital to enter the brain after intravenous administration. Thus, the clinician must be aware that prompt cessation of seizure activity may not occur and at least a 20-minute interval is advised before an additional 5 mg per kilogram dosage is repeated. If the patient is intubated the full loading dose can be given. The therapeutic serum level of phenobarbital is 20–40 mcg per cc but the level necessary for stopping status epilepticus is not known. The maintenance dosage of phenobarbital is 5 mg per kilogram per day given 12 hours after the initial loading dose is complete.

If diazepam, phenytoin and phenobarbital are unsuccessful in controlling status, the short-acting barbiturates, amobarbital, pentobarbital and thiopental should then be employed. An arterial line must be established so that blood pressure can be monitored simultaneously with drug infusion. If hypotension occurs, it is treated promptly with appropriate vasopressors such as dopamine. General anesthesia with halothane may be considered but offers no superiority to anesthesia with the shorter-acting barbiturates. Pavulon can be used as an adjuvant to assist ventilation in order to minimize the systemic effects of prolonged seizures, such as hypoxia, acidosis and hyperpyrexia. This nondepolarizing neuromuscular blocking agent has no effect on the continuing cerebral electrical discharges.

Paraldehyde is mentioned in all reviews and, indeed, was the drug of choice in the treatment of status epilepticus 30 years ago. The drug is now infrequently used because of the serious side effects of pulmonary edema, increased coagulability, thrombosis and metabolic acidosis. As with the other anticonvulsants, the drug must be given intravenously for treatment of status. Paraldehyde has a rapid distribution phase and slow elimination phase and thus has many of the problems of diazepam in preventing repetitive seizures. Paraldehyde is given in a loading dose of 200 mg per kilogram via a 5 minute infusion followed by a continuous infusion of 20 mg per kilogram per hour. This should produce a steady state serum level of 200 mcg per cc.[30] Paraldehyde should be diluted to a 4% solution (20 cc in 500 cc saline) and must be administered from a freshly opened vial since the drug deteriorates to acetaldehyde and acetic acid on exposure to light. The infusion rate is lowered every few hours until it is possible to discontinue infusion without resumption of seizure activity. Continuation of a longer-acting anticonvulsant maintenance dose is required.

Valproic acid is not available for parenteral use. The drug is rapidly absorbed after oral administration but this may be unreliable because of gastric stasis and ileus which accompanies status epilepticus. Vajda has administered valproic acid rectally as 200 mg lipid base suppositories.[31]

In addition to the treatment regime as outlined above, the treatment of other forms of status epilepticus described earlier in this chapter in *Clinical Presentation,* deserves mention. Myoclonic status is treated initially with diazepam followed by clonazepam given orally or via nasogastric tube. Valproic acid, phenytoin and phenobarbital can also be used. In absence and complex partial status epilepticus, diazepam is also the initial anticonvulsant drug. Ethosuximide, valproic acid and carbamazepine may then be added via oral administration. Focal motor status that is mild may be treated with oral anticonvulsants including primidone and carbamazepine. In the more severely affected patients with focal motor status, intravenous medication is required.

Conclusion

The physiology, pathology, clinical presentation and treatment of status epilepticus have been discussed. *Major motor status* is a major medical emergency and must be stopped quickly to avoid neurological sequelae and death. Treatment requires the facilities of a well staffed intensive care unit. The major goals of treatment are appropriate supportive care, prompt cessation of convulsant and nonconvulsant status, and accurate diagnosis of precipitating causes. Since the ideal drug for treating status has not been developed, the treating physician must be aware of the pharmacological concepts of volume distribution and elimination half-life as well as indications and contraindications for each of the drugs that he uses. Dosage regimes are only guidelines and anticonvulsant blood levels are required to insure drug levels in the upper therapeutic range and thus minimize therapeutic failure due to patient's rapid metabolism or drug nonavailability due to precipitation or degradation.

References

1. Commission for the control of epilepsy and its consequences (1977): *Plan for Nationwide Action on Epilepsy:* US Department of Health, Education and Welfare, Bethesda, Maryland.
2. Glaser G: Medical complications of status epilepticus. *In* Escueta AV, Wasterlain CG, Porter R, (eds): *Status Epilepticus.* New York, Raven Press, (In press.)
3. Meldrom BS, Vigouroux RA, Brierley JB: Systemic factors and epileptic brain damage: Prolonged seizures in paralyzed artificially ventilated baboons. *Arch Neurol* 29:82, 1973.
4. Borgstrom L, Chapman AG, Siesjo BK: Glucose consumption in the cerebral cortex of rat during bicuculline induced status epilepticus. *J Neurochem* 27:971, 1976.
5. Treiman DM, Delgado-Escueta AV: Status epilepticus. *In* Thompson RA, Green JR, (eds): *Critical Care of Neurologic and Neurosurgical Emergencies.* New York, Raven Press, 1980, pp 53–99.
6. Carnay LD, Tasaki I: Ion exchange properties and excitability of the squid giant axon. *In* Adelman W, (ed): *Biophysics and Physiology of Excitable Membranes.* New York, Van Nostrand Rheinhold, 1971, pp 379–422.
7. Westerlain CG, Graham S: Auto regulation of cerebral blood flow: An asset during single seizure, a liability during status epilepticus. *Ann Neurol* 8:94, 1980.
8. Meldrom BS, Nilsson B: Cerebral blood flow and metabolic rate early and late in prolonged epileptic seizures induced in rats by bicuculline. *Brain* 99:523, 1976.
9. Meldrom BS: Neuropathology and pathophysiology. *In* Laidlow J, Richens A, (eds): *A Textbook of Epilepsy.* Edinburgh, Churchill Livingstone, 1976, pp 314–354.
10. Wasterlain CG: Mortality and morbidity from serial seizures: An experimental study. *Epilepsia* 15:155, 1974.
11. Gross RA, Ferrendelli JA: Mechanisms of cyclic AMP regulation in cerebral anoxia and their relationship to glycogenolysis. *J Neurochem* 34:1309, 1980.
12. Wasterlain CG: Glucose and energy metabolism in the immature brain during status epilepticus. *International Symposium on Status Epilepticus.* Santa Monica, CA, 1980.
13. Norman RM: The neuropathology of status epilepticus. *Med Sci Law* 4:46, 1964.
14. Wasterlain, CG: Effects of epileptic seizures on brain ribosomes: Mechanism and relationship to cerebral energy metabolism. *J Neurochem* 29:707, 1977.
15. Delgado-Escueta AV, Wasterlain CG, Treiman DM, et al: Current concepts in neurology: Management of status epilepticus. *N Engl J Med* 306:1337, 1982.
16. Alcardi J, Chevne JJ: Convulsive status epilepticus in infants and children. *Epilepsia* 11:187, 1970.

17. Roger J, Lob H, Tassinari CA: Status epilepticus. *In* Magnos O, Lorentz DE, Hass AM, (eds): *Handbook of Clinical Neurology, The Epilepsies,* Vol 15, Amsterdam, North Holland Publishing Co, 1974, pp 145–188.
18. Kellaway P: Status epilepticus in neonates. *International Symposium on Status Epilepticus.* Santa Monica, CA, 1980.
19. Volpe J: Neonatal seizures. *Clin Perinatol* 4:43, 1977.
20. Coen RW, McCutchen C, Wermer D, et al: Continuous monitoring of the electroencephalogram following perinatal asphyxia. *J Pediatr* 100:628, 1982.
21. Wasterlain CG: Neonatal seizures and brain growth. *Neuropaediatric* 9:213, 1978.
22. Wasterlain C, Duffy T: Status epilepticus in immature rats. *Arch Neurol* 33:821, 1976.
23. Goldberg M, McIntyre H: Barbiturates in the treatment of status epilepticus. *International Symposium on Status Epilepticus.* Santa Monica, 1980.
24. Tassinari C, Dravet C, Roger C, et al: Tonic status epilepticus precipitated by intravenous benzodiazepine in five patients with Lennox-Gastaut syndrome. *Epilepsia* 13:421, 1972.
25. Booker H, Celesia G: Serum concentrations of diazepam in subjects with epilepsy. *Arch Neurol* 29:191, 1973.
26. Greenblatt D, Shader R: Prazepam and lorazepam, two new benzodiazepines. *N Engl J Med* 299:1342, 1978.
27. Rothner A, Erenberg G: Status epilepticus. Symposium on Pediatric Intensive Care. *Pediatr Clin North Am* 27:593, 1980.
28. Oppenheimer E, Rosman P: Seizures in childhood: An approach to Emergency Management. *Pediatr Clin North Am* 26:837, 1979.
29. Cranford R, Patrick B, Anderson C, et al: Intravenous phenytoin: Clinical and pharmacokinetic aspects. *Neurology* 28:874, 1978.
30. Bostrom B: Paraldehyde toxicity during treatment of status epilepticus. *Am J Dis Child* 136:414, 1982.
31. Vajda F, Mihaly G, Miles J, et al: Rectal administration of sodium valproate in status epilepticus. *Neurology* 28:897, 1978.

6

Management of Central Nervous System Infections In Infancy and Childhood

Stephen C. Aronoff, M.D.
William T. Speck, M.D.

Introduction

Prior to the availability of effective antimicrobial therapy, acute bacterial meningitis was uniformly fatal. With the utilization of sulfonamides followed by the penicillins and chloramphenicol, the mortality rate for uncomplicated bacterial meningitis was gradually reduced to less than 10%. Recently, the high mortality rate characteristic of Gram-negative enteric meningitis has also decreased due, in part, to the availability of the new, broad-spectrum, "third generation" cephalosporins. In addition to the availability of new and potent antibacterial agents, effective antiviral drugs have recently become a reality. More specifically, adenosine arabinoside usage has reduced the morbidity and mortality of Herpes simplex encephalitis, and acyclovir offers more promise as an effective antiviral agent. Amphotericin B, developed in the 1950s as the mainstay of systemic antifungal therapy, continues to be the drug of choice for fungal meningitis. However, 5-fluorocytosine has recently been shown to be a useful adjunct in selected patient populations.

In addition to specific anti-infective therapy for central nervous system infections, recognition of associated complications and the expectant management of these problems have contributed to the improved morbidity and mortality figures. Fluid therapy, hemodynamic monitoring, anticonvulsants, monitoring for and management of cerebral edema, have all improved the prognosis for CNS infections in children.

This chapter will focus on the treatment of central nervous system infections.

Anti-Infective Therapy

The bacterial, viral, and fungal agents commonly responsible for childhood CNS infections are listed in Table I.

Acute Bacterial Meningitis

Hemophilus influenzae. Following the neonatal period, *H. influenzae* is the principal pathogen responsible for bacterial meningitis in children.[20,109] Central nervous system infection with this microorganism often follows an upper respiratory tract infection and characteristically affects children less than five years of age.[20,27] *H. influenzae* meningitis is often associated with other infectious processes including bacteremia, otitis media, pneumonia, epiglottitis, cellulitis, arthritis and/or pericarditis.[109]

Ampicillin is the drug of choice for *H. influenzae* meningitis.[124] Originally recommended in high dosages (400 mg/kg/day), Greene and his colleagues demonstrated equal clinical efficacy with a low dose regimen.[37] At our institution, children with *H. influenzae* meningitis receive parenteral ampicillin in a dosage of 250–300 mgm/kg/day administered every four hours.

Central nervous system infections due to ampicillin-resistant strains of *H. influenzae* were initially described in 1974.[22,111,112] In many areas of the United States, these resistant microorganisms represent 10% of the clinical isolates of *H. influenzae.* Accordingly, chloramphenicol is now routinely included in the initial antimicrobial regimen for bacterial meningitis due to an unknown pathogen and discontinued only when microbiological studies demonstrate

Table I
Common Infectious Etiologies of the CNS in Children

Bacterial
Hemophilus influenzae, type b
Neisseria meningitidis
Streptococcus pneumoniae
Group B streptococcus
The *Enterobacteriaceae*
Listeria monocytogenes
Mycobacterium tuberculosis
Staphylococcus aureus
Staphylococcus epidermidis
Cornyebacterium
Viral
Coxsackie A, B
ECHO viruses
Enteroviruses
Arboviruses
Western Equine
Eastern Equine
St. Louis
California
Herpes simplex type 1, 2
Varicella zoster
Mumps virus
Rubeola virus
Rubella virus
Adenovirus
Lymphocytic choriomeningitis virus
Poliovirus
Fungal
Candida species
Cryptococcus neoformans
Coccidioides immitis
Histoplasma capsulatum

that the *H. influenzae* is ampicillin-sensitive.[1] (An alternative approach to the initial combination chemotherapy is to begin treatment with chloramphenicol and institute treatment with ampicillin in infections due to ampicillin-sensitive strains of *H. influenzae*.) Ampicillin resistance in *H. influenzae* is most often due to plasmid-mediated production of penicillinase, an extracellular enzyme which cleaves the beta lactam ring and inactivates the drug.[33] The major penicillinases produced by *H. influenzae* can be detected colorimetrically in most clinical laboratories, however, not all penicillinases can be detected by the commonly utilized assay, and ampicillin resistant *H. influenzae* have been identified which are penicillinase negative, i.e. resistance is chromosomally mediated and dependent upon the production of modified cell wall penicillin binding proteins. Accordingly, all clinical isolates of *H. influenzae* should be screened for penicillinase production and tested for ampicillin sensitivity with a disc diffusion assay before modifying the initial combination chemotherapy regimen. It is noteworthy that in any population of ampicillin-sensitive *H. influenzae* there may be ampicillin-resistant mutants.[53] Thus, most laboratories will simultaneously test several colonies for ampicillin resistance before reporting the clinical isolate as sensitive.

The conversion of parenterally administered chloramphenicol succinate to the active metabolite is erratic. More specifically, Kauffman and his colleagues demonstrated that following intravenous administration of chloramphenicol succinate, serum (and presumably CSF) concentrations of free chloramphenicol were unpredictable.[57] As a result, most authorities recommend that chloramphenicol succinate be used parenterally in an initial dosage of 100 mg/kg/day, that serum concentrations be routinely measured, and that peak levels of chloramphenicol be maintained below 25 mg/L.[57] In contrast to parenteral administration, orally administered chloramphenicol palmitate results in predictable serum and CSF concentrations of the active drug.[57,114] Thus, oral administration of chloramphenicol palmitate in a dose of 75 mg/kg/day is recommended in children with meningitis due to ampicillin-resistant *H. influenzae* when: (1) chloramphenicol sensitivity of the clinical isolate has been documented; (2) prolonged use of chloramphenicol is required; (3) clinical and microbiological response has occurred with parenteral chloramphenicol drug administration; (4) oral medications can be tolerated; and (5) patient response (including drug levels) and compliance is ensured by hospitalization.[114] Because of dose-related bone marrow toxicity, bone marrow function should be monitored periodically during therapy (complete blood count and platelet determinations on a biweekly basis). Total duration of therapy need not exceed 10–14 days.

Meningitis due to chloramphenicol-resistant strains of *H. in-*

fluenzae has recently been reported.[59,115] Chloramphenicol resistance in *H. influenzae* is due to plasmid-mediated production of an acetyl transferase enzyme capable of degrading chloramphenicol to an inactive intermediate. Treatment of central nervous system infections due to chloramphenicol and ampicillin-resistant strains of *H. influenzae* may become a problem in the near future. The third generation cephalosporin derivatives, e.g. moxalactam and cefotaxime, are not degraded by *H. influenzae* beta-lactamase, and are equally effective against both beta-lactamase-producing and non-producing strains.[63] There are no data on the sensitivity of chloramphenicol-resistant strains to these new cephalosporins; however, the dissimilarity of structure and mode of action between the newer cephalosporins and chloramphenicol suggests that plasmid mediated acetyl transferase production in chloramphenicol resistant strains will not inactivate these agents. Therefore, in the rare case where the responsible *H. influenzae* is resistant to both ampicillin and chloramphenicol, moxalactam in a dose of 150 mg/kg/day is recommended. Moxalactam is also indicated in infections due to ampicillin-resistant chloramphenicol-sensitive strains when chloramphenicol toxicity or the risk of toxicity precludes its use. Prophylaxis of household and day-care center contacts of children with *H. influenzae* meningitis is controversial. Rifampin is the drug of choice for prophylaxis (20 mg/kg/day) and is administered over four days.

Neisseria meningitidis. *N. meningitidis* is the second most common cause of acute bacterial meningitis in children.[42,109] Sulfonamides were the first agents to be used successfully in the treatment of meningococcal meningitis.[35] In 1944, Meads and associates demonstrated the efficacy of penicillin in meningococcal meningitis, and in 1951, McCrumb et al. successfully used oral and parenteral chloramphenicol to treat 15 adults and children with *N. meningitidis* meningitis.[75,76] Subsequently, in the 1960s a comparative study of sulfadiazine versus sulfadiazine plus penicillin demonstrated no difference in clinical efficacy.[61] As a result, many authorities considered sulfonamides to be the drug of choice in meningococcal meningitis.[42]

Sulfadiazine-resistant strains of *N. meningitis* were first isolated in naval recruits from San Diego in 1963.[78] Reports of resistant strains increased and by 1974, 23% of all clinical isolates were sulfonamide resistant.[32,51] The incidence of resistance for serogroups A and C was markedly higher.[51] As a result, penicillin is now considered to be the drug of choice for meningococcal meningitis. Thus, parenterally administered penicillin G is administered in a dose of 200,000 IU/kg/day every four hours and continued until the child has been afebrile for five days or until one week of therapy has been completed, whichever is longer.[93] Chloramphenicol succinate in a dosage of 100 mg/kg/day is the treatment of choice in penicillin-allergic patients. *In vitro* testing has demonstrated that the third-generation cephalosporins may also be useful in the therapy of meningococcal meningitis, however, clinical experience is lacking.[92]

Epidemics of meningococcal disease among military personnel have been reported since the First World War; however the first civilian epidemic may have been noted as early as 1802. Documentation of familial carriage and secondary cases in household contacts were first observed in Syracuse, New York, and more recently in Brazil.[38,82] Carriage rates for household contacts of children with meningococcal disease approach 24% and secondary cases of meningitis were noted in 2.6% of the siblings.[82] In addition to household contacts, secondary cases of meningococcal disease have recently been observed in children attending day-care centers.[52] As a result, household and day-care center contacts of index cases are at risk for asymptomatic carriage and/or the development of overt infection.

Sulfonamide prophylaxis was successfully used in 1942 to contain an epidemic of meningococcal disease in San Diego.[5] As previously mentioned, the emergence of sulfonamide-resistant strains of *N. meningitidis* limited the use of these drugs in clinical disease and as effective prophylactic agents. Minocycline and rifampin are two agents effective in eradicating the meningococcal carrier state, however, no data exist regarding their efficacy in preventing secondary cases.[40,81] The toxicity and side effects of minocycline (a tetracycline) precludes its use in young children and pregnant women. Rifampin is currently the drug of choice for household and day-care center contacts of children with meningococcal disease.[93] The dosage of rifampin for children under one year of age is 5 mg/kg every 12 hours for four doses. The dosage is doubled for older children with a maximum of 300 mg/dose in adult patients. Rifampin is contraindicated during the first trimester of pregnancy and use of soft contact lenses should be avoided during therapy.

The expense, toxicity, and problems of compliance with chemoprophylaxis have prompted research in the development of meningococcal vaccines. Effective vaccines for serogroups A and C are currently available and may be used to control endemic or epidemic infections due to these serotypes, however, these vaccines do not generate long lasting immunity in children under two years of age.[74,87] Presently, serogroup B is most often responsible for sporadic cases of meningococcal disease in children and to date there is no approved vaccine for this serogroup.[51]

Streptococcus pneumoniae. The pneumococcus is the most common cause of bacterial meningitis in adults.[20,109] Unlike *H. influenzae,* the incidence of pneumococcal meningitis remains fairly constant throughout infancy and childhood although mortality is greatest for children under one year of age.[65]

Prior to the advent of antimicrobial therapy, the mortality rate for pneumococcal meningitis approached 100%.[119] From 1940 to 1944, the use of sulfonamides in conjunction with pneumococcal anti-sera decreased the mortality to 60%.[96] In 1944, Ross and Burke used a combination of sulfadiazine and penicillin to treat pneumococcal meningitis; using this antibiotic combination, 84% of their patients recovered.[96] Schwartz and Dodge, in a subsequent comparative study, observed no difference between patients receiving penicillin alone or combined with sulfonamides.[109] The use of penicillin as a single agent for the treatment of pneumococcal meningitis was further supported by the observation that the growth of most isolates of *S. pneumoniae* was inhibited by less than 0.04 mg/L of penicillin.[60]

In 1967, a relatively penicillin-resistant isolate of *S. pneumoniae* was isolated.[45] This microorganism, although inhibited by achievable serum concentrations of penicillin, required a ten-fold greater concentration of penicillin for inhibition than observed with previous clinical isolates. Subsequently, numerous "relatively resistant" pneumococci have been isolated from both adults and children.[4,97] More disconcerting is a recent report of a penicillin-resistant pneumococcus isolated from a young girl.[21] This organism was sensitive only to chloramphenicol. Similar multiple-drug resistant strains of *S. pneumoniae* have been reported in South Africa. Effective treatment for these patients required the use of rifampin.

Despite the scattered reports of relatively-resistant *S. pneumoniae,* penicillin remains the drug of choice for pneumococcal meningitis. Heiber and Nelson demonstrated that bactericidal CSF concentrations of penicillin are achieved with a dosage of 250,000 IU/kg/day of penicillin G administered intravenously every four hours.[48] Higher dosages (up to 400,000 IU/kg/day) are recommended for the "relatively-resistant" strains. Chloramphenicol in dosages of 100 mg/kg/day administered every six hours is indicated in children allergic to penicillin and to treat infections caused by some penicillin-resistant strains. Rifampin and vancomycin have been used successfully in treating meningitis caused by multiple drug resistant strains. The total duration of antimicrobial therapy in pneumococcal meningitis is fourteen days.[93]

Group B Streptococcus (S. agalactiae). Historically associated with bovine mastitis, the group B streptococcus (GBS) is the leading cause of neonatal sepsis, meningitis, and osteomyelitis.[71] Classically, neonatal infections due to GBS are divided into two groups, early-onset and late-onset disease. Early-onset disease is acquired vertically from the colonized mother during the time of labor and delivery and characteristically presents with the signs and symptoms of septicemia and respiratory distress.[2,9,86] The onset of symptoms typically occurs within the first few days of life and is often associated with apnea and shock. There is typically a history of maternal obstetrical complications, e.g. premature labor, prolonged rupture of the amniotic membranes, and chorioamnionitis.[2,8,9,86]

Late-onset infection presents from ten days to two months of life and often presents with fever and signs and symptoms of central nervous system involvement. In one study, 62% of the infants had a full or bulging fontanelle on presentation and 19% had nuchal rigidity.[8] Epidemiologically, the serotype isolated from most children causing láte-onset disease is Type III.[8,86] The mortality rate from late-onset infection is 14%, significantly less than that of early-onset disease.[8]

Antibiotic prophylaxis of both colonized women and asymptomatic neonates has been investigated. Benzathine penicillin G or oral ampicillin administered to colonized pregnant women is not effective in eradicating the carrier state.[11,44] Presumably urethral colonization of the sexual partner(s) resulting in re-infection of the mothers and/or poor penetration of the mucosal membranes by the antimicrobial agents contribute to therapeutic failure.[11,85] However, intravenous administration of ampicillin to colonized women during labor will significantly decrease neonatal colonization with

GBS.[126] Siegal et al. investigated the use of a single prophylactic dose of penicillin G in preventing group B streptococcal disease among neonates.[102] Although the incidence of GBS infection decreased overall, an increase in the number of children with neonatal sepsis and meningitis due to penicillin-resistant organisms was noted. As a result, routine prophylaxis of neonates with parenteral penicillin G is not recommended. The suggestion that maternal antibodies to the various capsular types of GBS are protective to the infant has prompted attempts to immunize colonized mothers.[10] The cross-reactivity of Type III GBS with several pneumococcal antigens suggested the use of pneumococcal vaccine as a prophylactic agent, however, a large number of immunized women developed anti-B antibodies to red blood cells.[18] This phenomenon of cross reactivity probably represents contamination of the vaccine with a blood group A-like substance.[125]

Penicillin is the drug of choice for neonatal group B streptococcal meningitis. Ampicillin is also effective, however, drug concentrations needed for inhibition and killing are higher than penicillin. The recommended dosages and duration of therapy remains controversial. Schauf et al. and Allen and Sprunt demonstrated "tolerance" e.g. a discrepancy between the minimum inhibitory concentration and the minimum bactericidal concentration of drug of the GBS to penicillin.[3,99] This *in vitro* phenomenon may explain recurrence or relapse of infection in adequately treated patients.[19,31] As a result, the recommended dosages of penicillin G and ampicillin have been increased to 250,000 U/kg/day and 200 mg/kg/day respectively for GBS meningitis.[72] Therapy should be monitored with CSF bactericidal titers and continued for 14–21 days following sterilization of the CSF.[98]

The Enterobacteriaceae. Meningitis due to members of the Enterobacteriaceae family occurs in newborns, the immunosuppressed, the debilitated, and as a complication of head trauma. Cherubin et al. found in a series of 158 patients with Gram-negative meningitis in New York City, that 41% of the patients with *E. coli* meningitis were less than one month of age.[25] In other series, *E. coli,* particularly strains containing the K-1 antigen, remain the most common Gram-negative microorganisms responsible for neonatal meningitis, accounting for up to 70% of cases in some series.[46,71,73] *K. pneumoniae, Sr. marcesans,* Enterobacter spp. and Proteus spp. are infrequently encountered.

In spite of the availability of effective antimicrobial therapy, the mortality rate for neonatal Gram-negative meningitis approaches 50%.[25,69] In 1975, Chang and associates observed that parenterally administered aminoglycosides (e.g. gentamicin, amikacin, etc.) did not consistently achieve adequate CSF concentrations and that survival of neonates with coliform meningitis correlated with the susceptibility of the pathogen to concurrently administered ampicillin.[24] Accordingly, these authors recommended the use of chloramphenicol, an agent which achieves high CSF concentrations, for initial treatment of neonates with Gram-negative meningitis. More recently, Rahal and Simerkoff demonstrated a marked discrepancy between inhibitory and bactericidal concentrations (tolerance) of chloramphenicol for enteric microorganisms.[89] Cherubin et al. reported a decreased survival of patients with gram-negative meningitis receiving chloramphenicol.[25] Thus, the role of this antimicrobial agent in the treatment of Gram-negative meningitis remains unestablished.

The poor CSF concentrations achieved by parenterally administered aminoglycosides, the toxicity of chloramphenicol, and the *in vitro* "tolerance" of the Enterobacteriaceae spp. to chloramphenicol have resulted in numerous therapeutic approaches to patients with Gram-negative meningitis. Thus, Rahal and his associates demonstrated that intrathecally administered gentamicin achieved high lumbar concentrations eight hours after injection in adults.[88] However, several investigators noted treatment failures in infants with ventriculitis receiving gentamicin by the lumbar route. A large, multi-center study of neonatal Gram-negative meningitis comparing systemic with systemic and intrathecal aminoglycoside therapy found no significant difference in survival between the two patient populations.[71] They hypothesized that the poor results with intrathecal administration were due to inadequate aminoglycoside ventricular concentrations. In an uncontrolled study, Lee et al. treated 15 infants with Gram-negative meningitis by intraventricular administration of gentamicin, rifampin, penicillin, or erythromycin.[66] Although all of these infants survived, approximately half were neurologically impaired. In a second multi-center cooperative study, McCracken and his associates found a significantly higher mortality rate among neonates receiving direct intraventricular gentamicin compared with neonates receiving systemic therapy alone.[73] This observation has been refuted by others[110] although the method of intraventricular administration was not comparable i.e. direct intraventricular vs. installation through a ventricular reservoir. Although the older cephalosporin derivatives did not achieve adequate CSF concentrations the third generation cephalosporins, (cefotaxime and moxalactam), are active against the Enterobacteriaceae spp. and achieve bactericidal concentrations in the CSF. Accordingly, several authorities have recently recommended their usage in Gram-negative meningitis.[63,98] In 18 patients of various ages with Gram-negative meningitis many of whom failed therapy with traditional agents, 16 recoverd following parenteral treatment with moxalactam or cefotaxime.[63] Although comparative data of aminoglycoside versus the third generation cephalosporins in the treatment of Gram-negative meningitis are not yet available, preliminary data encourage the use of these agents in neonatal Gram-negative meningitis.

Our current recommendations for treatment of neonatal meningitis include initial management with ampicillin plus either moxalactam or cefotaxime. If the pathogen is sensitive to ampicillin, then the cephalosporin may be discontinued. Repeat lumbar punctures are useful in measuring bacteriologic response and CSF bactericidal titers. Peak bactericidal CSF titers during single agent therapy should exceed 1:10.[98] Treatment should be continued for three weeks.

Listeria monocytogenes. *Listeria monocytogenes* is an unusual cause of meningitis in infants and children. In addition to intrauterine infection and resultant abortion, Listeria causes clinical syndromes in newborns not unlike those seen with the group B streptococcus. Thus, an early onset clinical illness, due to microorganisms acquired vertically from the mother, presents within the first few days of life as overwhelming septicemia and respiratory distress. In addition, a delayed onset illness occurs following nosocomially acquired Listeria and presents at several weeks of age with central nervous system infection. Most cases of Listeria meningitis occur in the elderly and the immunosuppressed. Older children with ventriculoatrial shunts or exposure to infected gerbils have also been reported with Listeria meningitis.[117] Mortality rates in all age groups have ranged from 20%–62%.[117] High mortality rates occur when meningitis is associated with septicemia, treatment with chloramphenicol, severe hypoglycorrhachia and, in elderly and/or immunologically impaired individuals.[25,64,117] Antimicrobial therapy of Listeria meningitis has changed with time. Early studies of neonatal listeriosis compared the use of tetracycline, chloramphenicol, and penicillin singly and in combination.[91] Based on these studies several authors recommended the use of tetracycline. Battone and Sierra tested 21 isolates of *L. monocytogenes* with a number of agents and found no resistance to ampicillin or chloramphenicol,[17] however, three of 17 strains were resistant to penicillin. Lavetter and his colleagues found no difference in outcome in patients with ampicillin alone or in combination with aminoglycosides or chloramphenicol, however, benzyl penicillin proved ineffective when used singly or in combination with the aforementioned agents.[64] As noted earlier, Cherubin et al. found a higher fatality rate in Listeria meningitis patients receiving chloramphenicol either as a single agent or in combination with penicillin or ampicillin.[25] This phenomenon has been ascribed to the difference between inhibitory and bactericidal concentrations of chloramphenicol against *L. monocytogenes*.[25,98] *Listeria monocytogenes* has been found to be universally resistant to moxalactam.[62]

Thus, ampicillin is presently the drug of choice for patients with meningitis caused by *L. monocytogenes*. Penicillin has also been advocated. Despite *in vitro* studies demonstrating synergism with penicillin-aminoglycoside combinations, clinical studies have failed to demonstrate the advantage of an aminoglycoside.[79] Effective therapy with either single or a combination of agents should be continued for 14 days.

Mycobacterium tuberculosis. Although the incidence of tuberculous has declined over the past three decades, the recent influx of Southeast Asian refugees has increased the total number of cases of tuberculosis reported in the United States.[23] Tuberculous meningitis, while rare in the U.S., continues to be a problem in developing countries and among immigrants to the U.S.[90,108] Specific therapy for this disease falls into two categories: (1) the use of specific anti-tuberculous agents, and (2) the adjunctive use of corticosterioids.

Prior to 1947, no specific anti-tuberculous therapy was available. Lincoln and her colleagues reported 167 untreated and 74 treated children with tuberculous meningitis.[67] All of the untreated patients died. Anti-tuberculous therapy in this study consisted of intrathecal and intramuscular streptomycin or streptomycin plus isoniazid. Fifty of 74 children who received therapy survived, however, most had significant neurological sequelae. Sumaya et al. treated 59 children with tuberculous meningitis[106] with isoniazid, para-amino salicylic acid and streptomycin, and 21 patients survived. Sixty-two percent of these survivors had moderate or severe neurological deficits. Similar results have been reported by others utilizing the same therapeutic regimen.[50] One recent uncontrolled study demonstrated no difference between standard triple drug therapy (isoniazid, PAS, and streptomycin) and a two drug regimen consisting of isoniazid and rifampin. However, one controlled study in children found isoniazid plus rifampin to be superior to the triple drug regimen.[41,118] Not only was morbidity greatly reduced but 65% of the survivors were free of neurologic sequelae.

The emergence of isoniazid-resistant strains of *M. tuberculosis,* particularly in Southeast Asia, has complicated the therapeutic approach. Steiner and Portugalya reported three children infected with isoniazid resistant microorganisms.[105] One child died while receiving conventional three-drug therapy, but the other children survived after receiving isoniazid, streptomycin and two other drugs (cycloserine, ethionamide, or ethambutol).

Current therapeutic recommendations for tuberculous meningitis include the use of isoniazid (20 mg/kg/day) plus rifampin (15 mg/kg/day) as initial therapy.[103,108] Patients with known isoniazid-resistant strains or from areas with high resistance may also receive ethambutol (25 mg/kg/day) and/or streptomycin (20–40 mg/kg/day). Therapy is continued from nine to 18 months.

The use of corticosteroids in tuberculous meningitis was first suggested in 1958.[104] The routine use of steroids in tuberculous meningitis remains controversial since that report, however, in 1975 a controlled study suggested the efficacy of steroid therapy.[34] Furthermore, it was noted that low dose prednisone therapy (1 mg/kg/day) was as effective as high dosages. As a result, a one-month course of daily prednisone seems warranted as adjunctive therapy in the management of tuberculous meningitis.

Initial Antimicrobial Therapy for Acute Bacterial Meningitis

Acute bacterial meningitis is a medical emergency. The initial selection of antimicrobial agents (see Table II) should be broad to cover the most likely etiologic agents after considering the patient's

Table II

Recommended Dosages of Antimicrobial Agents for CNS Infections in Children

Drug	*Dosage (mg/kg/day)*	*Route*	*Frequency*	*Duration*
Adenosine Arabinoside	15	IV	daily	10–14 days
Amphotericin B	0.5–0.75	IV	daily	4–6 weeks
Ampicillin	200–300	IV	q 4 h	10 days–3 weeks
Chloramphenicol*	75–100	IV	q 6 h	10–14 days
	50–75	po	q 6 h	10–14 days
Ethambutol	15–25	po	q day	9–18 months
5-Fluorocytosine*	50–150	po	q 6 h	4–6 weeks
Isoniazid	15–20	po, IM	q day	9–18 months
Moxalactam	150–200	IV	q 8 h	10 days–3 weeks
Nafcillin	150–200	IV	q 6 h	2–3 weeks
Penicillin G	25,000-400,000 units	IV	q 4 h	10 days–3 weeks
Rifampin	15–20	po	q 12–24 h	3 weeks–18 months
Vancomycin	50	IV	q 6 h	2–4 weeks

*Levels must be monitored to avoid toxicity.

age and various risk factors. Following identification and antimicrobial sensitivity testing of the pathogen, the single most effective antimicrobial agent is continued until completion of therapy. Broad-spectrum coverage is often continued in cases of suspected bacterial meningitis when no pathogen is recovered e.g. partially-treated meningitis.

Neonates are at risk for CNS infection due to group B streptococci, the Enterobacteriaceae (particularly *E. coli* and *K. pneumoniae*), and *L. monocytogenes.* Selection of initial antimicrobial therapy should consider these organisms and provide bactericidal drug concentrations in the cerebrospinal fluid. Penicillin or ampicillin will provide excellent antibacterial activity against the principal Gram-positive organisms and a third-generation cephalosporin will provide excellent protection against the Enterobacteriaceae.

Beyond the neonatal period, *H. influenzae, N. meningitidis* and

S. pneumoniae are the primary meningeal pathogens in immunocompetent children. Penicillin and ampicillin are effective against the latter two pathogens. Beta lactamase-producing strains of *H. influenzae* and, to a lesser extent, penicillin-tolerant strains of *S. pneumoniae* have created major therapeutic problems. Chloramphenicol is usually effective against both of these organisms. Therefore, chloramphenicol alone or in combination with a penicillin derivative is used in the initial management of pediatric patients with bacterial meningitis. If no pathogen is recovered, chloramphenicol is continued as a single agent for a period of 10–14 days since prolonged exposure to combination therapy has been implicated in hearing loss in children with meningitis.[15]

CNS infections following disruption of the integrity of the skull, either by trauma or neurosurgical intervention may be caused by a variety of microorganisms. *S. epidermidis, S. aureus,* Corynebacterium spp. and the Enterobacteriaceae spp. are the major pathogens infecting CSF shunts.[100] Recommended treatment consists of systemically administered antimicrobial agents and removal of the infected appliance.[100] A semi-synthetic penicillinase-resistant is effective against most strains of Corynebacterium and *S. aureus,* however, a significant number of *S. epidermidis* isolates are methacillin-resistant. Rifampin and vancomycin have been utilized successfully in treating infections with this pathogen.[94,109] Prior to isolation of a pathogen, nafcillin plus a third-generation cephalosporin provide adequate initial coverage in patients with shunt infections. Following isolation and antibiotic sensitivity testing the single most effective antimicrobial agent is continued for the remainder of the treatment course.

Among immunocompromised children, bacterial meningitis may be caused by any of the typical childhood pathogens or by the Enterobacteriaceae spp.[25] As a result, penicillin or ampicillin plus a third-generation cephalosporin provide adequate initial coverage in this patient population. The single most effective agent is continued for the remainder of the treatment period.

CNS Infections of Viral Etiology

The incidence of viral infections of the central nervous system increases during the summer and fall months when enteroviral and arboviral epidemics occur throughout the United States.[23] The clinical presentation of aseptic meningitis is similar to that of acute bacterial meningitis. However, viral encephalitis differs in that meningeal signs are less frequently encountered and the prominent findings include changes in mental status. Prior to 1977, no specific antiviral therapy was available. Currently, the vast majority of patients with viral infections (enteroviral and arboviral infections) of the central nervous system require only supportive therapy. One exception to this therapeutic approach is encephalitis caused by Herpes Simplex Virus.

Herpes Simplex is a leading cause of sporadic viral encephalitis and is associated with high mortality and morbidity.[77,84] Idoxuridine, when used in biopsy proven cases of Herpes encephalitis in a double-blinded study with a placebo, failed to be effective.[16] Whitley and his associates in another recent placebo controlled study demonstrated a reduction in mortality and morbidity of Herpes encephalitis in adults receiving intravenous adenosine arabinoside (15 mg/kg/day).[121] Similar results were noted by the same authors in neonates with disseminated Herpes. Thus, adenosine arabinoside is currently recommended as specific antiviral therapy for CNS and disseminated infections caused by Herpes Simplex Virus. The poor solubility of the drug necessitates its administration in a large volume of fluid. As a result, the dosage of 15 mg/kg/day is often given over 8–12 hours. At this dosage, minimal toxicity has been observed.[121] Higher dosages may lead to encephalopathy.[12]

The decision to initiate antiviral therapy on clinical grounds or to perform a brain biopsy is difficult. Olsen and his colleagues clearly demonstrated the focal nature of neurological deficits in Herpes Simplex encephalitis.[84] Barza and Pauker emphasized the focal nature of Herpes encephalitis and do not suggest therapy or biopsy in the absence of such focal findings.[12] Focal changes limited to the temporal or frontal lobes by electroencephalography, brain scan or computed tomography are highly suggestive of Herpes encephalitis.[12,84] In such cases, prompt therapy without biopsy may be indicated. In the absence of laboratory or clinical evidence of focality, the diagnosis of herpes encephalitis is less certain and brain biopsy is invaluable in establishing the diagnosis.

Fungal Meningitis

Fungal infections of the CNS are unusual in healthy children. Advances in care of the premature infant, cancer chemotherapy, immunosuppression for chronic disease states and prolonged use of broad-spectrum antimicrobial agents have increased the risk for "opportunistic" fungal infections in the pediatric population. Central nervous system infections with Candida spp. are the most common causes of fungal meningitis in children and typically occur in premature infants requiring prolonged ventilatory and parenteral nutritional support and/or children with underlying lymphoreticular malignancies.[13,49,58,61,70] Meningitis due to *Cryptococcus neoformans* is unusual in children and typically occurs in the immunologically impaired.[54,83] Unlike CNS infections caused by Candida species or *Cryptococcus neoformans,* which typically occur in immunosuppressed children, coccidioidal meningitis occurs primarily in healthy children as a complication of disseminated coccidioidomycosis.[29,113] CNS infection with *Histoplasma capsulatum* is uncommon and occurs as a complication of disseminated infection in young children and in the immunocompromised.[39,56]

Amphotericin B remains the drug of choice for the treatment of systemic and CNS mycoses. Following a test dose of 0.1 mg/kg (maximum of 1 mg), amphotericin B is administered daily in dosages of 0.5–0.75 mg/kg intravenously over 4–8 hours. Total duration of therapy is from four to six weeks with cumulative dosages of 20–30 mg/kg administered over that period.

The systemic and renal toxicity of amphotericin B limit the frequency of administration. Fever, chills and nausea often accompany systemic administration of the drug and may be controlled by pre-treatment of the patient with meperidine or concomitant administration of 25–50 mg of hydrocortisone. Azotemia and hypokalemia also occur during therapy necessitating frequent monitoring of serum electrolytes and renal function. Potassium supplementation is often required. Alternate day administration of the agent is recommended for patients who develop significant elevations in serum creatinine and/or blood urea nitrogen.

Not recommended as for single drug therapy, flucytosine (5-fluorocytosine) is efficacious when used in combination with amphotericin B for the treatment of candidal or cryptococcal meningitis.[14,26,80] Flucytosine is administered orally in a dosage of 150 mg/kg/day in four divided doses. Myelosuppression, the major toxic side effect of flucytosine, is uncommon and may be avoided by maintaining peak serum concentrations at or below 100–125 mg/L.[30]

Ketoconazole, an orally administered imidazole, has been used in systemic mycoses. Although comparative studies with amphotericin B are not available, ketoconazole has been used successfully in a small number of patients with systemic candidiasis.[47] In view of its inability to achieve satisfactory CSF concentrations the drug is not currently recommended for CNS fungal infections.

Supportive Therapy

Aside from prompt administration of effective antimicrobial therapy, anticipatory management and prompt intervention in children with complications of CNS infection have contributed greatly to improve survival and reduced morbidity. The principles of management of shock, respiratory failure, and increased intracranial pressure have been discussed elsewhere in this volume. Similarly, anticonvulsant therapy has also been reviewed. These principles may be applied to the child with meningitis in the same fashion as they would be used in children with other life-threatening disease processes.

Inappropriate secretion of antidiuretic hormone is a unique problem in children with CNS infections. Manges and Lobeck described the syndrome of prolonged hyponatremia in children with CNS infections.[68] Kaplan and Feigin measured serum arginine vasopressin in normal children and in children with bacterial meningitis.[55] They demonstrated significantly higher concentrations of this hormone in the latter group. Excess antidiuretic hormone (ADH) promotes increased reabsorption of free water from the collecting tubules of the kidney. The end result is excretion of inappropriately concentrated urine and dilutional hyponatremia. The subsequent drop in serum oncotic pressure promotes free water uptake by the CNS causing cerebral edema and seizures. Inappropriate ADH secretion is managed prospectively. Fluid restriction during the early course of infection prevents the dilutional hyponatremia and its incumbent risks. Initial restriction of fluid intake to 800–1000 ml/M^2/day or by replacing insensible water loss (40–50 cc/100kcal/day) and urine output prevents hyponatremia.[55] Serial measurements of serum sodium, urinary specific gravity or serum and urinary osmolality provide adequate monitoring of the effect of ADH. Once the serum sodium has normalized and the urine has become dilute, fluid may be liberalized. In extreme cases of hyponatremia with seizures, rapid osmotic correction may be obtained by the administration of 3% sodium chloride and furosemide.[6,120]

Subdural effusions frequently occur following bacterial meningitis. The vast majority resolve spontaneously. Children with bacterial meningitis who develop focal neurological signs increasing head circumference or alterations in their level of consciousness should be evaluated by computed tomography. Transillumination and cranial ultrasonography are less reliable but may be used in unstable patients. Neurosurgical drainage is the treatment of choice for children with clinically significant collections of subdural fluid.

References

1. AAP Committee on Infectious Diseases. Ampicillin-resistant strains of *H. influenzae* type b. *Pediatrics* 55:145, 1975.
2. Ablow RC, Driscoll SG, Effmann EL, et al: A comparison of early-onset group B streptococcal neonatal infection and the respiratory-distress syndrome of the newborn. *N Engl J Med* 294:65, 1976.
3. Allen JL, Sprunt K: Discrepancy between minimum inhibitory and minimum bactericidal concentrations of penicillin for group A and group B-hemolytic streptococci. *J Pediatr* 93:69, 1978.
4. Anderson KC, Maurer MJ, Dajami AS: Pneumococci relatively resistant to penicillin: A prevalence survey in children. *J Pediatr* 97:939, 1980.
5. Awe CD, Babione RW, DeLamater JN: Meningococcic meningitis in San Diego area during 1942. *US Nav Med Bull* 41:625, 1943.
6. Ayus JC, Olivero JJ, Frommer JP: Rapid correction of severe hyponatremia with intravenous hypertonic saline solution. *Am J Med* 72:43, 1982.
7. Azimi PH, Cole KE: Ampicillin-resistant *Haemophilus influenzae* meningitis following an ampicillin-sensitive bacteremia in an infant. *Am J Dis Child* 131:812, 1977.
8. Baker CJ, Barrett FF, Gordon RC, et al: Suppurative meningitis due

to streptococci of lancfield group B: A study of 33 infants. *J Pediatr* 82:724, 1973.

9. Baker CJ, Barrett FF: Transmission of group B streptococci among parturient women and their neonates. *J Pediatr* 83:919, 1973.
10. Baker CJ, Kasper DC: Correlation of maternal antibody deficiency with susceptibility to neonatal group B streptococcal infection. *N Engl J Med* 294:753, 1976.
11. Baker CJ: Summary of the workshop on perinatal infections due to group B streptococcus. *J Infect Dis* 136:137, 1977.
12. Barza M, Pauker SG: The decision to biopsy, treat, or wait in suspected herpes encephalitis. *Ann Intern Med* 92:641, 1980.
13. Bayer AS, Edwards JE, Seidel JS, et al: Candida meningitis. *Medicine* 55:477, 1976.
14. Bennett JE, Dismukes WE, Duma RJ, et al: A comparison of amphotericin B alone and combined with flucytosine in the treatment of cryptococcal meningitis. *N Engl J Med* 301:126, 1979.
15. Berlow SJ, Caldarelli DD, Matz GJ, et al: Bacterial meningitis and sensorineural hearing loss: A prospective investigation. *Laryngoscope* 90:1445, 1980.
16. Boston Interhospital Virus Study Group and the NIAID-sponsored Co-operative Antiviral Clinical Study. Failure of high-dose 5′-iodo-2'deoxyuridine in the therapy of herpes simplex encephalitis. *N Engl J Med* 292:599, 1975.
17. Bottone EJ, Sierra MF: *Listeria monocytogenes:* Another look at the "cinderella" among pathogenic bacteria. *Mt Sinai J Med* 44:42, 1977.
18. Boyer KM, Theeravuthiahai J, Vogel CC, et al: Antibody response to group B streptococcus type III and AB blood group antigens induced by pneumococcal vaccine. *J Pediatr* 98:374, 1981.
19. Broughton DD, Mitchell WG, Grossman M, et al: Recurrence of group B streptococcal infection. *J Pediatr* 89:183, 1976.
20. Carpenter RR, Petersdorf RG: The clinical spectrum of bacterial meningitis. *Am J Med* 33:262, 1962.
21. Cates KL, Gerrard JM, Giebink GS, et al: A penicillin-resistant pneumococcus. *J Pediatr* 93:624, 1978.
22. Center for Disease Control. Ampicillin-resistant *Hemophilus influenzae* meningitis—Texas. *MMWR* 23:29, 1974.
23. Center for Disease Control. Annual summary 1980: Reported morbidity and mortality in the United States. *MMWR* 29:Supplement, 1981.
24. Chang MD, Escobedo M, Anderson DC, et al: Kanamycin and gentamicin treatment of neonatal sepsis and meningitis. *Pediatrics* 56:695, 1975.
25. Cherubin CE, Marr JS, Sierra MF, et al: Listeria and Gram-negative bacillary meningitis in New York City, 1972–1979. Frequent causes of meningitis in adults. *Am J Med* 71:199, 1981.
26. Chesney PJ, Justman RA, Bogdanowicz WM: Candida meningitis in newborn infants: A review and report of combined amphotericin B-flucytosine therapy. *Johns Hopkins Med J* 142:155, 1978.

27. Dajani AS, Asmar BI, Thirumoorthi MC: Systemic *Hemophilus influenzae* disease: An overview. *J Pediatr* 94:355, 1979.
28. Delaje G, DeClerck Y, Lescop J, et al: *Hemophilus influenzae* type B infections: Recurrent disease due to ampicillin resistant strains. *J Pediatr* 90:319, 1977.
29. Deresinski SC, Stevens DA: Coccidioidomycosis in compromised hosts: Experience at Stanford University Hospital. *Medicine* 54:377, 1974.
30. Diamond RD: "Fungal meningitis." *In* Feigin RD, Cherry JD, (eds): *Textbook of Pediatric Infectious Diseases,* Philadelphia, W.B. Saunders Co., 1981.
31. Dorand RC, Adams G: Relapse during treatment of group B streptococcal meningitis. *J Pediatr* 89:188, 1976.
32. Eickhoff TC, Finland M: Changing susceptibility of meningococci to antimicrobial agents. *N Engl J Med* 272:395, 1965.
33. Escamilla J: Susceptibility of *Haemophilus influenzae* to ampicillin as determined by use of a modified, one-minute beta-lactamase test. *Antimicrob Agents Chemother* 9:196, 1976.
34. Escoban JA, Belsey MA, Duenas A, et al: Mortality from tuberculous meningitis reduced by steroid therapy. *Pediatrics* 56:1050, 1975.
35. Fairbrother RW: Cerebrospinal Meningitis. *Br Med J* 2:859, 1940.
36. Feigin RD, Stechenberg BW, Chang JJ, et al: Prospective evaluation of treatment of *Hemophilus influenzae* meningitis. *J Pediatr* 88:542, 1976.
37. Greene GR, Overturf GD, Wehrle PF: Ampicillin dosage in bacterial meningitis with special reference to *Hemophilus influenzae. Antimicrob Agents Chemother* 16:109, 1979.
38. Greenfield S, Feldman HA: Familial carriers and meningococcal meningitis. *N Engl J Med* 277:497, 1967.
39. Goodwin RA, Shapiro JL, Thurman GH, et al: Disseminated histoplasmosis: Clinical and pathologic correlations. *Medicine* 59:1, 1980.
40. Guttler RB, Counts GW, Avent CK, et al: Effect of rifampin and minocycline on meningococcal carrier rates. *J Infect Dis* 124:199, 1971.
41. Haas EJ, Madhavan T, Quinn EL, et al: Tuberculous meningitis in an urban general hospital. *Arch Int Med* 137:1518, 1977.
42. Haggerty R, Zaia M: Acute bacterial meningitis. *Adv Pediatr* 13:129, 1964.
43. Haggerty RJ, Zaia M: Acute bacterial meningitis in children: A controlled study of antimicrobial therapy with particular reference to combinations of antibiotics. *Pediatrics* 25:742, 1960.
44. Hall RT, Barnes W, Krishman L, et al: Antibiotic treatment of parturient women colonized with group B streptococci. *Am J Obstet Gynecol* 724:630, 1976.
45. Hausman D, Bullen MM: A resistant pneumococcus. *Lancet* 2:264, 1967.
46. Heckmatt JZ: Coliform meningitis in the newborn. *Arch Dis Child* 51:569, 1976.

47. Heel RC, Brogden RN, Carmine A, et al: Ketoconazole: A review of its therapeutic efficacy in superficial and systemic fungal infections. *Drugs* 23:1, 1982.
48. Heiber JP, Nelson JD: A pharmacologic evaluation of penicillin in children with purulent meningitis. *N Engl J Med* 297:410, 1977.
49. Hughes WT: Systemic candidiasis: A study of 109 fatal cases. *Ped Infect Dis* 1:11, 1982.
50. Idriss ZH, Sinno AA, Kronfol NM: Tuberculous meningitis in childhood. *Am J Dis Child* 130:364, 1976.
51. Jacobson JA, Weaver RE, Thornsberry C: Trends in meningococcal disease, 1974. *J Infect Dis* 132:480, 1975.
52. Jacobson JA, Filice GA, Holloway JT: Meningococcal disease in day care centers. *Pediatrics* 59:299, 1977.
53. Jubelirer DP, Yeager AS: Simultaneous recovery of ampicillin-sensitive and ampicillin-resistant organisms in *H. influenzae* type B meningitis. *J Pediatr* 95:415, 1979.
54. Kaplan MH, Rosen PP, Armstrong D: Cryptococcosis in a cancer hospital—clinical and pathological correlates in forty-six patients. *Cancer* 39:2265, 1977.
55. Kaplan SL, Feigin RD: The syndrome of inappropriate secretion of anti-diuretic hormone in children with bacterial meningitis. *J Pediatr* 92:758, 1978.
56. Kauffman CA, Israel KS, Smith JW, et al: Histoplasmosis in immunosuppressed patients. *Am J Med* 64:923, 1978.
57. Kaufman RE, Thirumoorthi MC, Buckley JA, et al: Relative bioavailability of intravenous chloramphenical succinate and oral chloramphenical palmitate in infants and children. *J Pediatr* 99:693, 1981.
58. Keller MA, Sellers BB, Melish ME, et al: Systemic candidiasis in infants. *Am J Dis Child* 131:1260, 1977.
59. Kinmouth AL, Storrs CW, Mitchell RG: Meningitis due to chloramphenicol resistant *Haemophilus influenzae* type B. *Br Med J* 1:694, 1978.
60. Kislak JW, Razaui LMB, Daly AK, et al: Susceptibility of pneumococci to nine antibiotics. *Am J Med Sci* 250:261, 1965.
61. Klein JD, Yamauchi T, Horlick SP: Neonatal candidiasis, meningitis and arthritis: Observations and a review of the literature. *J Pediatr* 81:31, 1972.
62. Landesman SH, Corrado MC, Cherubin CE, et al: Activity of moxalactum and cefotaxime alone and in combination with ampicillin or penicillin against group B streptococci. *Antimicrob Agents Chemother.* 19:794, 1981.
63. Landesman SH, Corrado MH, Shah PM, et al: Past and current roles for cephalosporin antibiotics in treatment of meningitis. *Am J Med* 71:603, 1981.
64. Lavetter A, Leedom JM, Mathies AW, et al: Meningitis due to *Listeria monocytogenes. N Engl J Med* 285:598, 1971.
65. Laxer RM, Marks MI: Pneumococcal meningitis in children. *Am J Dis Child* 131:850, 1977.

66. Lee EL, Robinson MJ, Thong ML, et al: Intraventricular chemotherapy in neonatal meningitis. *J Pediatr* 91:991, 1977.
67. Lincoln EM, Sorclillo SVR, Davies PA: Tuberculous meningitis in children. *J Pediatr* 57:807, 1960.
68. Manges JA, Lobeck CC: Studies of sustained hyponatremia due to central nervous system infections. *Pediatrics* 34:503, 1954.
69. Mathies AW, Wehrle PE: Management of bacterial meningitis in children. *Pediatr Clin North Am* 15:185, 1968.
70. Mazumdar PK, Marks MI: *Candida albicans* infections in hospitalized children—survey of predisposing factors. *Clin Pediatr* 14:123, 1975.
71. McCracken GH, Mize SG: A controlled study of intrathecal antibiotic therapy in Gram-negative enteric meningitis of infancy. *J Pediatr* 89:66, 1976.
72. McCracken GH Jr: Editorial comment. *J Pediatr* 89:203, 1976.
73. McCracken GH, Mize SG, Threlkeld N: Intraventricular gentamicin therapy in Gram-negative bacillary meningitis of infancy. *Lancet* 1:787, 1980.
74. McCormick JB, Bennett JV: Public health considerations in the management of meningococcal disease. *Ann Int Med* 83:883, 1975.
75. McCrumb FR, Howard HE, Merideth AM, et al: Chloramphenicol in the treatment of meningococcal meningitis. *Am J Med* 10:696, 1951.
76. Meads M, Harris HW, Samper BA, et al: Treatment of meningococcal meningitis with penicillin. *N Engl J Med* 231:509, 1944.
77. Meyer HM, Johnson RT, Crawford FP, et al: Central nervous system syndromes of "viral" etiology: A study of 773 cases. *Am J Med* 29:334, 1960.
78. Millan JW, Geiss EE, Feldman HA, et al: *In Vivo* resistance to sulfadiazine in strains of neisseria meningitidis. *JAMA* 186:139, 1963.
79. Moellering R, Medoff G, Leech I, et al: Antibiotic synergism against *listeria monocytogenes. Antimicrob Agents Chemother* 1:30, 1972.
80. Montogomerie JZ, Edwards JE, Guze LB: Synergism of amphotericin B and 5-fluorocytosine for candida sepsis. *J Infect Dis* 132:82, 1975.
81. Munford RS, De Vasconelos ZJS, Phillips CJ, et al: Eradication of carriage of *Neisseria meningitidis* in families: A study in brazil. *J Infect Dis* 129:644, 1974.
82. Munford RS, Taunay AE, Morais JS, et al: Spread of meningococcal infection within households. *Lancet* 1:1275, 1974.
83. Newhauser EBD, Tucker A: The roentgen changes produced by diffuse torulosis in the newborn. *Am J Roentgenol* 59:805, 1948.
84. Olson LC, Buescha EL, Artenstein MS, et al: Herpesvirus infections of the human central nervous system. *N Engl J Med* 277:1271, 1967.
85. Paredes A, Wong P, Yow MD: Failure of penicillin to eradicate the carrier state of group B streptococcus in infants. *J Pediatr* 89:191, 1976.
86. Pass MA, Gray BM, Khare S, et al: Prospective studies of group B streptococcal infections in infants. *J Pediatr* 95:437, 1979.

87. Peltala H, Makela HP, Kayhty H, et al: Efficacy of group A meningococcal vaccine in young children. *N Engl J Med* 297:686, 1977.
88. Rahal JJ, Hyams PJ, Simberkoff MS, et al: Combined intrathecal and intramuscular gentamicin for Gram-negative meningitis. *N Engl J Med* 290:1394, 1974.
89. Rahal J, Simberkoff M: Bacteriocidal and bacteriostatic action of chloramphenical against meningeal pathogens. *Antimicrob Agents Chemother* 16:13, 1979.
90. Ramachandran RS, Ramanathan K, Indra G: Tuberculous meningitis: A review of 288 cases in children. *Indian J Pediatr* 37:85, 1970.
91. Ray CG, Wedgwood RJ: Neonatal listeriosis: Six case reports and a review of the literature. *Pediatrics* 34:378, 1964.
92. Reed MD, Bertino JS, Aronoff SC, et al: Clinical evaluation of moxalactam. *Clin Pharm* 1:124, 1982.
93. Report of the committee on infectious diseases, 18th ed. American Academy of Pediatrics, 1977.
94. Ring JC, Cates KL, Belami KK, et al: Rifampin for CSF shunt infections caused by coagulase-negative staphylococci: *J Pediatr* 95:317, 1979.
95. Roberts KB, Borzy MS: Fever in the first eight weeks of life. *Johns Hopkins Med J* 141:9, 1977.
96. Ross S, Burk FG: Pneumococcus meningitis in infants and children: A report on the use of combined sulfonamide and penicillin therapy. *J Pediatr* 29:737, 1946.
97. Saah AJ, Mallonee JP, Tarpay M, et al: Relative resistance to penicillin in the pneumococcus: A prevalence and case-control study. *JAMA* 243:1824, 1980.
98. Sande MA, Antibiotic therapy of bacterial meningitis: Lessons we've learned. *Am J Med* 71:507, 1981.
99. Schauf V, Deveikis A, Riff L, et al: Antibiotic killing kinetics of group B streptococcus. *J Pediatr* 89:194, 1976.
100. Schoenbaum SC, Gardner P, Shilito J: Infections of cerebrospinal fluid shunts: Epidemiology, clinical manifestations, and therapy. *J Infect Dis* 131:543, 1975.
101. Shackelford PG, Feigen RD: *Listeria* revisited. *Am J Dis Child* 131:391, 1977.
102. Siegel JD, McCracken GH, Threlkeld N, et al: Single-dose penicillin prophylaxis against neonatal group B streptococcal infections. *N Engl J Med* 303:769, 1980.
103. Sifantes JE: Editorial. Rifampin in tuberculous meningitis. *J Pediatr* 87:1015, 1975.
104. Smith MHD: The role of adrenal steroids in the treatment of tuberculosis. *Pediatrics* 22:774, 1958.
105. Steiner P, Portuguleza C: Tuberculous meningitis in children: A review of 25 cases observed between the years 1965 and 1970 at King's County medical center of Brooklyn with special reference to the problem of infection with primary drug-resistant strains of *M. tuberculosis*. *Am Rev Resp Dis* 107:22, 1973.
106. Sumaya CV, Simek M, Smith MHD, et al: Tuberculous meningitis

in children during the isoniazid era. *J Pediatr* 89:43, 1975.
107. Sutherland GE, Palitany EG, Marr JJ, et al: Sterilization of ommaya reservoir by instillation of vancomycin. *Am J Med* 71:1069, 1981.
108. Swart S: Tuberculous meningitis in asian patients. *Lancet* 2:15, 1981.
109. Swartz MN, Dodge PR: Bacterial meningitis—A review of selected aspects. *N Engl J Med* 272:725, 779, 1965.
110. Swartz MN: Intraventricular use of aminoglycosides in the treatment of Gram-negative bacillary meningitis: Conflicting views. *J Infect Dis* 143:293, 1981.
111. Thomas WJ, McReynolds JW, Mock CR, et al: Ampicillin-resistant *Hemophilus influenzae* meningitis—(letter). *Lancet* 1:313, 1974.
112. Tomeh MO, Starr SE, McGowan JE, et al: Ampicillin—resistant *Haemophilus influenzae* type B infection. *JAMA* 229:295, 1974.
113. Townsend TE, McKay RW: Coccidioidomycosis in infants. *Am J Dis Child* 86:51, 1953.
114. Tuomanen EI, Powell KR, Marks MI, et al: Oral chloramphenicol in the treatment of *Hemophilus influenzae* meningitis. *J Pediatr* 99:968, 1981.
115. Uchiyama N, Greene GR, Kitts DB, et al: Meningitis due to *Hemophilus influenzae* type B resistant to ampicillin and chloramphenicol. *J Pediatr* 97:421, 1980.
116. Van Klingeren B, van Embden JDA, Dessen-Kroon M: Plasma—mediated chloramphenicol resistance in *Haemophilus influenzae. Antimicrob Agents Chemother* 11:383, 1977.
117. Visintine AM, Oleske JM, Nahmias AJ: *Listeria Monocytogenes* infection in infants and children. *Am J Dis Child* 131:393, 1977.
118. Visudhiphan P, Chiemchanya S: Evaluation of rifampicin in the treatment of tuberculous meningitis in children. *J Pediatr* 87:983, 1975.
119. Waring AJ, Smith MHD: Combined penicillin and sulfanilamide therapy in the treatment of pneumococcic meningitis. *JAMA* 126:418, 1944.
120. Weizman Z, Goitein K, Amit Y, et al: Combined treatment of severe hyponatremia due to inappropriate antidiuretic hormone secretion. *Pediatrics* 69:610, 1982.
121. Whitley RJ, Soong SJ, Dolin R, et al: Adenosine arabinoside therapy of biopsy—proven herpes simplex encephalitis. *N Engl J Med* 297:298, 1977.
122. Whitley RJ, Nahmias AJ, Soong SJ, et al: Vidarabrine therapy of neonatal herpes simplex virus infection. *Pediatrics* 66:495, 1980.
123. Yeung CY: Intrathecal Antibiotic Therapy for Neonatal Meningitis. *Arch Dis Child* 51:686, 1976.
124. Yow MD: Ampicillin in the treatment of meningitis due to *Hemophilus influenzae:* An appraisal after 6 years of experience. *J Pediatr* 74:848, 1969.
125. Siber GR, Ambrosino DM, Gorgone BC: Blood group A like substance in preparation of pneumococcal vaccine. *Ann Intern Med* 96:580, 1982.
126. Yow MD, Mason EO, Leeds LS, et al: Ampicillin prevents intrapartum transmission of group B streptococcus. *JAMA* 241:1245, 1979.

Appendix 1

Guidelines for the Critical Care of Patients with Reye's Syndrome

Eliezer Nussbaum, M.D.

Definition

Reye's Syndrome is a severe encephalopathy with fatty infiltration of the viscera (mainly the liver) following recovery from a viral illness.

According to the Center for Disease Control (CDC),[1] the disease is linked to viral illness. In a recent report by the CDC, 75% of patients had respiratory symptoms prior to their illness, 15% had diarrhea, and 15% had chicken pox. The use of aspirin is currently discouraged in children with influenza B or varicella.[2–4]

Diagnosis

The criteria for the diagnosis of Reye's Syndrome as defined by the CDC[1] are that the patient must have an acute, noninflammatory encephalopathy with: (1) a microvascular, fatty metamorphosis of the liver confirmed by biopsy; or (2) SGOT, SGPT, or serum ammonia greater than three times normal.

If cerebrospinal fluid analysis is available, it should include no more than eight white blood cells per cubic ml.

In the differential diagnosis,[56] the following should be included: meningitis, diabetic ketoacidosis, renal failure, salicylate intoxication, encephalitis, and seizure disorder.

Age Distribution

According to a recent CDC[1] survey, 71% were between the ages of five and 14 years, 22% were less than four years, and 7% were 15 years or older.

For therapeutic purposes, Reye's Syndrome is divided into five stages:[6]

Staging of Reye's Syndrome

	Stages				
Signs	*I*	*II*	*III*	*IV*	*V*
Level of consciousness	Lethargy, follows verbal commands	Combative or in stupor; verbalizes inappropriately	Coma	Coma	Coma
Posture	Normal	Normal	Decorticate	Decerebrate	Flaccid
Response to pain	Purposeful	Purposeful or nonpurposeful	Decorticate	Decerebrate	None
Pupillary reaction	Brisk	Sluggish	Sluggish	Sluggish	None
Oculocephalic reflex (doll's eyes)	Normal	Conjugate deviation	Conjugate deviation	Inconsistent or absent	None

The electroencephalogram should correlate with the stages of coma. It should be remembered that in stages III-V, cerebral edema and increased intracranial pressure (ICP) are frequently observed.[7–12]

Treatment

Management for Stages I–II (All patients admitted to a Pediatric Intensive Care Unit.)

1. Fluid restriction to 50–70% normal maintenance fluid.
2. Elevate head to 30–45°.
3. Mannitol 0.5 g/kg intravenously over 30-minute period.
4. Decadron 1 mg/kg/day intravenously every six hours.
5. Vitamin K, 5 mg intravenously every day.
6. Administer hypertonic glucose (10–25% depending on patient's serum glucose) to prevent deepening coma due to glycogen depletion. Please note that the concentration of glucose in blood is usually normal especially in children four years of age and older.
7. Neomycin 50 mg/kg/day by nasogastric tube if blood ammonia (NH_3) exceeds 90 μmole/liter.
8. Obtain the following laboratory measurements: complete blood count, blood (arterial) ammonia, SGOT, SPGT, clotting profile (PT, PTT, fibrinogen), serum and urine osmolality, electrolytes determination, bilirubin, BUN, creatinine, serum calcium, phosphorus, amylase, acetaminophen, blood salicylate levels, viral studies, electroencephalogram (EEG), intake and output, and most important, serial determinations of serum glucose.

Management for Patients in Stages III–V[5,6,8–12]

1. Intubate and place on ventilator.
2. Induce muscle paralysis with Pavulon 0.1 mg/kg every 1–4 hours, as needed.
3. Use morphine intravenously 0.1 mg/kg every 4–6 hours, as needed. Titrate dose to pupillary response.
4. Hyperventilate with high concentration of inspired oxygen. Keep PaO_2 above 150 mm Hg and $Paco_2$ between 20–30 mm Hg.

5. PEEP should be used cautiously when exceeding 6 cm of water to prevent rise in intracranial pressure (ICP).
6. Monitor arterial blood gases via an arterial line.
7. Monitor intracranial pressure (ICP) using the Richmond Bolt or an intraventricular catheter.
8. If ICP is less than 10 mm Hg, perform lumbar puncture for CSF analysis and culture.
9. Proceed with all steps as recommended for the management of stage I and stage II.
10. Accomplish pulmonary artery catheterization using Swan-Ganz catheter, size 4-French or size 5-French (depending on the child's size) for monitoring of central venous pressure, pulmonary artery wedge pressure (PAWP), mean pulmonary artery pressure (PAP), cardiac output and cardiac index.
11. Establish hypothermia to 31°C using surface cooling.
12. Place a foley catheter and measure urine output serially. Urine output should be at least greater than 0.5 cc per kilogram per hour.
13. Maintain PAWP between 3–5 mm Hg. Provide more fluids if the level of PAWP is below 3 mm Hg providing that ICP is below 15 mm Hg.
14. Maintain serum osmolality between 290–310 mOsm per liter.
15. If ICP is greater than 15 mm Hg, hyperventilate, but if the level of ICP remains greater than 15 mm Hg, give a bolus of 0.5 g/kg Mannitol followed by Mannitol intravenous drip in the proper dose.
16. Electroencephalogram (EEG) should be obtained at least once a day and, if possible, on a continuous basis.
17. Stools must be checked for blood. Antacids should be provided whenever Decadron is used.
18. 10 mg of vitamin K in conjunction with fresh, frozen plasma should be considered if coagulation profile is abnormal.
19. If, in spite of all the above therapy, the ICP remains greater than 15 mm Hg for at least 30 minutes, induce pentobarbital coma.[7,10]
    - Barbiturate administration will begin with an IV dose of 3–5 mg/kg. The dose and the rate of administration

of the initial and subsequent doses of pentobarbital will be determined by the mean ICP and cerebral perfusion pressure (CPP):

$$CPP = BP - ICP$$

- BP = mean systemic blood pressure. Monitor barbiturate level every 12 hours.
- Pentobarbital will be given at an hourly dose of 2 mg/kg to maintain blood level between 2.5 and 4.0 mg%.
- Pentobarbital should be tapered if the mean arterial pressure is less than 60 mm Hg or if the blood barbiturate level is greater than 4.0 mg%.
- Pentobarbital therapy will be discontinued if the ICP remains below 15 mm Hg for 36 hours and CPP > 50 mm Hg.

20. Therapy will be continued until EEG pattern improves, blood ammonia levels approach normal. At this point, start gradual warming of patient. When the rectal temperature exceeds 35°C, discontinue Pavulon and morphine and observe ICP and clinical status very closely. Pay attention to neurological changes.
21. Observe patient for at least 36 hours before removing ICP monitor and arterial line or Swan-Ganz flow directed catheter.

Goals of Therapy

Prevent rise in ICP and save those neurons that are viable but severely insulted.

- Mean arterial pressure between 60–90 mm Hg.
- CPP greater than 50 mm Hg.
- ICP less than 15 mm Hg.

References

1. Morbidity-Mortality Weekly Report 29:321, July 11, 1980.
2. Starko KM, Ray CG, Dominguez LB, et al: Reye's Syndrome and salicylate use. *Pediatrics* 66:859, 1980.

3. Waldman RJ, Hall WN, McGee H, et al: Aspirin as a risk factor in Reye's syndrome. *JAMA* 247:3089, 1982.
4. Wilson JT, Brown RD: Reye Syndrome and aspirin use: The role of prodromal illness severity in the assessment of relative risk. *Pediatrics* 69:822, 1982.
5. Journal of the National Reye's Syndrome Foundation. Vol. 1, No. 2, 1980.
6. Medical Applications of Research: Diagnosis and Treatment of Reye's Syndrome. *JAMA* 246:2441, 1981.
7. Marshall LF, Shapiro HM, Rauscher A, et al: Pentobarbital therapy for intracranial hypertension in metabolic coma. *Crit Care Med* 6:1, 1978.
8. Hubbert CH: Critical care and anesthetic management of Reye's syndrome. *South Med J* 72:634, 1979.
9. Lansky LL, Kalavsky SM, Brackett CE, et al: Pressure monitoring in Stage IV Reye Syndrome. *J Pediatr* 90:639, 1977.
10. Frewen TC, Swedlow DB, Watcha M, et al: Outcome of severe Reye syndrome with early pentobarbital coma and hypothermia. *J Pediatr* 100:663, 1982.
11. Boutros A, Hoyt J, Menezes A, et al: Management of Reye's Syndrome: A rational approach to a complex problem. *Crit Care Med* 5:234, 1977.
12. Venes JL, Shaywitz BA, Spencer DD: Management of severe cerebral edema in the metabolic encephalopathy of Reye-Johnson syndrome. *J Neurosurg* 48:903, 1978.

Part II

Management of Acute Cardiovascular Disorders in Children

This part is composed of four chapters. The first chapter introduces modern technological concepts in cardiovascular monitoring. Subsequent chapters deal with cardiovascular insufficiency, CPR, and cor pulmonale in children. The first chapter deals with the basic concepts related to cardiovascular pathophysiology and serves as a conduit to the following chapters dealing with cardiopulmonary resuscitation and cor pulmonale in children. The clinical pharmacology in pediatric cardiology including the uses of inotropic agents, fluid management, and diagnostic modalities are discussed.

7

Pediatric Cardiovascular Monitoring

George S. Bisset, III, M.D.
Stephen S. Hirschfeld, M.D.

Introduction

The goals of hemodynamic monitoring in the critically ill child should focus on answering the questions: (1) which specific hemodynamic variables should be measured and why; and (2) will the risk/benefit ratio be acceptable? With the exponential growth of biomedical technology in recent years, one is faced with a multitude of choices in monitoring equipment. The advances in development of computer capabilities have resulted in a plethora of cardiovascular information potentially available to the physician.[3,4] Therefore, a certain degree of selectivity must be achieved. The purpose of this chapter is to acquaint the reader with basic hemodynamic monitoring and the goals of the various techniques.

There continues to be disagreement about the exact role of patient monitoring in an ICU setting. One end of the spectrum believes, "95% of useful information comes from talking with, seeing, smelling and feeling the patient."[8] The extensive monitoring systems may be injudicious if they remove physician-patient contact. The other extreme believes that there is nothing special about the physician's hands. If a mechanical device is trained to recognize certain patterns, then it will do so repeatedly. It seems logical that somewhere in between lies the truth. Certainly the monitoring devices cannot totally supplant the physician or the nurse. However, if they can assist in making important clinical decisions based on early subtleties, then they will serve their purpose.

Equipment

Basic, minimal monitoring consists of continuous electrocardiographic recording on an oscilloscope. A digital readout of heart rate and respiratory rate should also be accessible.

Other available parameters for monitoring are listed in Table I.

It is readily apparent in examining Table I and Table II that a great deal of information can be obtained at a great expense. A description of each of the parameters will follow.

Electrocardiographic Monitors

The typical 3-lead system with combined digital and hard copy readout is essential to the management of any ICU patient. This important tool will result in rapid identification of changes in sinus rate, atrioventricular conduction and arrhythmias. More sophisticated diagnoses, however, should not be made until a standard 12-lead ECG is performed. The lead placement during monitoring is not standard, thereby, making diagnostic inferences incorrect in many cases.

Table I

Parameters for Monitoring

Body temperature (continuous display)
Urine output
Accurate body weights
Arterial blood gases
Arterial pressure (indwelling cannula)
Pulmonary arterial and capillary wedge pressures
Central venous pressure
Cardiac output (thermodilution)

Table II

More Elaborate Monitoring Equipment Available in Some Units

Fluoroscopy
M-mode, two dimensional and Doppler echocardiography
Computers with differentiation capabilities (calculate LV dp/dt)
Transcutaneous PO_2 and PCO_2 monitoring
Portable nuclear cameras
Doppler/microprocessor systems (for noninvasive calculation of cardiac output)
Metabolic measurement systems

Body Temperature

Continuous monitoring of skin and core (rectal or esophageal) temperatures may be very useful in preventing wide swings in metabolic demand. Electrically controlled thermocouples are connected to thermistor probes at appropriate sites to provide continuous temperature readouts.

The importance of skin temperature cannot be overemphasized. In 1969, an excellent correlation was demonstrated between cardiac output and temperature of the great toe.[5] If toe temperature was less than 27° C or the difference between toe and ambient temperature was greater than 2° C, there was a high correlation with subsequent mortality. Recently it was reported that pedal skin temperature and pedal pulses were better predictors of mortality than actual measurements of cardiac index in infants following cardiac surgery.[6]

As divergence of peripheral extremity and core temperatures takes place, peripheral vasoconstriction is progressing. A fall in core temperature represents an ominous sign, indicating a failing circulation and decreased body metabolism.

Urine Output

Catheterization of the urinary bladder, with continuous measurement of urinary output is another sensitive indicator of cardiac output. As cardiac output falls, the glomerular filtration rate will likewise decrease. If no intrinsic renal disease is present, an accurate assessment of blood volume and fluid balance is available. A minimum urine volume of 1 ml/Kg/hr should be maintained, if adequate renal perfusion is to be assured.

Body Weight

A meticulous weight chart should be an integral part of every child's intensive care record.[7] Subtle fluctuations in fluid balance and metabolic rate may be detected, particularly in smaller children. In children where bladder catheterization is not feasible, or where leaks develop around these catheters, this may provide the only reliable estimate of total fluid output.

Evaluation of certain types of therapeutic intervention can be performed more readily when accurate weights are available, i.e. diuretic therapy, dietary changes, etc. With the use of bed or sling scales, patients can be weighed with a minimum of disruption.

Arterial Blood Gases

Cannulation of a peripheral artery for sampling of arterial blood gases and continuous arterial pressure monitoring have become important parts of intensive care. In children, the radial, temporal or dorsalis pedis arteries may be selected for cannulation. Techniques for insertion are well described in other publications; therefore further attention will not be devoted to this skill.

Monitoring of serial arterial blood gas samples is essential in evaluating the effectiveness of ventilation and perfusion. An estimate of cardiac output is based upon the knowledge that decreased tissue perfusion results in lactic acidemia (secondary to anaerobic metabolism). Progressive acidosis will then provide an indication of falling cardiac output.

The values obtained also indicate differences between predominantly metabolic and predominantly respiratory problems. Oxygen saturations can be utilized to calculate cardiac outputs via the Fick method.

Normal blood gas values vary slightly with age.[11,13] In the neonate from 1–3 days of age, the pH will vary from 7.38–7.41, the

P_{CO_2} between 34 and 38 torr and the normal bicarbonate level between 23 and 26. The arterial P_{O_2} during this period of time varies from 60–90 torr. Beyond this period, the pH ranges from 7.35–7.45, the P_{CO_2} between 35 and 45 torr and the bicarbonate level still between 23 and 26. The P_{O_2} normally ranges from 85–110 in children.

Arterial Pressure

An indwelling arterial catheter may also be used for continuous monitoring of arterial blood pressure. Although a standard sphygmomanometer and stethoscope provide an adequate indirect monitoring technique in most children, they are of little benefit in critically ill children where hemodynamic changes may occur very rapidly.

Three parameters of arterial blood pressure need to be considered: (1) mean arterial pressure; (2) systolic arterial pressure; and (3) diastolic pressure.

The *mean pressure* is the average pressure in the systemic arterial circuit during a single cardiac cycle. This pressure reflects the elastic properties of the arterial tree and the mean volume of blood in the system. The measurement of mean pressure is useful in calculating peripheral vascular resistance (R). This resistance is equal to the difference between the mean systemic arterial pressure and the mean right atrial pressure (CVP) divided by the cardiac output ($R = P_{sa} - P_{ra}$/cardiac output). As peripheral resistance increases, one can see by the equation that central venous pressure (P_{ra}) and cardiac output must decrease. Therefore, one can use this measure of resistance to judge the need for afterload reduction to increase cardiac output. The normal systemic vascular resistance varies from 15–30 units (mm Hg/L/min/m^2) in children.[11,13]

The *systolic arterial pressure* reflects information about stroke volume, cardiac contractility and elasticity of the major arterial vessels. The *diastolic blood pressure* provides indirect assessment of the peripheral runoff, following ejection of blood into the major elastic arteries during systole.

Normal blood pressures in children are shown in Table III.

It is important when considering the normal pressures that they be interpreted in light of the clinical examination. Blood pres-

Table III
Normal Blood Pressures in Children*

	B.P.	*+25.0*
Newborn (full-term)	65–75/50	
1–6 months	80/50	±15/15
6–12 months	90/60	±30/10
1–2 years	95/65	±25/25
2–6 years	100/65	±25/25
6–10 years	105/60	±15/8
10–18 years	120/70	±15/10

*The above values are for males. Females range approximately 5% lower for corresponding age levels.[7]

sure may be well maintained in children despite rather catastrophic clinical situations. In point of fact, a fall in blood pressure tends to be a late, ominous sign in children in shock.

Pulmonary Arterial and Capillary Wedge Pressures

Because accurate assessment of cardiovascular function is of critical importance in many severely ill children, more invasive monitoring techniques have been designed. With the use of pulmonary arterial and capillary wedge pressure (PCWP) monitoring, information concerning left ventricular filling pressures and pulmonary vascular resistance can be obtained.[2,14]

Balloon flotation catheters are generally inserted into basilic, femoral or internal jugular veins, and with the use of continuous electrocardiographic and pressure monitoring are advanced into the pulmonary artery. If the catheter is advanced more distally, a wedge pressure may be obtained. In this position, the tip of the catheter (distal to the balloon) senses the "back" pressure transmitted through the pulmonary venous system from the left atrium. This, in turn, is reflective of the left ventricular end diastolic pressure (providing there are no mitral valve abnormalities). The normal mean values in older children range from 5–10 mm Hg and from 3–6 mm Hg in infants. If a balloon catheter is not utilized, the pulmonary artery end diastolic pressure is usually representative (1–2 mm Hg higher) of the mean PCWP. This holds true only in patients with normal pulmonary vascular resistance.

Higher filling pressures generally indicate decreased left ventricular distensibility, as may be seen in hypervolemia, left ventricular failure and/or cardiac tamponade. Low PCWP readings almost invariably indicate hypovolemia. A great deal of information may become available in patients with sepsis, respiratory failure, congenital heart disease, etc. with the use of these monitoring techniques.

Several complications may result from utilization of these catheters.[12] A common, but generally benign problem, is that of atrial or ventricular ectopy. As the tip of the catheter contacts the endocardial surface, a superficial "irritability" is evoked. When the catheter is withdrawn, the problem is generally resolved. Other complications include myocardial perforation, catheter knotting, valve rupture, thromboembolism, and in small children, balloon obstruction of right ventricular inflow or outflow. Other longer-term complications include infection and bleeding (particularly around the site of catheter insertion).

In each child the risk:benefit ratio must be weighed prior to insertion of a central catheter. It must also be emphasized that removal of the catheter at the earliest possible time may prevent some of the serious late complications.

Central Venous Pressure (CVP)

Just as PCWP and/or mean left atrial pressure reflect the left ventricular end diastolic pressure, the CVP is an accurate predictor of the right ventricular end diastolic pressure. This basically means that the CVP measures the ability of the right ventricular myocardium to handle the available systemic venous return.

A CVP catheter can be placed with a minimum of skill. Usually the tip of the catheter (or the proximal port of a pulmonary arterial catheter) is positioned in the right atrium. The normal mean CVP values are as follows: infants: 1–4 mm Hg, older children: 2–7 mm Hg. These values are valid only in patients with normal tricuspid valves.

Interpretation of the CVP must be done with a great deal of thought, as errors are common. Certainly, a low CVP reading in a child in shock is an indication of hypovolemia. Fluid management may be guided by monitoring the CVP. A high reading, however, may be less specific. It may indicate hypervolemia, right ventricular dysfunction, high intrathoracic pressures (as may be seen in a child on a ventilator), or even left ventricular dysfunction, which has caused a "back-up" of pressure.

Complications related to CVP catheter placement are similar to those associated with pulmonary artery cannulation.

In general, although several problems in interpretation may occur, the measurement of CVP provides a useful guide to fluid management. In combination with measurement of skin temperature, urine output and systemic blood pressure, this represents a basic core of information in management of the critically ill child.

Cardiac Output

Since improvement in myocardial function is one of the ultimate goals in treating critically ill children, a functional assessment of myocardial performance is necessary, usually in the form of cardiac output calculation. Cardiac output can be calculated invasively by three methods:[10] (1) direct Fick method; (2) thermodilution method; and (3) dye dilution method. All require central line placement.

An understanding of some basic cardiovascular physiology is required prior to discussion of techniques.[11,13] When an indicator substance is introduced into a volume of fluid, this volume can be calculated if the concentrations of the indicator are known before and after the addition. The amount that is removed is proportional to the amount consumed by the organ.

The *Fick principle* utilizes oxygen as the indicator substance. Many articles have dealt with this technique in the past. The basic equation is as follows:

$$\text{Cardiac output} = \frac{V\text{O}_2}{C\text{AO}_2 - C\text{VO}_2}$$

where $V\text{O}_2$ is the oxygen consumption, $C\text{AO}_2$ is the arterial oxygen content, and $C\text{VO}_2$ represents the mixed venous (pulmonary artery) oxygen content.

Problems associated with cardiac output calculation are generally related to technique. Subtle changes in injection speeds or time sequences of sampling may lead to major errors in calculation of output. It must also be emphasized that these techniques are partially based on assumed variables which may change in certain hemodynamic states, resulting in up to 25% error in actual flow calculation. For this reason, the greatest value of cardiac output calculation may be in observing trends in a single patient.

Fluoroscopy

Portable fluoroscopy units provide valuable tools in facilitating placement of central catheters. Although these units are quite expensive, they save a great deal of time regarding patient management.

Certain precautions must be considered prior to the use of this type of equipment. Since fluoroscopy results in a significant amount of radiation exposure, adequate protection of adjacent patients must be ensured. Also, gonadal shielding must be utilized for optimal patient and personnel protection. Fluoroscopy time should be kept to a minimum.

M-Mode, Two-Dimensional and Doppler Echocardiography

Over the last six to ten years, echocardiography has had a great deal of impact on the management of children with congenital cardiac defects.[14] Recently, the study of dynamic cardiac function has been applied to the pediatric critical care situation.

The basic principle of echocardiography is that ultrasonic waves, which are generated by a transducer, are directed into human tissue. At interfaces between two different types of tissue (i.e. blood and heart) a reflected echo will arise. The transducer then receives the reflected image, which is processed and displayed on an oscillographic scope. A plethora of literature has been devoted to the physics of ultrasound. The reader should refer to these excellent references for more information.

M-mode echocardiography reprcsents a single "ice-pick" view of the cardiac structures. It is most useful for quantifying dimensions, function and time intervals. A hard copy recording can be used to evaluate myocardial performance (i.e. ability of the left ventricle to contract), anatomical defects, intracardiac masses, valvar vegetations and pericardial effusions. By examining the aortic and pulmonic valves with simultaneous time markers, an estimate of left and right ventricular afterload may be obtained.

Two-dimensional echocardiography portrays cardiac anatomy as a "pie-slice" view. This type of study utilizes multiple rotating, array-type or a single "rocking" transducer to depict anatomical structures. Two-dimensional echocardiography may be used effectively to position catheters, obtain a general overview of myocardial function, look for effusions, guide needle placement for pericardiocentesis and to diagnose specific congenital defects.

A much newer technique available in some pediatric intensive care units is *pulsed Doppler echocardiography.*[1] This technique utilizes ultrasound to study blood flow patterns. Information about velocity, flow disturbances and direction of flow may be obtained. Doppler echocardiography is generally combined with two-dimensional echocardiography, so that accurate positioning of the Doppler flow detection sampler is attained. This device may be used to roughly quantitate the significance of various organic mumurs, to distinguish innocent from pathologic murmurs and to identify the origins of various heart sounds and murmurs. However, Doppler echocardiography is more than just an "intracardiac stethoscope." If certain constants are determined, such as the vessel lumen area and the angle between the ultrasound beam axis and the flow vector, an accurate measurement of rate of flow can be made (e.g. cardiac output, if aortic flow is sampled).

Newer, simpler devices incorporate pulsed and continuous wave Doppler ultrasound to measure cardiac output quickly and noninvasively. The transducer can be placed in the suprasternal notch and aimed at the aortic root. A microprocessor system uses flow, angle, and cross-sectional area information to calculate cardiac output. These techniques do not require two-dimensional imaging system, thus making it less expensive and easier to use.

Other Ancillary Monitoring Devices

Computers are now being utilized, in conjunction with arterial and venous catheters, to calculate various parameters of left ventricular function.[9] The differentiation capabilities of these devices permit early detection of changes in left ventricular pressure wave forms and contractility (dp/dt).

Over the last 8 to 10 years, *transcutaneous monitors* have been developed for providing continuous measurement of Po_2, Pco_2, and tissue pH. Correlation coefficients have suggested a nearly linear correlation between transcutaneous and aortic blood Po_2s in most patients. The benefits of continuous sampling need not be overemphasized, since the importance is obvious in following patient trends. Since $tcPo_2$ reflects peripheral oxygen delivery, it would stand to reason that this technique will be useful in noninvasively determining localized blood flow. This may be useful in children with decreased cardiac output.

An excellent correlation also exists between $tcPco_2$ and arterial Pco_2. Following an initial response time lag, the results are accurate, regardless of patient body habitus, age or cardiac output. Ventilatory status and the effects of interventions may be accurately monitored.

Monitoring continuous skin pH has also been a useful, newly developed technique. Correlations between skin and arterial pH have been excellent. The use of these electrodes has been restricted, so far, to younger infants. It should be noted that this technique involves a more invasive procedure, in that the electrode must be transcutaneously inserted.

Portable nuclear cameras have introduced another new technique in intensive care monitoring. Following injection of various radionuclide materials into peripheral vessels, ejection fractions, ventricular volumes and myocardial perfusion can be evaluated. Also, cardiac shunt detection can be roughly quantitated. These studies can be performed with little disturbance to the patient or disruption of patient care.

Another result of modern research has led to the development of a *metabolic measurement system.* This is a mobile device which allows for immediate assessment of respiratory, metabolic and cardiac indices. In an intensive care setting, measurements can be made, noninvasively, of oxygen consumption, carbon dixoide production, minute and tidal volumes, R/Q ratios, end tidal O_2 and CO_2, cardiac output and shunt calculations. The measurements may be made on-line through a ventilator or via an appropriately fitted mask or mouthpiece. The values obtained may be very useful in managing ventilator settings, calculating energy expenditures (permitting calculation of hyperalimentation needs), assessing cardiac output and measurement of other physiological parameters related to the process of respiration.

Conclusion

Several monitoring systems are becoming available now, and only the test of time will provide information regarding the value of these techniques. Intensive care in the pediatric population still remains in a logarithmic growth phase. However, with the rapid advances in technology, an important perspective must be kept in mind—that still the greatest amount of information is gained by the observations of a skilled observer, who is trained in recognizing early signs of danger.

References

1. Baker DW: The present role of Doppler techniques in cardiac diagnosis. *Prog Cardiovasc Dis* 21:79–91, 1978.
2. Buchbinder N, Ganz W: Hemodynamic monitoring: Invasive techniques. *Anesthesiology* 45:146–155, 1976.
3. Edmonds JF, Barker GA, Conn AW: Current concepts in cardiovascular monitoring in children. *Crit Care Med* 8:548–553, 1980.
4. Finer NN: Newer trends in continuous monitoring of critically ill infants and children. *Pediatr Clin North Am* 27:553–566, 1980.
5. Joly HR, Weil MH: Temperature of the great toe as an indication of the severity of shock. *Circulation* 39:131–138, 1969.
6. Kirlin JK, Blackstone EH, Kirlin JW, et al: Intracardiac surgery in infants under age 3 months: Predictors of post-operative in-hospital cardiac death. *Am J Cardiol* 48:507–512, 1981.
7. Lowry GA: *Growth and Development of Children.* Sixth Edition. Chicago. Year Book Medical Publishers, 1975.
8. Maloney JV: The trouble with patient monitoring. *Ann Surg* 168: 605–619, 1968.
9. Midgley FM: Recent advances in the post-operative care of the pediatric cardiac surgical patient. *Crit Care Med* 8:559–561, 1980.
10. Moodie DS: Measurement of cardiac output by thermodilution in pediatric patients. *Pediatr Clin North Am* 27:513–523, 1980.

11. Nadas AS, Fyler DC: *Pediatric Cardiology*. Third Edition. Philadelphia. W.B. Saunders Co, 1972.
12. Puri VK, Carlson RW, Bandor JJ, et al: Complications of vascular catheterization in the critically ill—a prospective study. *Crit Care Med* 8:495–499, 1980.
13. Rudolph AM: *Congenital Diseases of the Heart*. Chicago. Year Book Medical Publishers, 1974.
14. Wetzel RC, Rogers MC: Pediatric hemodynamic monitoring. *In* Shoemaker WC, Thompson WL, (eds): *Critical Care*. Society of Critical Care Medicine, Fullerton, California, 1–77, 1981.

8

Diagnosis and Management of Circulatory Insufficiency and Shock

Stephen S. Hirschfeld, M.D.
George S. Bisset, III, M.D.

Introduction

Shock is a syndrome of circulatory insufficiency characterized clinically by hypotension, pallor, diaphoresis and oligemia. At the tissue level, shock implies an inadequate or maldistributed supply of blood which leads to irreversible cellular damage from hypoxia and acidosis. These circulatory abnormalities are dynamic, may be paradoxical and evolve with time. The complex cardiovascular derangements make careful, usually invasive, physiological monitoring necessary to evaluate and treat the hemodynamic, respiratory and metabolic abnormalities.

Classification and Etiology

Conventionally, shock has been classified according to a precipitating disease, causative agent, or etiologic event. Hypovolemic, cardiogenic or endotoxic shock account for the majority of cases of circulatory insufficiency in children. Hypovolemia, which is usually secondary to hemorrhage or dehydration, ranks as the most common cause of shock in pediatric patients. Failure of the pumping action of the heart, or cardiogenic shock, has recently been recognized with increased frequency in the pediatric population.[1] The low cardiac output state which may follow open heart surgery is a major cause of mortality following cardiopulmonary by-pass. Asphyxiated newborns have been recognized to have cardiogenic shock.[2] The syndrome may also occur secondary to myocarditis, dysrhythmias and advanced septic shock. Septic, or endotoxic, shock has assumed increased importance because of the large number of children requiring immunosuppressive therapy.[12] Although Gram-negative enteric bacilli and the meningococcus have been the major pathogens in septic shock, all organisms, including Gram-positives, anerobes and fungi may produce a similar state of circulatory collapse.[13]

Other factors may rarely result in sudden vascular collapse. These include hypersensitivity reactions or anaphylaxis, severe central nervous system injuries, endocrine failure and mechanical obstruction to the circulation by cardiac compression (i.e., pericardial tamponade) or pulmonary embolism.

Pathophysiology

The unifying circulatory defect in all shock states is an inadequate blood supply at tissue level. In hypovolemic states this is produced by an insufficient intravascular volume caused by loss of blood or fluid. In cardiogenic shock, the myocardial contractility results in pump failure and low cardiac output.[9]

Septic shock is quite a complex process characterized by inappropriate loss of vasomotor tone and vasodilatation which produce a state of relative hypovolemia.[12] Although cardiac performance and output are usually increased, there is, nevertheless, an insufficient blood supply to tissues. The complex and somewhat paradoxical circulatory derangements documented in septic shock are the result of a complex interaction of endotoxin with the cardiovascular, hematologic and metabolic systems.[9,12]

Endotoxins are located in the outer layers of the bacterial cell wall and are a lipid-polysaccharide-peptide macromolecule. The polysaccharide component of endotoxin activates the complement system which in turn leads to leukocyte and platelet aggregation and the release of vasoactive amines. These amines, which include histamine, serotonin and kinins, produce local vasoactive effects on the microvasculature resulting in endothelial cell cytotoxicity. This effect combined with hypoxia produces capillary leaks. Along with the capillary leaks, other major hemodynamic abnormalities that are produced are decreased blood pressure secondary to the diminished peripheral arterial resistance and increased venular tone. Redistribution of blood volume results and a sizable portion of the patient's total circulatory volume becomes pooled in venous capacitance vessels and the capillary bed. Arteriolar-venular shunting occurs and the capillary beds of many tissues may be by-passed. The pathophysiology of septic shock is thus mediated through several factors including relative hypovolemia, abnormal vascular tone and relative myocardial insufficiency.[10,12]

Early cardiorespiratory adjustments are common to most patients in shock regardless of the etiology of the circulatory insufficiency. Shock is usually diagnosed by clinical examination after development of hypotension, but major adjustments begin immediately after the precipitating insult and well before the onset of hypotension. There is increased activity of the sympathetic nervous system, creating an out-pouring of catecholamines, which produces increased heart rate, myocardial contractility, myocardial oxygen consumption, in addition to vasoconstriction and enhanced alveolar ventilation.

This early phase of shock commonly passes undetected because of the minimal or absent hypotension. In early septic shock, there is usually enhanced myocardial function and, even, enhanced peripheral perfusion. This early phase is often termed "hot shock," because of the increased cardiac output without perfusion failure. In early cardiogenic shock, the myocardium has limited ability to improve its performance, so that the effect of adrenergic activity is often intense vasoconstriction, with little or no increase in cardiac output. The increased afterload produced by intense vasoconstriction may preserve the blood pressure, but will be detrimental by increasing the workload of the already failing myocardium. The intense arteriolar and venular constriction may be beneficial in hypovolemic shock because of the shifting of interstitial fluid into the circulatory volume. Provided the loss of intravascular volume is not overwhelming, hypotension and reduced cardiac output may be avoided.

Subsequent phases of shock reflect the uneven organ and microcirculatory blood flow as well as tissue ischemia from cessation of adequate oxygenation. Once adequate circulation can no longer be supplied to all organs, flow is diverted from the kidneys, gastrointestinal tract, liver and skin and shunted preferentially to the brain and heart. As significant tissue hypoxia occurs, metabolic products, such as lactic acid, accumulate. Precapillary blood vessels lose their responsiveness to vasoconstriction and there is loss of fluid into the interstitial space.

Capillaries of the pulmonary circulation are readily injured and permit escape of water, electrolytes and protein into the interstitium and alveolar space. A ventilation-perfusion abnormality results which further compromises oxygenation. The etiology of this entity, which has been termed "shock lung" or adult respiratory distress syndrome (ARDS), is debatable. Intense systemic vasoconstriction, present in the early phases of shock, may force volume into the pulmonary circulation and accentuate leakage of capillaries. These capillaries may have been previously damaged by endotoxin directly or by an indirect reaction involving capillary endothelium, activated complement and neutrophils.

Diffuse intravascular coagulation may further aggravate the circulatory insufficiency by reducing nutrient blood flow to tissues. The intravascular coagulation is probably caused by an interaction of endotoxin and vascular endothelium or sludging of red blood cells during a period of low cardiac output.

A prolonged period of inadequate tissue oxygenation leads to irreversible damage of mitochondria and disruption of cell membranes. Damage to tissues is irreversible at this point. Cardiac function, often enhanced early in septic and hypovolemic shock, deteriorates rapidly in the face of hypotension and acidosis. The coronary circulation may be so compromised that areas of subendocardial infarction may occur. The brain tolerates any degree of hypoxia very poorly. The blood flow to the cerebral cortex is reflexly preserved in the face of moderate reduction in cardiac output, but if hypotension and diminished tissue flow persist, cerebral anoxia and death ensue.

Clinical Presentation

Most children or neonates with septic or cardiogenic shock will have a history of previous illnesses, open heart surgery or complicated birth. In such a patient, findings of unexplained metabolic acidosis, cool extremities or peripheral edema should suggest circulatory insufficiency and impending vascular collapse. Suspicion of hypovolemia as the etiology of shock should be aroused by a history of vomiting, diarrhea, gastrointestinal bleeding, or severe trauma.

In children at risk for the development of sepsis and endotoxic shock, the onset of reduced urine production, edema or metabolic acidosis should always suggest early circulatory insufficiency. The patient may not have cool extremities at this time, but may actually be warm with evidence of enhanced cardiac output.

In general, on physical examination, there are signs of increased sympathetic activity with cool, diaphoretic skin, tachycardia and apprehension. The coolness, quantified as reduced great toe temperature, has been an excellent clue to diminished perfusion.[6] Hypotension occurs in the middle stage of shock, but may be absent or minimal in the early stages of circulatory compromise. Children with septic shock frequently have peripheral edema, differentiating them from hypovolemic patients, who may have loss of skin turgor or dry mucous membranes.

Careful examination of the abdomen often suggests an intra-abdominal etiology of sepsis or blood loss. Rales and wheezes may be auscultated in the lungs and often indicate the presence of pulmonary edema. A gallop rhythm indicates the presence of myocardial dysfunction.

Physiological and Laboratory Monitoring

Shock is a devastating illness; from onset to death the course is usually less than 48 hours in duration. In several reported series of adult patients, survival did not occur, regardless of treatment, if a substantial lactic acidosis was present. For these reasons, critical therapeutic decisions must be made rapidly, and physiological responses evaluated quickly. The development of a balloon-tipped catheter has permitted measurement of cardiac output by thermodilution techniques, as well as measurement of central venous or right atrial pressure, pulmonary arterial pressures and calculation of pulmonary vascular resistance.[11] These Swan-Ganz thermodilution catheters (Edwards Laboratories) are balloon-tipped and flow directed. This monitoring system may be inserted from the femoral, subclavian, jugular or brachial veins; may be inserted by percutaneous techniques or cutdown; and can be guided at the bedside with little or no fluoroscopy. In children with septic or cardiogenic shock, this sophisticated hemodynamic monitoring is recommended. In patients with hypovolemic shock, a simple central venous pressure catheter is usually adequate.

The pulmonary artery wedge pressure may be used to assess left ventricular (end-diastolic) filling pressure in patients with myocardial dysfunction, as often occurs in septic or cardiogenic shock. The pulmonary artery wedge pressure, or pulmonary artery diastolic pressure in cases where pulmonary hypertension is absent, must be used as the guide for intelligent administration of fluids and therapy with vasoactive medications. The central venous or right atrial pressure is not an adequate reflection of left ventricular filling status and should not be employed as a reliable guide for managing the circulation of patients in septic or cardiogenic shock.

A cannula should be routinely inserted into the radial artery for monitoring blood pressure, calculating systemic vascular resistance and evaluating acid-base and respiratory status from arterial blood gases. Mixed venous blood gases, obtained from the superior vena cava or pulmonary artery are invaluable in assessing the circulatory state. An increased mixed venous Po_2 or percent hemoglobin saturation with a reduced arteriovenous oxygen difference is generally observed early in septic shock and results from increased cardiac output with arteriovenous shunting. Reduced mixed venous Po_2 or oxygen saturation with an increased arteriovenous difference reflects a low cardiac output present with cardiogenic and advanced septic shock.

The electrocardiogram should be recorded on a continuous basis to monitor cardiac rhythm and electrical activity. The M-mode echocardiogram permits assessment of left ventricular contractility by measurement of systolic time intervals and changes in dimension from diastole to systole. The chest X-ray is of value for assessing gross cardiac size and indicating the presence of pulmonary edema as is seen in patients with "shock lung."

Quantity of urine output should be measured and necessitates insertion of a urinary catheter. Adequate renal perfusion and cardiac output are suggested by a urine production of at least 1 ml/kg/hr. The presence of red blood cells and casts indicate evidence of renal injury, such as tubular necrosis. Renal function should be assessed by measurement of BUN and creatinine. At times it will be necessary to determine whether diminished renal function is a result of poor cardiac output or renal injury. A urine/serum nitrogen ratio of less than 20:1 or a fractional excretion of sodium greater than 3% suggests acute renal failure.

Although vital signs are routinely monitored, they have little prognostic importance and often will not differentiate a normal patient from one in a compensated shock state. Heart rate, blood pressure, temperature, and respiratory rate should nevertheless be sequentially evaluated. The difference between core or rectal temperature and distal or great toe temperature may be employed as a clinical guide to the level of cardiac output. The larger the gradient between rectal and great toe temperature, the poorer the circulation to the periphery; sequential changes in this temperature gradient have been useful in evaluating therapy.

Shock is a multisystem disease and requires extensive bacteriologic and laboratory evaluation. Complete bacteriologic workups should include blood cultures, lumbar puncture, urine culture, and evaluation for abdominal sources of infection. The CBC should be evaluated for absolute white blood cell count, as diminished numbers of neutrophils often forebode an ominous prognosis. The coagulation system should be assessed for evidence of intravascular coagulation by measurement of platelet count, fibrinogen level, and prothrombin and partial thromboplastin times.

Serum potassium, sodium, albumin and calcium must be measured. Potassium increases with cellular damage or renal insufficiency, whereas sodium decreases as hypoxic cell membranes lose their integrity. Serum albumin decreases as it leaks through damaged capillary endothelium. Albumin should be administered to maintain intravascular oncotic pressure and retard capillary fluid losses. Calcium may be depressed and should be maintained at normal levels to prevent reduction of cardiac function.

The liver and pancreas are often damaged by circulatory insufficiency. Serum enzymes such as SGOT, SGPT, LDH, and amylase should be obtained. Significant bleeding may occur from intestinal lesions that result from ischemia. Hemoglobin levels must be maintained to insure adequate oxygen carrying capacity.

An elevated arterial lactic acid level is consistent with the presence of anerobic metabolism. Lactic acid levels that are significantly elevated generally portend a poor prognosis. Serum glucose levels should be followed closely. Glucose levels are often elevated because of the increased adrenergic activity but as shock progresses, glycogen stores are depleted and hypoglycemia may result.

Therapy

The goals of therapy are: to maximize blood volume and cardiac loading; to improve cardiac performance by pharmacological agents; to relieve respiratory insufficiency; to identify and treat the underlying disorders producing shock; and to diagnose organ damage resulting from tissue hypoxia.[8,12]

Emergency monitoring and treatment should be started as soon as the presence of shock is suspected. In the emergency phase of therapy, basic monitoring such as blood pressure, great toe temperature and urine monitoring are all that are necessary to guide fluid administration and inotropic support. In patients with suspected hypovolemic and septic shock, large volumes of intravenous fluids may be necessary to restore arterial blood pressure.

Once the patient has been brought to an intensive care area, hemodynamic monitoring by a Swan-Ganz catheter and measurement of cardiac output will facilitate assessment of the cardiovascular system. If the central venous pressure is less than 5–8 mm Hg and a pulmonary arterial wedge pressure is less than 10 mm Hg, a further push of 10 cc/Kg of intravenous fluid should be administered. The type of fluid that is administered is often dictated by necessity. Sodium rich crystalloids generally have short-lived effects as the fluid is lost from the vascular space into the interstitium. In patients with septic shock, zealous administration of crystalloids may accentuate pulmonary capillary leakage and edema. If available, plasma, albumin or blood should be employed for volume expansion. These colloids improve mean arterial pressure and cardiac output to a far greater degree than crystalloids and the benefits are prolonged. In advanced shock, even the colloids may leak from the vascular space.

During fluid loading, repeated cardiac output and blood pressure measurements will indicate optimal cardiac filling pressures for each patient. In general, fluids may be administered until central venous pressure is 10–12 mm Hg and wedge pressure is 16–18 mm Hg. It should be remembered that each patient's response may vary, depending on such factors as myocardial contractility, lung compliance, or level of mechanical ventilation.

During fluid loading, depressed myocardial function may be unmasked. If the filling pressure of the heart increases, but there is no significant increase in cardiac output, then myocardial function is depressed and inotropic support with sympathomimetic amines is suggested. In cardiogenic shock, digitalis glycosides may also be administered, but in general, when electrolyte status and renal function are unstable, the use of digitalis should be discouraged. This would be especially true in septic shock. The slow onset of action and long half-life are also distinct disadvantages to the use of digitalis.

Sympathomimetic amines have enjoyed popularity in the treatment of shock because of their rapidity of onset, accurate dosage administration, and ultra-short half-lives.[5] The most commonly employed amines are isoproterenol, epinephrine, dopamine and dobutamine.

Isoproterenol stimulates purely beta adrenergic receptors to produce an inotropic and chronotropic effect in addition to dilatation of skeletal muscular vascular beds. Isoproterenol may actually be detrimental to myocardial perfusion and oxygenation because of the chronotropic effect and vasodilatation. The increased heart rate and decreased mean blood pressure will reduce coronary blood flow and predispose to myocardial ischemia and arrhythmias. The usual dose range of isoproterenol is 0.05–3.0 μg/Kg/min but extreme care and careful monitoring are necessary before dosage changes can be made. In newborn animals, isoproterenol is the only agent capable of producing a hemodynamic response regardless of neonatal age.

Epinephrine has the advantage of being strongly inotropic and has a dose-dependent dual vascular response. In the lower dosage ranges (0.1–0.5 μg/Kg/min) vasodilator effects of epinephrine predominate along with some inotropic effect. At large doses (1.0–3.0 μg/Kg/min) there is further enhancement of myocardial function along with rather potent vasoconstriction.

Over the past decade, epinephrine and isoproterenol have given way to dopamine and dobutamine in the therapy of circulatory insufficiency. Dopamine is a naturally occurring precursor of norepinephrine, which activates adrenergic receptors in a dose-dependent fashion.[3,7] At very low dosage (0.5–2.0 μg/Kg/min) dopamine has a so-called "dopaminergic" effect which is uniquely specific and which causes renal and splanchnic vasodilatation. This effect may be employed to enhance renal blood flow and urine production. In the moderate dosage range (3.0–10.0 μg/Kg/min) inotropic effects predominate and there is mild or little vasoconstriction, while in the upper dose levels (15.0–30.0 μg/Kg/min) there is marked vasoconstriction with the still present inotropic effects. Dopamine has been found useful in treating septic and cardiogenic shock and has recently been found to be of value in treating pre-term and full-term neonates with asphyxial syndromes. Dopamine's only drawback is the tendency to produce tachycardia and vasoconstriction at higher doses. Its use is quite safe, generally free of side effects and may be employed with little more monitoring than urine output and blood pressure. Dopamine must be administered in simple electrolyte solutions without sodium bicarbonate. The bicarbonate solutions will inactivate the drug.

A new, and very safe inotrope is dobutamine, which was synthesized from isoproterenol, but without the peripheral vasodilatation and tachycardia. Although dobutamine is a strong inotrope, there are few peripheral vascular effects and large doses may be used without peripheral vasoconstriction. The dose range of dobutamine is similar to that of dopamine, but dobutamine does not have the renal vasodilatory effects at low doses. Dobutamine is particularly suitable in patients with low cardiac output but increased peripheral vascular resistance, while the higher dose levels of epinephrine and dopamine are recommended in hypotensive patients.[4,7]

Another approach to the treatment of myocardial failure, in association with elevated septemic vascular resistance, is the use of a vasodilator such as sodium nitroprusside.[1] Nitroprusside has no effect on cardiac muscle, but acts by relaxing vascular smooth muscle. This vasodilator is particularly applicable to patients with septic or cardiogenic shock who demonstrate increased cardiac filling pressures, normal or elevated blood pressure, and depressed cardiac output. Nitroprusside should not be used without measurement of intravascular pressures. An arterial cannula is an absolute necessity and pulmonary arterial diastolic or wedge pressures are almost always essential.

The usual dosage level of nitroprusside is 0.5–3.0 μg/Kg/min.

At doses above this, or in patients with impaired renal function, metabolic breakdown products should be measured for potential toxicity. The metabolic product responsible for toxicity is thiocyanate. Toxic symptoms begin to appear at plasma thiocyanate levels of 5–10 mg/100/ml. The administration of nitroprusside may be tricky as the drug is light sensitive. The intravenous solutions should be covered with aluminum foil, and solutions several hours old should be discarded. The drug should be given in a central line as sloughing of skin may occur if the fluids infiltrate.

A word of caution should be given about the administration of either inotropes or vasodilators. The intravenous infusion should not be interrupted, nor should the lines be employed for withdrawing blood samples or pushing antibiotics. Interrupting infusions will result in rebound effects, especially for nitroprusside, and pushing medications will result in a bolus of these vasoactive agents with disastrous effects.

Acidosis further depresses myocardial function and will inhibit the circulatory response to the inotrope. A pH above 7.25 should be maintained, if possible. Calcium chloride may also be administered and often has a striking, although short-lived, inotropic effect.

The use of corticosteroids, such as methylprednisone and decadron, remains controversial in septic shock. If given early, in pharmacologic doses, they have been reported to stabilize lysosomal membranes, improve oxygen transport in peripheral tissues, and improve hemodynamics.

Most patients with cardiogenic and septic shock will require mechanical ventilation. Patients should be ventilated early as the "work of breathing" will be reduced and low cardiac output may be better tolerated by reducing the patient's oxygen consumption. At a Po_2 of less than 60–80 torr, despite an enrichment of the inspired oxygen, mechanical ventilation should begin. If loss of fluid into the alveolus has occurred, levels of positive end expiratory pressure (PEEP) 10 cm H_2O or greater may be necessary to achieve adequate ventilation. With very high levels of PEEP (15 cm H_2O or greater), the venous return may be impaired and cardiac output reduced. The use of "super PEEP" (levels 20–40 cm H_2O) has been necessary in special circumstances, and monitoring of cardiac output and filling pressures are necessary to insure adequate cardiac performance.

Conclusion

The challenge of treating shock can be readily appreciated but even with optimal care mortality is disappointingly high. Because the shock evolves with time, therapy must be aggressive. The ultimate goal of therapy is to minimize the circulatory insufficiency and irreversible tissue damage by maximizing intravascular volume, inotropic support, and mechanical ventilation. These objectives may be achieved by a sound understanding of pathophysiology and appropriate hemodynamic monitoring.

References

1. Dillon TR, Janos GG, Meyer RA, et al: Vasodilator therapy for congestive heart failure. *J Pediatr* 96:623–629, 1980.
2. Di Sessa TG, Leitner M, Ching CT, et al: The cardiovascular effects of dopamine in the severely asphyxiated neonate. *J Pediatr* 99: 772–776, 1981.
3. Driscoll DJ, Gillette PC, McNamara DG: The use of dopamine in children. *J Pediatr* 92:309–314, 1978.
4. Driscoll DJ, Gillette PC, Duff DF, et al: Hemodynamic effects of dobutamine in children. *Am J Cardiol* 43:581–585, 1979.
5. Driscoll DJ, Pinsky WW, Entman ML: How to use inotropic drugs in children. *Drug Therapy (Hosp.)* 39–51, 1979.
6. Joly RH, Weil MH: The temperature of the great toe as an indication of the severity of shock. *Circulation* 39:131–136, 1969.
7. Leier CV, Heban PT, Huss P, et al: Comparative systemic and regional hemodynamic effects of dopamine and dobutamine in patients with cardiomyopathic heart failure. *Circulation* 58:466–475, 1978.
8. Shine KI: Aspects of the management of shock. *Ann Intern Med* 93:723–734, 1980.
9. Shoemaker WC: Pathophysiology, monitoring and therapy of shock syndromes. *In* Shoemaker WC, Thompson WL, (eds): *Critical Care.* Society of Critical Care Medicine, Fullerton, CA, 1980.
10. Siegal JH, Greenspan M, Del Guerico LPM: Abnormal vascular tone, defective oxygen transport and myocardial failure in human septic shock. *Ann Surg* 165:504–517, 1967.
11. Sise MJ, Hollingsworth P, Brimm JE, et al: Complications of the flow-directed pulmonary artery catheters: A prospective analysis in 219 patients. *Crit Care Med* 9:315–320, 1981.
12. Weil MH: Current understanding of mechanisms and treatment of circulatory shock caused by bacterial infections. *Ann Clin Res* 9: 181–191, 1977.
13. Wiles JB, Cerra FB, Siegel JH, et al: The systemic septic response: does the organism matter? *Crit Care Med* 8:55–60, 1980.

9

Pediatric Cardiopulmonary Resuscitation (CPR)

Stephen S. Hirschfeld, M.D.
George S. Bisset, III, M.D.

Introduction

Only two decades have passed since the introduction of external chest compression and the institution of the modern practice of cardiopulmonary resuscitation (CPR). Initially, the practice of CPR was confined to the hospital environment, but over the past ten years there has been widespread standardization of the techniques by the American Heart Association. Training in CPR has reached such complete acceptance that competency in proper techniques is recommended not only for health care professionals, but for the general population as well.[1,9]

The literature dealing with CPR relates primarily to the adult. Children differ greatly from adults, however, in terms of etiology for CPR and in the actual mechanics of CPR.[11] This chapter will stress the unique aspects of cardiac arrest and resuscitation in children. Recent research has reopened the question of the mechanism of forward blood flow in CPR.[2,12] The new theories of blood flow deserve special consideration since they may one day change CPR techniques.[13] Management of a pediatric cardiac arrest, including rational use of fluids and cardioactive drugs will be discussed. The team approach to CPR, as well as complications of a cardiac arrest will also be emphasized.

Cardiac Arrest in Childhood

There are several fundamental differences between cardiac arrest in childhood and adulthood. In adults, cardiac arrest is usually secondary to an arrhythmia, following myocardial infarction or progressive congestive heart failure. Most adult cardiac arrests are sudden in onset and occur outside the hospital. Cardiac arrest in childhood is generally secondary to progressive respiratory failure and rarely due to circulatory insufficiency.[11] It is unusual for cardiac arrest to occur outside the hospital. These instances generally occur in association with trauma, drowning, foreign body aspiration, or swelling of tissues of the airway by infection, burns and allergies.

Because most pediatric cardiac arrests are precipitated by progressive respiratory failure, the implication is that they could have been prevented by proper evaluation and monitoring. Those situations in which cardiac arrest occurs are predictable and include: changes or withdrawal of respiratory support; suctioning of the airways; chest physiotherapy; sedation for procedures; and restraining of a patient for lumbar puncture. Vagal stimulation may produce extreme bradycardia during such procedures as lumbar puncture or passage of nasogastric and endotracheal tubes. Other children at high risk for cardiopulmonary arrest include those with unstable cardiovascular states, rapidly progressive pulmonary disease or coma. Children with artificial airways and in the immediate postoperative state must also be carefully monitored.

There are several cardinal clinical signs which should suggest impending cardiac arrest. Often there is a change in mental status, such as somnolence, irritability, or combativeness. Signs of a worsening severe respiratory distress, such as cyanosis, sternal retractions and use of accessory respiratory muscles, may forebode impending arrest. Just prior to a cardiac arrest, heart rate changes are usually noted. Initially, there may be tachycardia, but far more ominous is the bradycardia that immediately precedes cessation of cardiac activity or ventricular fibrillation.

Mechanisms of Blood Flow During CPR

In the past few years, investigation has reopened the question of how forward blood flow occurs during chest compression.[15] The classical concept theorizes that forward flow occurs because of compression of the heart between the sternum and spine. In smaller children (less than 7–10 kilograms) this may well be the mechanism of propelling blood through the heart. In older infants and children, recent evidence points away from direct cardiac compression as the event producing blood flow. In 1976, it was demonstrated that coughing, by raising intrathoracic pressure, could produce circulation during early cardiac arrest.[5] Direct cardiac compression was not necessary to generate circulation. Measurement of intracardiac and intravascular pressures also suggested that direct compression was not occurring during chest compression.[13] If cardiac compression were the mechanism of blood flow, higher pressures would be expected in the arterial vessels and ventricles, with low pressure in the atria. However, pressures in the left ventricle, aorta, right atrium and pulmonary artery were essentially identical during chest compression and equal to the generated intrathoracic pressure. Equivalent elevations of atrial and arterial pressures are inconsistent with selective ventricular compression or atrioventricular valve closure.

More recent studies with two-dimensional echocardiography and cine-angiography during cardiac arrest and chest compression appear to confirm the concept that the left heart is a conduit, not a pump, during CPR.[10,17] It has also been demonstrated that the mitral valve is wide open during chest compression. The left atrial and left ventricular cavities also undergo little distortion or compression during CPR. The thoracic cage appears to be the functioning pump with the heart acting as a conduit.

Net forward intravascular flow occurs because there is a venous valving mechanism at the junction of the bradiocephalic veins and the jugular venous system.[13,17] With chest compression, the venous valves close and prevent backflow from the right atrium and superior vena cava. Systemic arterial vessels are resistant to collapse at the thoracic outlet, jugular venous pressure is consistently less than aortic pressure, so that compression will produce antegrade flow through the aorta and its tributaries.

There is no comparable valving mechanism in the inferior vena cava, so pressures are similar to aortic pressures. Little net flow occurs into the lower body during CPR and some investigators think the impulses palpated in the inguinal region are not arterial in origin but regurgitant caval waves.

Cardiac output during conventional CPR falls to 25–30% of control levels. With proper technique, the cerebral circulation is maintained at close to normal levels. The preferential perfusion of the brain is probably related to low arterial resistance, which occurs when cerebral vessels dilate in response to increased P_{CO_2}. The heart, kidneys, small intestine and endocrine organs are extremely compromised during CPR, because there is little pressure gradient or flow across these vascular beds.[3,4]

Recent attempts to augment cardiac output during CPR have been made by elevating intrathoracic pressure during chest compression.[3,4] This is accomplished by maintaining end expiratory pressure and ventilating at high airway pressure, while simultaneously performing chest compression. In animal experimentation, this "new" CPR produced substantial increases in aortic and carotid pressures and blood flow. Velocity of aortic flow increased significantly, but the coronary arterial system continues to remain underperfused and myocardial ischemia is a significant postarrest complication.

Management of a Cardiac Arrest

The principles for management of a pediatric cardiac arrest are broken down in the mnemonic ABCD, where A = airway, B = breathing, C = circulation and D = drugs.[11] The *airway* must first be opened and its patency assured. Tilting the head backwards and lifting the chin will usually throw the tongue out of the posterior pharynx and clear the airway of an unconscious patient. An absence of respiratory effort should be documented by observing chest movement, checking the nose and mouth for movement of air, and listening for the quality of breath sounds. If no air is being exchanged, then a seal should be established over the mouth and mouth-to-mouth ventilation begun. There is usually the need to inflate the lungs with one or two forceful breaths, but after this the force of ventilation may be regulated by observing the chest for adequacy of movement. In the small child, the volume of air in the rescuer's mouth will provide adequate volume for ventilation but it is necessary to exhale in order to adequately inflate the lungs of an older child. The optimal rate of ventilation is 20–30/min for infants and 15–20/min for children.

Next the child should be examined for adequate *cardiac activity*. An arterial pulse is best palpated in the axillary or brachial region. An absence of pulses or a slow pulse with weak cardiac activity requires immediate external cardiac massage. The heart's position is more cephalad in the infant and child than in the adult, so that external pressure should be applied at mid-sternal level. Because of the cartilaginous nature of the child's sternum, the fingers, rather than heel of the hand, are adequate for applying compression. An optimal rate of compression is 100 bpm for infants and 80–90 bpm for children. The compression/breath ratio should be 4–5:1 and compression should occupy about 50% of the cardiac cycle so that filling may occur during the relaxation phase.[1]

On occasion the child may have adequate *circulation* but stridorous or noisy breathing suggests foreign body aspiration, infection of the airway (i.e. croup or epiglottitis) or trauma. The safest policy is not to agitate the patient by airway examination and manipulation until a controlled hospital environment and expert technical help are available.

Although *intubation* is not required immediately following a cardiac arrest, the passage of an endotracheal tube should be placed if the event is going to last more than a few minutes. In the case of impending arrest, the endotracheal tube should be passed by the most experienced person available, lest undue airway trauma be inflicted on a hypoxic, agitated patient. Once unconsciousness occurs, the tissues relax and successful intubation can be performed by most people with some experience at intubation. The endotracheal tube varies from 4.5–6.0 mm with the smaller tube recommended for small infants and the larger tube being adequate for children up to age seven years. Any patient who requires intubation or prolonged mask ventilation should have a nasogastric tube placed to relieve gastric distention.

If a *foreign body* is suspected on the basis of historical information, the airway should be inspected and the object removed if it is easily accessible to the fingers. Blind sweeps should not be performed as the foreign body may be pushed into an inaccessible position. Chest thrusts and back blows are also effective in dislodging foreign substances and should be employed in combination. It should be remembered that maneuvers which are initially ineffective may later become successful as hypoxic tissues relax.

An intravenous line should be inserted quickly so that circulating volume can be increased. This is critical as pooling of vascular volume usually occurs in the lower extremities and sufficient blood may not be present for cardiac filling. Colloids, such as plasma or albumin, appear to be more effective in restoring vascular volume than crystalloids, such as saline or Ringer's lactate. In controlled studies, patients given colloids had shorter resuscitation times and responded more rapidly and completely to CPR than those given crystalloids. Administration of fluids and drugs should take place through an upper extremity route, because filling of the heart during CPR takes place predominantly from superior vena caval return.

Although a myriad of *medications* may be given in the course of CPR, only a few of the major ones will be discussed in detail. These are atropine, epinephrine, sodium bicarbonate, calcium chloride or gluconate and lidocaine. In children with bradycardia, particularly of sinus origin, atropine in a dose of 0.01 mg/kg (maximum = 0.5 mg) should be given intravenously and may be repeated every 5–10 minutes. If no intravenous route is available, the medication may be given through an endotracheal tube into the airways. Atropine is particularly useful in instances where extreme vagal stimulation has precipated the cardiac arrest.

Epinephrine in a dosage of 0.1 cc/kg of a 1:10,000 solution may be given intravenously, in an endotracheal tube or by an intracardiac route. The dose may be given every five minutes or as a continuous infusion at a rate of 0.5–2.0 μg/kg/min. The vasoconstriction and improvement in cardiac contractility are the central mechanisms of action of epinephrine. Systemic vasoconstriction increases the intracardiac blood volume and improves cardiac output. Although other agents such as dopamine and dobutamine (see *Diagnosis and Management of Circulatory Insufficiency and Shock*) are available, epinephrine appears to be the most efficacious during cardiac arrest because of its significant systemic vasoconstrictive effects.

Administration of sodium bicarbonate is guided by blood gas parameters and is given in a dosage of 1–2 mEq/kg intravenously, administered not more frequently than every ten minutes. However, vigorous therapy with sodium bicarbonate is contraindicated as hypernatremia may be produced. The acidosis of cardiac arrest is usually respiratory and effective ventilation, rather than large amounts of bicarbonate, will correct the imbalance. Medications such as epinephrine and dopamine are inactivated by alkaline solutions and should be given at separate times.

Calcium chloride (dose = 20–30 mg/kg, maximum = 0.50 grams) may be given in children with heart rates above 80 bpm and poor myocardial contractility or hypotension. Calcium gluconate (dose = 100–200 mg/kg, maximum = 1.0 grams) is an acceptable alternative and either preparation may be repeated every 10–15 minutes. Calcium is indicated in patients with electromechanical dissociation, namely an electrocardiographic complex with an absence of mechanical cardiac activity. Calcium solutions are contraindicated in the presence of suspected digitalis toxicity or bradycardia.

Lidocaine has limited value since ventricular tachycardia is rarely responsible for cardiac arrest, except in the postoperative cardiac patient. The dose is 1 mg/kg given as a bolus and maintained as a continuous infusion of 20–50 μg/kg/min.

Direct current countershock is occasionally necessary in the pediatric age group because of ventricular tachycardia or fibrillation.[6–8] It may be difficult to differentiate ventricular fibrillation from asystole, and cardioversion is recommended even when asystole is suspected. The dose of electricity should be 1–2 watt/sec/kg, with the initial shock in the lower dose range.[7] If too much current is employed, skin burns and myocardial injury may result. Care must be taken that the paddles are placed at the base and apex of the heart and that skin contact is optimal, using saline sponges or abrasive paste. When paddles are placed too close together, a substantial amount of current shunts between the electrodes and an insufficient amount reaches the heart. Adequate spacing of the paddles allows electrical current to reach and depolarize the left ventricle. The size of the paddles should be relatively large to decrease electrical resistance.[8] Defibrillation should be performed in the expiratory phase of respiration as the rate of successful cardioversion is dramatically improved when the lungs are deflated.

If previous defibrillation attempts are unsuccessful, it may not be necessary to increase electrical output on subsequent attempts.

Prior shocks decrease transthoracic impedence without necessarily accomplishing defibrillation of the mass of the heart.[8] Subsequent shocks may take advantage of this reduction in impedence and facilitate cardioversion. Once ventricular fibrillation, ventricular tachycardia or asystole are noted, defibrillation should be performed immediately. The duration of the arrhythmia is inversely proportional to the maximum achievable success of countershock therapy and directly related to the energy requirements for conversion. Hypoxia, acid-base and electrolyte derangements increase with the duration of circulatory insufficiency and make cardioversion progressively more difficult.

The scene of a cardiac arrest, whether in or out of the hospital, is often utter chaos. The functions to be performed can be delineated as follows: (1) airway management and ventilation; (2) chest compression; (3) procurement of intravenous lines; (4) monitoring of the electrocardiogram and performing defibrillation; (5) distributing medications and intravenous fluids; and (6) directing and recording keeping. A single person should take control of the CPR. This person should be responsible for determining when to administer medications and the proper dosage; the timing and dosage of defibrillation; defining any additional maneuvers to be undertaken; and determining when resuscitative efforts cease.

A simple flow sheet usually suffices for monitoring. The graphics should record time, pulse rate and strength, pupillary response, level of neurological response, respiratory rate, EKG, blood gases, fluid therapy, and medications.

The decision to terminate CPR efforts should be made when the cardiovascular system is no longer responsive to basic external compressions and cardioactive medications. A reliable assessment of brain recoverability is difficult, if not impossible to make in the midst of CPR efforts. Failure of properly applied resuscitative efforts to re-establish effective cardiovascular function, should be the basis for the decision to terminate efforts.

In children with chronic, terminal illnesses where death is not unexpected, the performance of CPR is usually not indicated. When a decision is made not to provide CPR, it should be stated in the patient's chart and order sheet. The family and medical team should be in agreement with this difficult decision.

Complications of CPR

In general, the complications of CPR are similar to those of circulatory insufficiency. The brain is the most susceptible organ to anoxic damage.[14,16] Cerebral tissue will rarely tolerate circulatory arrest for periods longer than five minutes, unless hypothermia has been present, as may be seen during a near-drowning episode. The neurological outlook for children who remain comatose longer than 18 hours after resuscitation is dismal as is that for children whose arrest occurs outside the hospital. Reliable prognostic information may be obtained by clinical assessment within 12 hours.

Persistence of coma, motor unresponsiveness, absent pupillary light reflexes and absent cold caloric responses forebode a dismal prognosis.

Other organ systems may be damaged by anoxia. The heart is particularly susceptible to circulatory insufficiency, but injuries to the gastrointestinal tract, kidney, adrenal and pituitary glands are all very likely. After a cardiac arrest, all patients should be observed for seizure activity and adequate urine output.

Trauma is frequently caused by the physical process of resuscitation. The placement of the endotracheal tube must be verified. There may be direct trauma to the lungs by sternal compression or fracture of the sternum and ribs. Liver or abdominal viscera may be lacerated by abdominal thrusts or compression over the xyphoid process. The heart may be contused or punctured by sternal compressions or the intracardiac injection of medications. Pericardial tamponade is a relatively rare occurrence after CPR. Needless to say, meticulous monitoring in a pediatric intensive care unit is necessary in all children, following CPR.

References

1. American Heart Association. Standards and guidelines for cardiopulmonary resuscitation (CPR) and emergency cardiac care (ECC). *JAMA* 244:453–509, 1980.
2. Babbs CF, Redding JS, Safar P, et al: Cardiopulmonary resuscitation. *Crit Care Med* 8:119–195, 1980.

3. Chandra N, Rudikoff M, Weisfeldt ML: Simultaneous chest compression and ventilation at high airway pressure during cardiopulmonary resuscitation (CPR) in man. *Circulation* 58:II–203, 1978. (Abstract)
4. Chandra N, Weisfeldt ML, Tsitlik J, et al: Augmentation of carotid flow during cardiopulmonary resuscitation by ventilation at high airway pressure simultaneous with chest compression. *Am J Cardiol* 48:1053–1063, 1982.
5. Criley JM, Blaufuss AH, Kissel GL: Cough-induced cardiac compression. *JAMA* 236:1246–1250, 1982.
6. Ewy GA: Defibrillating cardiac arrest victims. *J Cardiovasc Med* 7:28–49, 1982.
7. Gutgesell HP, Tacker WA, Geddes LA, et al: Energy dose for ventricular defibrillation of children. *Pediatrics* 58:898–901, 1976.
8. Kerber RE, Jensen SR, Grayzel J, et al: Elective cardioversion: Influence of paddle-electrode location and size on success rates and energy requirements. *N Engl J Med* 305:658–662, 1981.
9. Kouwenhoven WB, Jude JR, Knickerbocher GG: Closed chest cardiac massage. *JAMA* 173:1064–1067, 1960.
10. Niemann JT, Rosborough JP, Hausknecht M, et al: Pressure-synchronized cine-angiography during experimental cardiopulmonary resuscitation. *Circulation* 64:985–991, 1981.
11. Orlowski JP: Cardipulmonary resuscitation in children. *Pediatr Clin North Am* 27:495–512, 1980.
12. Redding JS: Second Wolf Creek Conference on CPR. *Crit Care Med* 9:357–435, 1981.
13. Rudikoff MT, Maughan WL, Effron M, et al: Mechanics of blood flow during cardiopulmonary resuscitation. *Circulation* 61:345–352, 1980.
14. Seshia SS, Chow PN, Sankarau K: Coma following cardiorespiratory arrest in childhood. *Develop Med Child Neuro* 21:143–153, 1979.
15. Silverberg RA, Weil MH: Changing concepts in cardiopulmonary resuscitation. In McIntosh HD, (ed): *Cardiology Series*. Baylor College of Medicine, Princeton, NJ, 1982.
16. Snyder BD, Ramirez-Lassepas M, Lippert M: Neurologic status and prognosis after cardiopulmonary arrest. *Neurology* 27:807–811, 1977.
17. Werner JA, Greene HL, Jawko CL, et al: Visualization of cardiac valve motion in man during external chest compression using two-dimensional echocardiography: Implication regarding the mechanisms of blood flow. *Circulation* 63:1417–1421, 1981.

10

Cor Pulmonale in Children

Beverly Morgan, M.D.

Introduction and Definition

Pulmonary heart disease or *cor pulmonale* is the least familiar of the many diseases that commonly affect the heart. The World Health Organization[1] defines chronic cor pulmonale as "hypertrophy of the right ventricle resulting from diseases affecting the function and/or the structure of the lung, except when these pulmonary alterations are the result of diseases that primarily affect the left side of the heart or congenital heart disease." Acute cor pulmonale is defined as "right heart strain or overload without hypertrophy," but pulmonary hypertension is basic to both the acute and chronic form.

Cor pulmonale is caused by many disease states with diverse etiologies (see Table I) which have as the only common denominator a disturbance of pulmonary hemodynamics. The term cor pulmonale does not necessarily imply heart failure.

Pathophysiology

In the fetus and in the very young infant, the right ventricle is larger and heavier than the left. As the infant grows normally, the left ventricle becomes dominant; in older children and adoles-

Table I

Etiology and Relative Incidence of Cor Pulmonale in Infants and Children

Etiology	*Common*	*Less Common*	*Rare*
Pulmonary parenchymal diseases	Cystic fibrosis, Broncho-pulmonary dysplasia, Wilson-Mikity syndrome	Pulmonary hemosiderosis	Hamman-Rich syndrome
Airway obstruction	Hypertrophied tonsils and adenoids, Pierre-Robin syndrome	Asthma (severe), Bronchiectasis, Laryngomalacia, Tracheomalacia	
Poor ventilatory drive		Obesity (Pickwickian syndrome), Neuromuscular disorders	Primary alveolar hypoventilation (Ondine's curse), Sleep hypoxia
Abnormal chest wall		Kyphoscoliosis (severe), Pectus excavatum (severe)	Asphyxiating thoracic dystrophy
Pulmonary vascular disease	Persistent fetal circulation (primary or secondary), High altitude	Collagen disease	Primary pulmonary hypertension, Pulmonary lymphangiectasis
Multiple pulmonary emboli		Sickle cell anemia, Ventriculoatrial shunt	Nephrotic syndrome, Schistosomiasis, Infective endocarditis

cents, the right ventricular wall is relatively thin and has a characteristic crescentic configuration.

Angiocardiographic studies have revealed that in infants the end-diastolic volume of the right ventricle is generally larger than the left ventricle,[2] while as the child grows there is a relative decrease in right ventricular size.

In chronic lung disease the right ventricle must assume an increased pressure load and an increased volume load. In adults the volume load is caused by an increase in total blood volume; however, this point is not fully documented in infants and children. The determinant of the pressure load is increased resistance of the pulmonary vascular bed. Resulting alterations in right ventricular function also contribute to the pathophysiology.

Pulmonary hypertension is a prerequisite for cor pulmonale. The increase in vascular resistance may be anatomic or vasomotor in origin, but often both mechanisms are involved. In the normal individual, the pulmonary circulation is a highly distensible low resistant circuit accommodating the same blood flow as the systemic circulation at approximately one-fourth the mean blood pressure. During moderate exercise, tripling of the blood flow elicits only slight increase in pulmonary arterial pressure. Even after removal of one lung the residual pulmonary vascular bed accepts considerable increments in pulmonary blood flow with only slight increases in pulmonary artery pressure as long as the remaining lung is normal. However, when pulmonary vascular reserve has been exhausted by a progressive reduction in the extent and the distensibility of the pulmonary vascular tree, even modest increases in blood flow associated with normal activity may elicit marked pulmonary hypertension. The essential component of this vulnerability is a decrease in the cross sectional area of the pulmonary resistance vessels. The restricted vascular bed results from wide spread narrowing and obstruction of small pulmonary arteries and arterioles usually accompanied by a decrease in the distensibility not only of the vessels but of the adjacent lung.[3]

The most potent stimulus for pulmonary vasoconstriction is alveolar hypoxia which acts directly on adjacent small pulmonary arteries and arterioles. In chronic hypoxia these effects may be intensified by increased viscosity of the blood due to secondary polycythemia.[3]

The effects of carbon dioxide (CO_2) on pulmonary circulation may be due to the acidosis it generates rather than a direct action on pulmonary vessels. Despite uncertainty regarding the mechanism, studies in animals and human subjects suggest that hypercarbia causes an increase in pulmonary artery pressure. Heart failure in cor pulmonale is often associated with respiratory insufficiency and the management of that insufficiency generally determines the prognosis; therefore, the noncardiac effects of hypercarbia are important.

Severe acidosis also elicits pulmonary vasoconstriction. The metabolic acidosis resulting from hypoxemia and the respiratory acidosis of hypercarbia result in acidemia which contributes to the pulmonary vasoconstriction.[3]

Carbon dioxide retention is self-perpetuating. On the one hand, hypercapnia blunts the responsiveness of the respiratory center to the CO_2 stimulus and on the other hand it promotes retention of bicarbonate by the kidney. Patients with chronic hypercapnia are particularly vulnerable to the effects of sedatives or oxygen breathing, both of which may cause serious increases in the degree of hypercapnia: sedatives, by depressing the respiratory centers in the brain, and oxygen, by abolishing the hypoxic drive to ventilation.[3] It is usually in the severely hypoxic hypercapnic patient that right-sided heart failure occurs.

Alveolar ventilation is an important component in the pathogenesis of cor pulmonale. Recognition of this fact is necessary since elimination of the initiating mechanism may reverse the alveolar hypoventilation and, unless alveolar ventilation is improved, other therapeutic maneuvers are not likely to be effective.

Pulmonary hypertension is the *sine qua non* of cor pulmonale. At sea level, two distinct patterns characterize cor pulmonale. The first is episodic and the second is progressive unremitting pulmonary hypertension and cor pulmonale leading inevitably to right-sided heart failure. Although relief of hypoxia may restore pulmonary arterial pressure to normal or near normal levels, with each subsequent attack the pulmonary vascular tree seems to lose some of its adaptability and the patient moves a little closer to persistent cor pulmonale.

In the patient who develops cor pulmonale, pulmonary hypertension first appears either when blood flow is increased or during bouts of acute hypoxia. The highest pulmonary arterial pressures occur in pulmonary vascular and interstitial disease.

Pressures are less impressive and fixed in chronic obstructive lung disease. At first, pulmonary hypertension during exercise or hypoxia is associated with normal end-diastolic pressure in the right ventricle. As pulmonary hypertension is prolonged or becomes more severe, end-diastolic (filling) pressure in the right ventricle increases and is associated with right ventricular dilatation and/or diminished ventricular compliance and hypertrophy. Cardiac output may still be normal at rest and increased during exercise (cor pulmonale without heart failure). Ultimately, the onset of right-sided heart failure is identified by abnormally high end-diastolic pressure in the right ventricle; the cardiac output may still be normal at rest but fails to increase during exercise and the systemic veins are engorged reflecting the inability of the right ventricle to empty normally.[3]

At sea level, cor pulmonale is not associated with left ventricular enlargement as long as arterial hypoxemia is modest in degree. If it is severe, left as well as right ventricular enlargement and malfunction may occur. Left ventricular involvement is more likely to occur in the adult patient with independent diseases of the left ventricle, such as arteriosclerotic heart disease and is less likely to be present in infants and children.

Clinical Presentation and Evaluation

Cor pulmonale does not imply right ventricular failure, although right ventricular failure develops with severe cor pulmonale. Acute or subacute cor pulmonale usually includes some degree of right ventricular failure.

Chronic cor pulmonale presents as a slowly progressive complication of a respiratory disorder. The severity of the underlying disease is a major contributing factor since the degree of hypoxia and hypoventilation are the important determinants of cardiac involvement. Chronic cor pulmonale may be unrecognized as long as the heart is compensated. Therefore, incipient cor pulmonale must be suspected on all longstanding conditions that predispose to this complication. The most common of these in childhood is severe cystic fibrosis.[4]

In general, cardiac involvement can be established clinically only in its advanced form. An accentuated pulmonary second sound is a helpful diagnostic finding when present, but may be absent because of muffling by overlying emphysematous lung. On roentgenograms, enlargement of the pulmonary arteries may be the only evidence of chronic cor pulmonale. Cardiomegaly is usually a late manifestation.

Cor pulmonale in the severe form is characterized by clinical evidence of heart failure with cardiac enlargement. Heart failure may be difficult to recognize because cyanosis, dyspnea and tachycardia are common features of severe respiratory disease without cardiac involvement. Hepatomegaly may be misleading because it can be a manifestation of depression of the diaphragm secondary to underlying pulmonary disease rather than true enlargement of the liver. Measurement of liver span rather than of depression below the costal margin may help in this differentiation, and the presence of true hepatomegaly (together with pitting edema) is strongly suggestive of heart failure in the patient with cor pulmonale. A progressive enlargement of the heart on serial roentgenograms as well as hepatomegaly and peripheral edema are reliable clinical signs of cardiac failure with cor pulmonale.[4]

When acute cor pulmonale is suspected the following studies should be obtained:[4]

Roentgenograms of the Chest. These permit evaluation of pulmonary parenchyma, heart size and nasopharyngeal tract. In the absence of pericarditis, definite cardiomegaly is strong evidence of heart failure.

Electrocardiogram. In the acute form of cor pulmonale, recordings may show only tall peaked P waves documenting right atrial enlargement. With cor pulmonale of longer duration there is likely to be evidence of right ventricular hypertrophy.

Vectorcardiogram. Some observers believe that the vectorcardiogram is more trustworthy than the electrocardiogram in the clinical recognition of cor pulmonale,[5] but this clinical tool is not as widely available as the electrocardiogram.

Blood Gases. Respiratory failure has been defined as a state of impaired respiratory function with arterial Po_2 of less than 60 mm of mercury (without intracardiac right to left shunting) and with arterial Pco_2 above 50 mm of mercury.[6] These levels should raise suspicion of possible or impending cor pulmonale.

Echocardiogram. Despite the technical difficulties which may be encountered in obtaining echocardiograms on infants and children with lung disease, with skill and experience it is possible to obtain adequate studies in the majority of patients. While it is possible that two-dimensional echocardiographic studies may prove useful in evaluating patients with obstructive lung disease, currently, the M-mode technique is utilized routinely in patients with cor pulmonale. A considerable volume of information is available regarding M-mode echocardiographic findings in cor pulmonale.[7] Most studies have demonstrated that even early in the disease right ventricular wall hypertrophy is often present and is more severe in patients with advanced disease. The right ventricular cavity dimension is also greater than normal and the increase is generally greatest in patients with advanced disease. Right ventricular wall and cavity changes are probably secondary to elevated pulmonary arterial pressure. Other progressive cardiac changes include septal and left ventricular thickness in later stages of the disease. At all stages of the disease the left ventricle is somewhat smaller than normal, probably due to secondary septal indentation into the left ventricle. In the late states of the disease, the aorta is quantitatively larger than would be expected in a normal population. Functional and anatomic alterations are detected by M-mode echocardiography.[7]

Right ventricular systolic time intervals as determined echocardiographically have been used to assess the pulmonary vascular bed[10] and echocardiographic changes in children with pulmonary hypertension secondary to upper airway obstruction have been described.[9] The association between elevated pulmonary artery (PA) pressure and alterations in the pulmonic valve echocardiogram has been described. Measurement of the right ventricular pre-ejection (RPEP) and right ventricular ejection time (RVET) in pediatric patients undergoing cardiac catheterization demonstrated a correlation between PA diastolic pressure and the RPEP/RVET ratio. The utility of RPEP/RVET has been confirmed in sequential data on patients in whom alterations in RPEP/RVET accurately reflected the changing PA diastolic pressure. When measured from the pulmonary valve echocardiogram, a RPEP/RVET ratio of greater than 0.35 has been associated with elevated PA diastolic pressure and increased pulmonary vascular resistance.[9]

Cardiac Catheterization. Cardiac catheterization is not ordinarily required to diagnose cor pulmonale. Indications for catheterization include congestive heart failure without obvious cause, and possible association of other cardiac diseases with cor pulmonale.

Radionuclide Cardiac Angiography. This technique has been used recently to study patients with cor pulmonale. However, reports to date are somewhat conflicting.[8]

Differential Diagnosis of Underlying Disease

While cystic fibrosis has long been considered the most common cause of cor pulmonale in pediatric patients, bronchopulmonary dysplasia is becoming an increasingly important cause of this disease. Other relatively common causes of cor pulmonale include high altitude, upper respiratory tract obstruction, parenchymal restrictive lung disease, sickle cell anemia, and ventriculoatrial shunts. Less common causes include kyphoscoliosis, neuromuscular disease, obesity, severe asthma and collagen diseases. Uncommon causes of cor pulmonale in infants and children include primary pulmonary hypertension, pulmonary veno-occlusive disease, primary alveolar hypoventilation (Ondine's curse), alveolar proteinosis, and Alpha-1-antitrypsin deficiency.[4] Recently, sleep hypoxia has been implicated.

Therapy

Many pharmacologic agents have been used in the treatment of cor pulmonale including inotropic agents, diuretics and pulmonary vasodilators.[8] When congestive heart failure is present in cor pulmonale, decongestive measures are recommended, including the use of the diuretic furosemide and the inotropic agent, digoxin. If rapid action is necessary, these drugs should be given intravenously.

Patients with cor pulmonale may be particularly sensitive to digitalis because of their altered metabolic state. The prophylactic use of digitalis for patients with severe cor pulmonale without heart failure is controversial.[8]

Oxygen is often required but should be administered with awareness of the potential for oxygen toxicity worsening the pulmonary problem. In addition, oxygen may interfere with the hypoxic drive to ventilation.

If superimposed pulmonary infection is present, appropriate antibiotics should be administered. This is of particular importance in patients with cystic fibrosis.

The use of pulmonary vasodilators is often considered. However, most of the cases of cor pulmonale in infants and children do not have underlying lung disease which is likely to be responsive to such therapy. Pulmonary vasodilators which have been considered for the treatment of high pulmonary vascular resistance include antihistamines, diazoxide and tolazoline. However, it has been demonstrated in laboratory animals that vascular resistance in collapsed lungs is reduced by pulmonary vasodilators; therefore, their use in cor pulmonale might be counterproductive because the increased flow through nonventilated lungs would accentuate the right to left shunt and increase hypoxemia.[8]

There is increasing evidence however, that therapeutic measures aimed at the heart can best be considered as a delaying action, and that the most important aspect of reversing the process is relieving the pulmonary hypertension, since this is the basis of the cor pulmonale. Therefore, therapeutic attention should be directed mainly to the pulmonary problem and associated hypoxemia rather than to the heart.

Therefore, specific therapy of cor pulmonale will be specific therapy for the underlying disease. For example, in the patient with cystic fibrosis, relief of bronchial obstruction and hypoxemia, together with therapy for intercurrent pulmonary infections are indicated. Upper respiratory tract obstruction can be relieved once it is recognized. The increasing incidence of cor pulmonale in infants with bronchopulmonary dysplasia represents a difficult therapeutic problem, but in general, the management of these patients is similar; in the small premature infant particularly careful fluid management may be required also.

Prognosis

Prognosis is dependent entirely on the etiology of the cor pulmonale. If a readily curable cause is found, such as upper airway obstruction, the prognosis is excellent. If, on the other hand, the patient has a potentially lethal and inevitably progressive disease such as cystic fibrosis, the prognosis is poor.

Prevention is a complex issue, since cor pulmonale is not a primary disease process but rather a complication of another underlying pathophysiologic state. Therefore, prevention would require elimination of the underlying disease (i.e. prenatal diagnosis for cystic fibrosis, prevention of prematurity which is commonly complicated by bronchopulmonary dysplasia).

Summary

Cor pulmonale is a state of altered anatomy and physiology of the right heart secondary to diseases affecting the lung. The pathophysiology has been reviewed, the clinical presentation described, and a plan for diagnostic evaluation outlined. A differential diagnosis of the underlying etiologies has been presented. Therapy has been discussed, with emphasis on treating the underlying lung disease as well as the associated heart failure. For an indepth discussion of the subject the reader is referred to two excellent reviews.[4,10]

References

1. World Health Organization Expert Committee. Chronic cor pulmonale. *Circulation* 27:594, 1963.
2. Mathew R, Thilenius OG, Arcilla RA: Comparative response of right and left ventricles to volume overload. *Am J Cardiol* 38:203, 1976.
3. Fishman AP: *Harrison's Principles of Internal Medicine.* New York, McGraw-Hill, 1977, Pages 1406–1412.
4. Monset-Couchard M, Mason CV, Moss AJ: Cor pulmonale in children. *Current Problems in Pediatrics,* Vol 5, No 4, February 1975.
5. Siassi B, Moss AJ, Dooley RR: Clinical recognition of cor pulmonale in cystic fibrosis. *J Pediatr* 78:798, 1971.
6. Koerner SK, Malovany RJ: Acute respiratory insufficiency and cor pulmonale: Pathophysiology, clinical features and management. *Am Heart J* 88:115, 1974.
7. Goldberg SJ, Allan HD, Sahn DJ: *Pediatric and Adolescent Echocardiography.* Second Edition, Chicago, Yearbook Medical Publishers, 1980, page 396.

8. Riggs T, et al: Assessment of the pulmonary vascular bed by echocardiographic right ventricular systolic time intervals. *Circulation* 59:939, 1978.
9. Nussbaum E, et al: Echocardiographic changes in children with pulmonary hypertension secondary to upper airway obstruction. *J Pediatr* 93:931, 1978.
10. Moss AJ: The cardiovascular system in cystic fibrosis. *Pediatrics.* (In press.)

Part III

Pulmonary Failure and Disorders of the Respiratory Tract

Part III is composed of seven chapters covering the entire spectrum of the respiratory tract from upper to lower airways. The part begins with an overall introduction to emergencies of the respiratory tract in infants and children. Diagnosis is a key element in dealing with the respiratory tract; therefore, radiological approach to airways in children receives maximal attention. The second chapter provides the reader with an overview of the pathophysiology of respiratory failure in children. Essential concepts in oxygen transport are emphasized. The third and fourth chapters deal with common disorders of the respiratory tract which are considered emergencies in pediatrics. The third chapter meticulously covers the topic of acute epiglottitis and croup, and the fourth chapter provides an excellent practical approach to the child with status asthmaticus. The fifth chapter deals with a relatively new entity termed *adult respiratory distress syndrome*, which has been recognized only recently in children. Reports dealing with this issue have been mounting over the past three years, and it was felt that this chapter should therefore be included. The sixth chapter deals with a common issue in pediatrics, namely, pleural effusion. The concluding chapter outlines the respiratory care of the pediatric patient. This essential chapter provides insight into mechanical ventilation, oxygen therapy, and respiratory monitoring in children.

11

Radiologic Evaluation of Emergencies of the Respiratory Tract in Infants and Children

Barry S. Yulish, M.D.
Stuart C. Morrison, M.B.

Obstructive Airway Lesions

Lesions which produce acute respiratory problems in infants and children frequently produce symptoms because of obstruction of the major airways. They may be congenital or acquired, inflammatory, neoplastic or traumatic, and include aspirated or ingested foreign bodies.

The symptoms and signs produced by obstructing lesions of the respiratory tract commonly point toward the level of obstruction, and may aid in radiologic diagnosis. Nasal and pharyngeal airway obstruction produce stertorous breathing, a coarser and more gutteral sound than true stridor, which can be altered by crying or change in position.[1] Inspiratory stridor with soft tissue retraction usually means obstruction at or above the glottis; biphasic stridor usually means that the obstruction is subglottic or in the extrathoracic portion of the trachea while expiratory stridor and wheeze accompany obstructing airway lesions of the intrathoracic portion of the trachea.[1] Hoarseness points toward glottic or paraglottic lesions; dysphagia and drooling can occur with obstructive lesions associated with impaired pharyngeal and/or esophageal function as with epiglottitis and retropharyngeal abscess. Expiratory stridor and wheeze with dysphagia may occur secondary to intrathoracic lesions such as vascular rings and masses which compress both the airway and the esophagus.[1]

Anatomic Considerations

The pediatric airways of the child are smaller than the adult; the skeleton and soft tissues of the pediatric larynx are softer and more compressible than in the adult, and the laryngeal vestibule is relatively small.[1] The AP diameter of the glottis of a newborn is 7 mm, and it has been estimated that 1 mm of mucosal edema of the glottic region will reduce the airway to 35% of normal.[2] The subglottic region of the airway is the narrowest, measuring 5–7 mm in diameter, and is the least expandable because it is surrounded by the complete cricoid cartilage.[1] These features in conjunction with a loosely attached mucosa make the subglottic portion of the airway prone to significant obstruction with only mild inflammatory or edematous changes. The high position of the newborn larynx and proximity of the epiglottis to the palate help to make the infant a preferential nasal breather.[2] These anatomic differences mean that obstructive airway problems in infants and children are more acute and severe than in the adult.

Radiologic Evaluation of Obstructive Airway Disease

Emergency examination should include conventional films, frontal and lateral, of the upper airways and chest. These are best performed in the radiology department but can be done using portable technique, although film quality may then be suboptimal. Supplementary examinations frequently used include inspiration/expiration films of the chest and airways, and fluoroscopy with barium swallow. Airway films made with high kilovoltage, magnification and special filtration can be useful for detection of airway foreign bodies and minor changes in caliber of the airways.[3] Depending upon the urgency and availability, computerized tomography can provide valuable additional information. The lateral view of the neck should include the nasopharynx and should be made in inspiration and extension except in suspected cases of epiglottitis. Since air is the contrast medium used in outlining the airways, it can be appreciated that a film made in expiration or during the act of swallowing, can produce displacement of air from the airways and create the appearance of pathology when none is present. Furthermore, the infant trachea is a mobile structure so that a film made in expiration and flexion will cause the trachea to buckle forward, and the retropharyngeal soft tissues to bulge forward again creating the appearance of a mass when none is present. If there is any question whether the appearance on the lateral neck radiograph is due to an artefact of the examination, fluoroscopy utilizing inspired air as the contrast medium and supplemented by a barium swallow as needed, can prove or disprove the presence of a mass. (See Figs. 1A, 1B, 2, 3A, and 3B for normal anatomy and variations in appearance of the upper airways.)

The Nasopharynx

Choanal Atresia

Choanal atresia is the result of failure of the bucconasal membrane to rupture during the seventh week of gestation, thereby preventing communication between the nasal cavity and pharynx.[4] The lesion is more commonly unilateral with female preponderance; in 90% the vestigial plate is bony while in 10% it is membranous.[4] The obstruction may be complete (atresia) or incomplete (stenosis). Although not common, bilateral choanal atresia is a neonatal emergency. Since the newborn is a preferential nasal breather, death can result from asphyxia if the lesion is not recognized.

Diagnosis is suspected because of respiratory distress at birth alleviated by crying or insertion of an oral airway, nasal discharge and inability to pass a small feeding tube through the nostrils.[4]

Radiographic studies are confirmatory. Following suction of nasal secretions, oily Dionosil (usually less than 2 cc) is instilled sequentially into each nostril under fluoroscopic control. If the opaque medium enters the nasopharynx, atresia but not stenosis

Text continued on page 180

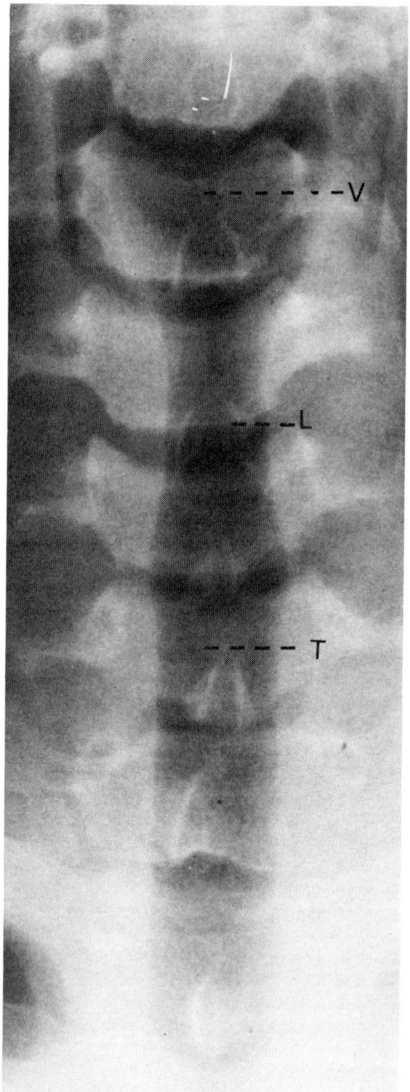

Figure 1A. AP view of the neck in an adolescent male, made in inspiration. Vestibule (V), airway at the level of the vocal cords (L) and trachea (T). In inspiration the cords are abducted and the airway at the level of the vocal cords is wide open and nearly the same size as the trachea.

Illustration continued on the opposite page

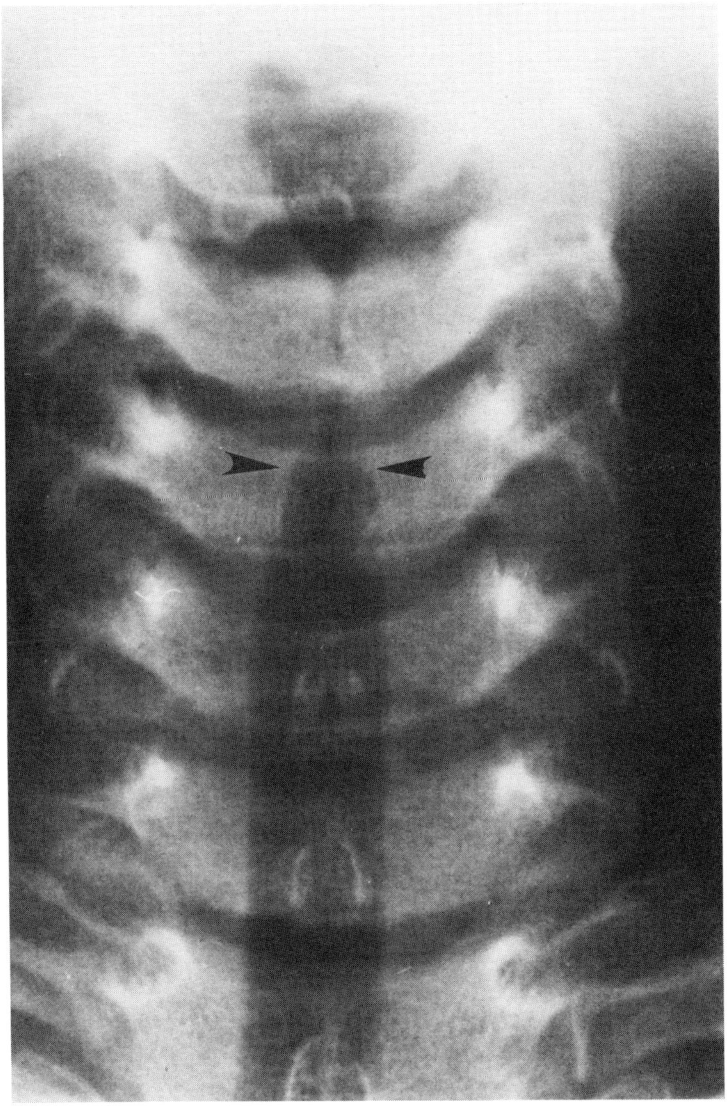

Figure 1B. AP view of the neck during a Valsalva maneuver. The vocal cords are adducted, air is displaced from the glottic region and the superior lateral margins of the subglottic portion of the airway are smoothly rounded and resemble "shoulders" (arrowheads). The subglottic area should never be tapered or asymmetrical.

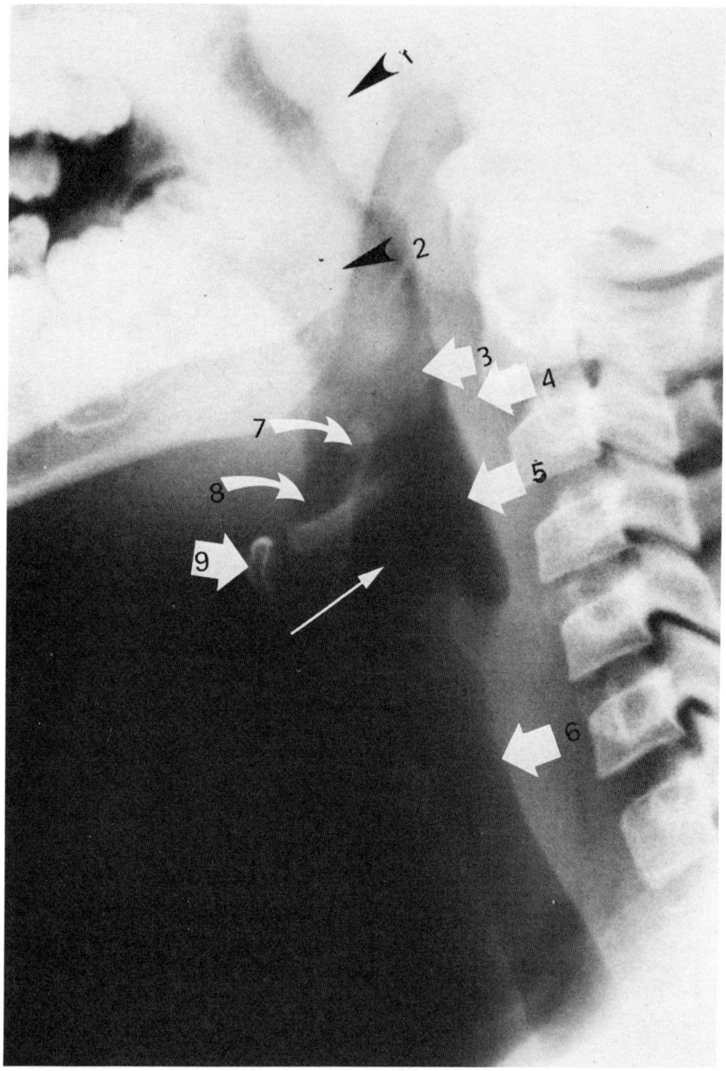

Figure 2. Lateral view of the neck of a normal child made during inspiration and in extension. (1) Nasopharynx containing adenoid tissue; (2) region of the uvula; (3) tonsils; (4) retropharyngeal space; (5) pyriform sinuses; (6) normally radiolucent subglottic portion of the airway; (7) normal thin epiglottis; (8) valleculae; and (9) hyoid bone. The thin white arrow points to thin, normal, ary-epiglottic folds (not well seen).

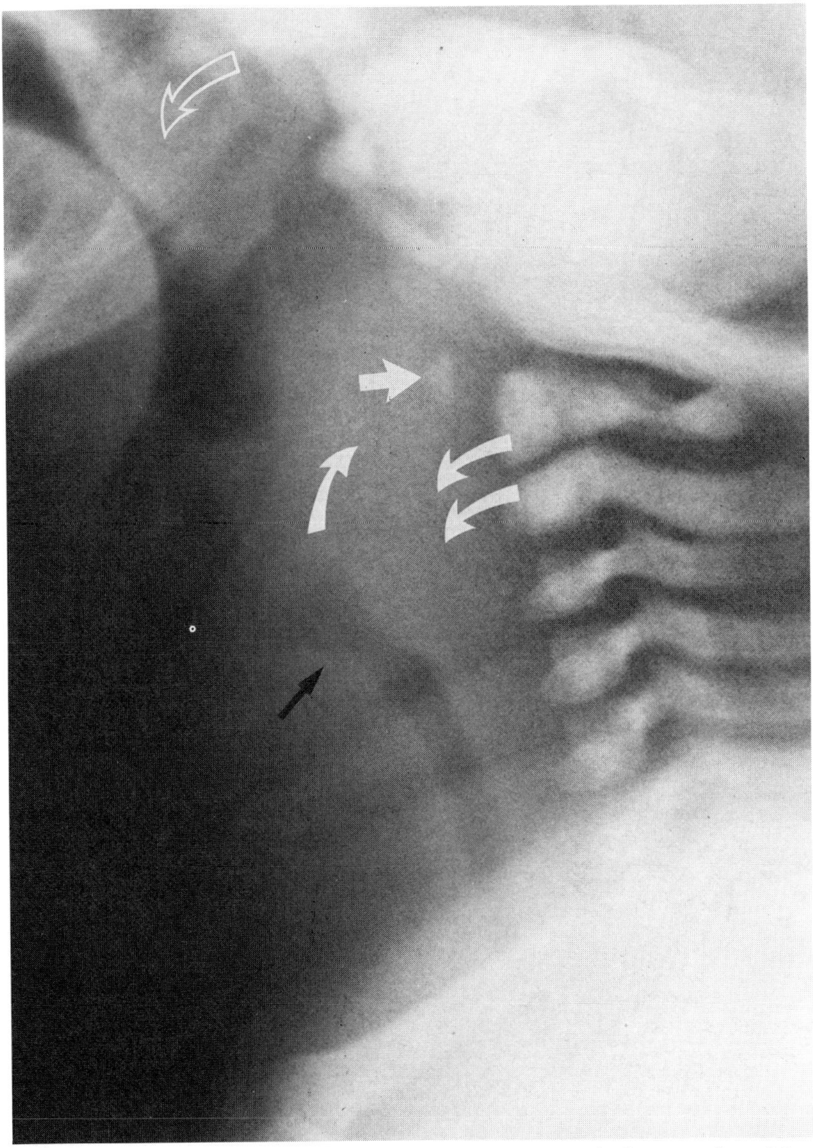

Figure 3A. Lateral view of the neck in a young infant made with the neck in slight flexion and in expiration. The nasopharynx (curved open arrow) is devoid of air. The trachea is buckled forward (black arrow). The retropharyngeal space is enlarged (curved white arrows). These findings suggest a retropharyngeal and nasopharyngeal mass but are due to the film being made during expiration and in flexion. (Compare with Fig. 3B.) The short white arrow points to the anterior arch of C-1.

Illustration continued on the following page

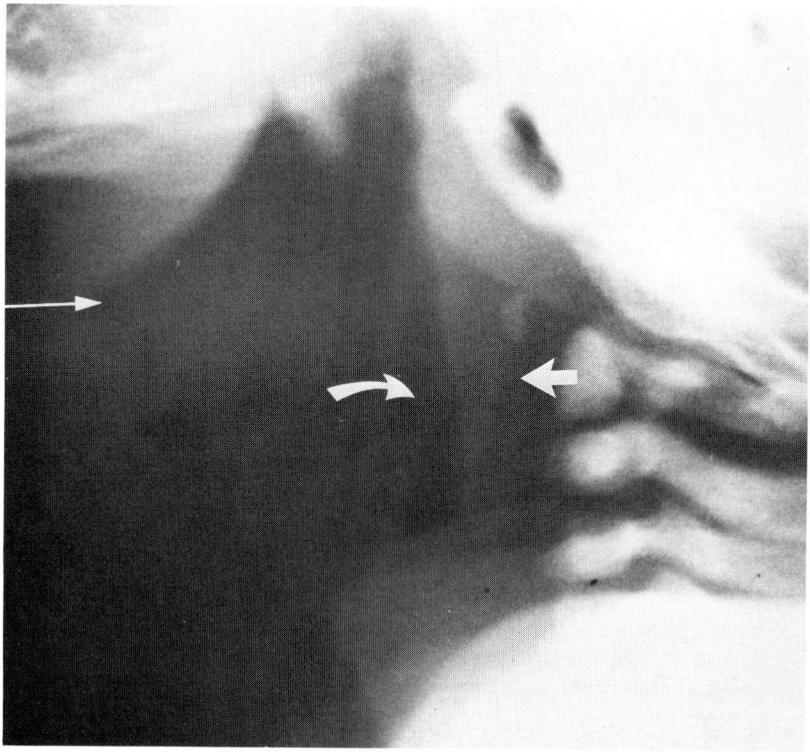

Figure 3B. The same infant as in Figure 3A. A lateral view of the neck made during inspiration and with slight extension. The short straight arrow points to a normal retropharyngeal space without evidence of a mass. The curved white arrow points to the hypopharyngeal airway and pyriform sinus. The long straight arrow points to normal valleculae. The "retropharyngeal mass" seen in Figure 3A disappears on a film made with extension and inspiration. This demonstrates the importance of evaluating the airway in an infant by means of a lateral film of the neck with full inspiration and extension.

can be excluded. Failure of passage of the dye implies atresia (Fig. 4). A recent report[5] illustrates the usefulness of computed tomography in the evaluation of choanal atresia. The site of obstruction, thickness, height and bony nature of the plate were all demonstrated. Such information is undoubtedly useful to the operating surgeon.

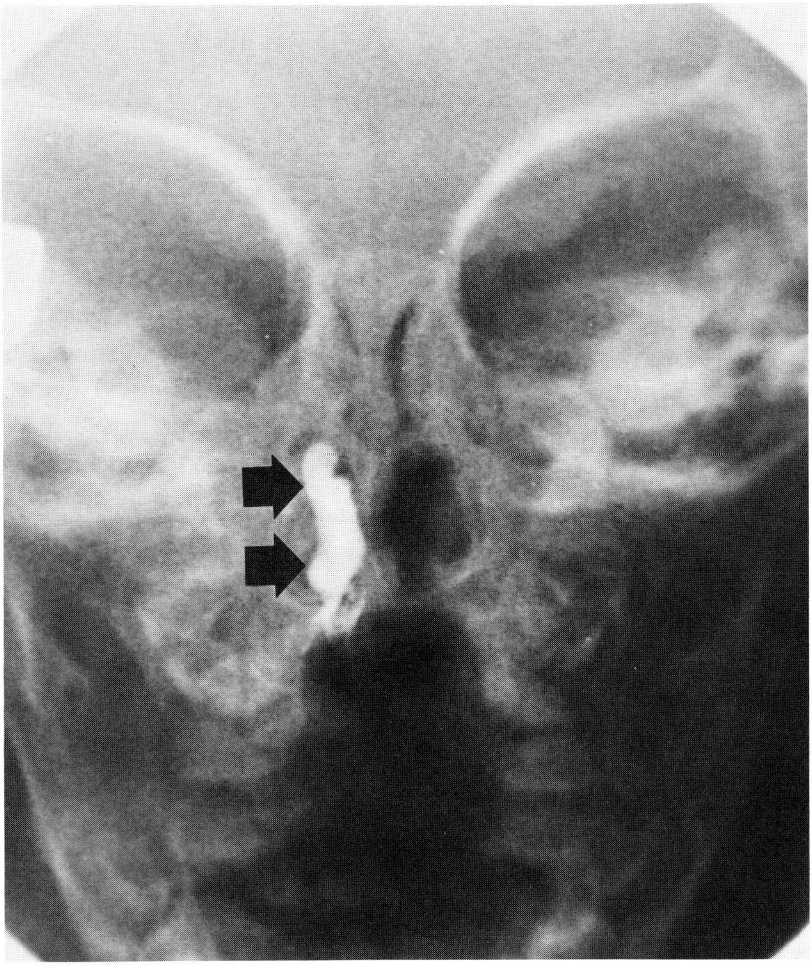

Figure 4. Unilateral choanal atresia in a 3-month-old female. Dye was instilled into the right nostril under fluoroscopic control (arrows) but did not enter the nasopharynx.

Other obstructive lesions of the nasopharynx in children are usually due to masses. These are best demonstrated by a lateral view of the neck and nasopharynx made in extension and inspiration. The most common "mass" in the nasopharynx of a child is normal lymphoid tissue (adenoids). Adenoid tissue is not radiographically demonstrable before one month of age.[6] Between the age of one and six months, two-thirds of children should have visible adenoid tissue and after six months of age, all children should have radiographically demonstrable adenoid tissue.[6] The absence of adenoid tissue after six months of age should lead one to suspect immunologic deficiency.[6] Enlargement of adenoids and tonsils can be seen by two years and can become quite pronounced in childhood, but in the majority of children produces no symptoms. In some children, enlargement of the adenoids and tonsils can lead to chronic respiratory obstruction. Symptoms and signs may be most pronounced during sleep and may include snoring, stertorous respirations, apneas, disturbed nocturnal sleep, somnolence with daytime sleepiness and mouth breathing. Early diagnosis of airway occlusion by hypertrophied lymphoid tissue is important because in some children enlargement of adenoids and tonsils can lead to chronic upper respiratory obstruction, cor pulmonale and pulmonary edema.[7–11] Chronic upper respiratory obstruction can lead to alveolar hypoventilation, resulting in hypoxia, hypercapnia, respiratory acidosis; and in susceptible individuals, hypoxia causes pulmonary arteriolar constriction, pulmonary artery hypertension and right-sided failure.[8–11] The mechanism of the pulmonary edema is not completely elucidated. Other lesions causing chronic upper airway obstruction may also lead to cor pulmonale and pulmonary edema. These include Down's syndrome, Pierre-Robin syndrome, and choanal atresia.[12,13] Massive enlargement of tonsils and adenoids together with prevertebral soft-tissue swelling can occur in infectious mononucleosis, and can lead to severe upper airway obstruction requiring emergency measures to maintain the airway.[14,15] We have seen pulmonary edema, secondary to enlargement of tonsils and adenoids, in a child with infectious mononucleosis. Enlarged obstructing tonsils and adenoids have also been reported to cause or contribute to the sleep-apnea syndrome.[16]

Marked enlargement of tonsils and adenoids with narrowing of the nasopharyngeal air column, can be seen in asymptomatic children. Radiographic examination can only confirm the presence of large adenoids and tonsils and help exclude other causes of upper airway obstruction in symptomatic children (Fig. 5). Chest films may demonstrate cardiac enlargement and possibly pulmonary edema in children with the cardiorespiratory syndrome secondary to upper airway obstruction (Fig. 6). Relief of the upper respiratory obstruction leads to clinical improvement and return of cardiac size to normal.

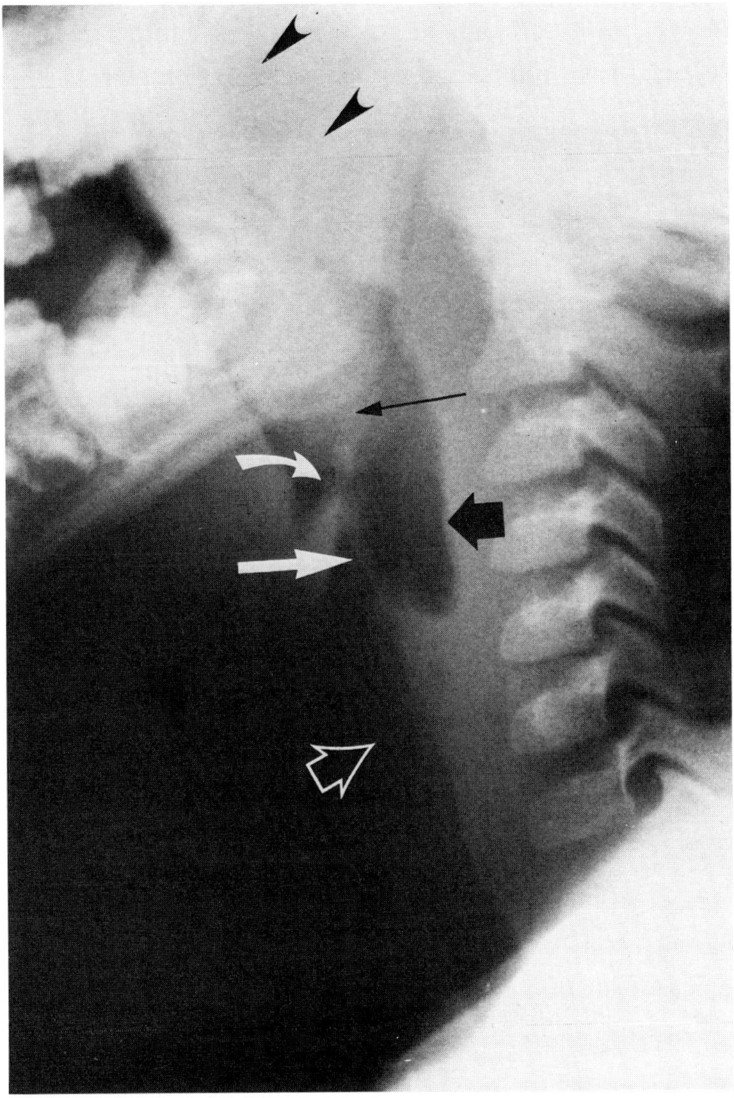

Figure 5. Enlarged Tonsils and Adenoids. A lateral view of the neck in a child with signs of upper respiratory tract obstruction, disturbed sleep and daytime somnolence. The nasopharynx is completely occluded by the adenoids (arrowheads). The tonsils are enlarged (thin black arrow). The pyriform sinus (short black arrow), epiglottis (curved white arrow), aryepiglottic folds (straight white arrow), and subglottic portion of the airway (open arrow) are all normal in appearance.

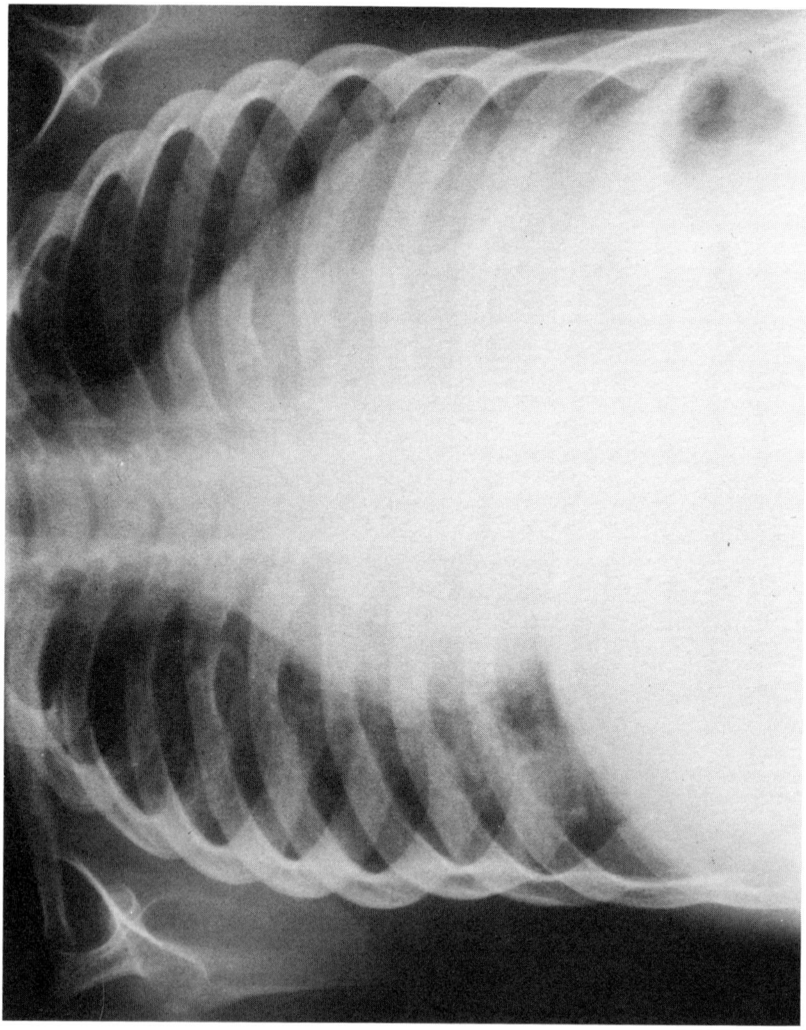

Figure 6. A frontal chest film shows massive cardiomegaly and mild congestive changes. This child, with achondroplasia, developed upper respiratory tract obstruction secondary to a thick tongue, and huge tonsils and adenoids. He was admitted in congestive failure. After tonsillo-adenoidectomy, clinical signs and symptoms disappeared and the heart rapidly became normal in size.

True neoplasms of the nasopharynx may be difficult to distinguish from adenoid tissue radiographically since they may present with respiratory obstruction, and a lateral radiograph may simply demonstrate a nasopharyngeal mass indistinguishable from adenoid tissue. Radiographic demonstration of invasion of adjacent structures such as sinuses and nasal cavity, or destruction of bone are important differential features since normal adenoids do not cause bone destruction. Since there is no adenoid tissue in the nasopharynx of the newborn less than one month of age, a nasopharyngeal mass in the newborn should be regarded as due to encephalocele, hemangioma or other tumor.[6,17] A variety of tumors can occur in the nasopharynx of the older child.

Lymphoma may involve the lymphoid tissue of the nasopharynx and unless there is obvious bone destruction shown on a plain lateral radiograph, one frequently cannot distinguish lymphoma of the nasopharynx from enlarged adenoids (Fig. 7). Rhabdomyosarcoma may involve the nasopharynx but unless there is destruction of adjacent bony structures, demonstration of rapid growth or distant metastases, radiographically it may be difficult to distinguish this tumor from adenoid tissue. Plain tomography and CT scanning are invaluable for the demonstration of invasion of adjacent structures or bony destruction, and frequently may enable the diagnosis of a malignant neoplasm to be made.

The juvenile nasopharyngeal angiofibroma requires special mention because it is a very vascular tumor and biopsy can produce uncontrollable hemorrhage. This may be avoided if the diagnosis from plain films can be suspected. This tumor is usually seen in adolescent males; it may regress after the age of 20–25 years or when sexual maturity is reached.[18] The tumor does not metastasize but can grow and erode the base of the skull and sinuses. Presenting symptoms are usually nasal obstruction, sinus disease and epistaxis which, together with the age and sex, should alert the clinician to the possibility of this lesion.[7] This tumor has a rather typical radiographic appearance on the lateral film, which is of a nasopharyngeal mass producing anterior bowing and displacement of the posterior walls of the maxillary antra, which are normally convex posteriorly[7,18] (Fig. 8—compare with Fig. 7). If this tumor is suspected from plain films, angiography should be done.

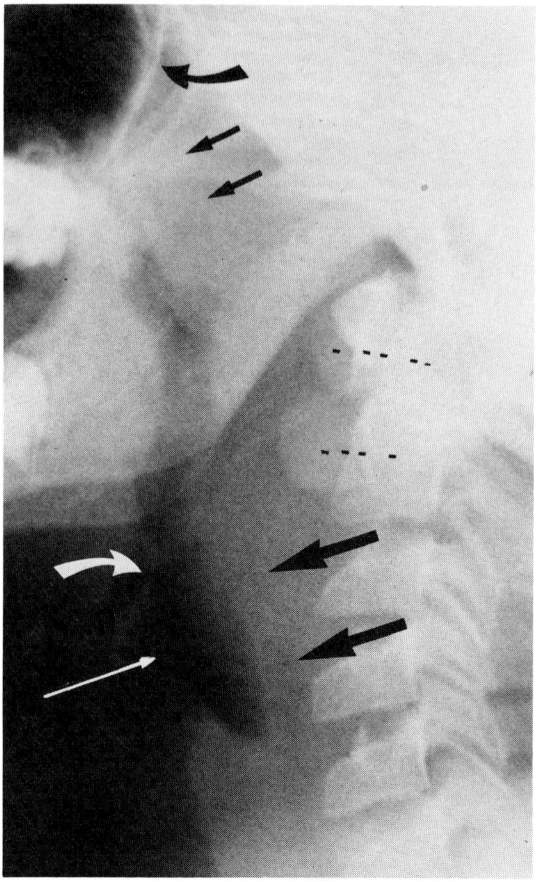

Figure 7. Non-Hodgkin's lymphoma. This child had symptoms and signs of upper respiratory tract obstruction and palpable supraclavicular lymph nodes. The lateral view of the neck shows a nasopharyngeal mass (thin straight black arrows) which cannot be distinguished from adenoid tissue. (Compare with Fig. 5.) There was also a retropharyngeal mass (thick black arrows) compressing the posterior aspect of the pyriform sinuses. The nasopharyngeal and retropharyngeal masses were due to non-Hodgkin's lymphoma. Note the normal posterior walls of the maxillary antra which are convex posteriorly (curved black arrow), a normal thin epiglottis (curved white arrow) and the normal thin aryepiglottic folds (thin white arrow). The rounded densities (dotted lines) are the earlobes.

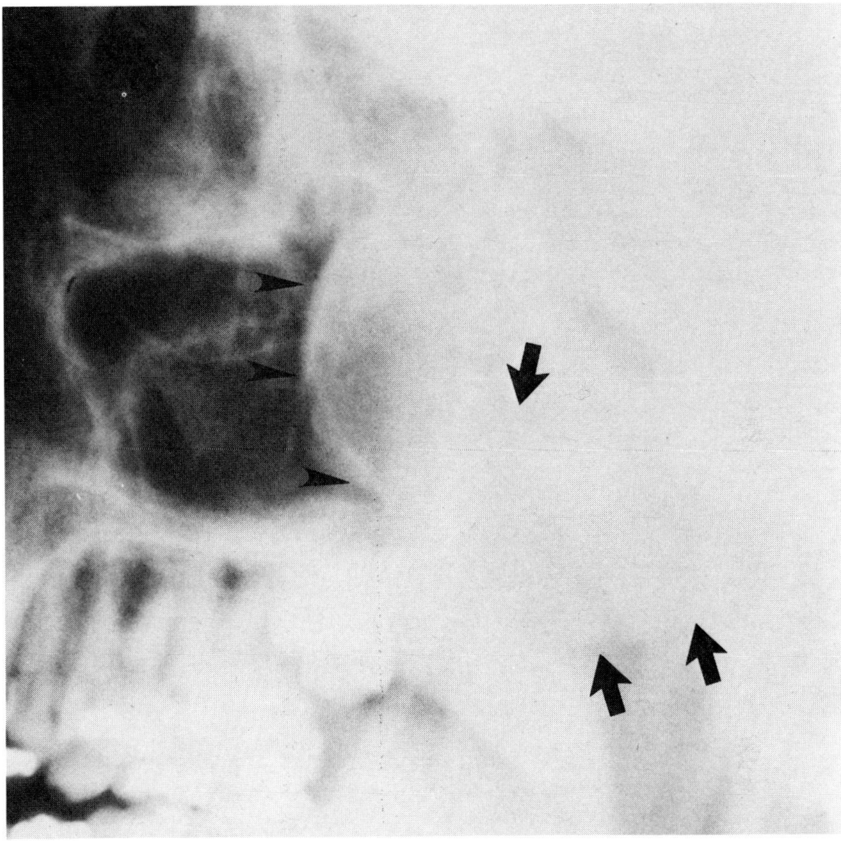

Figure 8. Juvenile nasopharyngeal angiofibroma. A lateral view of the nasopharynx in this prepubertal boy shows a large nasopharyngeal mass (thick black arrows). The anterior extent of the mass is shown by anterior bowing of the posterior walls of the maxillary antra (black arrowheads). (Compare with Fig. 7.) These findings are rather specific for juvenile nasopharyngeal angiofibroma and taken in the context of the child's age and sex, and the presenting clinical symptomatology of upper respiratory tract obstruction and epistaxis, should enable the diagnosis of juvenile nasopharyngeal angiofibroma to be made from the lateral film of the nasopharynx. It is important to recognize this tumor to avoid biopsy and uncontrollable bleeding.

Oral Cavity and Pharynx

Macroglossia can produce respiratory distress and can be seen with hypothyroidism, Beckwith-Wiedemann syndrome and infiltration of the tongue by cystic hygroma.[19] Micrognathia with displacement of the mandible and tongue posteriorly into the pharynx can produce severe respiratory distress as seen in Pierre-Robin syndrome.[7,19,20] While these diagnoses can be made clinically, a lateral radiograph can demonstrate the degree of obstruction and exclude other causes.

Enlargement of the uvula, secondary to angioneurotic edema[19] or tumor can produce respiratory obstruction; enlargement of the uvula can be demonstrated radiologically (Fig. 9A and 9B). Thyroglossal cysts and ectopic thyroid at the base of the tongue can produce severe respiratory distress and difficulty in swallowing as they enlarge.[19–21] These lesions can be recognized on a lateral radiograph as a mass at the base of the tongue filling the valleculae and displacing the epiglottis.[20,21]

Retropharyngeal Space

Lesions of the retropharyngeal space by virtue of their size can produce airway obstruction secondary to displacement and compression of the airways. Their recognition depends upon demonstration of increased thickness of the retropharyngeal space, shown on a lateral film of the neck and nasopharynx made in inspiration and extension. In the infant and neonate, the prevertebral soft tissue space above the larynx can be up to one and one-half times the width of the neighboring cervical vertebral bodies, while in the older child, this distance is seldom more than 3 mm.[19] The prevertebral soft tissue thickness measured at about the level of the larynx may be twice the thickness of the retropharyngeal soft tissues because the esophagus separates from the airway at the level of the larynx.[19] Lesions which can produce enlargement of the retropharyngeal space include tumors such as cystic hygroma (the most common), retropharyngeal goiter, neurogenic tumors, prevertebral soft tissue swelling due to significant cervical spine injury, hypothyroidism, inflammation and abscess formation.[7,19,22] Of these, enlarging tumors and abscesses can produce displacement and distortion of the airways and lead to respiratory distress. Retropharyngeal abscess usually results from suppuration of retropharyngeal lymph nodes secondary to infection of the nasopharynx, although occasionally trauma from a foreign object is the cause. The clinical course may include fever, stiff neck, dysphagia and possibly signs of upper respiratory obstruction following an upper respiratory tract infection in a child usually four years old or younger.[7,19,23] A lateral film of the neck may show retropharyngeal soft tissue thickening, possibly with air bubbles within an abscess cavity, and displacement of the airway[7,19,23] (Figs. 10A and 10B). Not all abscesses or tumors will be so obvious, however, and fluoroscopy with barium swallow may be necessary to show that the retropharyngeal space is thickened due to an actual lesion rather than to an artefact of the examination.

Larynx

Many lesions of the larynx can produce respiratory distress because of respiratory obstruction.

Vocal cord paralysis may be unilateral or bilateral, complete or incomplete and can cause stridor and severe respiratory distress. Cord movement can be detected at fluoroscopy[20,24] and shown on films. (See Figs. 1A and 1B.)

Laryngomalacia is the most common cause of stridor in the neonate and is worse when the infant is breathing quietly. It is said that laryngomalacia can be diagnosed at fluoroscopy as the supraglottic structures (epiglottis and aryepiglottic folds) collapse into the laryngeal lumen.[19,20]

Respiratory papillomas may cause obstructive symptoms and frequently can be seen as soft tissue masses on airway films. If the lesion seeds the respiratory tract, lung infiltrates and masses sometimes with cavitation, can be seen and death can result from respiratory failure.[19,23]

Subglottic hemangioma produces symptoms early in life and is accompanied by intermittent obstruction. The usual radiographic finding is an eccentric mass or deformity of the subglottic airway.[19] Many of these children have cutaneous hemangiomas which can be a clue to the diagnosis.

Aryepiglottic cysts may be seen radiologically as a mass density frequently deforming the aryepiglottic fold and producing respi-

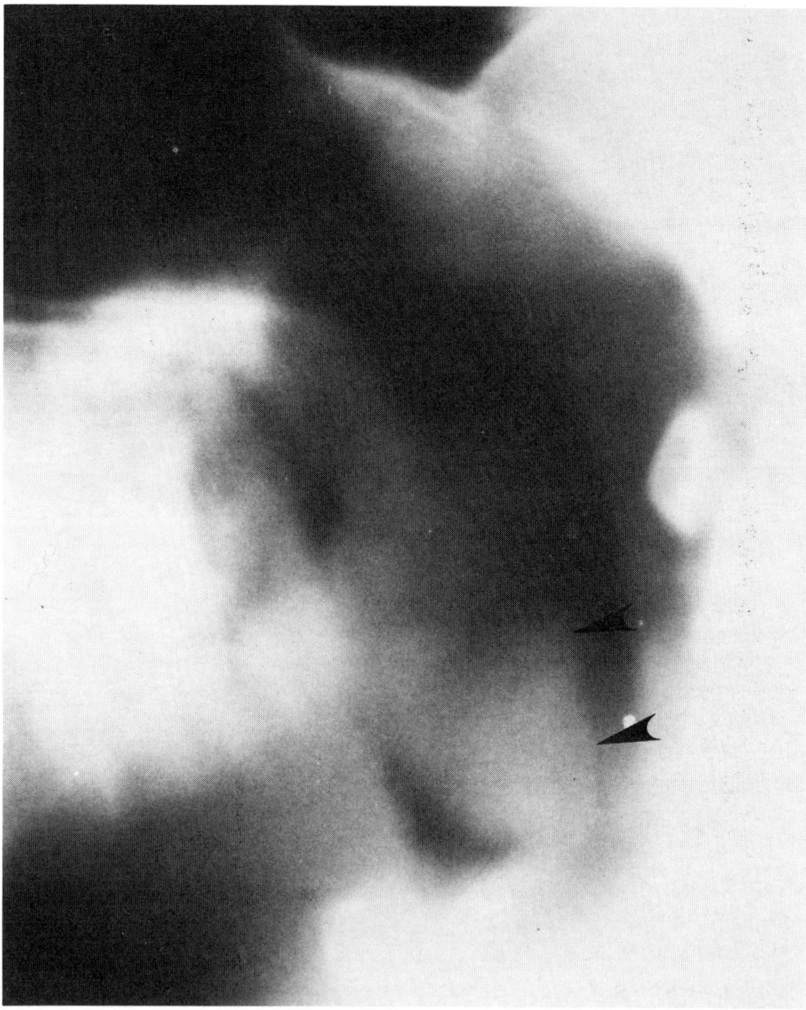

Figure 9A. Rhabdomyosarcoma of the uvula (black arrowheads). This child had increasing upper respiratory tract obstruction. The mass involving the uvula is shown on a lateral tomogram of the oropharynx. (See also Fig. 9B.)

Illustration continued on the opposite page

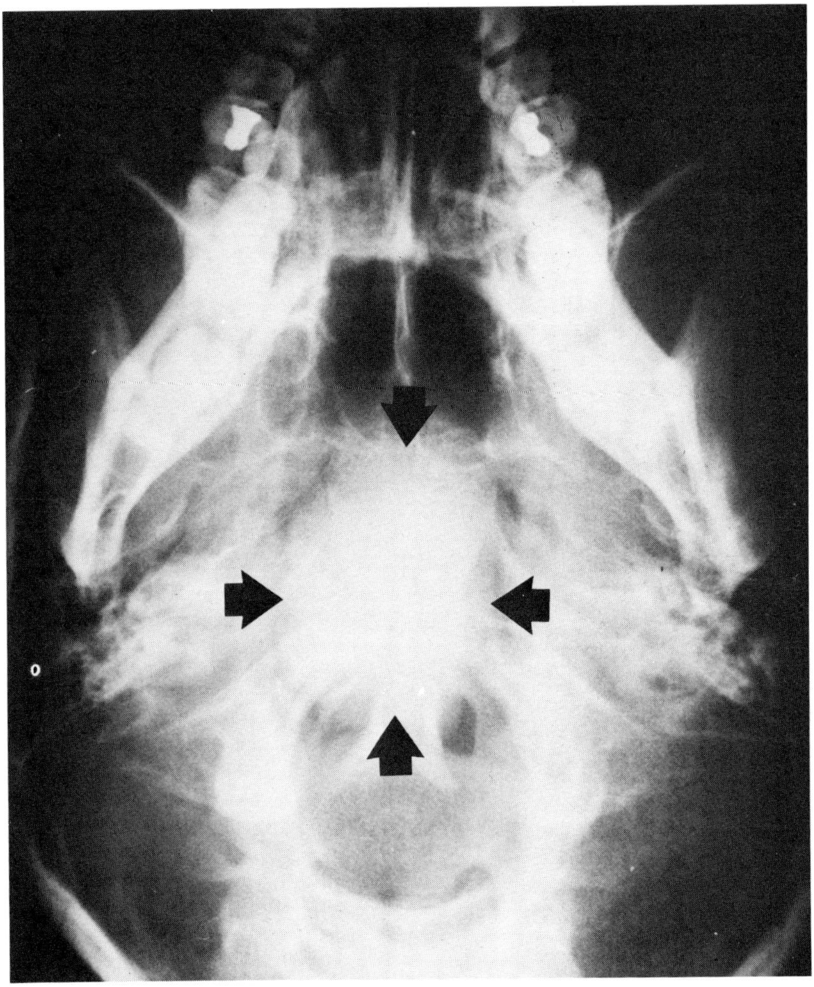

Figure 9B. The rhabdomyosarcoma (black arrows) is shown as a mass on a submentovertical film of the skull. Normally the uvula is much smaller than this enormous tumor.

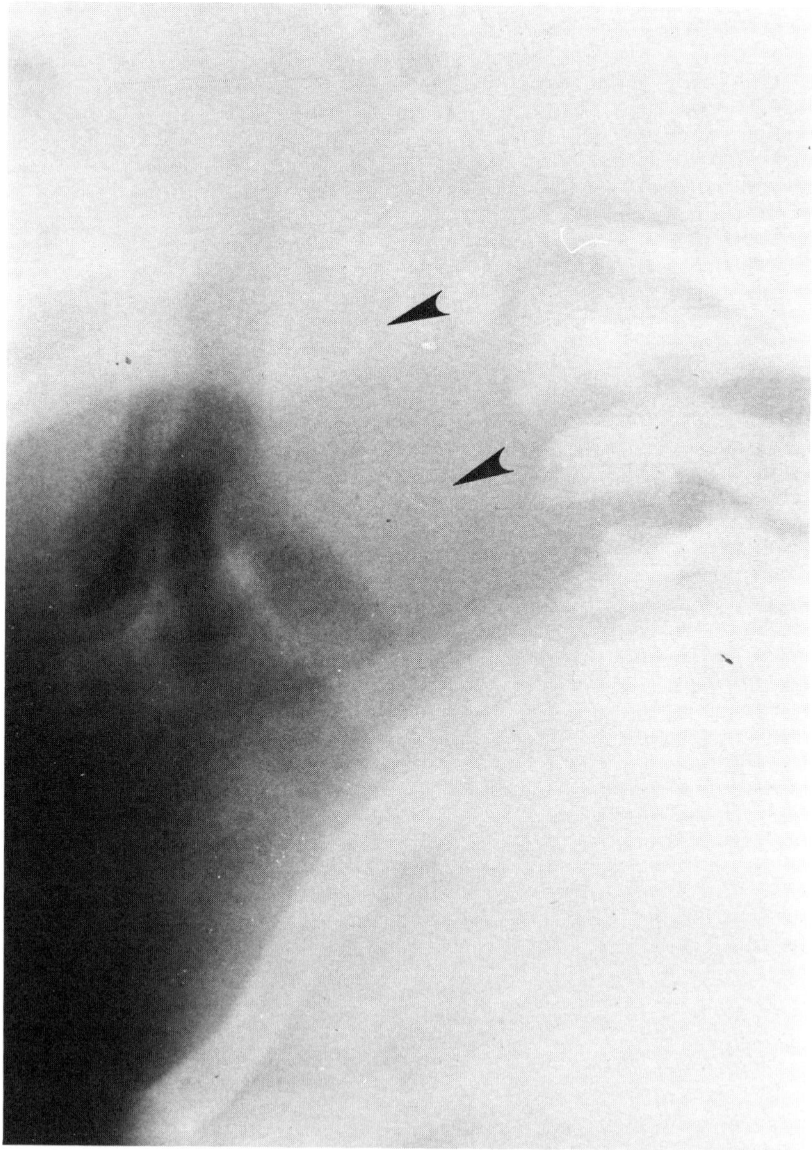

Figure 10A. A retropharyngeal mass (black arrowheads) is suspected on a flexion lateral view of the neck. There is compression of the posterior aspect of the pharyngeal air column. (See also Fig. 10B.)

Illustration continued on the opposite page

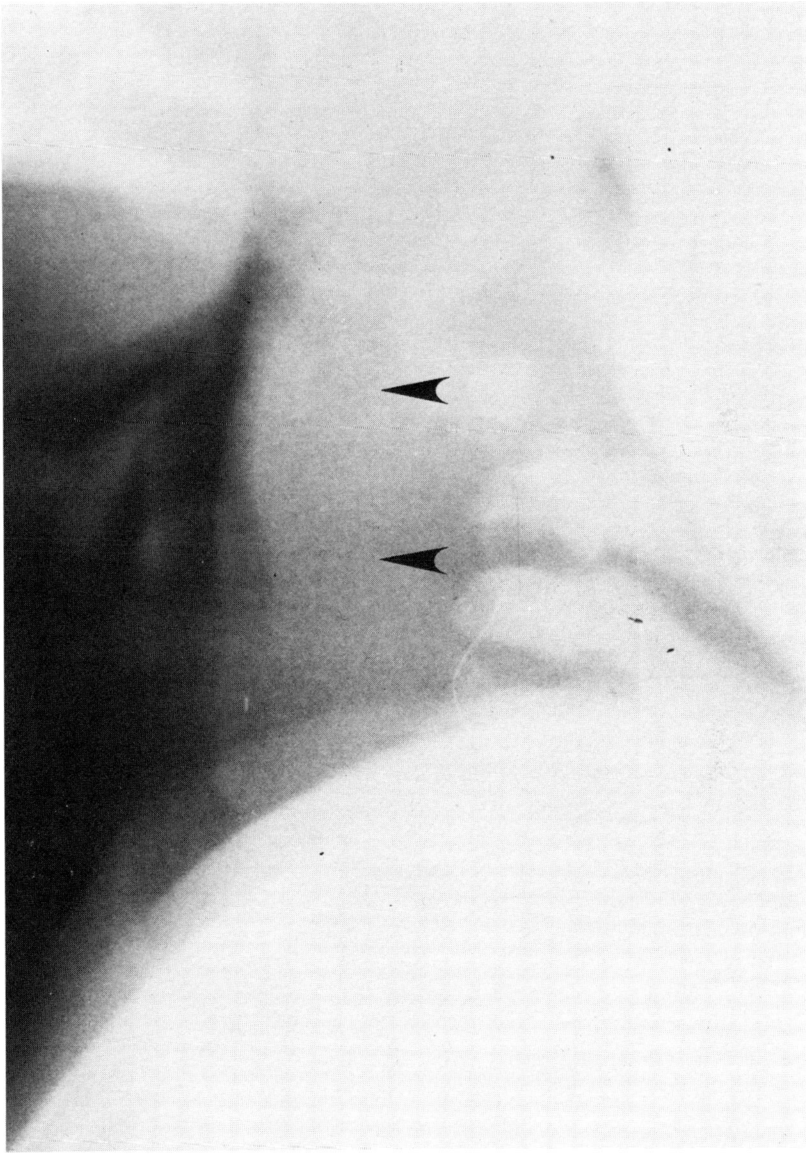

Figure 10B. A lateral view of the neck in extension, (the same child as in Fig. 10A) demonstrates that the retropharyngeal thickening is constant (black arrowheads). This was a retropharyngeal abscess in a 7-month-old child who had symptoms which included those of upper respiratory tract obstruction.

ratory distress.[20] The appearance may not be pathognomonic as other lesions may involve the aryepiglottic fold area.

Subglottic stenosis may be congenital or may occur secondary to intubation. The radiographic findings are similar to those seen in croup and will be discussed under that heading.

Croup

Croup is a common cause of upper respiratory obstruction, usually affecting children six months to three years of age and is of a viral etiology. Symptoms include barking cough, stridor (sometimes biphasic) and soft tissue retractions. The glottis and subglottic portion of the airway are the most severely involved. The usual radiologic evaluation consists of AP and lateral views of the neck and nasopharynx, in inspiration. The radiographic findings are best appreciated on an AP view of the neck. The lateral view is useful to exclude other causes of airway obstruction such as foreign body and epiglottitis. On the AP view in inspiration, one sees slit-like funnel-shaped narrowing of the subglottic and glottic portions of the airway. The slit-like lumen at the glottic level is due to edema and spasm of the vocal cords. The subglottic narrowing is due partly to edema and partly to paradoxical narrowing of this portion of the airway during inspiration.

During inspiration with glottic obstruction, the intraluminal subglottic tracheal pressure is reduced allowing the trachea to collapse and narrow. With expiration the subglottic narrowing may become less. This is an important differential point with subglottic stenosis since the radiographic appearance of subglottic stenosis can mimic croup except that with subglottic stenosis, the subglottic narrowing tends to be fixed and does not disappear on expiration.[19,20,23,25] A lateral view may show hypopharyngeal overdistension, subglottic narrowing, perhaps indistinct vocal cords and an unusually dense subglottic portion of the airway[23,25] (Figs. 11A, 11B and 11C).

Acute Epiglottitis (Supraglottitis)

Acute epiglottitis is an inflammatory lesion affecting the entire supraglottic portion of the larynx (false cords, arytenoid cartilages,

Text continued on page 200

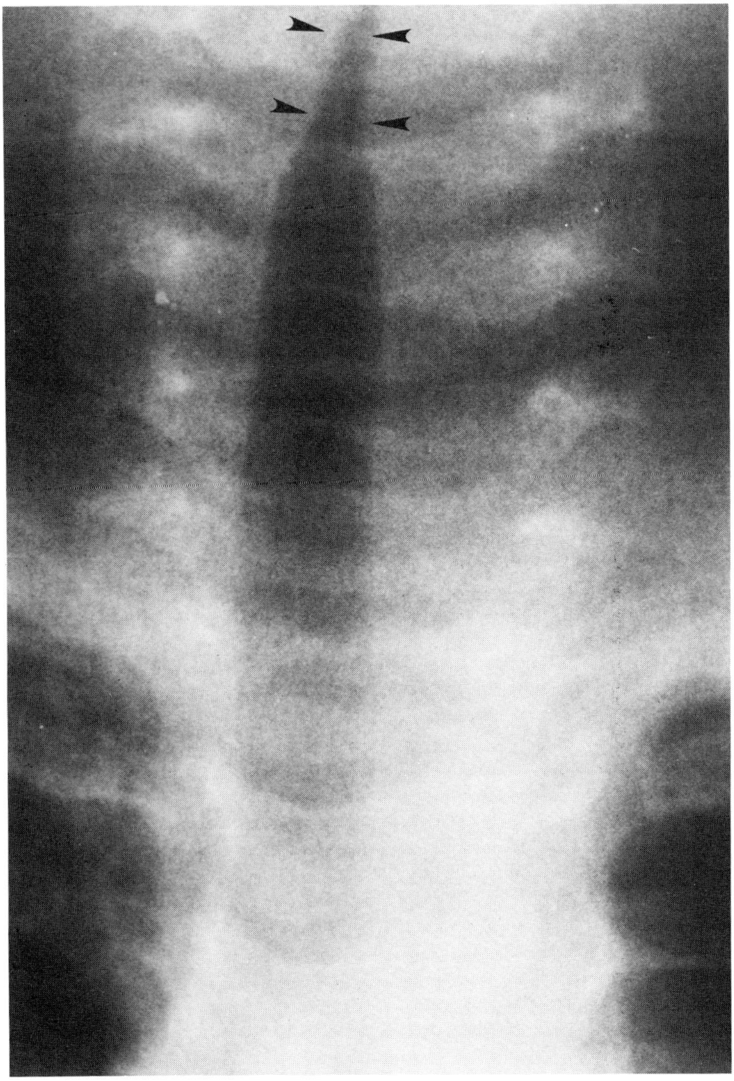

Figure 11A. Croup. This is an AP view of the neck during inspiration in a 14-month-old female with inspiratory stridor. There is moderate, funnel-shaped narrowing of the subglottic and glottic portions of the airway (black arrowheads). In inspiration, with the cords abducted, the airway should be wide open and never tapered as in this instance. (Compare with Fig. 1A.)

Illustration continued on the following page

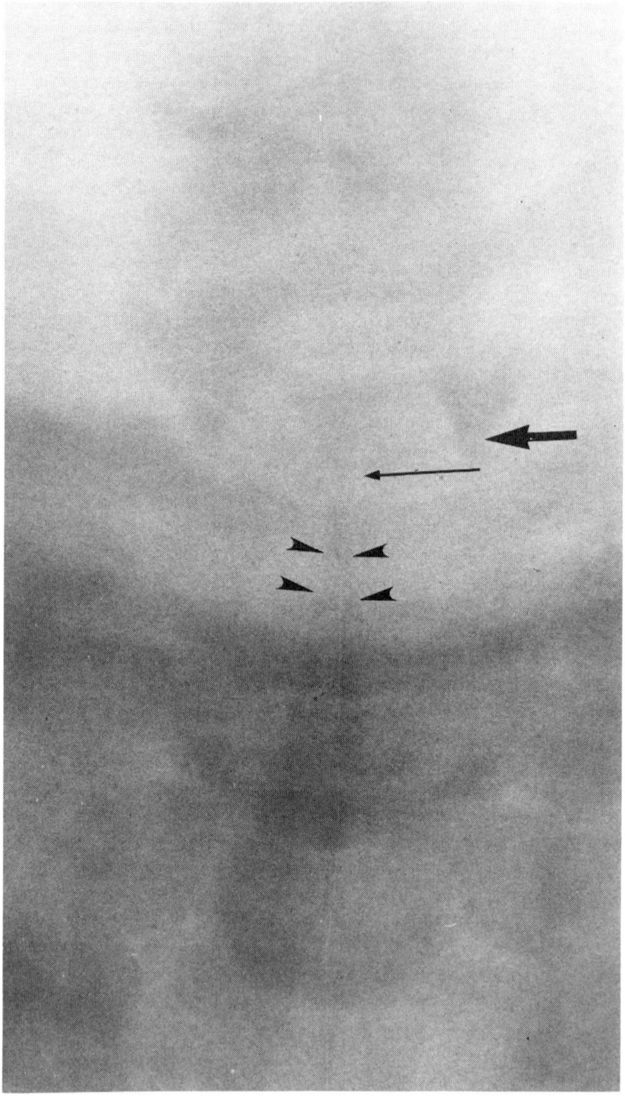

Figure 11B. Croup. This is a 5-month-old female with inspiratory stridor. There is marked funnel-shaped narrowing of the subglottic portion of the airway (black arrowheads) and of the glottic region (long black arrow). There is distension of the hypopharynx. The tip of the pyriform sinus (thick black arrow) is at the level of the glottis. This marked glottic and subglottic narrowing should never be seen during inspiration. (Compare with Figs. 11A and 1A.)

Illustration continued on the opposite page

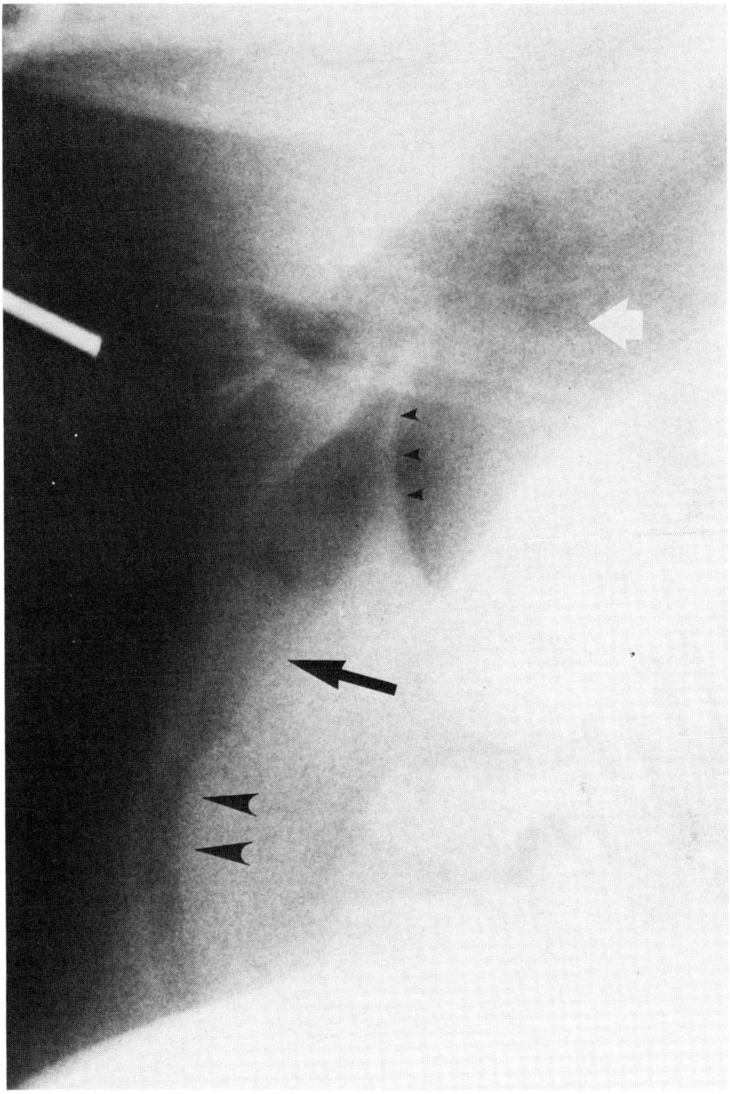

Figure 11C. Croup. The lateral view of the neck in inspiration demonstrates hypopharyngeal distension (white arrow), subglottic tracheal narrowing (large black arrowheads) and an unusually dense appearance of the subglottic portion of the airway (thick black arrow). (Compare with Fig. 2.) Normal thin aryepiglottic folds are shown (small black arrowheads). The subglottic density is due to edema, while the subglottic narrowing of the trachea is probably due to negative intraluminal pressure secondary to the paraglottic obstruction. This film enables one to exclude radiopaque foreign body and epiglottitis as a cause of inspiratory stridor.

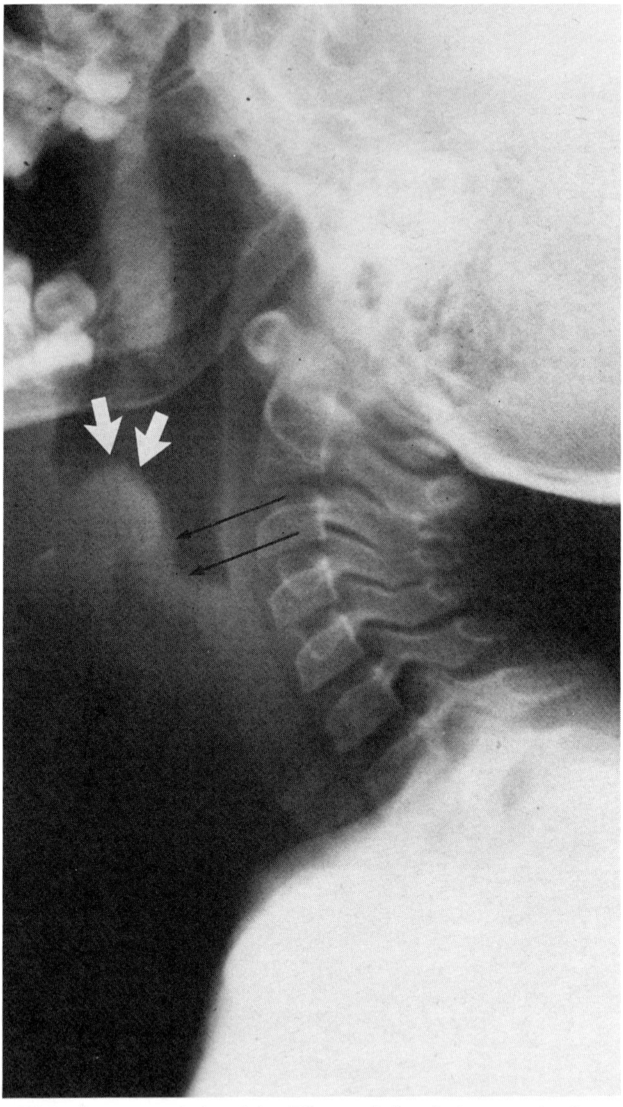

Figure 12A. Acute epiglottitis. The epiglottis is massively enlarged and resembles a mass (white arrows). The aryepiglottic folds (black arrows) are very thick. (Compare with Figs. 2, 5, 7, and 11C.) This is the rather typical appearance of acute epiglottitis. The aryepiglottic folds are invariably involved and may be thicker than the epiglottis. (See Fig. 12B.) Note the deficiency of adenoid tissue. This was a 6-year-old girl with repeated infections due to immunologic deficiency. Absence of adenoid tissue after 6 months of age should alert the physician to the possibility of immunologic deficiency.

Illustration continued on the opposite page

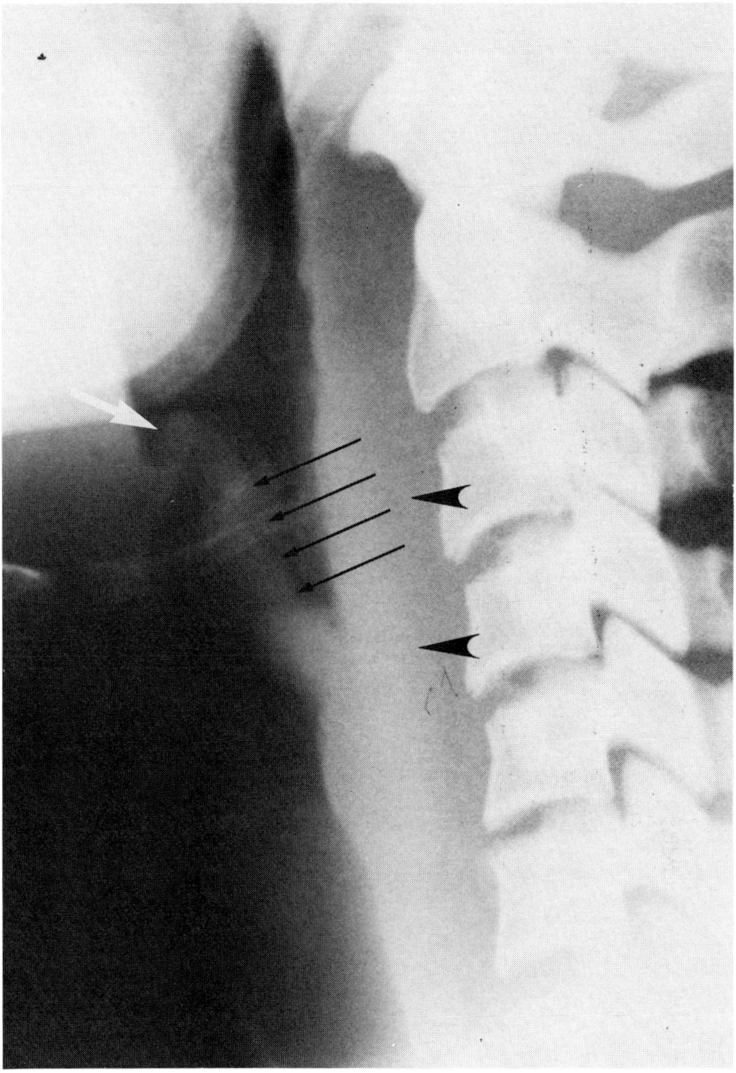

Figure 12B. Acute epiglottitis. The epiglottis (white arrow) is not nearly as involved as in Figure 12A. The aryepiglottic folds (thin black arrows) are moderately thickened. The prevertebral space is moderately thickened (black arrowheads), an uncommon finding with acute epiglottitis. This case in a 15-year-old boy points out that the disease can occur at any age and that the aryepiglottic folds can be more extensively involved by the disease than the epiglottis. Note also that the hypopharynx is not usually as distended as it is with croup.

aryepiglottic folds, epiglottis and occasionally pharyngeal walls).[23] It is a life-threatening emergency most commonly affecting children between two and six years of age, but it has been reported in infants and adults as well.[26,27] The offending organism is nearly always Hemophilus influenzae type B. The onset is abrupt and the clinical course is very rapid beginning with fever, sore throat, difficulty swallowing, drooling and progressing to symptoms of respiratory obstruction with inspiratory stridor, muffled voice, restlessness, anxiety, air hunger and cyanosis.[26,27] The child may assume a tripod position with the head in the "sniffing dog" position or sit up and lean forward with wide open mouth, protruding tongue and hyperextended neck.[26,27,28] Early diagnosis and treatment is mandatory, lest death occur. If the diagnosis can be made clinically radiographs are not necessary. If a radiograph is needed to make the diagnosis, radiographic technique in these children must be modified; a single lateral film of the neck made in the position of comfort for the child usually upright is all that is necessary. No attempt shold be made to extend the neck to obtain a film as this may produce total occlusion of the airway by the epiglottis. A child with suspected acute epiglottitis should always be accompanied to the radiology department by a physician or team capable of establishing an emergency airway.

The radiographic appearance of acute epiglottitis on a lateral radiograph of the neck can vary from massive inflammatory edema obliterating all the supraglottic structures to mild to moderate thickening of the epiglottis and aryepiglottic folds[7,19,20,23,25–29] (Fig. 12A). A rather constant finding is thickening of the aryepiglottic folds which may be even more pronounced than the thickening of the epiglottis (Fig. 12B).

The epiglottis may appear enlarged for a number of reasons other than acute infectious epiglottitis. The "omega" epiglottis can present difficulties in diagnosis since it is a normal epiglottis which appears thickened because the lateral flaps turn down more than usual.[25] With the "omega" epiglottis, the aryepiglottic folds are not thickened whereas they are invariably involved in acute epiglottitis. Pathologic enlargement of the epiglottis and aryepiglottic folds has been reported with angioneurotic edema, ingestion of caustic substances and chronic epiglottitis.[7,24,25,30] An enlarged epiglottis and normal aryepiglottic folds have been reported with the presence of a foreign body,[30] and we have seen it secondary to invasion by cystic hygroma (Figs. 13A and 13B). Pathologic entities which produce enlargement of the epiglottis can produce significant respiratory obstruction and may be difficult to differentiate radiologically from acute infectious epiglottitis, especially if the aryepiglottic folds are also thick but clinical differentiation is usually possible. Some patients with acute epiglottitis have been reported to have subglottic airway narrowing on AP neck radiographs, a little known feature of the disease.[24,28,31] The subglottic narrowing has been shown to disappear after therapy.[24]

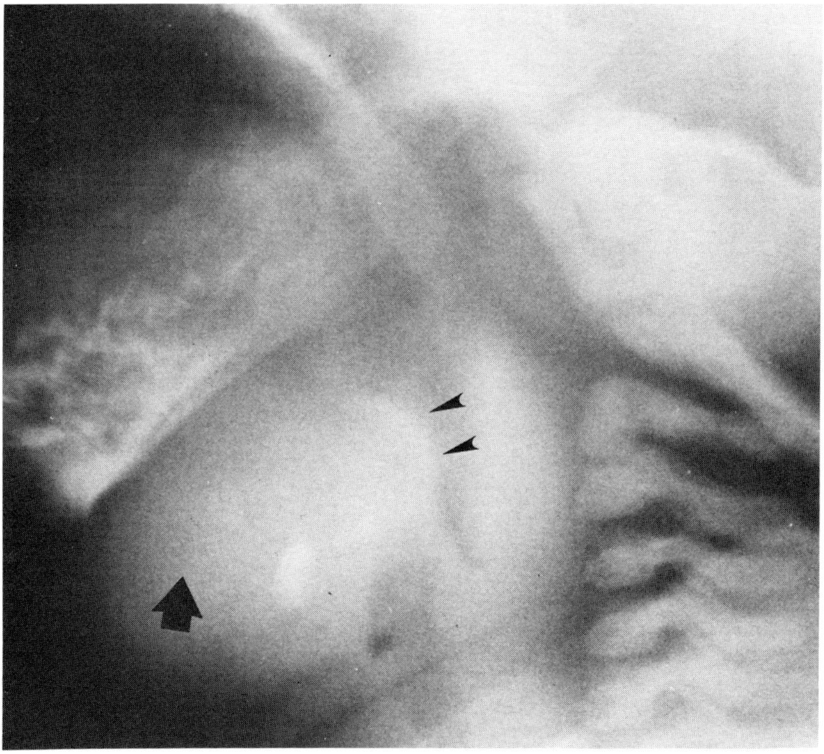

Figure 13A. Cystic hygroma. The lateral film of the neck in a 3-week-old female shows a large submandibular tumor (thick black arrow) which was part of a cystic hygroma. The epiglottis (small black arrowheads) is massively enlarged because of infiltration of the epiglottis by the cystic hygroma. The tongue was also involved in this child.

Illustration continued on the following page

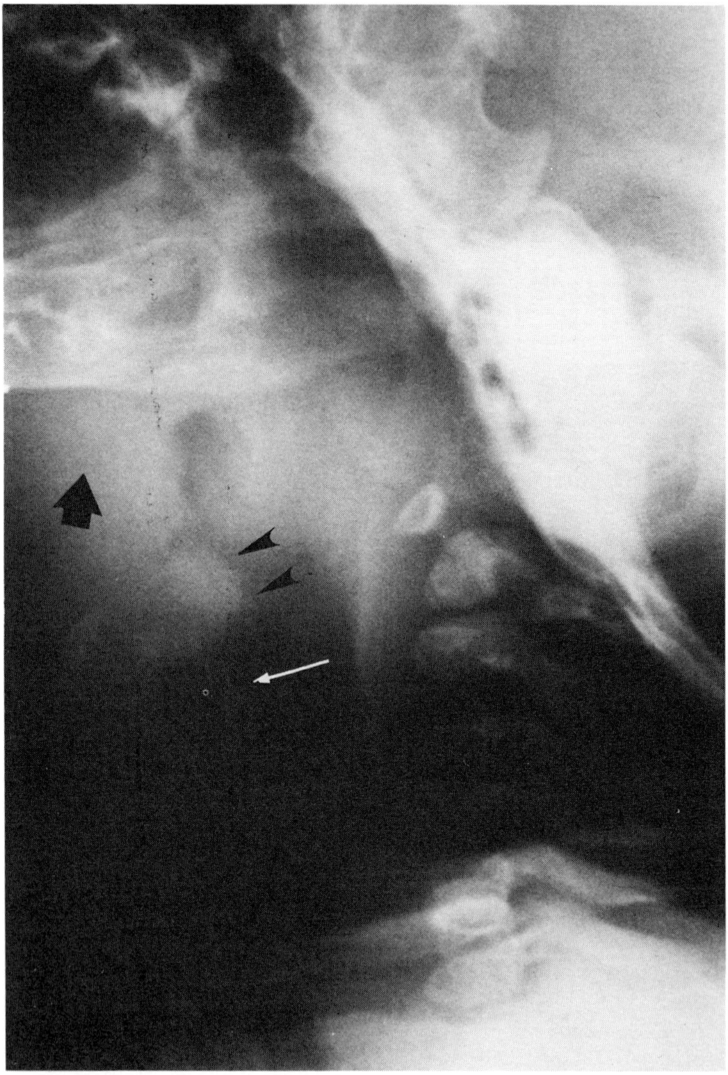

Figure 13B. Cystic hygroma. This was a 3-month-old male with a large submandibular cystic hygroma (thick black arrow) and nodular enlargement of the epiglottis (small black arrowheads) because of infiltration by the cystic hygroma. The neck was also extensively involved. The aryepiglottic folds (white arrow) are normal. The presence of normal aryepiglottic folds, with an enlarged epiglottis, should alert the physician to the possibility of an etiology other than acute infectious epiglottis as the reason for the enlarged epiglottis.

Tumors

Tumors growing adjacent to the airway can by virtue of their enlargement displace and compress the airway, especially the trachea, and produce stridor and respiratory distress. Such tumors may reach a very large size before symptoms of respiratory embarrassment occur and they also frequently displace the esophagus so that dysphagia may be an accompanying feature. Plain films supplemented by barium swallow, magnification high KV special filtration films and CT as needed will ordinarily demonstrate the lesion (Figs. 14 and 15).

Vascular Ring

A true vascular ring encircles and narrows both the trachea and esophagus, and can produce respiratory distress, stridor, wheezing, cyanosis, poor feeding and dysphagia in the infant. The most common types of vascular rings are the double aortic arch, and the complex of right aortic arch, left ligamentum arteriosum and aberrant left subclavian artery.[23,32] The diagnosis of a vascular ring can be suspected from the symptom complex and plain chest films. The trachea normally descends to the right of the midline and in the infant may make a fairly sharp buckle to the right at the thoracic inlet.[33] Any deviation from the right sided trachea is abnormal. A frontal chest film may show the trachea narrowed and displaced toward the left with compression along its right side, which should suggest a right aortic arch. The right sided aortic arch and descending right aorta may be seen as soft tissue structures to the right of the spine. A lateral chest film may show an impression on the anterior surface of the trachea as well as forward bowing of the trachea.[23,32] Confirmation can be obtained by a barium swallow which will demonstrate a large pressure defect on the posterior surface of the esophagus (Figs. 16A, 16B and 16C).

Anomalous Pulmonary Artery (Pulmonary Sling)

This refers to the left pulmonary artery arising from the right pulmonary artery and passing between the trachea and esophagus to the left side. This lesion has been implicated as a cause of respiratory distress with air trapping or collapse in either lung.[32]

Text continued on page 209

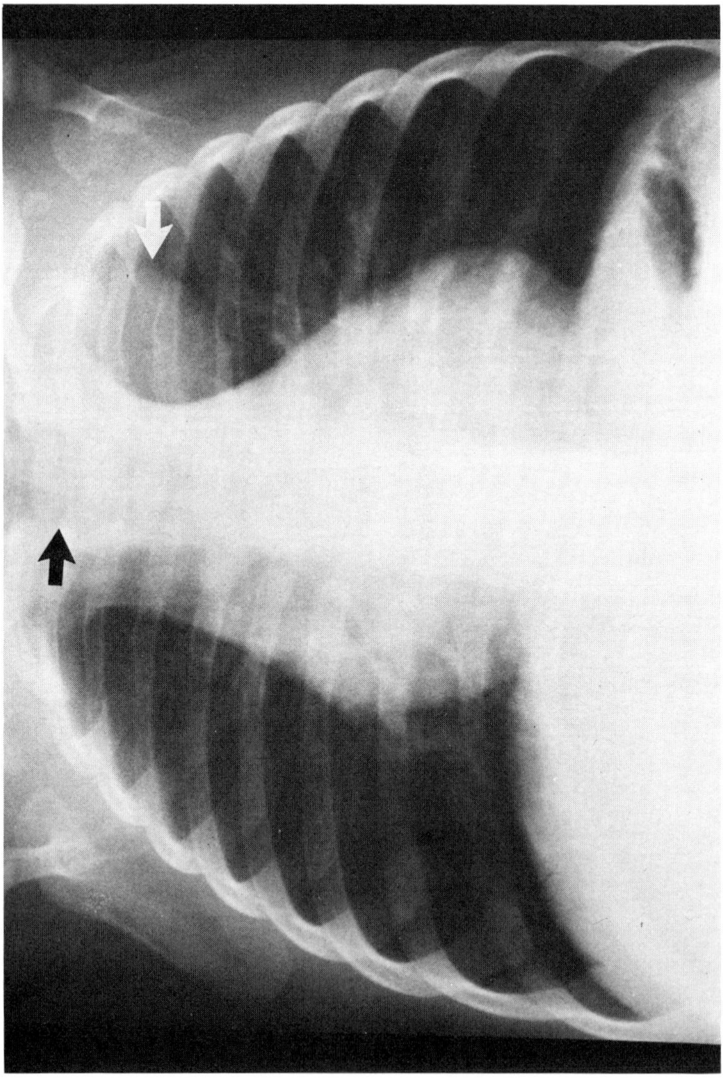

Figure 14. Neuroblastoma. Chest films were obtained because this 9-month-old male, with persistent wheezing, was thought to have asthma. The large mass in the left upper chest (white arrow) was a neuroblastoma producing pressure along the left side of the trachea (black arrow).

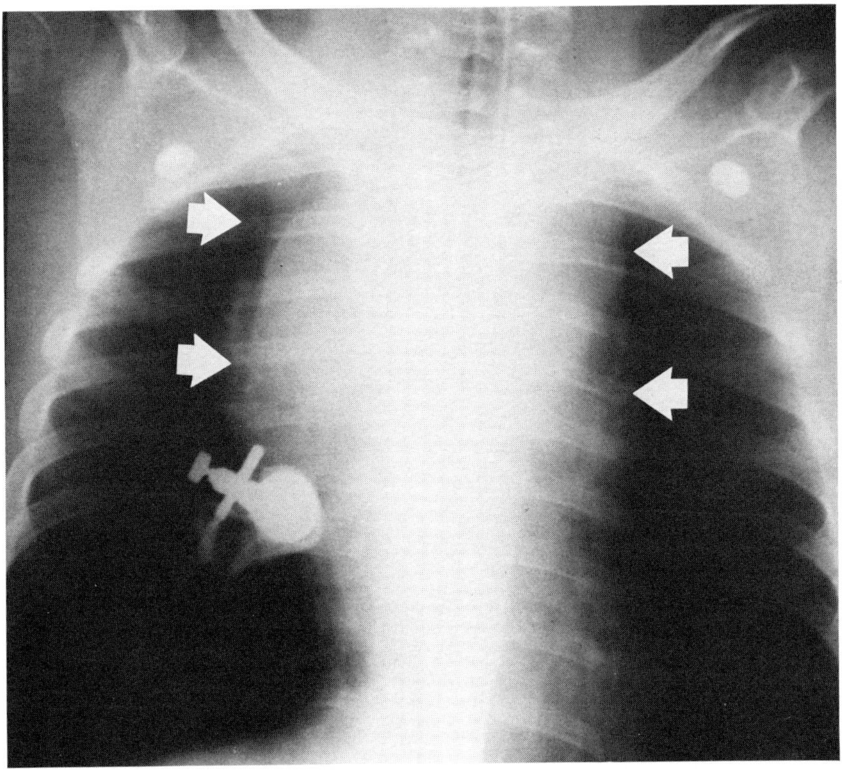

Figure 15. Non-Hodgkin's lymphoma. The frontal chest film of an older child demonstrates a huge mediastinal mass (white arrows) extending up into the neck with displacement of the endotracheal tube to the left. This child was brought to the emergency room in respiratory arrest and was asymptomatic previously. This illustrates the enormous size which a mass can reach before producing significant respiratory tract obstruction. The mass resolved quickly during therapy.

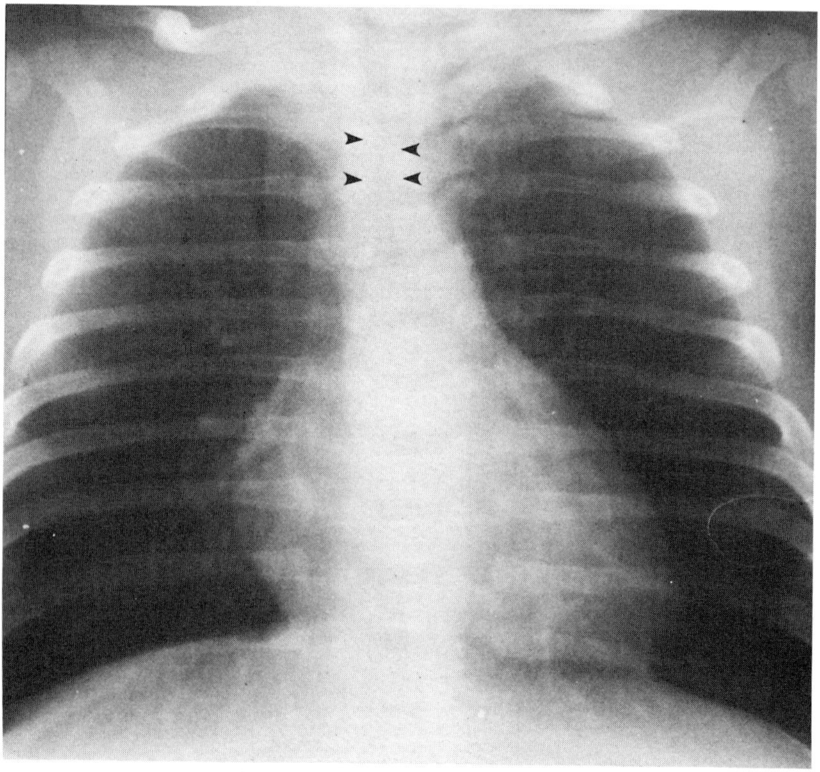

Figure 16A. Vascular ring. This is a frontal chest film of a 3-month-old boy with noisy respiration, respiratory distress, dysphagia, and failure to thrive since birth. This child was very ill at admission. The frontal chest film shows overinflated lungs bilaterally. The trachea (small black arrowheads) is nearly in the midline and irregularly narrowed. Even though a right aortic arch and descending right aorta cannot be seen on this film, probably because of a little rotation, the displacement of the trachea and narrowing should always lead one to suspect a right-sided aorta and a vascular ring.

Illustration continued on the opposite page

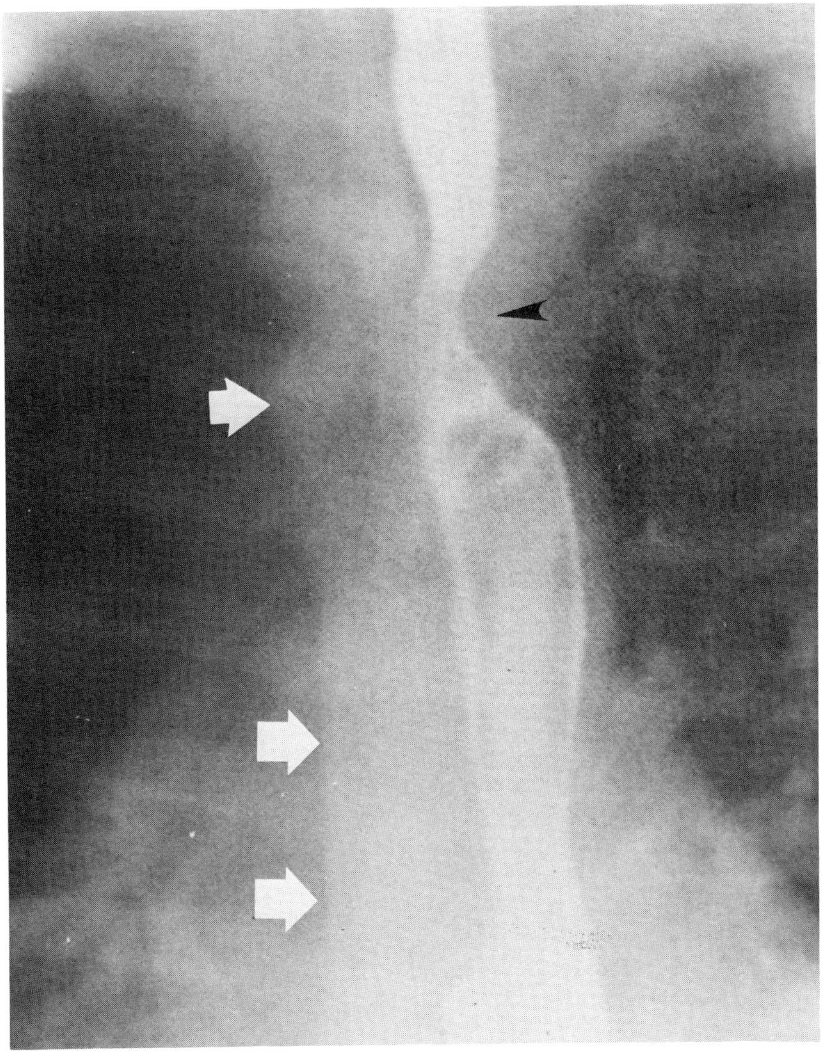

Figure 16B. This is a spot film at fluoroscopy in the AP position during a barium swallow. One can see a right-sided aortic arch and right descending aorta (white arrows). The esophagus is irregularly narrowed (black arrowhead) since it too is encircled by the vascular ring.

Illustration continued on the following page

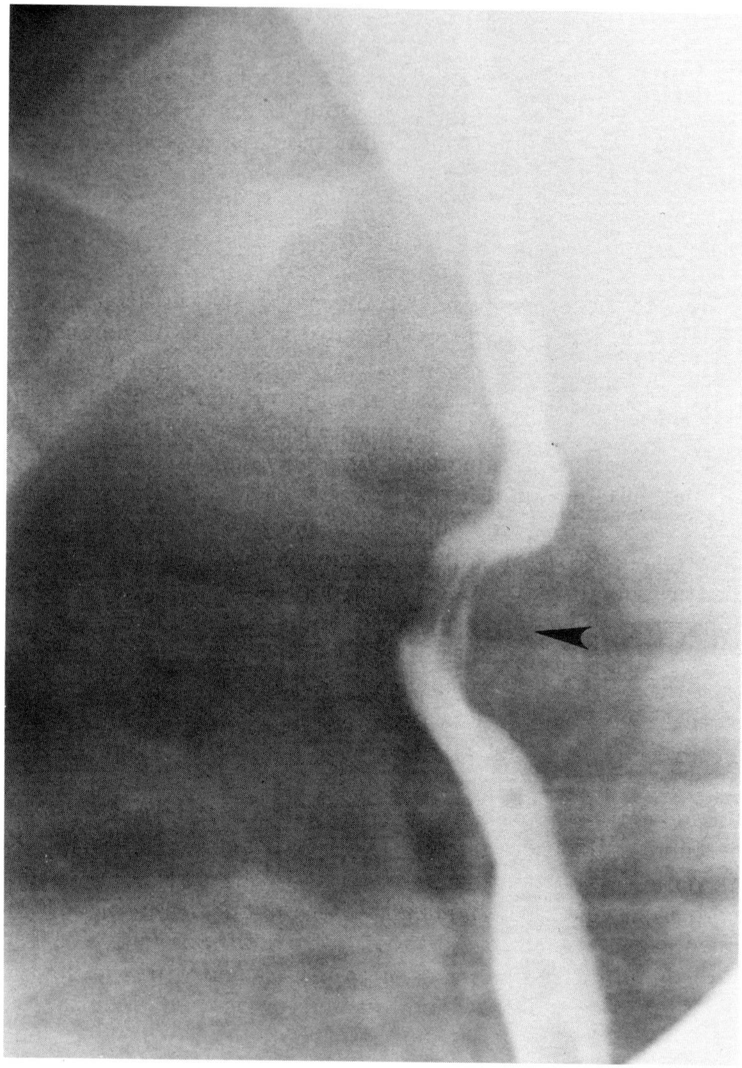

Figure 16C. This is a lateral spot film from the barium swallow. There is a large posterior impression upon the esophagus with narrowing (black arrowhead) typical for an encircling vascular ring. At surgery, a double aortic arch was found. The displacement and narrowing of the trachea and compression and narrowing of the esophagus account for the combination of respiratory distress and dysphagia. A trachea which does not descend to the right of the midline is abnormal and should lead one to suspect a mass displacing the trachea or more commonly, a right-sided aortic arch. Barium swallow can then be done to confirm the diagnosis of a vascular ring.

There have been reported, however, associated stenoses of the trachea and major bronchi in areas other than those of the anomalous vessel so that the replacement of the left pulmonary artery may not relieve the obstructive airway abnormality.[23] Evaluation of such a lesion can be done with a barium swallow. Since the anomalous vessel passes between the trachea and the esophagus above the carina, it will produce an indentation on the posterior surface of the trachea and on the anterior surface of the esophagus with separation of these structures.

Trauma

A fracture of the larynx usually results from direct trauma to the neck resulting in compression of the larynx between the object and the cervical spine.[34] Clinically, there may be dysphonia and pain on deglutition and radiographically, subcutaneous emphysema may be seen.[34] Since the pediatric airway is cartilaginous and relatively pliable up until the age of approximately 20 years, laryngeal fracture is rarely seen in children. Cervical subcutaneous emphysema, therefore, should prompt evaluation of the esophagus and chest for other injuries.

Fractures of the face can compromise the airway because of obstruction by blood, secretions or soft tissues. CNS injuries may also be accompanied by airway compromise either due to obstructing soft tissue or central depression of respiration. The role of radiology in these instances is to determine grossly the extent of skeletal injury and evaluate the intracranial contents as needed.

Foreign Bodies

Respiratory symptoms can occur either from aspirated or ingested foreign bodies. Aspirated foreign bodies remain a serious cause of morbidity and mortality in young children. Clinical findings depend upon the site of impaction and the size of the foreign body. Initially, aspiration may be followed by coughing, perhaps gagging and vomiting and varying degrees of respiratory distress. With partial obstruction of the larynx at the glottis, one may see inspiratory stridor and soft tissue retractions. If the foreign body impacts in the distal trachea, signs and symptoms may be those of both upper and lower tract obstruction, that is, inspiratory stridor, soft tissue retractions and wheezing.[20] If the foreign body is aspirated distal to the carina into the bronchial tree, the clinical findings will more likely be cough, decreased air entry, wheezing and dyspnea.[35] Radiographic detection of an aspirated foreign body depends on the size and radiopacity of the foreign body. Metallic objects are plainly visible. The majority of aspirated foreign bodies in children are, however, nonradiopaque (food stuff such as peanuts and vegetables) and, therefore, may be visible only as filling defects within the air column.

Radiologic examination should consist of AP and lateral views of the neck and nasopharynx, frontal views of the chest in inspiration and expiration, a lateral view of the chest and occasionally a film of the abdomen. Magnification, high KV, special filtration films are useful to supplement conventional films for detection of airway foreign bodies, particularly of the larynx and trachea.[3] If the foreign body cannot be directly visualized by film technique, its presence may be inferred by its impact on respiratory dynamics, as seen at fluoroscopy.

Hypopharyngeal Foreign Bodies

If these foreign bodies are of sufficient size, they can produce significant occlusion of the hypopharyngeal airway, altough if they do not they may be clinically silent after the initial coughing episode[36] (Fig. 17).

Laryngo-Tracheal Foreign Bodies

Fortunately, laryngo-tracheal foreign bodies are a relatively small percentage of the cases of aspirated foreign bodies in childhood since they are associated with a greater morbidity and mortality than endobronchial foreign bodies and are difficult to diagnose radiologically if they are not radiopaque. Such foreign bodies may present with severe respiratory distress and can result in death if they produce total occlusion of the laryngo-tracheal airway.[36] One may resort to fluoroscopy if laryngo-tracheal foreign bodies cannot be seen on radiographs. A partially obstructing foreign body in the larynx or trachea may cause exaggeration of normal

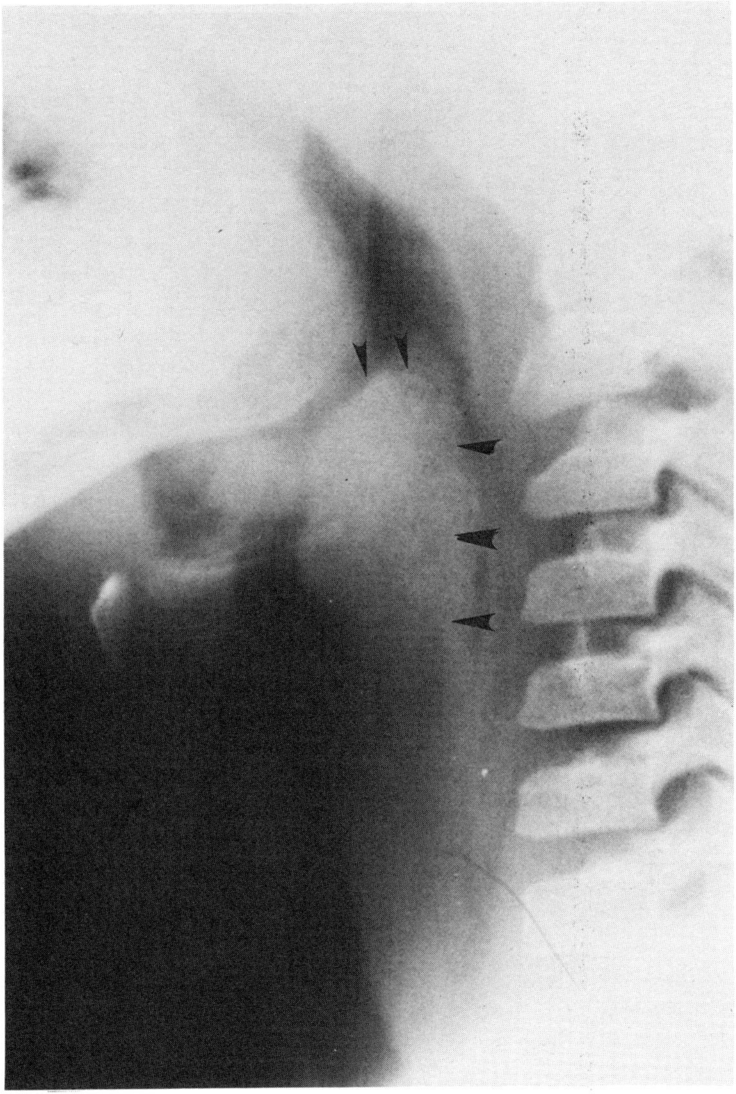

Figure 17. Foreign body in the hypopharynx. A lateral view of the neck shows a large mass density within the pyriform sinus (black arrowheads). This film is of a 5-year-old boy who choked while eating and came to the emergency room with signs of upper respiratory tract obstruction. Just before endoscopy, he coughed up a piece of meat, swallowed it and became immediately asymptomatic. Hypopharyngeal foreign bodies can produce significant respiratory obstruction if they are large enough to occlude the airway as in this instance. The pyriform sinus is normally radiolucent and when replaced by a density such as in this case, should lead one to consider a tumor as well as a foreign body. (Compare with Fig. 2.)

intra-alveolar and intra-pleural pressures leading to mediastinal widening in inspiration and mediastinal narrowing in expiration, the reverse of normal.[37]

Unfortunately, this sign is frequently not present with partially obstructing laryngo-tracheal foreign bodies and is nonspecific since it can be seen with any anatomic lesion producing partial obstruction of the laryngo-tracheal airway. If the foreign body lodges in the distal trachea, fluoroscopy may also show prolonged and difficult inspiration and expiration.[20] If conventional studies do not demonstrate a foreign body, computed tomography has been reported to be useful.[38]

Endobronchial Foreign Bodies

Aspirated endobronchial foreign bodies are usually easier to diagnose radiologically since they usually produce asymmetric changes in the lungs.

Total occlusion of a bronchus may produce densities and volume loss distal to the occlusion. Radiographic findings may consist of varying degrees of opacity of the obstructed lung, shift of the mediastinum toward the obstructed lung and secondary signs of volume loss such as elevation of the ipsilateral diaphragm and change in position of the pulmonary fissures. If total collapse of the lung secondary to bronchial occlusion occurs, the affected lung will be completely dense and airless and the mediastinum will shift sometimes entirely into the obstructed side, so that the heart will not be visible (Figs. 18, 19A and 19B). The unaffected lung may be compensatorily overinflated. If total collapse of the lung occurs rapidly, cyanosis and syncope can result because one lung becomes functionless and kinking and obstruction of the great veins may be produced by the abrupt mediastinal shift.[36] One may also see pneumomediastinum and pneumothorax which can result from rupture of either the obstructed or compensatorily overdistended normal lung.[36]

More commonly, the bronchus is not totally obstructed by the foreign body, and the radiologic findings are those of obstructive emphysema. Obstructive emphysema occurs because there is physiologic dilatation of the airway during inspiration permitting air to flow into the lung distal to the foreign body, and physiologic collapse of the airway during expiration, trapping the inspired air

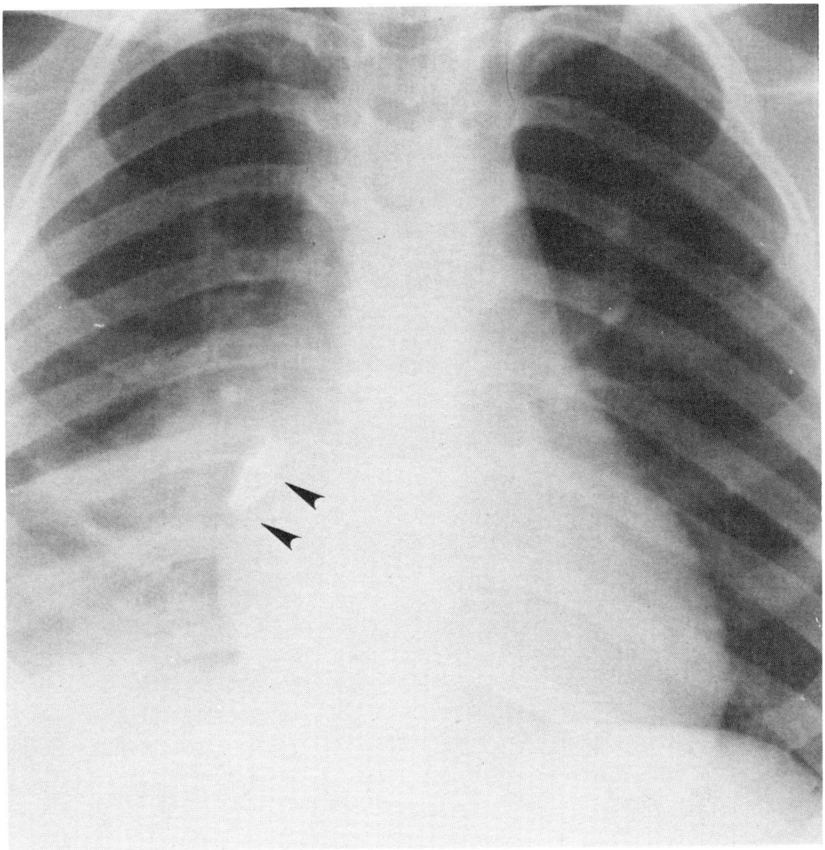

Figure 18. Endobronchial foreign body. The cap of a pen (black arrowheads) superimposes over the right side of the heart. This endobronchial foreign body produced consolidation and volume loss in the lung distal to it. The lung cleared rapidly following removal of the foreign body.

within the lung distal to the foreign body. With obstructive emphysema, the obstructed lung appears larger and more radiolucent than the normal lung. The radiolucency is probably a combination of both air trapping and decreased perfusion because of pulmonary vasoconstriction secondary to endobronchial obstruction and regional alveolar hypoxia. This effect is the basis for the use of perfusion lung scans in the diagnosis of endobronchial foreign bodies.[36,39,40,41]

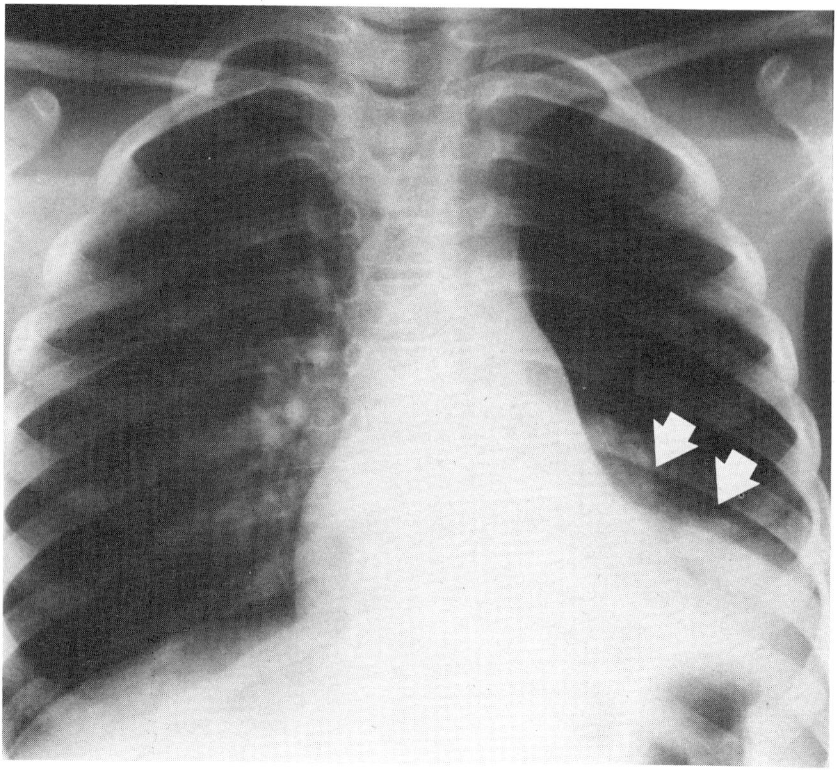

Figure 19A. Left lower lobe consolidation and loss of volume due to endobronchial foreign body. This child had symptoms and signs of pneumonia. The frontal chest film shows left lower lobe consolidation and loss of volume (white arrows) with overinflation of the left upper lobe. She was treated with antibiotics and quickly became asymptomatic. She returned for follow-up films after 3 weeks to document clearing of her pneumonia (See also Fig. 19B.)

Illustration continued on the opposite page

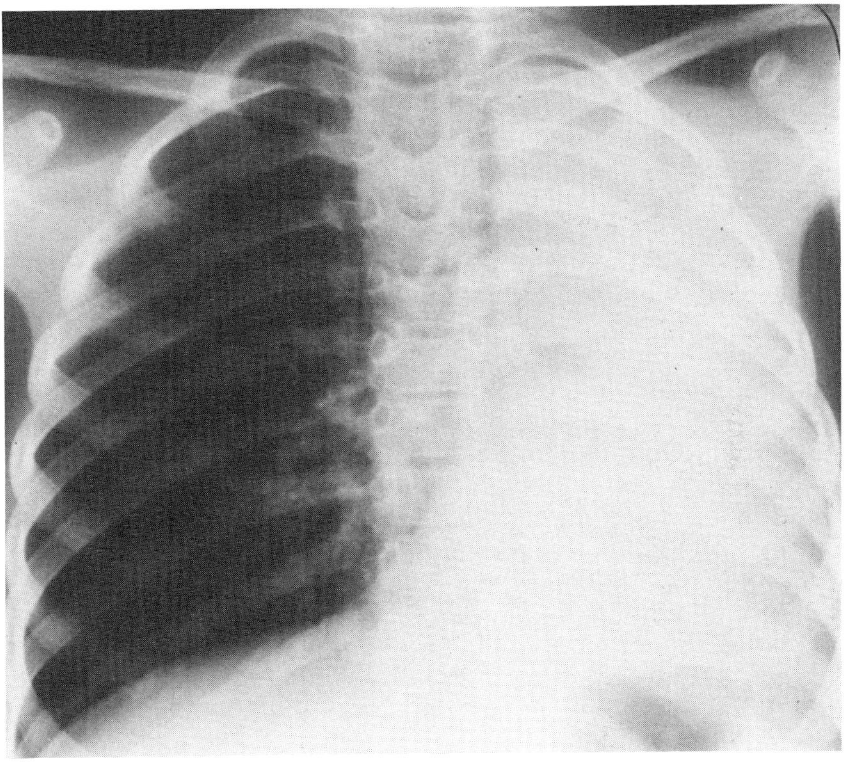

Figure 19B. Complete collapse of the left lung due to chronic endobronchial foreign body. There is opacification of the left hemithorax and shift of the heart entirely into the left side of the chest with displacement of the trachea to the left. The cause of the original lobar loss of volume (Fig. 19A) which progressed to complete loss of volume of the left lung, was a pencil eraser which was removed from the left mainstem bronchus at bronchoscopy. No symptoms of aspiration could be elicited even in retrospect. This case illustrates the importance of documenting clearing of pneumonia particularly with volume loss, and of being suspicious of significant lung volume loss in children. Non-clearing infiltrates, progressive or significant volume loss, unexplained areas of emphysema and persistent symptoms, should lead one to suspect aspirated foreign body.

The key to the diagnosis of obstructive emphysema is the frontal chest film in expiration. With obstructive emphysema, the obstructed lung will not empty during expiration, remaining large and radiolucent with a depressed ipsilateral hemidiaphragm. The normal, unobstructed contralateral lung will deflate and become smaller. The mediastinum will shift away from the obstructed nonemptying lung toward the normal deflating lung. On inspiration as the normal lung fills, the mediastinum will shift back toward the obstructed lung as the pressures equalize so that the inspiratory film may be nearly normal in appearance (Figs. 20A, 20B, 21A and 21B). If good inspiration and expiration films cannot be obtained in the young child, a lateral decubitus film can be useful in the diagnosis of obstructive emphysema. With a lateral decubitus film the dependent lung should be deflated. The obstructed lung, when dependent, will not deflate.[42]

We find it expeditious and informative to fluoroscope children with a history suggestive of aspirated foreign body in whom the preliminary films in inspiration and expiration are either normal or equivocal. At fluoroscopy, one sees the respiratory dynamics such as the mediastinal shift, differences in diaphragmatic mobility and differences in emptying of the lungs. These images may be recorded on videotape for future review. If radiographic and fluoroscopic studies are equivocal, perfusion lung scans have been used to detect obstructing endobronchial foreign bodies.[39,41]

Chronically present foreign bodies which are unrecognized will, over time, lead to pulmonary infiltration and loss of volume. The appearance of pulmonary infiltrates is more rapid if the foreign body is organic, such as a peanut, and somewhat delayed with inorganic foreign bodies such as plastic or metal.[36] One must also be aware that foreign bodies can shift within the tracheobronchial tree and, as they change locations, symptoms and signs as well as radiographic findings may change.

A high index of suspicion is necessary to avoid missing aspirated foreign bodies. Clinically, persistent wheeze, stridor or cough should raise the suspicion of aspirated foreign body. Radiologic findings of focal emphysema, pneumonia which does not clear following adequate therapy and significant or progressive loss of volume on chest radiographs should alert the radiologist to the possibility of an aspirated foreign body. If radiographic studies and fluoroscopy are normal but the clinical situation is suspicious, bronchoscopy should be done since the presence of a foreign body can never be completely excluded by radiologic means.[40,43]

Text continued on page 221

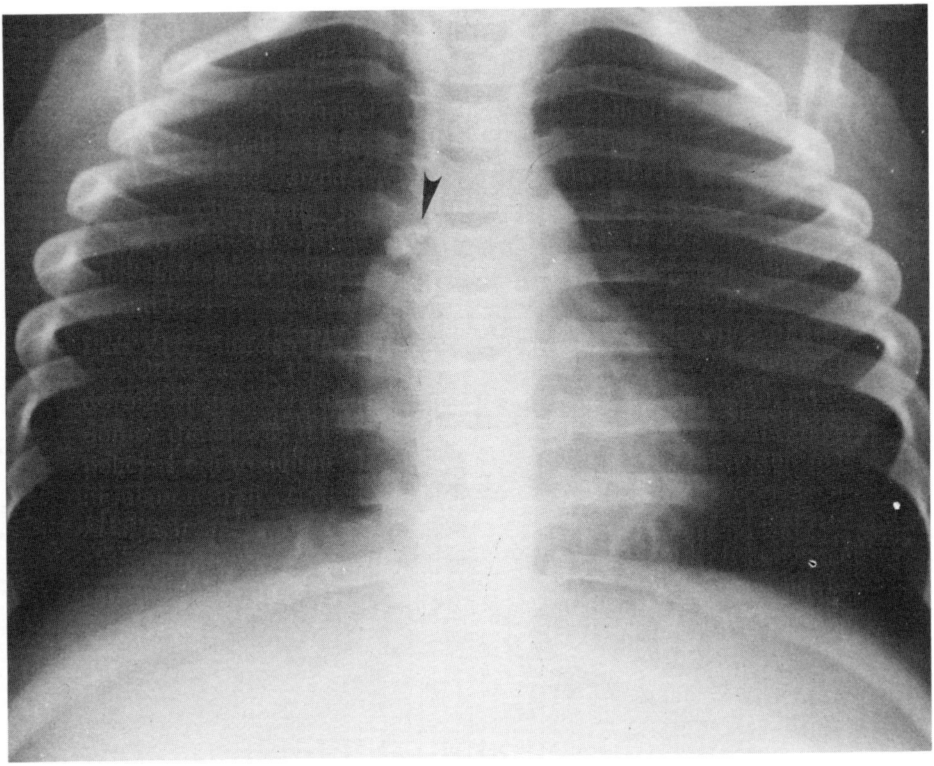

Figure 20A. Endobronchial foreign body. Figure 20A is a frontal film of the chest in inspiration showing overaerated lungs and a calcific appearing density (black arrowhead) in the region of the right hilum. (See Fig. 20B.)

Illustration continued on the following page

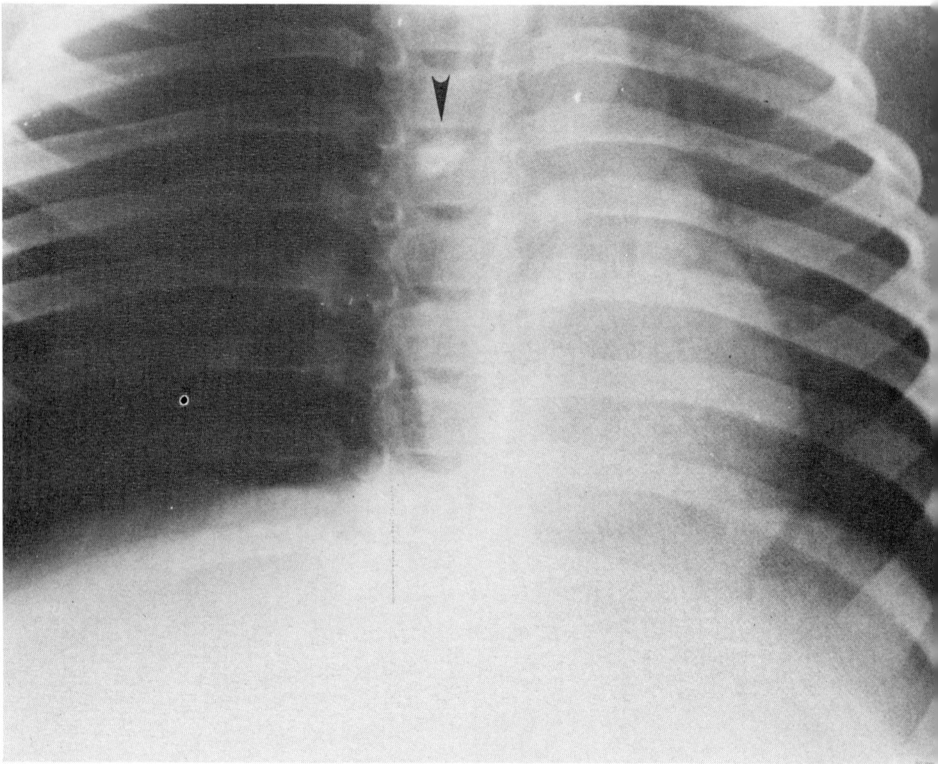

Figure 20B. Obstructive emphysema due to an endobronchial foreign body. A frontal film of the chest in expiration shows the calcific density (black arrowhead) and obstructive emphysema of the right lung. In expiration, the right lung does not empty and the mediastinum shifts toward the normal deflating left lung. This child had a cough for one week which began when he was playing near a fireplace. The "calcific density" was a cinder aspirated into the right mainstem bronchus and removed at bronchoscopy. Figs. 20A and 20B show the importance of a film made in expiration to demonstrate obstructive emphysema.

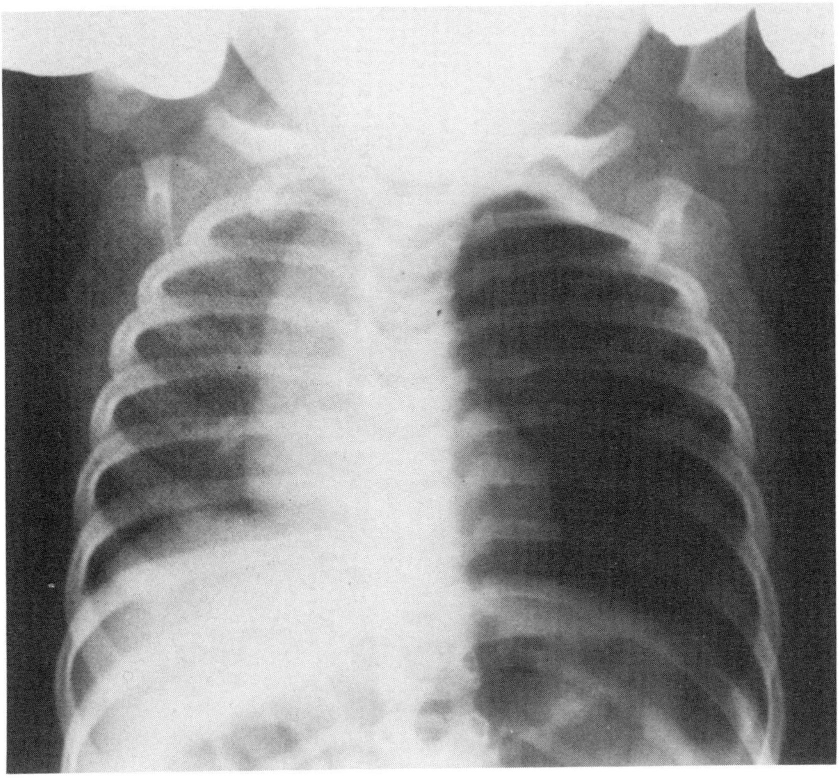

Figure 21A. Endobronchial foreign body. This is a frontal chest film in inspiration which shows pulmonary overinflation and a midline mediastinum. (See Fig. 21B.)

Illustration continued on the following page

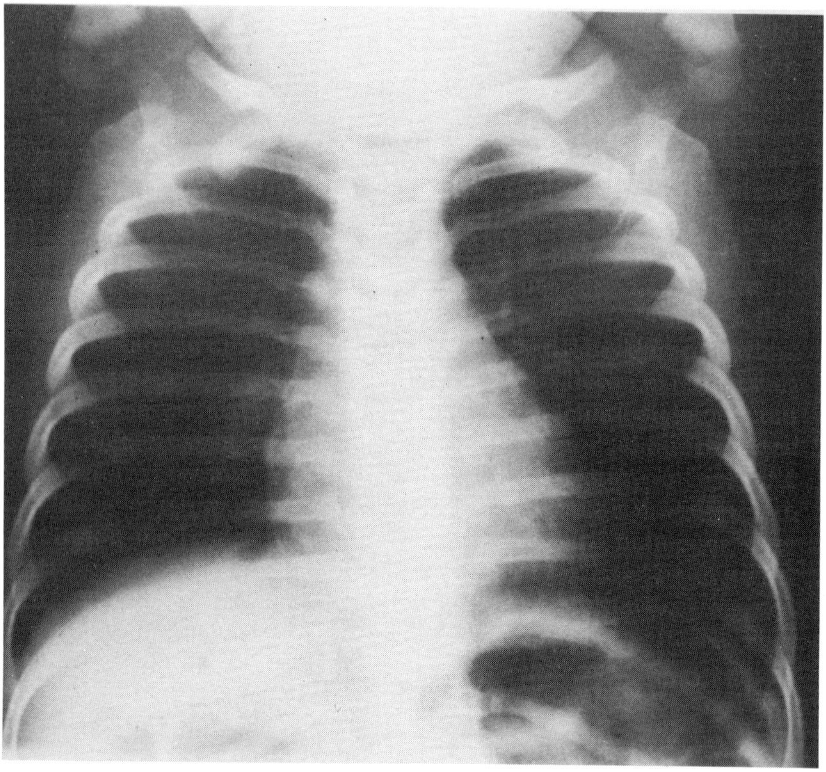

Figure 21B. Obstructive emphysema due to an endobronchial foreign body. This is a frontal film of the chest in expiration (the same child as in Fig. 21A), which shows obstructive emphysema of the left lung. The left lung does not empty and the mediastinum is displaced toward the normal deflating right lung. The cause of the left-sided obstructive emphysema was a peanut in the left mainstem bronchus. This case emphasizes the necessity for good expiration films in cases of suspected aspiration of a foreign body, especially when the foreign body is not radiopaque. If satisfactory films cannot be obtained, fluoroscopy should be done.

Esophageal Foreign Bodies as a Cause of Respiratory Distress

Initial symptoms of the presence of esophageal foreign bodies may include cough, excessive drooling, poor feeding and dysphagia. These symptoms may soon subside and be followed by a relatively symptomless interval in which there is no dysphagia in a young child, and diet is formed mainly of liquids or soft foods which may pass around an incompletely obstructing esophageal foreign body.[44] Respiratory symptoms such as stridor, wheezing or findings of chronic pneumonia may then occur early or late and cause one to focus initial attention on the respiratory tract as the cause of the symptoms rather than to consider retained esophageal foreign body.[44,45] The most frequent site of impaction of foreign bodies of the esophagus is just below the crico-pharyngeus muscle.[44,45]

Respiratory symptoms in infants and children due to esophageal foreign bodies may occur because of direct mechanical compression by the esophageal foreign body against the posterior wall of the adjacent trachea, paraesophageal inflammation and abscess formation producing compression and displacement of the adjacent trachea, direct extension of the inflammatory process into the trachea or larynx, aspiration and pneumonia secondary to esophageal obstruction by the foreign body, or tracheoesophageal fistula secondary to ulceration of the esophagus.[44–47] Esophageal inflammatory disease (moniliasis) has been reported to produce sufficient periesophageal inflammation to compress the trachea and cause respiratory symptoms.[46]

Radiographic evaluation usually depends upon the clinical situation. It is not uncommon to find an esophageal foreign body on chest and neck radiographs made in children for evaluation of asthma or inspiratory stridor. Frontal and lateral views of the neck and chest should be obtained and a film of the abdomen should probably be included if there is a history of ingestion of foreign body. If the foreign body is radiopaque, a satisfactory set of films should demonstrate it. If the foreign body is not radiopaque, secondary signs of its presence may be inferred from compression and anterior displacement of the adjacent trachea or the presence of soft tissue gas if perforation of the esophagus has occurred (Figs. 22, 23 and 24). If the plain radiographs are normal or show

Text continued on page 225

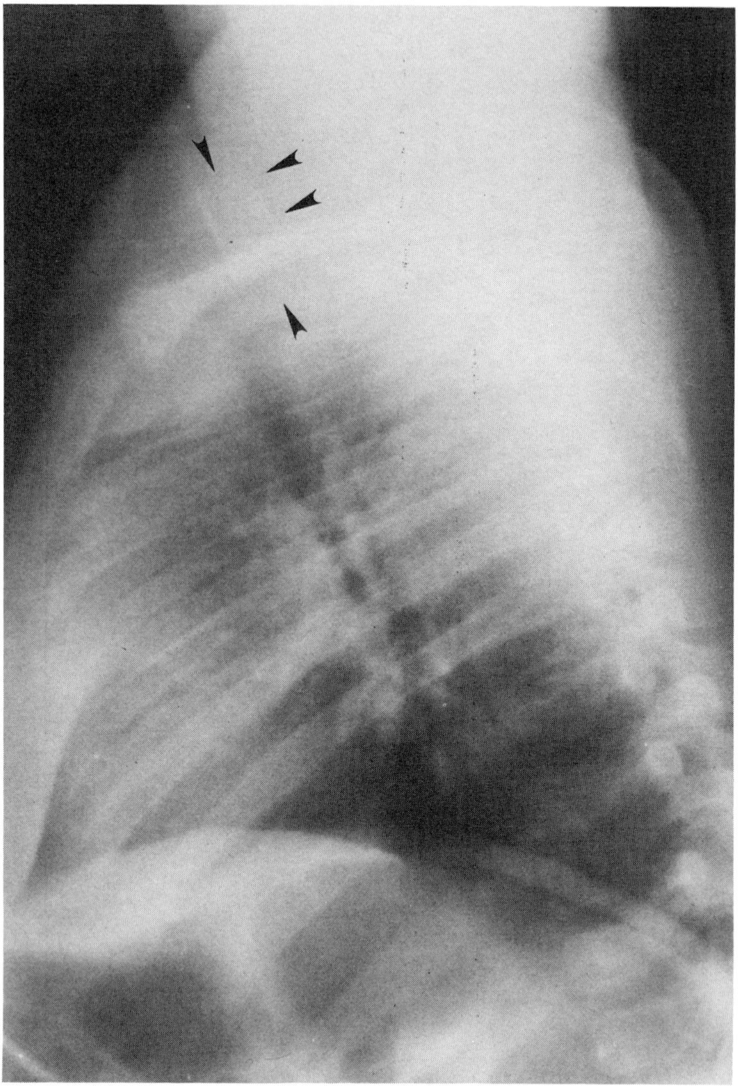

Figure 22. Esophageal foreign body. A lateral view of the chest in an infant shows a faintly radiopaque esophageal foreign body (black arrowheads). This was an aluminum pull tab from the top of a can of pop. There was a history of approximately 2 months of stridor; dysphagia was minimal or absent and there was no weight loss. These foreign bodies are particularly troublesome since they are not very radiopaque.

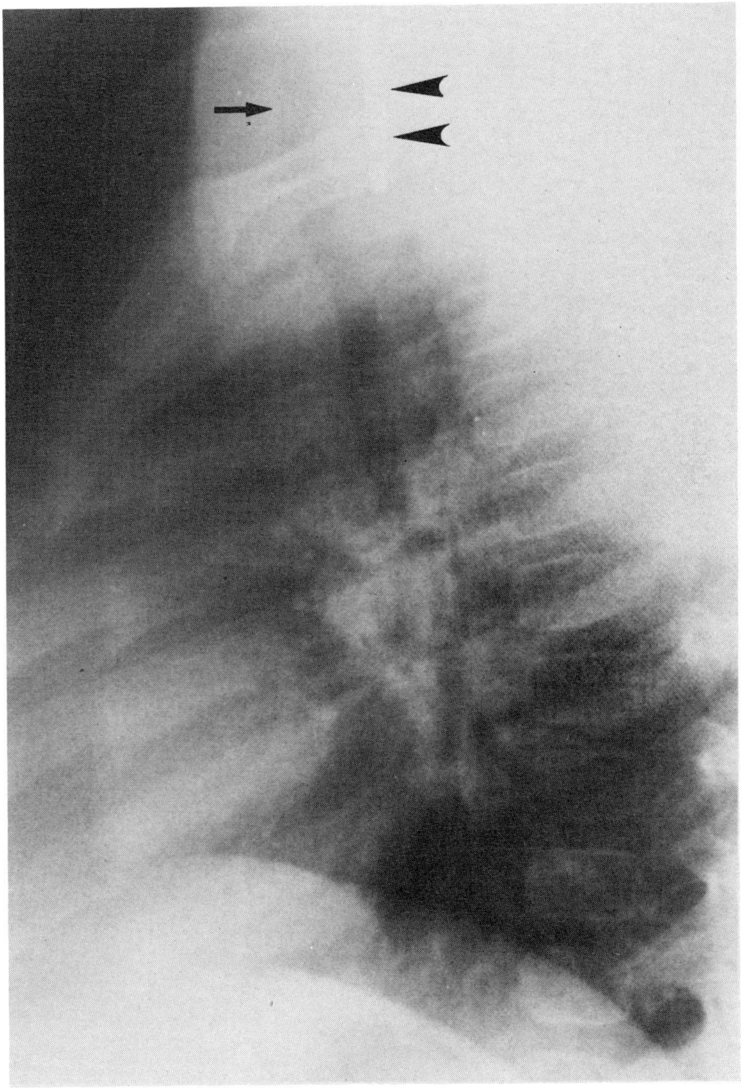

Figure 23. Esophageal foreign body. A lateral film of the chest shows a coin in the esophagus (black arrowheads). Note the anterior displacement of the trachea (black arrow) and the pressure along its posterior surface. Stridor was present.

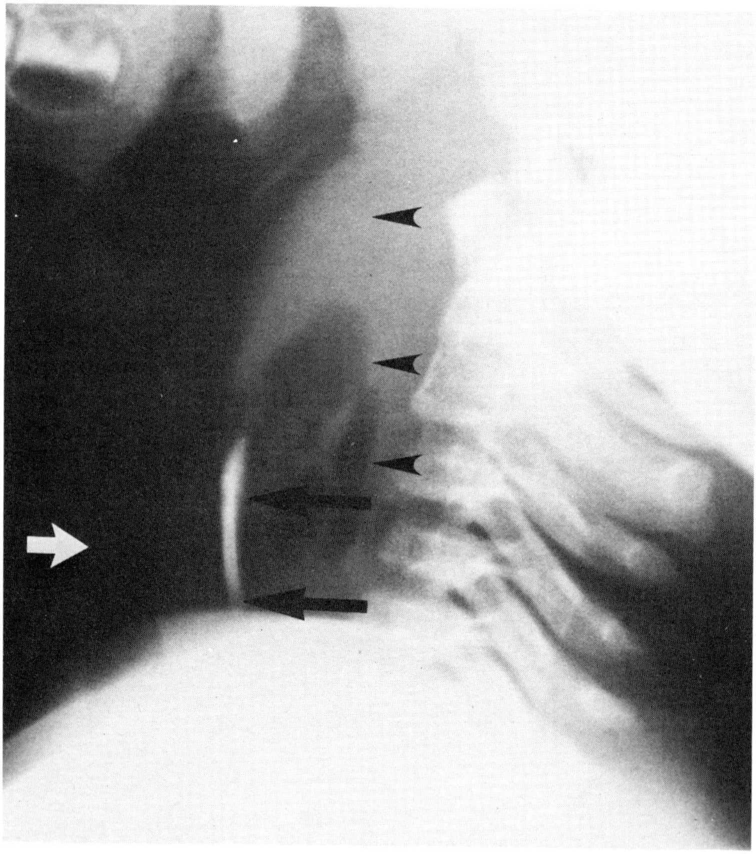

Figure 24. Esophageal foreign body. A lateral view of the neck shows a dense foreign body (thick black arrows). The foreign body is glass in the esophagus. The retroesophageal soft tissue thickening with air collections and the retropharyngeal soft tissue thickening (black arrowheads) were due to abscess formation secondary to esophageal perforation. Note the anterior displacement of the trachea (white arrow). Respiratory distress was present in this 1-year-old boy.

secondary signs of the presence of a nonradiopaque esophageal foreign body, a barium swallow will confirm its presence.

The physician must be aware that an esophageal foreign body and esophageal inflammatory disease may produce significant respiratory symptomatology which may mask esophageal symptoms. One should not hesitate to obtain a barium swallow in a child with unexplained respiratory symptomatology and normal plain film studies.

The Thorax

All lines and catheters used in the hospital should be radiopaque. Before analyzing the chest X-ray one should follow every catheter and line throughout its course. By doing this, one will not miss many of the iatrogenic complications of inserting these tubes and lines (Figs. 25 and 26).

Pulmonary Edema

On a normal chest X-ray the "lung markings" are almost all due to blood vessels.[48] Bronchi may be seen "end on" toward the center of the lung but are not visualized in the greater part of the lung unless they are surrounded by consolidation. The margins of the pulmonary vascularity are sharply defined.

In the normal erect position, the bases show the greatest perfusion and the apices the least perfusion. This is reflected radiologically in the size of the pulmonary vascularity. The lower lobe vessels are slightly larger than those of the upper lobes and there is a greater density of vascular branching in the lower lung. With a normal patient supine, the upper lobe vessels enlarge with more small branches becoming visible. This is an important point to remember as many films taken on sick patients are taken portable and supine.

Pulmonary edema is an abnormal extravascular accumulation of transudated fluid in the pulmonary tissues. This fluid may collect initially in the interstitial compartment and later be identified in the alveolar compartment of the lung. However, in many cases of pulmonary edema, transudated fluid is initially identified in the alveolar compartment.

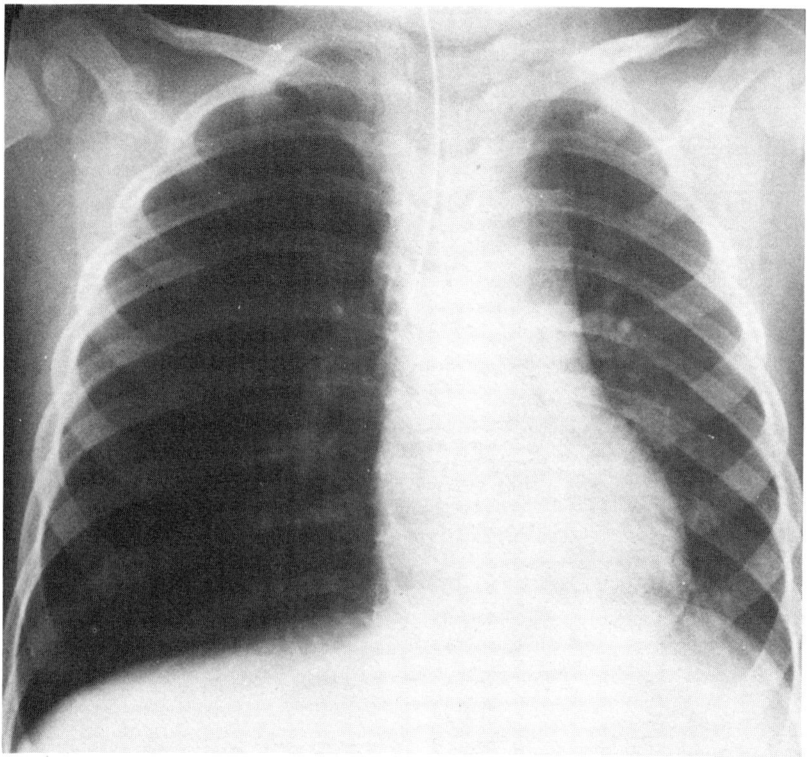

Figure 25. Endotracheal tube is in the right mainstem bronchus. Note the overinflation of the right lung with mediastinal shift toward the left. The left hemithorax by comparison is small. A nasogastric tube can also faintly be visualized in the upper esophagus.

Pulmonary edema can be divided into two broad categories. The first is due to increased pulmonary capillary pressure. Causes of this would be left-sided heart failure, pulmonary venous obstruction, increased intravascular volume, or pulmonary lymphatic obstruction. Increased permeability between the alveolus and capillary is the second cause. Examples of this would be inhalation of noxious agents. Clearly, one cannot usually distinguish these two causes on a chest X-ray.

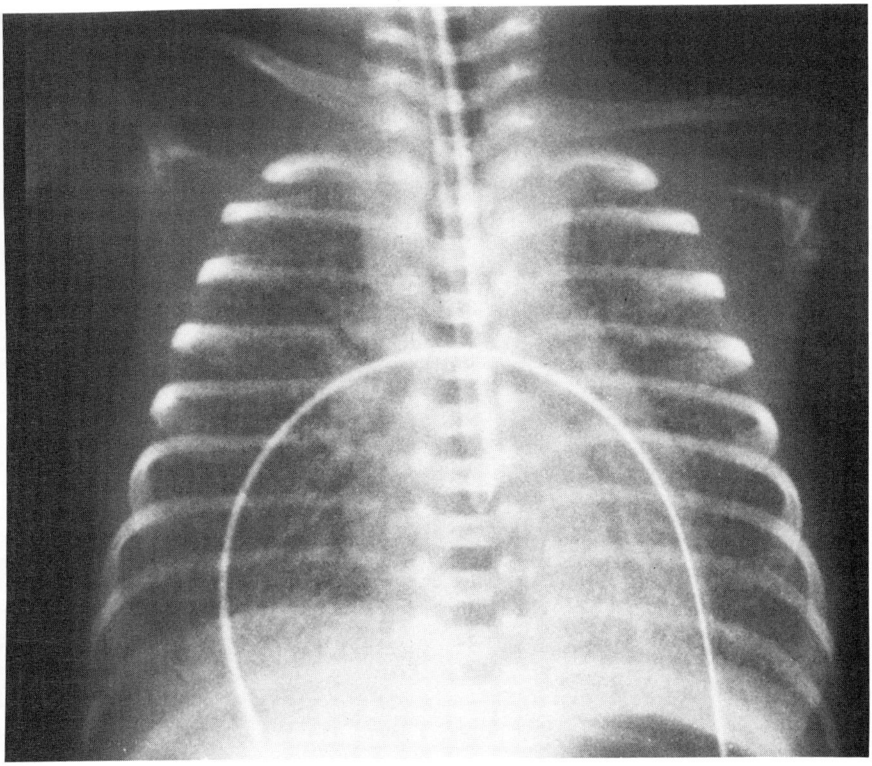

Figure 26. Endotracheal tube is identified with its tip at the level of the T6,7 disc space. Clearly this cannot be in the trachea and lies within the esophagus. Curved tubing overlying the lower thorax is on the patient's skin. This premature infant has respiratory distress syndrome.

Interstitial Edema

Kerley initially described three types of linear shadows related to interstitial edema. *Kerley A* lines are thin, nonbranching lines several inches long radiating from the hila (Fig. 27). They do not follow the course of either arteries, veins or bronchi. *Kerley B* lines are short, thin linear shadows arranged in a horizontal stepladder pattern. These are best seen in the costophrenic angles and on the lateral view of the chest just behind the sternum. They are perpendicular to the pleural space and are thought to represent fluid in the interlobular septa. *Kerley C* lines are fine interlacing lines seen throughout the lung. These lines are all thought to represent fluid in the lymphatic spaces.

Interstitial edema can also be identified on the chest X-ray by obscuration of the normally sharp edges to the pulmonary vascularity. One must be very careful, however, in dealing with a chest X-ray of sufficient inspiration.

Thickening of the bronchial walls can also occur with interstitial edema.

Alveolar Edema

Transudate into the alveolar spaces produces the typical radiographic appearance of an alveolar infiltrate. This is a confluent density in the lungs with poorly defined edges (Fig. 28). The appearance of air bronchograms is diagnostic of an alveolar infiltrate (Fig. 29). Although pulmonary edema is classically said to give a butterfly distribution around the pulmonary hila, this is a rare finding. An alveolar infiltrate secondary to pulmonary edema cannot be distinguished from that due to exudate or hemorrhage into the alveolar spaces.

Adult Respiratory Distress Syndrome

Adult respiratory distress syndrome is a clinical entity of pulmonary insufficiency, impaired gas exchange, decrease in lung compliance and diffuse pulmonary infiltrates on a chest X-ray resulting from a variety of nonpulmonary insults including shock, trauma and sepsis.

Text continued on page 232

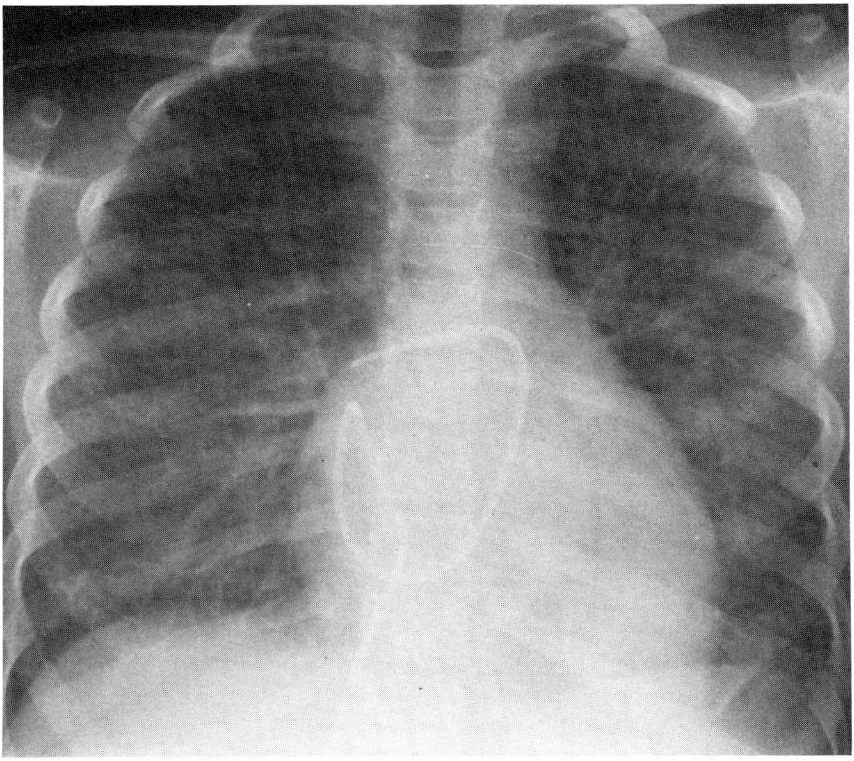

Figure 27. Interstitial pulmonary edema. Kerley A lines can be identified radiating from the hilum into the lungs in this patient who was fluid overloaded. A Swan-Ganz catheter is identified with its tip in the right main pulmonary artery.

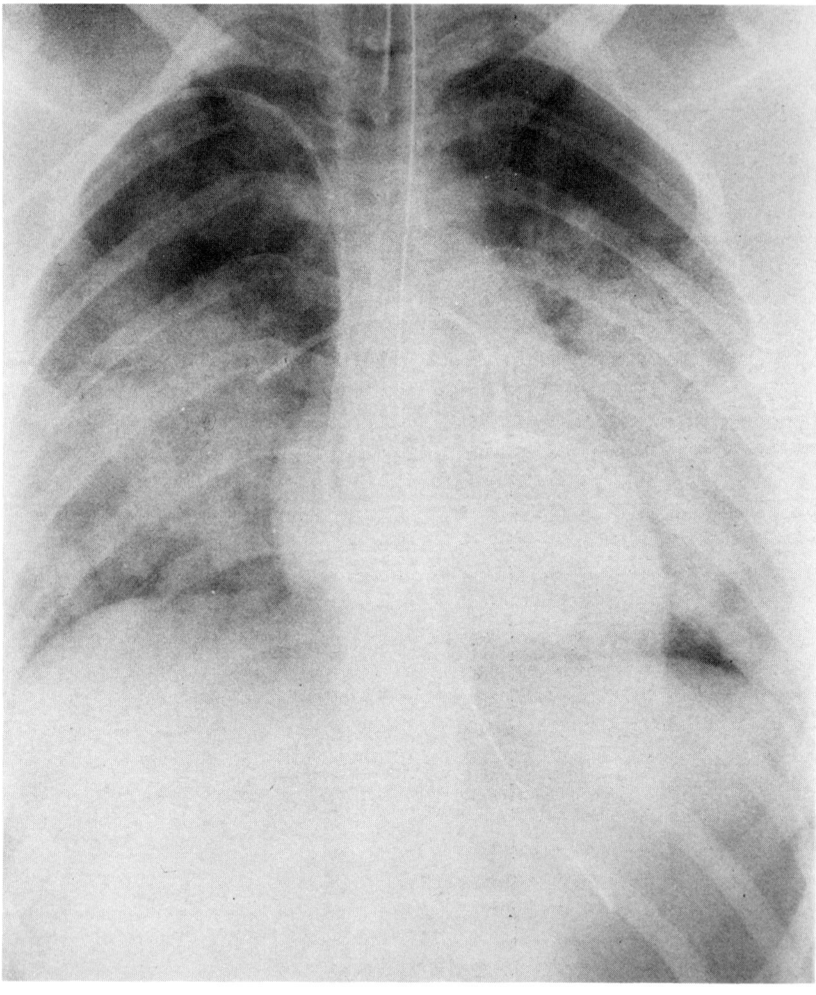

Figure 28. Alveolar pulmonary edema. Near-drowning in an adolescent girl produced this extensive bilateral alveolar disease, secondary to pulmonary edema. The patient is intubated and a Swan-Ganz catheter is identified with its tip in the right inferior pulmonary artery.

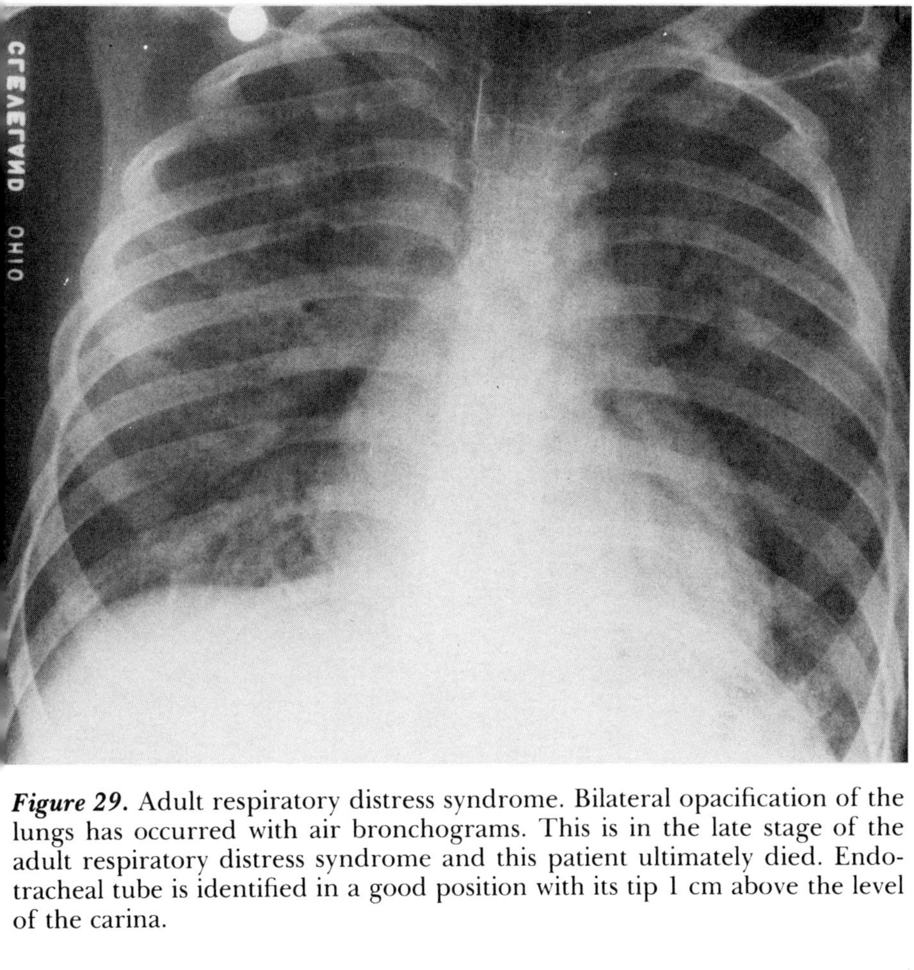

Figure 29. Adult respiratory distress syndrome. Bilateral opacification of the lungs has occurred with air bronchograms. This is in the late stage of the adult respiratory distress syndrome and this patient ultimately died. Endotracheal tube is identified in a good position with its tip 1 cm above the level of the carina.

This disease entity was first described in 1967[49] although it had been appreciated previously as the "wet lung" in war casualties and also as respiratory distress following cardiopulmonary bypass and hemodialysis. Many synonyms for this entity exist:

- Adult hyaline membrane disease
- Adult respiratory insufficiency syndrome
- Oxygen toxicity
- Post-perfusion lung
- Pump lung
- Respirator lung
- Shock lung
- Wet lung

Although initially described in adults, this disease complex does occur in pediatric patients following the same nonspecific insults to the lung that precipitate the disease complex in adults.[50] Initially, similarities to neonatal respiratory distress syndrome and cardiogenic pulmonary edema were emphasized. Indeed, Petty and Ashbaugh suggested that this syndrome may be secondary to defective surfactant synthesis as is found in the infant respiratory distress syndrome.[51] Although abnormality of sufactant is found in these patients, this is not now thought to be the primary cause. It is thought that these abnormalities of surfactant are another marker of lung injury.

The damaged capillary endothelium of the lungs allows a protein-rich exudate to appear in the interstitial lung compartment and later in the alveoli. This increased capillary permeability is thought to be one of the basic underlying physiological defects. This may be induced by granulocyte aggregation which causes activation of the complement cascade. Complement activation generates C5a which causes leukocyte aggregation in the lung. These aggregated neutrophils injure the endothelial cells by the generation of toxic oxygen radicals. Further damage occurs from intravascular coagulation and fibrinolysis together with platelet aggregation. Microvascular obstruction by thrombi has been demonstrated both in autopsy specimens[52] and at the bedside in patients with acute respiratory failure.[53]

Corticosteroids are, therefore, both theoretically and practically useful. Steroids will reverse many of the previously described pathophysiological abnormalities. However, no controlled clinical trials in children have yet been reported. Mechanical ventilation with positive end-expiratory pressure improves survival with ARDS and is now widely used.[54]

In the early stage, the chest x-ray will be clear. However, profound pathophysiological events are occurring but are not evident on the chest x-ray. The patient will usually be hyperventilating with a moderate respiratory alkalosis at this stage. Often there is little or no hypoxemia. The lungs will show decreased compliance and although interstitial edema secondary to endothelial damage is occurring, this is not yet visible on the x-ray.

With increasing disruption of the capillary integrity, more protein-rich exudate spills over into the alveoli. The patient is now more agitated as hypoxia, cyanosis and increased respiratory distress develop. The chest x-ray now shows patchy alveolar infiltrates and "interstitial" edema. Functionally, there is now a marked decrease in lung compliance and in functional residual capacity. Mismatch of ventilation and perfusion in the lungs is also becoming exaggerated as alveoli fill with fluid.

The densities on the chest x-ray next progress, becoming more confluent until there may be a complete "whiteout" of the lungs. (See Fig. 29.) Clinically, there is now severe hypoxemia and respiratory failure requiring mechanical ventilation. Barotrauma from mechanical ventilation may now become a complication of treatment. At this stage also, there is endothelial leak of fibrinogen into the alveoli resulting in the formation of hyaline membranes.

Finally, the chest x-ray may slowly improve, resulting eventually in a completely normal chest x-ray. However, the mortality from this syndrome is very high,[55] with reported mortality rates of between 50 and 60%. Death is often due to a central nervous system complication rather than lung disease.[56] While the chest x-ray may return to normal, there may also be changes of residual fibrosis and even pulmonary arterial hypertension.

Pneumothorax

Large collections of air in the pleural space are easily recognized on chest x-rays taken on erect patients (Fig. 30).

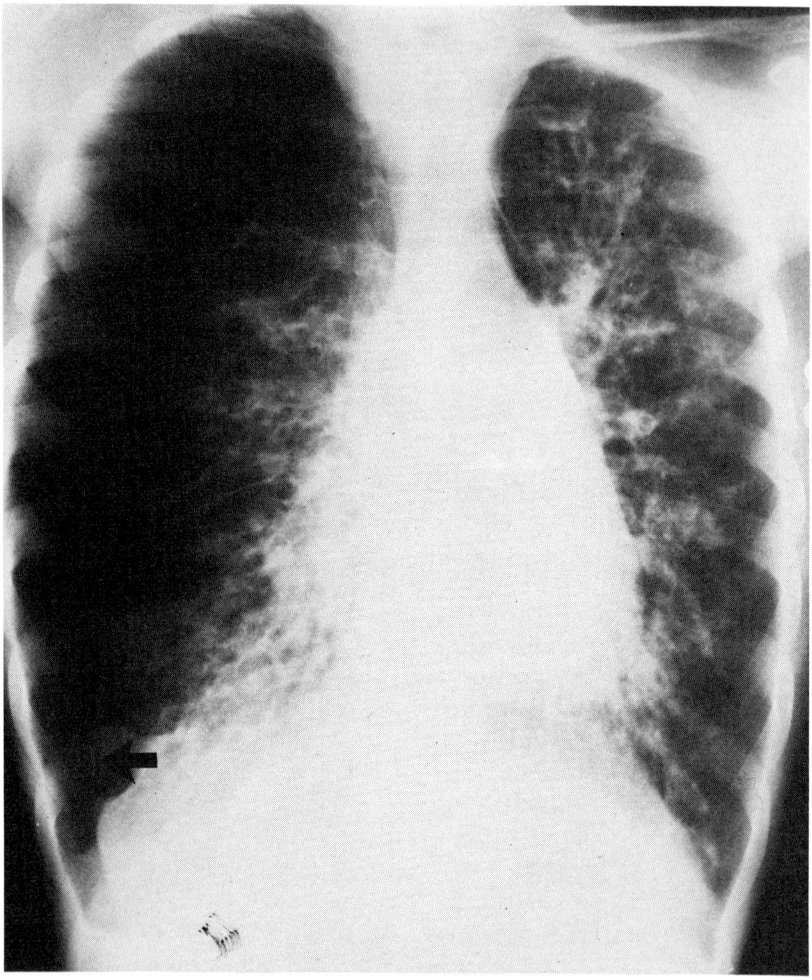

Figure 30. Tension pneumothorax in a patient with cystic fibrosis. Bilateral severe bronchiectatic and bullous changes of cystic fibrosis are identified. A large right pneumothorax is identified which is under tension and has displaced the mediastinum to the left. The right lung is unable to collapse any further because of the underlying cystic fibrosis. Note the thin white line of visceral pleura identified at the edge of the pneumothorax (arrow).

However, when the pneumothorax is small, an expiration view, lateral decubitus or cross-table lateral view may be very helpful in making the pneumothorax more obvious radiographically. A tension pneumothorax is diagnosed by displacement of the mediastinum away from the pneumothorax. Other signs include diaphragmatic depression and ribcage expansion on the side of the tension pneumothorax (Fig. 31). The degree of lung collapse is not a reliable sign for or against a tension pneumothorax.[57]

In the supine patient, air tends to collect anteriorly and inferiorly. This may produce X-ray appearances which are not immediately obvious as the free edge of the visceral pleural is not identified on the X-rays.[58,59]

One should then look very carefully for any areas of hyperlucency especially along the diaphragmatic surface or adjacent to the cardiac outline. Often these structures will have "sharper" edges because of the free air.[60] A lateral decubitus or cross-table lateral view of the chest may be particularly helpful in this situation.

Artefacts from tubing can usually easily be separated from the edge of a pneumothorax. However, in supine patients, skin folds can occasionally give misleading lines and be confused with a pneumothorax.[61] Often the skinfold line can be traced outside the thorax and then one is confident that one is not dealing with a pneumothorax. The thin visceral pleura of a pneumothorax will also parallel the course of the chest wall over its whole length. This is rarely true of a skin fold. The density of a skin fold also increases progressively to the edge of the skin fold. This is a completely different density profile from that of a pneumothorax where the lucent lung and pneumothorax are interrupted by a thin white line which represents visceral pleura. (See Fig. 30.)

Congenital lobar emphysema shows hyperlucency involving an upper lobe and by this distribution, can usually be differentiated from a pneumothorax.

Pneumomediastinum

In contrast to pneumothorax, pneumomediastinum is rarely symptomatic. In fact, it is often not appreciated on PA films of the chest and only identified on a lateral view (Fig. 32). Air is identified

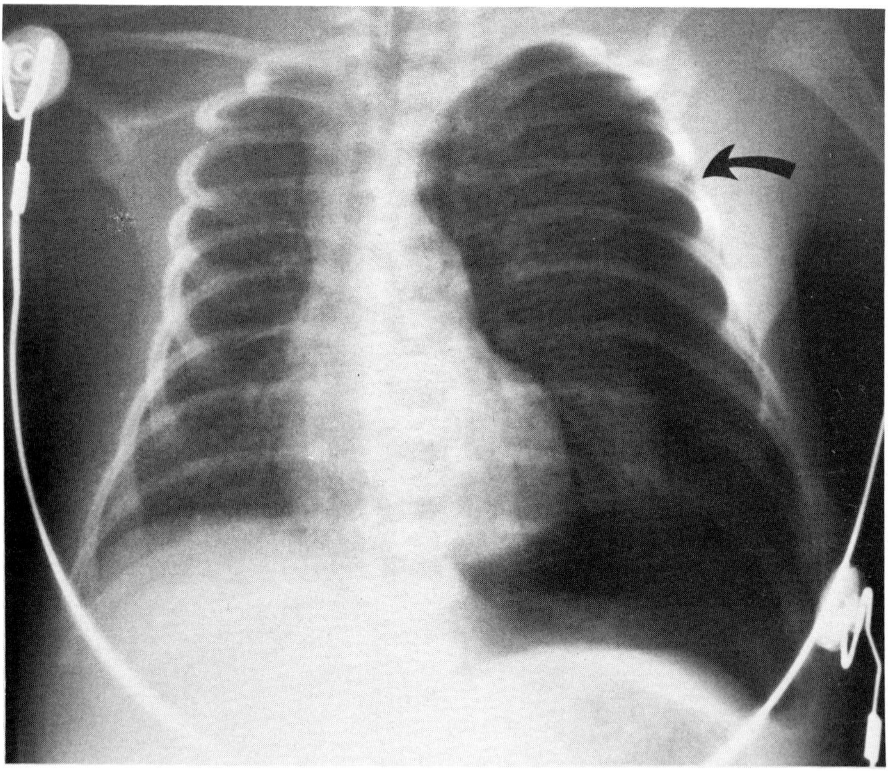

Figure 31. Tension pneumothorax in a premature infant with respiratory distress syndrome. Although there is some mediastinal shift to the right from the left-sided tension pneumothorax, this may not occur in patients who are on positive-end expiratory pressure ventilators. Then one must look at compliant areas for evidence of a tension pneumothorax. Notice the bulging of the intercostal pleura (arrowhead) and the flattening of the left hemidiaphragm. These are two compliant areas that must always be checked for signs of a tension pneumothorax.

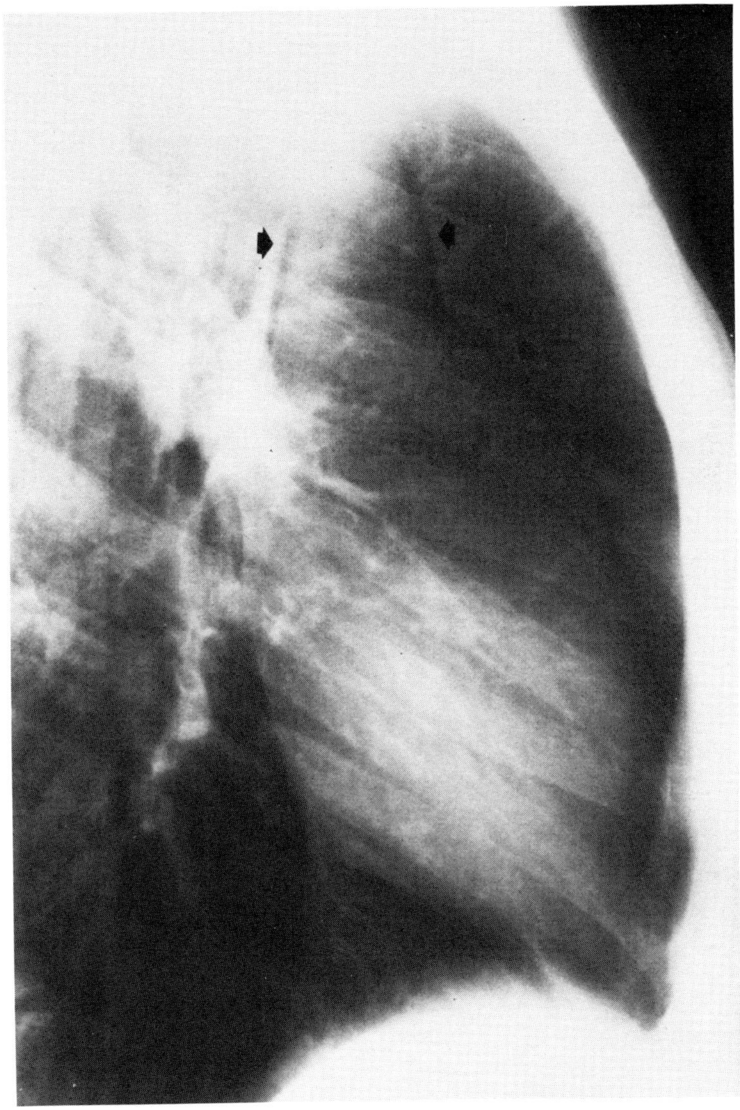

Figure 32. Pneumomediastinum. The PA film on this patient with asthma appeared normal. However, on inspection of the lateral view as well as recognizing overinflation in this asthmatic, linear gas collections can be identified outlining the mediastinal structures (arrowheads). This represents a pneumomediastinum and on the following day, subcutaneous emphysema could be palpated in the patient's neck.

outlining the mediastinal structures. Linear collections of air are identified outlining the aorta, pulmonary artery and thymus. The thymus in younger children may be elevated and outlined by air, producing a so-called "spinnaker sign".[62] This mediastinal air may also dissect up into the soft tissues of the neck and superior mediastinum.

Air from a pneumomediastinum may also outline the heart and difficulties may arise in distinguishing this pneumomediastinum from a medial pneumothorax or even a pneumopericardium. With pneumopericardium, air should completely surround the heart (Fig. 33). To distinguish a pneumomediastinum from a medial pneumothorax may be difficult and a cross-table view of the chest is essential. In the supine patient, a medial pneumothorax should be seen anteriorly. If one sees a linear gas shadow outlining a mediastinal structure, one can therefore exclude a pneumothorax. If possible, decubitus views are also very helpful for distinguishing a pneumothorax from a pneumomediastinum.

Pleural Fluid

Initially, small amounts of pleural fluid collect in the dependent parts of the pleural space. Lateral decubitus views may be helpful to visualize small pleural fluid collections. Usually the earliest sign of pleural fluid is blunting of the costophrenic angles. This can be seen laterally on the PA view of the chest and posteriorly on the lateral view. Classically, there is a curved or sloping upper surface to the pleural fluid. Because of underlying lung collapse, mediastinal shift may not occur.

When the patient is X-rayed supine, the pleural fluid layers posteriorly and produces an opacification of that hemithorax on the chest X-ray. This is often not appreciated in the severely ill patient. If pleural fluid collections are bilateral, this makes the interpretation even harder.

Another area where pleural fluid collections are missed is when the fluid collects in the subpulmonic space. The fluid in this space is free to move and again lateral decubitus views may be very helpful. Initially, one may think that the hemidiaphragm is elevated on this side, but closer inspection will often exclude this possibility. The shape of the subpulmonic fluid collection is dif-

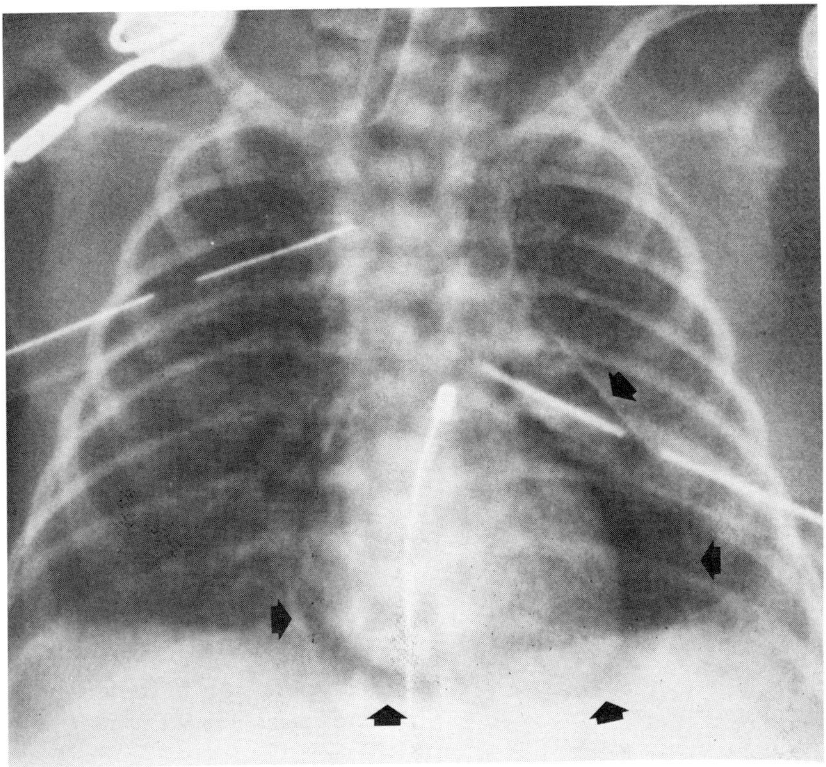

Figure 33A. Pneumopericardium causing cardiac tamponade. This child with respiratory distress syndrome suddenly deteriorated and a film shows a pneumopericardium (arrowheads outline the parietal pericardium). Cardiac size is decreased and following pericardiocentesis, there was marked improvement. The heart was being tamponaded by the air collection in the pericardial cavity.

Illustration continued on the following page

ferent from that of the normal diaphragmatic contour. On the left side there may be widening of the distance between the gastric air bubble and the lung.

Obviously the nature of the pleural fluid collections on the chest x-ray cannot be ditinguished. Whether the pleural fluid is an exudate or a transudate or whether this represents a hemothorax or empyema, is impossible to tell.

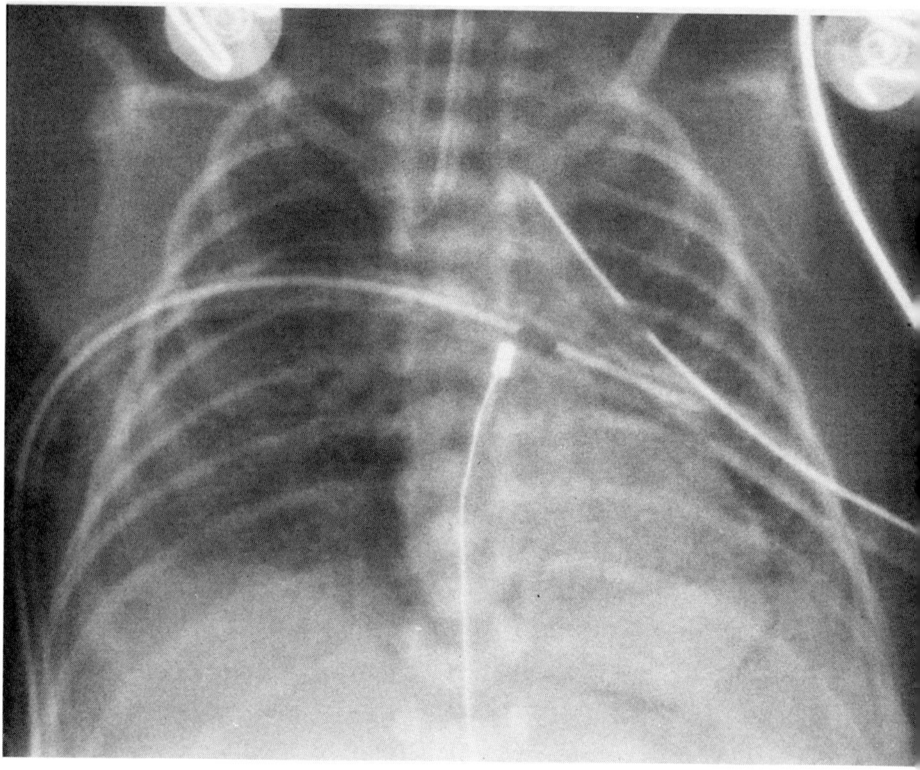

Figure 33B. Heart size has now returned to normal following pericardiocentesi The thoracostomy tubes have been changed in position and the right thoraco tomy tube has herniated across the midline into the left lung posteriorly. Th tip of the left thoracostomy tube is now pointing more superiorly. An umbilic artery catheter is noted in the thoracic aorta with its tip at the level of the 7t thoracic vertebral body.

Lung Infections

Viruses are by far the most common cause of lower respiratory tract infections in children.[63] These can produce several patterns on a chest X-ray which are reasonably specific.[36] These include a picture of overinflation as is seen in bronchiolitis, an interstitial lung pattern, and the most common of all, an increased density in the hilar region which is peribronchial. Less commonly, viruses can produce an alveolar lung parenchymal pattern.

Bacterial lung infections, however, produce a different pattern giving a parenchymal opacification. While no single pattern is specific for any organism, there are certain common patterns seen more commonly and these may help in management of these patients and selection of antibiotics before laboratory studies are available.

Acute streptococcal pneumonia may be seen in infants and neonates. It should always be thought of when the radiographic pattern of hyaline membrane disease is asymmetrical and particularly when it just involves one lobe. Rarely, acute streptococcal pneumonia may present with a bilateral reticulo-granular pulmonary pattern identical to that seen in hyaline membrane disease.[64] Streptococcal pneumonia is, however, an infection of mature infants and this is another important distinguishing feature.

Chlamydial pneumonia also produces a characteristic X-ray appearance (Fig. 34) of overinflation and diffuse infiltrates which often look radiographically worse than the patient would appear clinically.[65] This occurs typically between ages 2–14 weeks. The patients present with a cough often described as a "staccato cough". There is a lack of fever, but there is frequently eosinophilia and elevated serum immunoglobulins (IgM and IgG). Pleural fluid and lobar consolidation are never seen.

Chlamydial pneumonia is not a rare disease, representing 27% of infants less than six months of age admitted to a hospital with lower respiratory tract disease and 45% of those with a diagnosis of pneumonia.[66] It has been estimated that infants born to infected mothers have a 40–50% risk of developing conjunctivitis and a 10% risk of pneumonia.[67]

Staphylococcal infection of the lungs typically gives a localized area of consolidation associated with a pleural fluid collection. Empyemas commonly develop as do pneumatoceles (Fig. 35).

Text continued on page 243

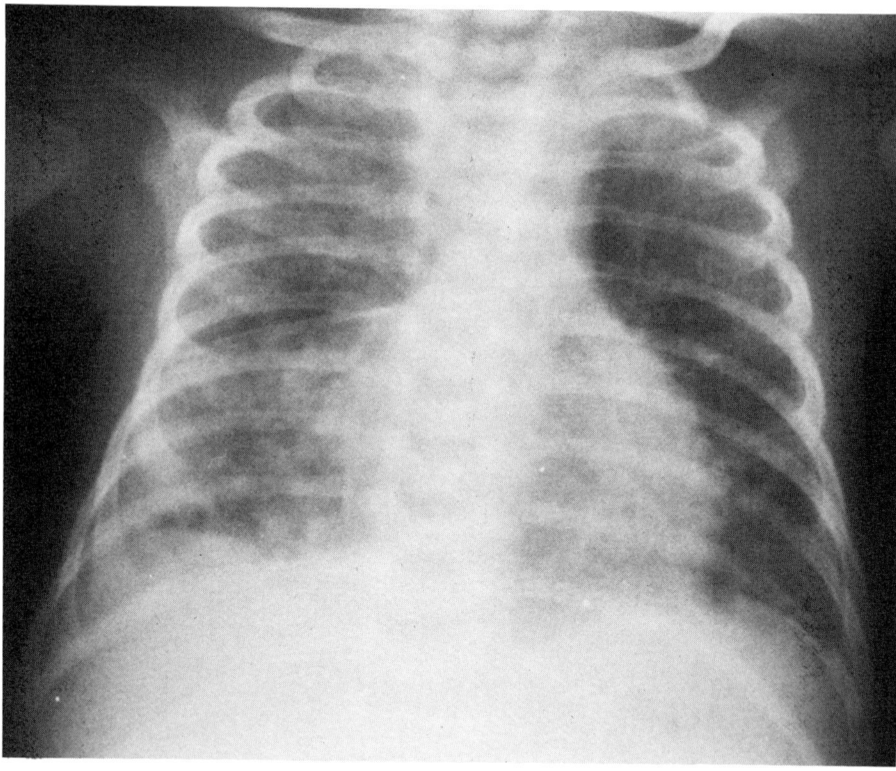

Figure 34. Chlamydial pneumonia. This 6-week-old child presented with a cough and an x-ray was performed. The extent of the bilateral infiltrate surprised everyone as the child was not as sick as the x-ray appeared to show. This is very typical of chlamydial pneumonia and following a course of erythromycin, the lung infiltrates eventually cleared completely.

Pneumococcal infection in the lung can present with a typical lobar distribution. However, in children a peculiar rounded infiltrate may be identified with sharp borders. This appearance is not unlike that seen in the peripheral solitary tumors of the lung in adults. This so-called "round pneumonia" is very typical for a pneumococcal infection.[68]

Primary pulmonary tuberculosis may show a peripheral infiltrate with an associated unilateral hilar or paratracheal adenopathy. Other fungal diseases, such as histoplasmosis, can produce a similar pattern.

A miliary pattern on a chest x-ray again may be secondary to tuberculosis or another fungal infection (Fig. 36). Tuberculosis is a disease that should not be forgotten and is particularly common in immigrants from Southeast Asia and the Caribbean.

Aspergillosis can produce several different lung patterns.[69] Invasive aspergillosis occurs almost solely in the immunologically compromised host. A necrotizing bronchopneumonia often associated with blood vessel invasion and vascular occlusion occurs. Most commonly on the x-ray one identifies multiple peripheral rounded lung opacities with progression to cavitation. A mycetoma or fungus ball may develop in a preceding cavitary lesion of the chest. It has been described most commonly in previous tuberculous cavitary disease but is also identified in bronchiectatic cavities and lung cysts. Allergic bronchopulmonary aspergillosis is characterized by asthma, eosinophilia and recurrent pulmonary densities. There is an immediate skin reactivity to aspergillus antigen. This is a type I hypersensitivity reaction to noninvasive aspergillus growing in the bronchial tree. On the x-ray, one often sees transient lung opacities and proximal bronchiectasis. Mucoid impaction giving a so-called "gloved finger" appearance is also a characteristic x-ray appearance (Fig. 37). This is an important x-ray pattern to recognize as corticosteroids are the standard treatment for allergic bronchopulmonary aspergillosis.

Asthma

Usually the diagnosis of asthma is known and radiographs are obtained to look for complications. However, one must never forget that a foreign body may present with asthmatic symptoms. (See Fig. 21A.)

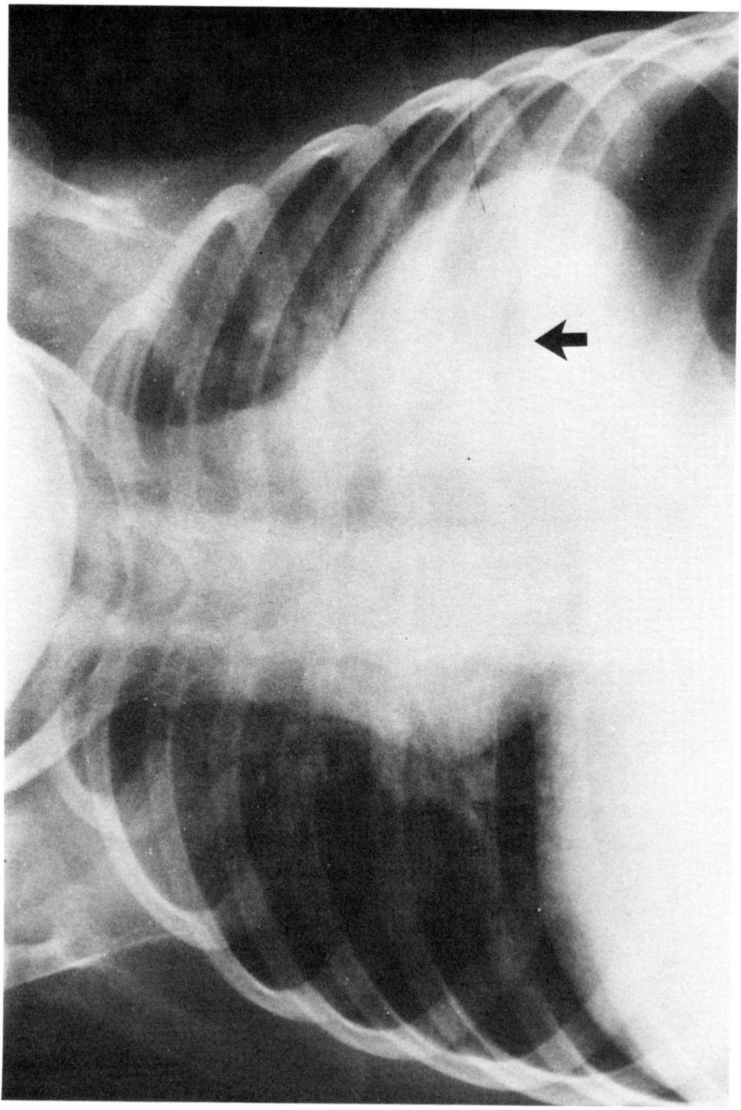

Figure 35A.

Illustration continued on the opposite page

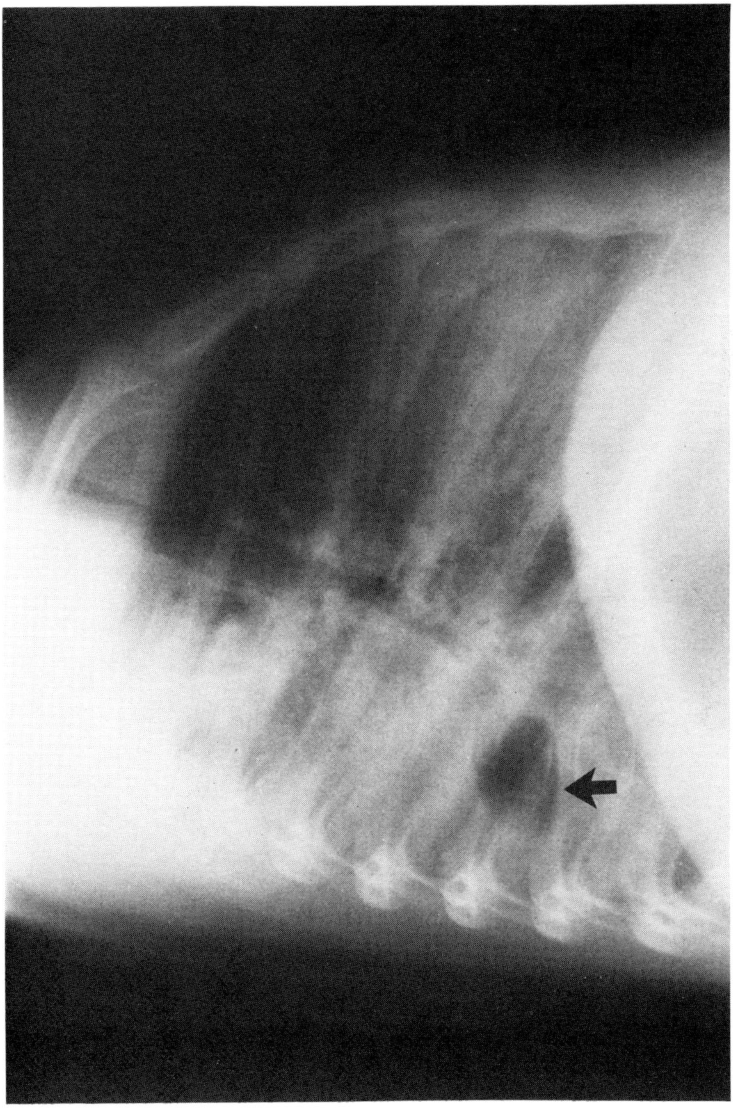

Figures 35A and B. Staphylococcal pneumonia. An infiltrate is identified in the left lower lobe with a fluid level. Arrow shows the fluid level on the PA and lateral views.

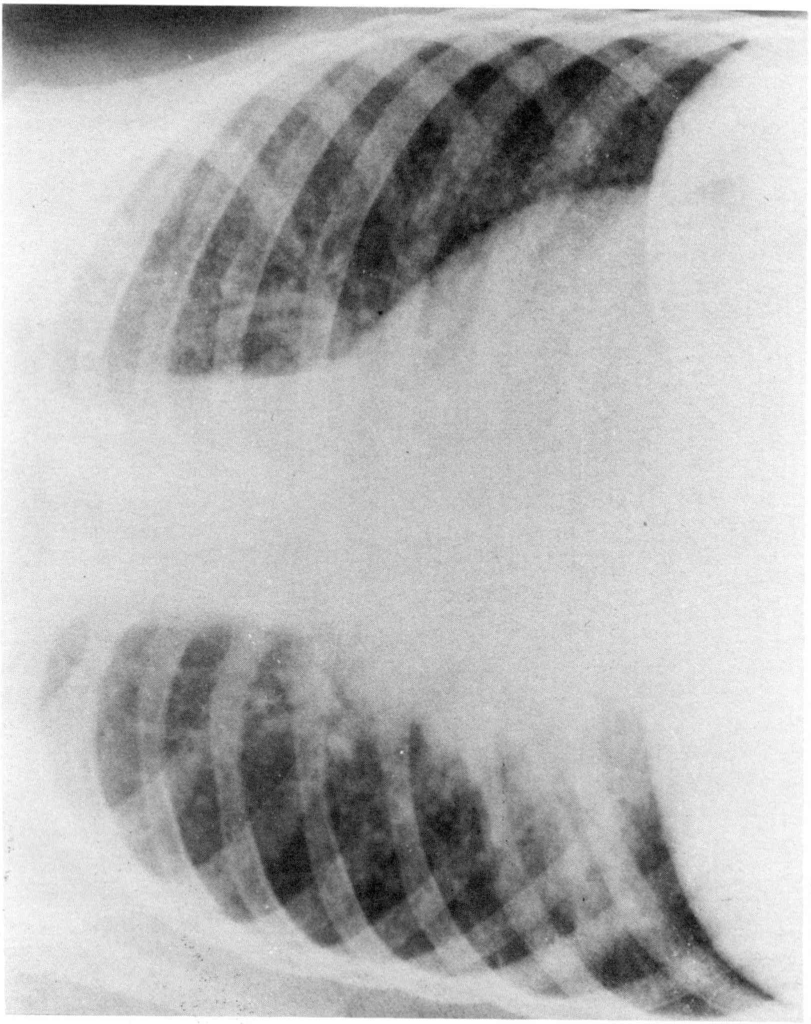

Figure 36. Miliary tuberculosis. Multiple small nodules are identified throughout the lungs. These nodules are evenly and widely distributed. Note the re-infection tuberculosis of the right middle lobe.

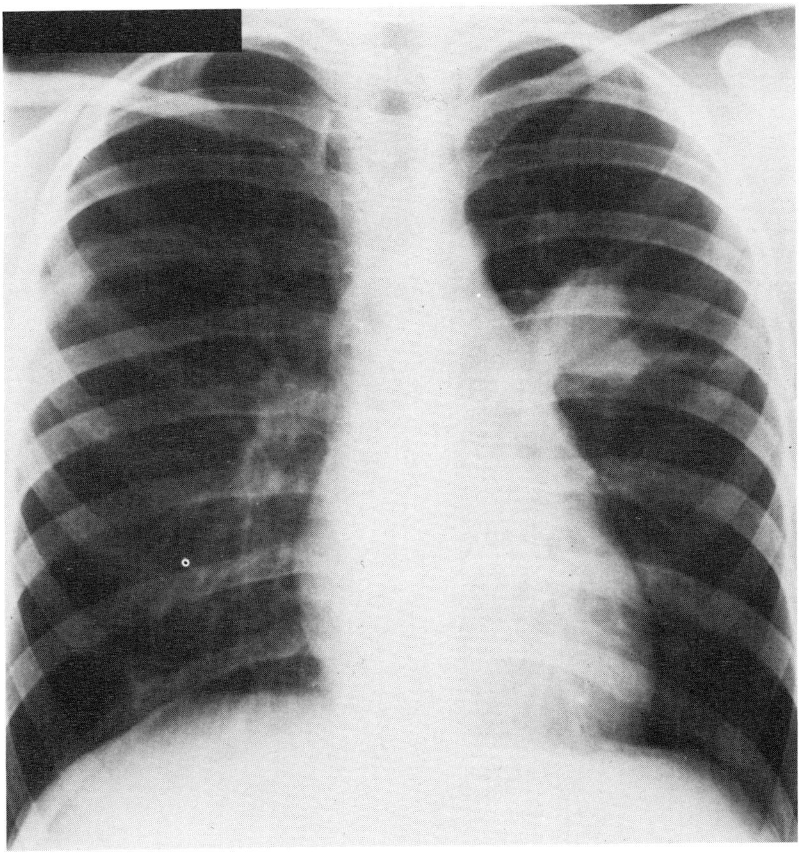

Figure 37. Mucoid impaction secondary to aspergillosis. A lobulated opacity is noted just lateral to the left hilum. This is sometimes likened to a gloved finger, although in this case only 2 fingers are present! Right 5th rib shows postoperative changes secondary to previous invasive aspergillosis.

The lungs and chest wall are usually overinflated. The lungs appear hyperlucent. The cardiac size appears small. Often the overinflation of the lungs is best appreciated on a lateral view of the chest when the diaphragm is identified as being flattened and even sometimes everted.

Complications of Asthma

Atelectasis. Tenacious mucoid sputum together with bronchial spasm and dehydration all contribute to a very high frequency of areas of collapse. These areas may be subsegmental, segmental or even occasionally lobar. Often these areas of collapse are interpreted as areas of infiltrates, secondary to infection and antibiotics are needlessly given to these patients. Often these patients, however, do have a viral lower respiratory tract infection. This may be a precipitating event in the attack of asthma.

Segmental areas of atelectasis are the most common pattern identified on an X-ray.[70] Often these are best appreciated as areas of collapse by their rapid change and improvement on serial X-rays (Figs. 38 and 39).

Rarely, areas of mucoid impaction can occur in the bronchi of asthmatics. While this may just represent areas of dried mucus within the bronchial tree, one should always be suspicious for mucoid impaction secondary to aspergillosis. (See Fig. 37.) Usually allergic bronchopulmonary aspergillosis occurs in patients who have already been diagnosed as having asthma for many years. Precipitating antibodies are present in the patient's serum.

Extraventilatory Air. Pneumomediastinum is more commonly seen than pneumothorax in asthmatics. However, it is not often appreciated until a lateral view of the chest is obtained. (See Fig. 32.) Usually it produces little in the way of symptoms.

Pneumothorax, however, will often produce marked symptoms. Although the pneumothorax may not radiographically appear very large in a patient who is already dyspneic due to asthma, this can be a disasterous complication. Physical examination on these patients is often unable to detect these pneumothoraces.

Gastroesophageal Reflux. While not the cause of asthma, gastroesophageal reflux can certainly exacerbate a patient's known asthma. This is often compounded by the patient's medication such

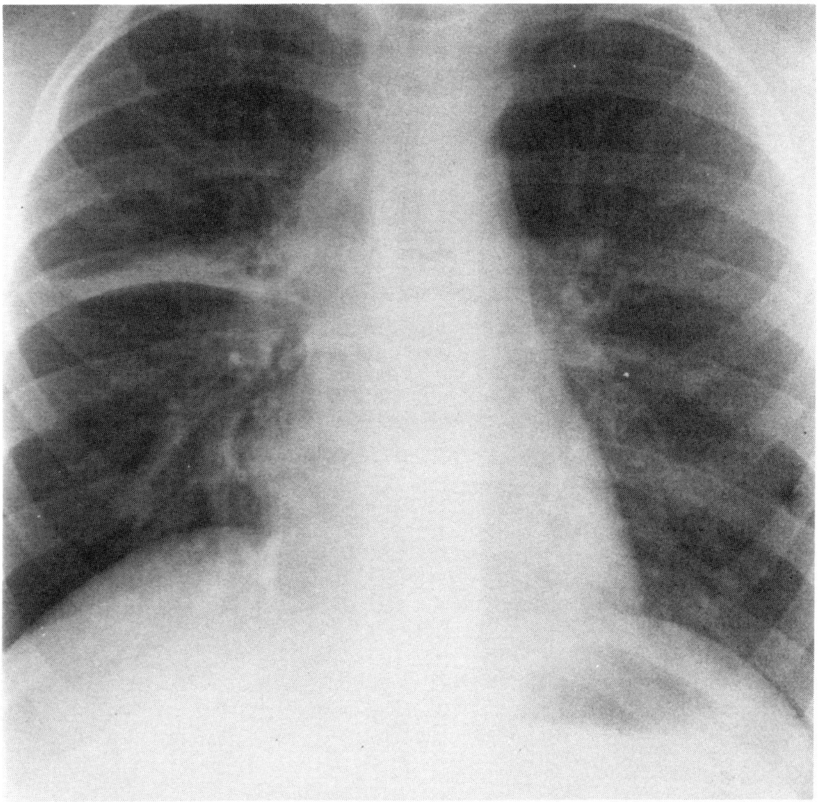

Figure 38A. Multiple areas of atelectasis in an asthmatic.
Illustration continued on the following page

as aminophylline, anticholinergics, and beta-adrenergic agents all of which decrease the lower esophageal sphincter tone.[71] Often these patients are asymptomatic otherwise from their gastroesophageal reflux.

Lobar Collapse

When there is complete collapse of a lobe, there are certain classical radiographic appearances on the PA and lateral chest x-ray.[72]

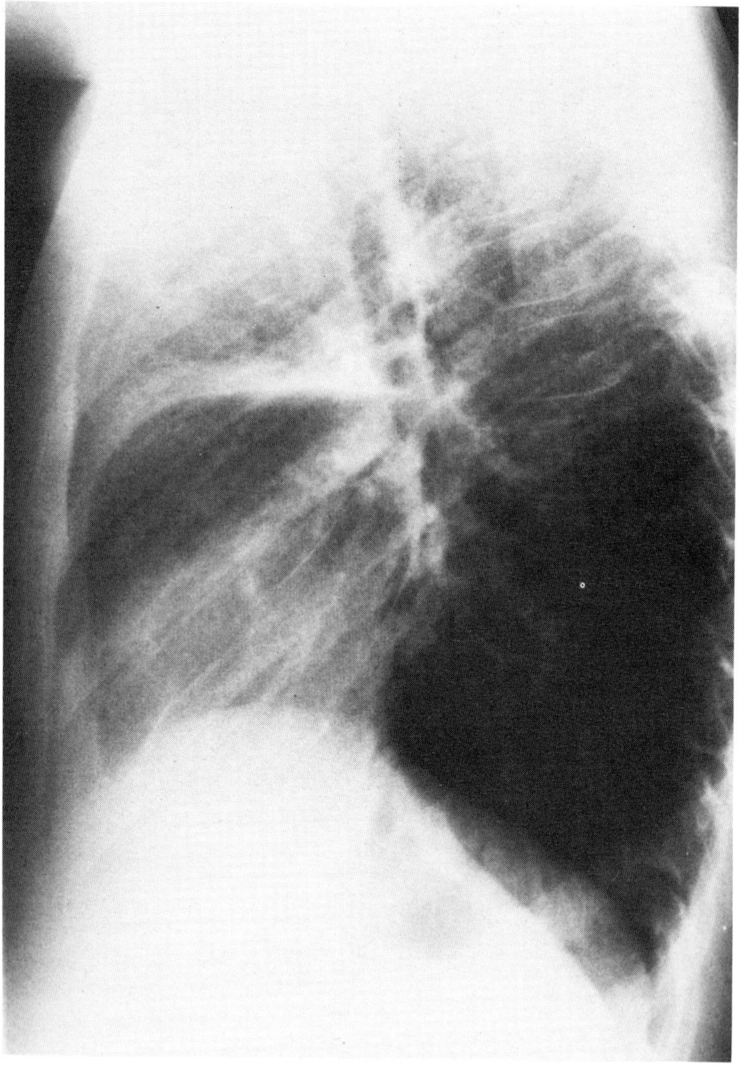

Figures 38A and B. Multiple areas of atelectasis in an asthmatic. This known asthmatic presented to the emergency room with worsening of his wheezing and a productive cough. Chest X-ray shows a "platelike" infiltrate just above the right minor fissure anteriorly. Note the loss of the right cardiac border secondary to right middle lobe disease.

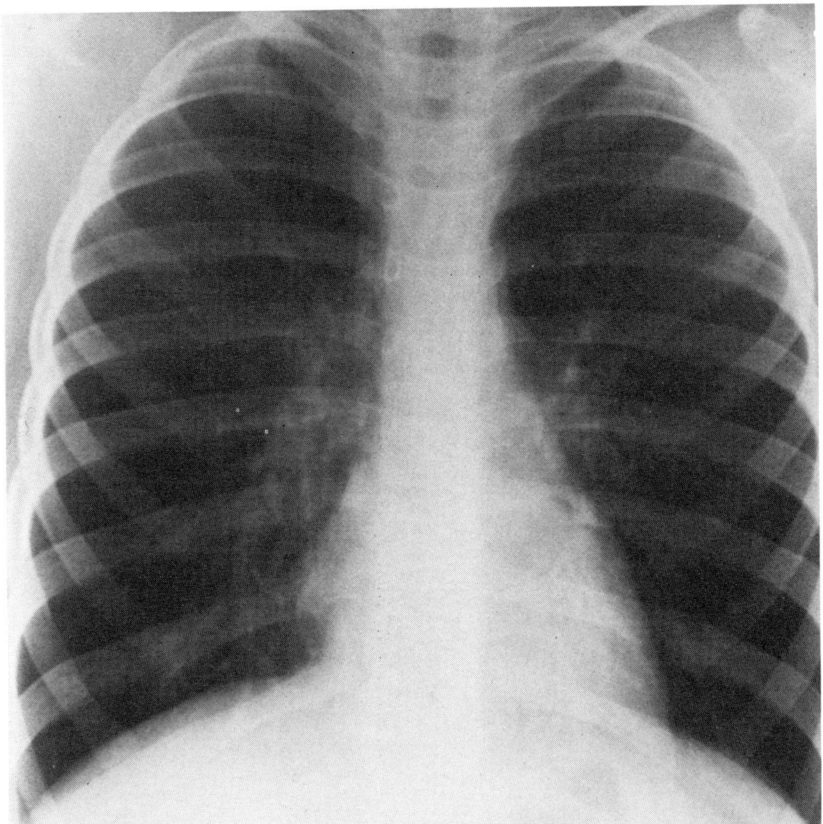

Figure 39. The same asthmatic patient 24 hours later shows complete clearing of the previously noted infiltrates and these must have, therefore, been areas of atelectasis. Note the "reappearance" of the right cardiac border. Such rapid resolution of infiltrates is very typical of the areas of collapse in asthmatics.

Lower lobe collapse gives a triangular density in the lower paraspinal areas as seen on the PA view of the chest. On the left side, this triangular density may not be appreciated "through" the cardiac silhouette. (See Fig. 19A.) One should always look very carefully in this area, particularly in postoperative patients. On the lateral view there is increased density over the posterior lower chest.

Lingular and right middle lobe collapse can be thought of similarly. These will cause silhouetting of the corresponding heart border and on the lateral view will show a triangular density extending from the hilum toward the anterior lower sternum.

Upper lobe collapse is dissimilar on the two sides. When there is left upper lobe collapse, an increased density is noted on the PA chest x-ray causing silhouetting of the entire left cardiac border. This density has a poorly defined lateral border and increases from lateral to medial. On the lateral view of the chest x-ray, the major fissure is displaced anteriorly toward the sternum. This displaced major fissure stays approximately parallel to the outline of the sternum (Fig. 40). The right upper lobe collapses, however, in a different manner. The right minor fissure can be identified as elevated and increased density is noted in a triangular shape over the right upper lung. On the lateral view of the chest, a triangular area of increased density is noted over the upper lung.

Diaphragmatic Hernia

While most diaphragmatic hernias present in the newborn period, they may occasionally be delayed in their presentation.[73] Another cause of delayed appearance is a previous group B streptococcal infection of the newborn which is associated with right diaphragmatic hernia.[74]

The more common Bochdalek-type of congenital diaphragmatic hernia occurs more commonly on the left side (Fig. 41). This is thought to be because the liver acts as a "plug". Traumatic diaphragmatic hernias are often missed at the time of trauma and in one large series, 94% were not appreciated initially.[75] The average interval from time of injury to time of recognition was 4–5 years.

The finding of bowel gas in the thorax makes the diagnosis easy. However, less common x-ray findings may include a single air-containing structure with an air-fluid level in the hemithorax.

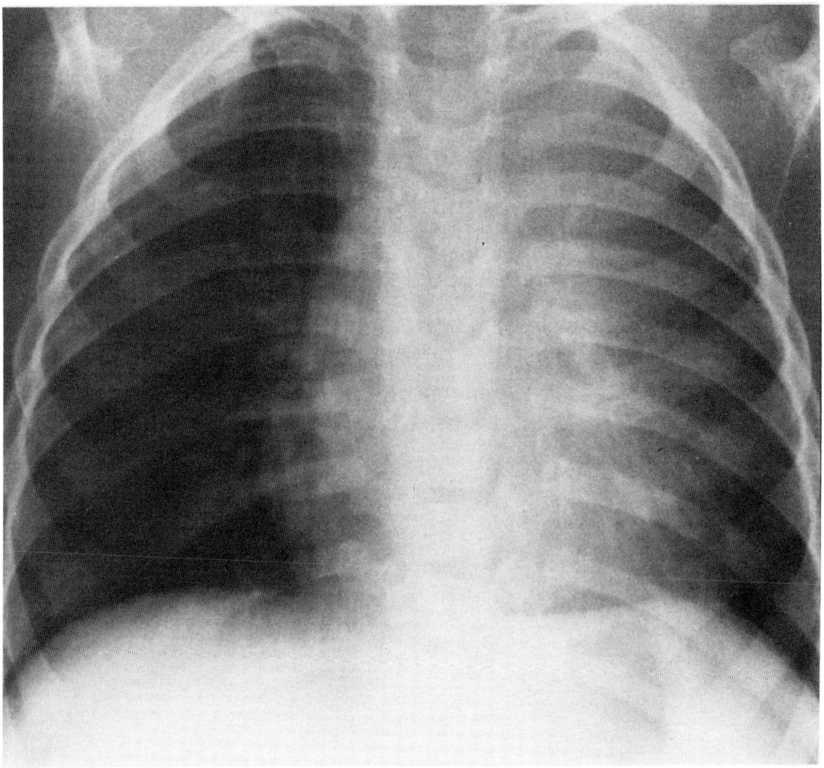

Figure 40A. Left upper lobe collapse. There is increased density in the left hemithorax with loss of the left cardiac border. Notice that this density increases from lateral to medial.

Illustration continued on the following page

This can even be mistaken for a hydropneumothorax. This single dilated loop of bowel often represents a volvulus of the stomach. Loops of bowel in the thoracic cavity may be completely fluid-filled and again this would give a misleading X-ray appearance. The differential diagnosis would then include cystic adenomatoid malformation.

Lung Trauma

Accidents are a leading cause of death in children one to 14 years of age.[76] Forty-seven percent of all deaths in children in this

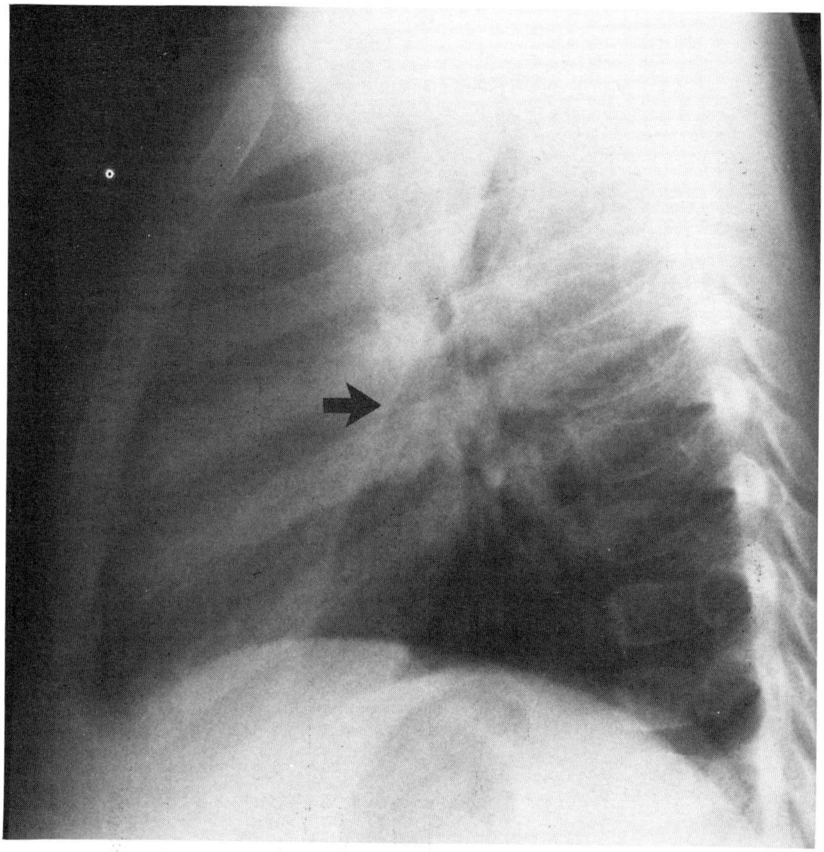

Figure 40B. Left upper lobe collapse. The opacified left upper lobe can be identified in front of the left major fissure (arrow).

age group are related to accidents. Acute trauma to the chest contributes significantly to this large figure. Chest radiography is obtained in the vast majority of these patients.

Lung Contusion

Lung contusion is produced by the rupture of alveoli and blood vessels producing an alveolar and interstitial hemorrhage with edema. This is the most common x-ray abnormality found in survivors of blunt chest trauma.[77] These x-ray changes usually develop within six hours from the injury. An initial period of clinical

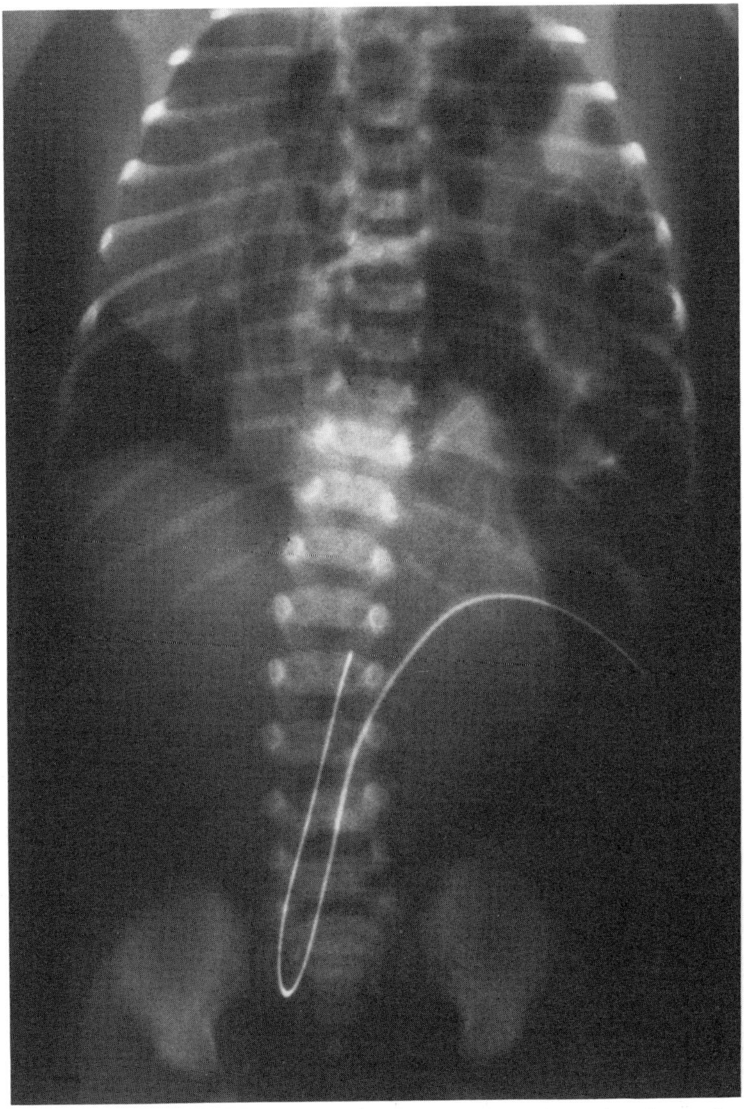

Figure 41. Congenital diaphragmatic hernia. There has been herniation of the bowel through a foramen of Bochdaleck. Note the lack of bowel contents in the abdomen which, clinically, is described as scaphoid. The mediastinum and nasogastric tube are displaced toward the right. Note the tip of the nasogastric tube in the stomach lies in the region of the left hemithorax. An umbilical artery catheter is identified with its tip at the level of the disc space between the 1st and 2nd lumbar vertebral bodies.

symptomatology with a normal X-ray is common. Hypoxemia frequently precedes the appearance of the pulmonary contusion. Also the size of the alveolar-arterial oxygen gradient and the magnitude of the physiological shunt are often larger than the X-ray opacity appears. Presumably much of the shunting that occurs following the trauma is not visible on the chest X-ray.

The lung contusion shows as a poorly defined area of increased density (Fig. 42). The size will depend on the extent of the trauma and contracoup injury is not uncommon. Clearing of the pulmonary contusion usually begins between 2–3 days following the injury. The contusion is usually completely cleared within 1–3 weeks. This temporal relationship to the time of the injury is very helpful in the diagnosis of pulmonary contusion. Certainly, if no clearing has occurred by 72 hours following the initial injury, then some other cause of the pulmonary density should be entertained.

Lung Hematoma

A lung hematoma is a macroscopic collection of blood within the lung usually following a pulmonary laceration. Initially the hematoma is often not visible roentgenographically because of the surrounding area of contusion. As the contusion clears, the lung hematoma becomes more obvious. A lung hematoma has sharply defined borders. It is commonly ovoid in shape because of the lung elasticity although other more bizzare shapes are often seen. A lung hematoma is commonly subpleural or mediastinal in position (Fig. 43).

The lung hematoma will not start to disappear until several weeks after the injury. It may persist as a nodule of diminishing size for up to a year. One must be aware of this possibility when confronted with a solitary pulmonary nodule. Often the patient or physician will have forgotten a previous history of trauma.

Pulmonary Laceration

The lung may be torn by the cutting edge of a penetrating object or the edge of a broken rib. The lung could also be torn from a blunt injury when the concussion wave can be of sufficient

Text continued on page 260

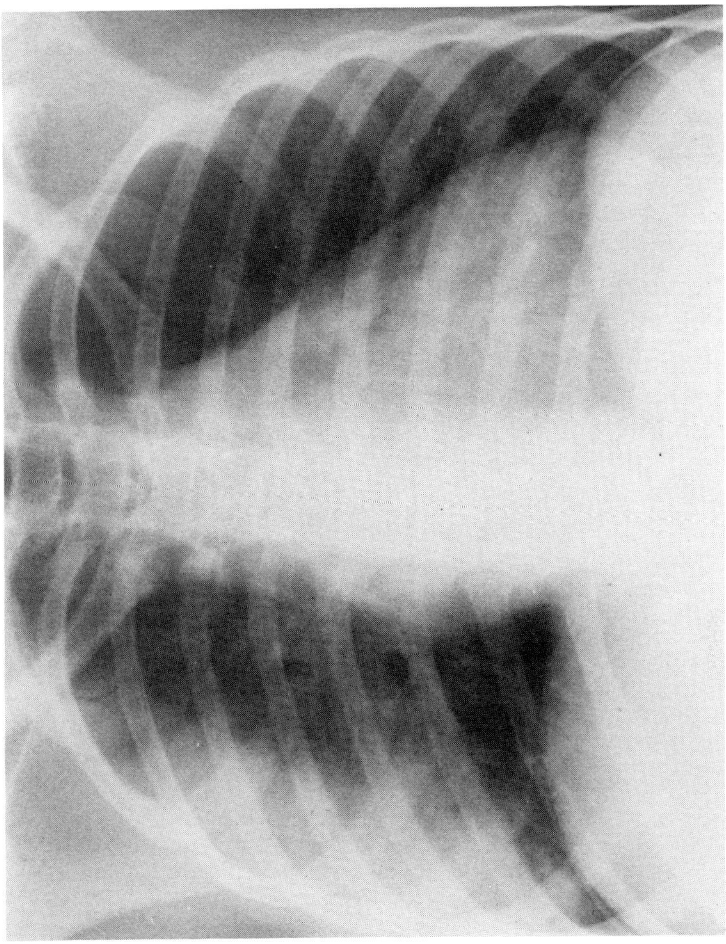

Figure 42A. Pulmonary contusion. Right-sided blunt chest injury was sustained by this patient. This film was obtained six hours later. Note the diffuse opacification of the right lateral lung secondary to the pulmonary contusion.

Illustration continued on the following page

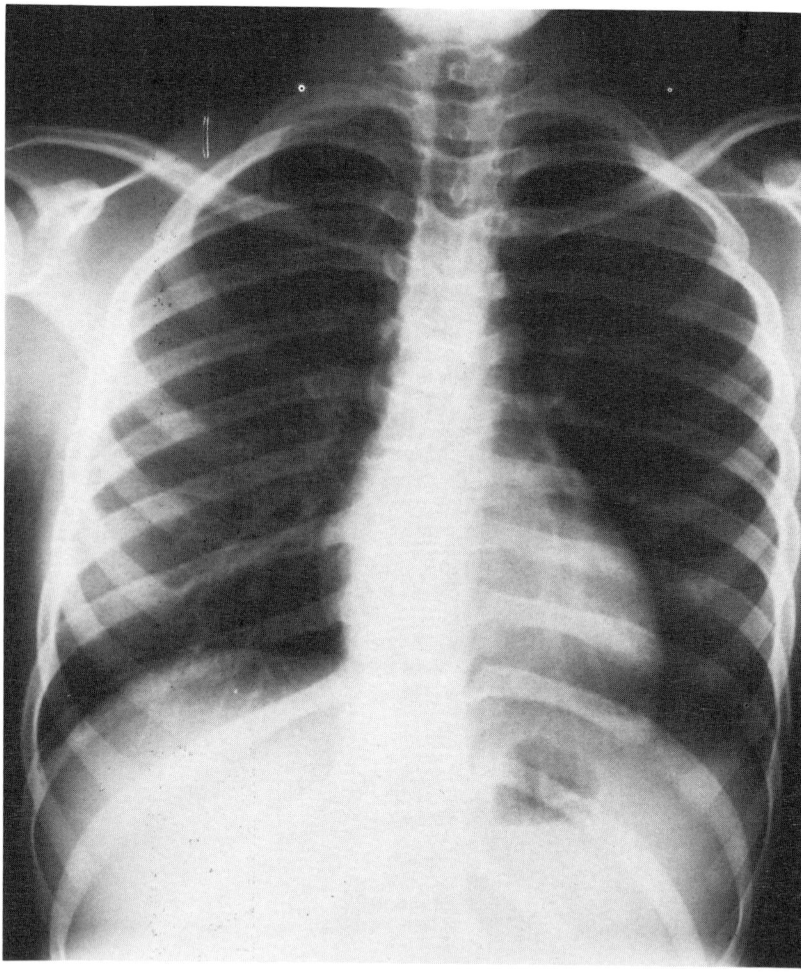

Figure 42B. Pulmonary contusion. Forty-eight hours later shows almost complete clearing of the previously noted right lateral chest wall opacification. Also note the fracture of the superior aspect of the right first rib anteriorly.

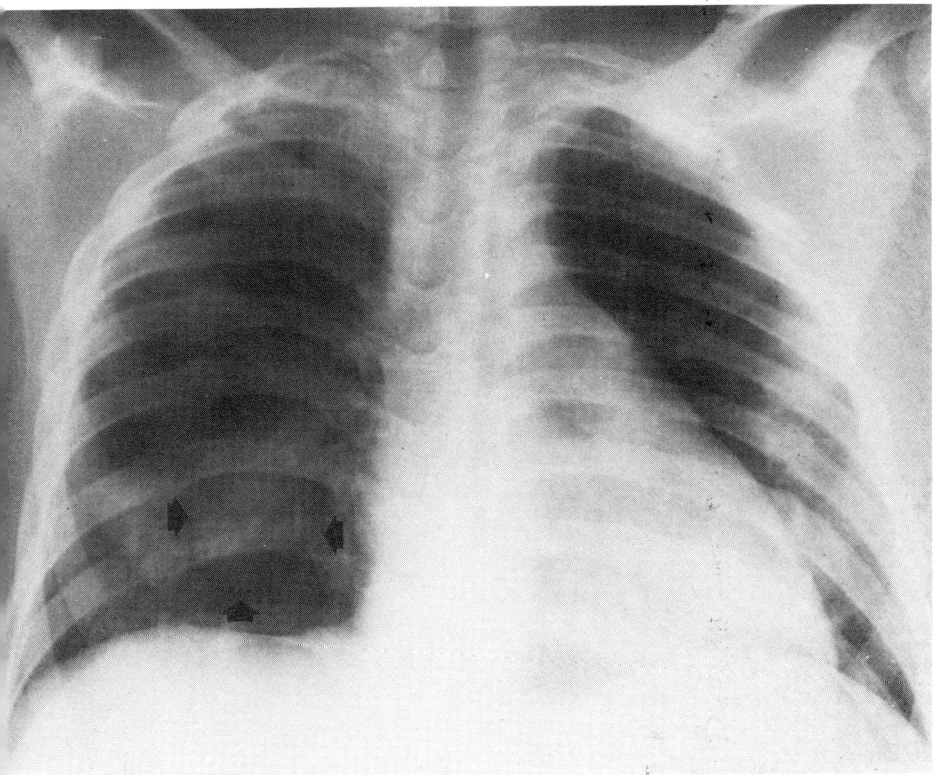

Figure 43. Pulmonary hematoma. This 10-year-old boy was involved in a motor vehicle accident and sustained severe injury to both lungs. Initially, there were bilateral pulmonary contusions. This film was obtained approximately one month following the initial trauma. Note the well circumscribed density in the right lung outlined by arrowheads. This only appeared on the x-ray following the resolution of the pulmonary contusion. This represents a pulmonary hematoma. Also notice the bilateral rib fractures with callus formation. The rib fractures extend from the 1st rib on the right side. There was also a fracture of the left clavicle. Incidental note is made of bilateral cervical ribs. This pulmonary hematoma took several months to clear radiographically.

magnitude to produce a shearing stress and tear the lung. An associated hydropneumothorax is frequent. The X-ray appearance of a pneumothorax and hemothorax must take account of the affect of gravity on the distribution of gas and fluid within the pleural space. Many of these patients are X-rayed on portable machines in the supine position.

A tension pneumothorax is diagnosed when there is displacement of intrathoracic structures. This is best appreciated by shift of the mediastinum. An important caveat is that patients who are on mechanical ventilators may have marked tension pneumothoraces, but only show minor degrees of mediastinal shift. This is because the positive airway pressure on the opposite side tends to counterbalance the tension pneumothorax. One should, therefore, look at compliant areas for evidence of a tension pneumothorax. The diaphragm and intercostal pleura will often show shift secondary to a tension pneumothorax when the mediastinum remains central. (See Fig. 31). Pneumothorax which does not respond to chest tube suction should raise the suspicion of a bronchial tear.

Pneumatocele

The transmitted force of a blunt chest injury may compress one area of lung, closing off a segment of its peripheral bronchial tree. This may be severe enough to produce an explosive-like bursting pressure within the lung distal to the occluded bronchus. Because of this, alveolar walls are ruptured. This acute traumatic pneumatocele is thus composed mainly of remnants of adjacent alveoli into which the air has dissected. The frequently associated air-fluid level is secondary to concomitant rupture of small vessels within the alveolar walls (Fig. 44). The traumatic lung space may be filled with blood (hematoma) or air (pneumatocele). Lacerations of lung adjacent to the inferior pulmonary ligament result in a characteristic X-ray appearance.[78] On the AP view of the chest, the air collection is noted medially and posterior to either side of the spine (Fig. 45). On the lateral radiographs, it is identified over the lower dorsal spine.

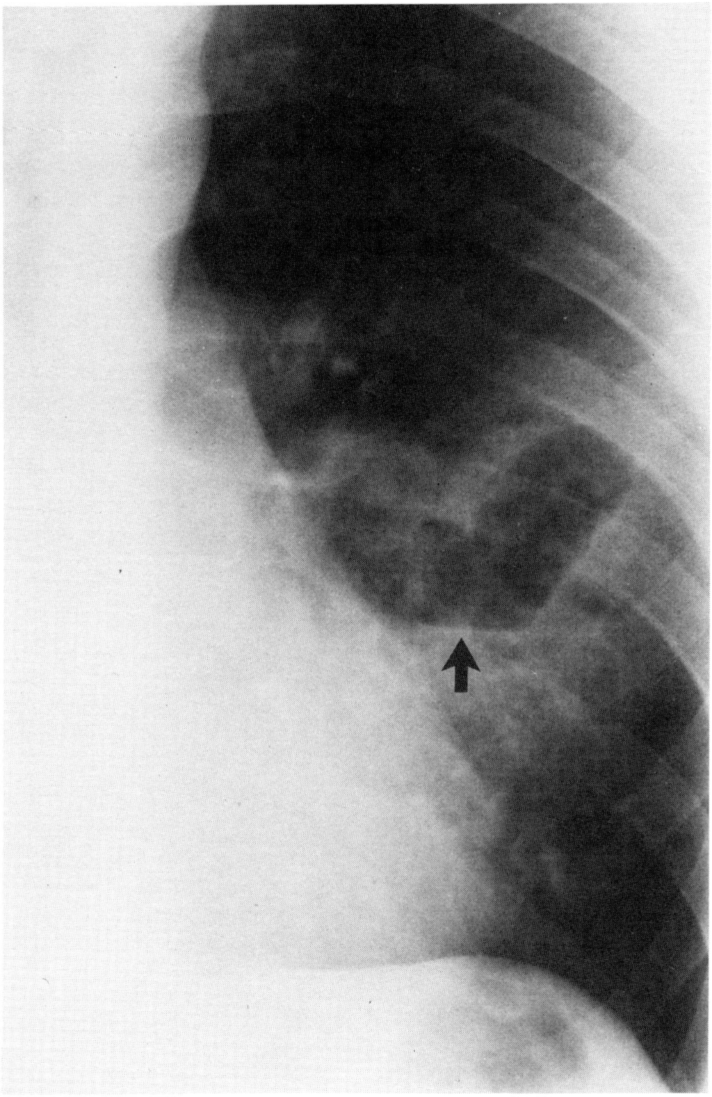

Figure 44. Traumatic parenchymal pneumatocele. Note the air-fluid level (arrow) which occurred in this patient following hemoptysis a day following blunt injury to the chest wall.

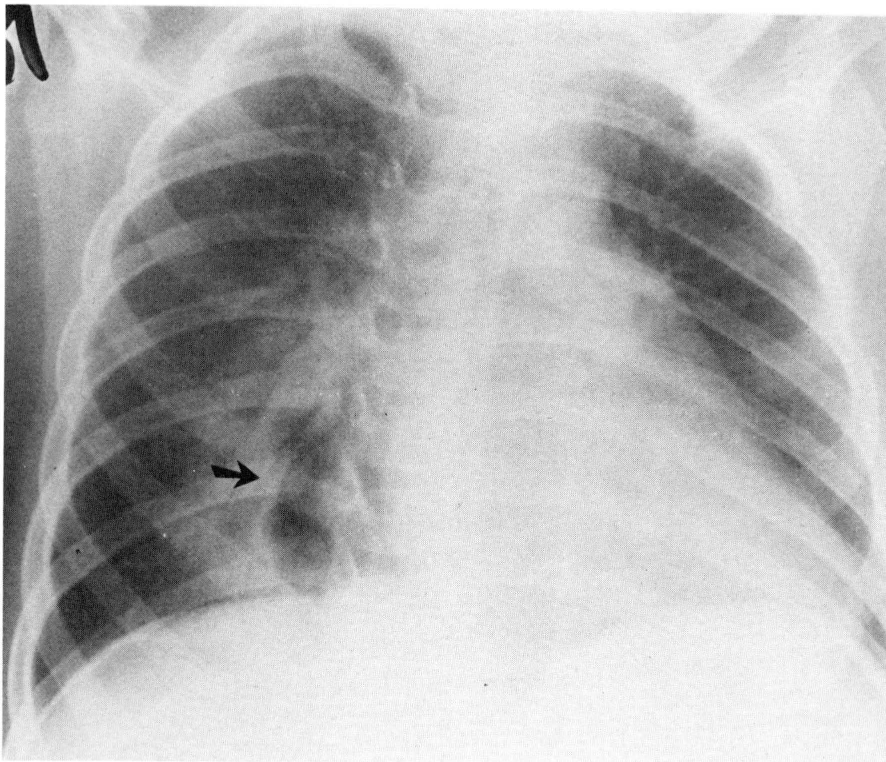

Figure 45. Traumatic pneumatocele of the right inferior pulmonary ligament. The arrow points to the pneumatocele localized in the right inferior pulmonary ligament. Lateral view of the chest showed this collection of air to lie posteriorly overlying the dorsal spine. A surrounding opacity is secondary to a lung contusion.

Rib Fractures

Rib fractures are uncommon in children because of the resilience of their chests. Rib fractures are often missed on the initial x-ray and only identified on follow-up films when callus is noted. (See Fig. 43). If rib fractures are identified on the initial x-ray, they should alert the clinician to the severity of the injury and also by their distribution make one aware of associated injuries. Fractures of the first 3 ribs may be associated with injuries to the aorta and brachiocephalic vessels. Fractures of the lower ribs posteriorly should alert one to the possibility of renal trauma. Anterior and lateral fractures of the lower thoracic area should make one suspicious for trauma to the liver and spleen.[36]

Bronchial Fracture

Fractures of the major bronchi usually occur several centimeters distal to the level of the carina.[79] Whenever one sees massive atelectasis, one should always be aware of the possibility of a bronchial fracture. When the bronchus is totally torn, the lung may separate and lie in the dependent position in the thorax. A pneumothorax is commonly associated with this severe injury.

Occasionally, these children may present much later with bronchial stenosis. It is thought that the connective tissue sheath around the torn bronchus remains intact at the time of the injury. Scarring occurs and these children present with air trapping or repeated infections. This complication should always be kept in mind in children who have undergone major thoracic trauma.

Aortic Tear

With rapid deceleration, the aorta can be torn at its two fixed points. These are the aortic root and the aortic arch just distal to the left subclavian artery. Mediastinal widening may occur, although this is a difficult radiographic sign to interpret. Most of these films are taken in the AP supine position and in children with a normal visible thymus. If any clinical suspicion exists, then an aortogram is recommended.

Radiographic features which would point towards a traumatic aortic rupture include displacement of the nasogastric tube and endotracheal tube to the right, a fluid collection over the left apex of the lung (the so-called apical cap), loss of definition of the aortic arch and widening of the upper mediastinum.

Injury to the Diaphragm

Diaphragmatic rupture occurs in 4–5% of patients involved in multiple injuries following blunt trauma.[75] The left hemidiaphragm is ruptured much more frequently than the right. Eighty-eight percent of ruptures occur on the left and only 11% are right-sided. The force required to rupture the diaphragm nearly always produces other serious visceral injuries. Because of this, the ruptured diaphragm is sometimes overlooked. When the tear is large, there may be massive herniation of abdominal viscera into the thorax.

Radiographic signs of diaphragmatic tear include pseudoelevation of the hemidiaphragm with obscuring of the left hemithorax by a mixture of gas and soft-tissue densities. Nasogastric tubes which enter the left hemithorax are virtually diagnostic of a diaphragmatic tear.

Cardiac Injury

Cardiac injuries result from blunt trauma to the chest compressing the heart between the sternum and spine. Most commonly, these contusions are frequently overlooked because of other, more obvious, injuries. Injury may occur to the pericardium, myocardium, valves or coronary arteries.[80] Cardiac tamponade can result before there has been significant change in the cardiac silhouette on x-ray. Ultrasound and EKG monitoring should be performed on all patients with blunt injury to the chest which may involve the heart.

Acknowledgment

We would like to thank Mrs. Bess Ficken for her secretarial work in the manuscript preparation and Daniel Yulish for his aid in research.

References

1. Sellars SL: Obstruction of the pediatric airway. *Ear Nose Throat J* 58:20, 1979.
2. Tucker JA: Obstruction of the major pediatric airway. *Otol Clin North Am* 12:329, 1979.
3. Joseph PM, Berdon WE, Baker DH, et al: Upper airway obstruction in infants and small children. *Radiology* 121:143, 1976.
4. Maniglia AJ, Goodwin WJ Jr: Congenital choanal atresia. *Otol Clin North Am* 14:167, 1981.
5. Shirkhoda A, Biggers WP: Choanal atresia. A case report illustrating the use of computed tomography. *Radiology* 142:93, 1982.
6. Capitanio MA, Kirkpatrick JA: Nasopharyngeal lymphoid tissue: Roentgen observations in 257 children two years of age or less. *Radiology* 96:389, 1970.
7. Capitanio MA, Kirkpatrick JA Jr: Upper respiratory tract obstruction in infants and children. *Radiol Clin North Am* 6:265, 1968.
8. Luke MJ, Mehrizi A, Folger GM Jr, et al: Chronic nasopharyngeal obstruction as a cause of cardiomegaly, cor pulmonale, and pulmonary edema. *Pediatrics* 37:762, 1966.
9. Levy AM, Tabakin BS, Hanson JS, et al: Hypertrophied adenoids causing pulmonary hypertension and severe congestive heart failure. *N Engl J Med* 277:506, 1967.
10. Gerald B, Dungan WT: Cor pulmonale and pulmonary edema in children secondary to chronic upper airway obstruction. *Radiology* 90:679, 1968.
11. Cayler GG, Johnson EE, Lewis BE, et al: Heart failure due to enlarged tonsils and adenoids. The cardiorespiratory syndrome of increased airway resistance. *Am J Dis Child* 118:708, 1969.
12. Rowland TW, Nordstrom LG, Bean MS, et al: Chronic upper airway obstruction and pulmonary hypertension in Down's syndrome. *Am J Dis Child* 135:1050, 1981.
13. Jeresaty RM, Huszar RJ, Basu S: Pierre Robin syndrome. Cause of respiratory obstruction, cor pulmonale, and pulmonary edema. *Am J Dis Child* 117:710, 1969.
14. Sato Y, Dunbar JS: Abnormalities of the pharynx and prevertebral soft tissues in infectious mononucleosis. *AJR* 134:149, 1980.
15. Wolfe JA, Rowe LD: Upper airway obstruction in infectious mononucleosis. *Ann Otol* 89:430, 1980.
16. Kravath RE, Pollak CP, Borowiecki B: Hypoventilation during sleep in children who have lymphoid airway obstruction treated by nasopharyngeal tube and T and A. *Pediatrics* 59:865, 1977.
17. Strauss M, Widome MD, Roland PS: Nasopharyngeal hemangioma causing airway obstruction in infancy. *Laryngoscope* 91:1365, 1981.
18. Holman CB, Miller WE: Juvenile nasopharyngeal fibroma. Roentgenologic characteristics. *AJR* 94:292, 1965.
19. Swischuk LE, Smith PC, Fagan CJ: Abnormalities of the pharynx and larynx in childhood. *Semin Roentgenol* 9:283, 1974.
20. Dunbar JS: Upper respiratory tract obstruction in infants and children. *AJR* 109:227, 1970.

21. Paez P, Warren WS, Srouji MN: Stridor as the presenting symptom of lingual thyroglossal duct cyst in an infant. *Clin Pediatr* 13:1077, 1974.
22. Grunebaum M, Moskowitz G: The retropharyngeal soft tissues in young infants with hypothyroidism. *AJR* 108:543, 1970.
23. Kushner DC, Harris GBC: Obstructing lesions of the larynx and trachea in infants and children. *Radiol Clin North Am* 16:181, 1978.
24. Slovis TL, Haller JO, Berdon WE, et al: Noninvasive visualization of the pediatric airway. *Curr Probl Diagn Radiol* 8:1, 1979.
25. Swischuk LE: Acute respiratory distress in the infant. *Radiol Clin North Am* 16:77, 1978.
26. Lazoritz S, Saunders BS, Bason WM: Management of acute epiglottitis. *Crit Care Med* 7:285, 1979.
27. Cavanaugh RM Jr, Newsum JK: Supraglottitis in children: Evaluation and management. *South Med J* 73:1353, 1980.
28. Battaglia JD, Lockhart CH: Management of acute epiglottitis by nasotracheal intubation. *Am J Dis Child* 129:334, 1975.
29. Poole CA, Altman DH: Acute epiglottitis in children. *Radiology* 80:798, 1963.
30. Watts FB Jr, Slovis TL: The enlarged epiglottis. *Pediatr Radiol* 5:133, 1977.
31. Shackelford GD, Siegel MJ, McAlister WH: Subglottic edema in acute epiglottitis in children. *AJR* 131:603, 1978.
32. Berdon WE, Baker DH: Vascular anomalies and the infant lung: Rings, slings, and other things. *Semin Roentgenol* 7:39, 1972.
33. Chang LWM, Lee FA, Gwinn JL: Normal lateral deviation of the trachea in infants and children. *AJR* 109:247, 1970.
34. Kirchner JA: Cervical mediastinal emphysema. *Arch Otolaryngol* 106:368, 1980.
35. Blazer S, Naveh Y, Friedman A: Foreign body in the airway. A review of 200 cases. *Am J Dis Child* 134:68, 1980.
36. Swischuk LE: *Emergency Radiology of the Acutely Ill or Injured Child.* Baltimore. Williams and Wilkins Co., 1979.
37. Grunebaum M, Adler S, Varsano I: The paradoxical movement of the mediastinum. A diagnostic sign of foreign-body aspiration during childhood. *Pediatr Radiol* 8:213, 1979.
38. Berger PE, Kuhn JP, Kuhns LR: Computed tomography and the occult tracheobronchial foreign body. *Radiology* 134:133, 1980.
39. Kassner EG, Solomon NA, Steiner P, et al: Persisting perfusion defects after bronchoscopic removal or spontaneous expulsion of aspirated foreign objects. *Radiology* 121:139, 1976.
40. Reed MH: Radiology of airway foreign bodies in children. *J Can Assoc Radiol* 28:111, 1977.
41. Vered IY, Rosen G: Foreign bodies of the lower respiratory tract in children. *Ear Nose Throat J* 58:57, 1979.
42. Capitanio MA, Kirkpatrick JA: The lateral decubitus film. An aid in determining air-trapping in children. *Radiology* 103:460, 1972.
43. Blumhagen JD, Wesenberg RL, Brooks JG, et al: Endotracheal foreign bodies. Difficulties in diagnosis. *Clin Pediatr* 19:480, 1980.

44. Smith PC, Swischuk LE, Fagan CJ: An elusive and often unsuspected cause of stridor or pneumonia (the esophageal foreign body). *AJR* 122:80, 1974.
45. Newman DE: The radiolucent esophageal foreign body: An often forgotten cause of respiratory symptoms. *J Pediatr* 92:60, 1978.
46. Kirks DR, Merten DF: Stridor in infants and children due to esophageal inflammatory disease. *Gastrointest Radiol* 5:321, 1980.
47. Humphry A, Holland WG: Unsuspected esophageal foreign bodies. *J Can Assoc Radiol* 32:17, 1981.
48. Milne ENC: Correlation of physiologic findings with chest roentgenology. *Radiol Clin North Am* 11:17, 1973.
49. Ashbaugh DG, Bigelow DB, Petty TL, et al: Acute respiratory distress in adults. *Lancet* 2:319, 1967.
50. Rinaldo JE, Rogers RM: Adult respiratory-distress syndrome. Changing concepts of lung injury and repair. *N Engl J Med* 306:900, 1982.
51. Petty TL, Ashbaugh DG: The adult respiratory distress syndrome. Clinical features, factors influencing prognosis and principles of management. *Chest* 60:233, 1971.
52. Pinet F, Tabib A, Clermont A, et al: Post-traumatic-shock lung: Postmortem microangiographic and pathologic correlation. *AJR* 139:449, 1982.
53. Greene R, Zapol WM, Snider MT, et al: Early bedside detection of pulmonary vascular occlusion during acute respiratory failure. *Am Rev Respir Dis* 124:593, 1981.
54. Ashbaugh DG, Petty TL, Bigelow DB, et al: Continuous positive-pressure breathing (CPPB) in adult respiratory distress syndrome. *J Thorac Cardiovasc Surg* 57:31, 1969.
55. Holbrook PR, Taylor G, Pollack MM, et al: Adult respiratory distress syndrome in children. *Pediatr Clin North Am* 27:677, 1980.
56. Lyrene RK, Truog WE: Adult respiratory distress syndrome in a pediatric intensive care unit: Predisposing conditions, clinical course, and outcome. *Pediatrics* 67:790, 1981.
57. Greene R, McLoud TC, Stark P: Pneumothorax. *Semin Roentgenol* 12:313, 1977.
58. Ziter FMH Jr, Westcott JL: Supine subpulmonary pneumothorax. *AJR* 137:699, 1981.
59. Schulman A, Dalrymple RB: Subpulmonary pneumothorax. *Br J Radiol* 51:494, 1978.
60. Riggs W Jr, Tonkin ILD: Lingular collapse with medial pneumothorax: Puzzling image in children. *AJR* 136:919, 1981.
61. Fisher JK: Skin fold versus pneumothorax. *AJR* 130:791, 1978.
62. Moseley JE: Loculated pneumomediastinum in the newborn. A thymic "spinnaker sail" sign. *Radiology* 75:788, 1960.
63. Smith CB, Overall JC Jr: Clinical and epidemiologic clues to the diagnosis of respiratory infections. *Radiol Clin North Am* 11:261, 1973.
64. Weller MH, Katzenstein AA: Radiological findings in group B streptococcal sepsis. *Radiology* 118:385, 1976.
65. Radkowski MA, Kranzler JK, Beem MO, et al: Chlamydia pneumonia in infants: Radiography in 125 cases. *AJR* 137:703, 1981.

66. Tipple MA, Beem MO, Saxon EM: Clinical characteristics of the afebrile pneumonia associated with chlamydia trachomatis infection in infants less than 6 months of age. *Pediatrics* 63:192, 1979.
67. Schachter J: Chlamydial infections. *N Engl J Med* 298:428/490/540, 1978.
68. Rose RW, Ward BH: Spherical pneumonias in children simulating pulmonary and mediastinal masses. *Radiology* 106:179, 1973.
69. Greene R: The pulmonary aspergilloses: Three distinct entities of a spectrum of disease. *Radiology* 140:527, 1981.
70. Eggleston PA, Ward BH, Pierson WE, et al: Radiographic abnormalities in acute asthma in children. *Pediatrics* 54:442, 1974.
71. Cohen S: Motor disorders of the esophagus. *N Engl J Med* 301:184, 1979.
72. Lubert M, Krause GR: Further observations on lobar collapse. *Radiol Clin North Am* 1:331, 1963.
73. Siegel MJ, Shackelford GD, McAlister WH: Left-sided congenital diaphragmatic hernia: Delayed presentation. *AJR* 137:43, 1981.
74. McCarten KM, Rosenberg HK, Borden S, et al: Delayed appearance of right diaphragmatic hernia associated with group B streptococcal infection in newborns. *Radiology* 139:385, 1981.
75. Wise L, Connors J, Hwang YH, et al: Traumatic injuries to the diaphragm. *J Trauma* 13:946, 1973.
76. Leading causes of death among children aged 1–14, both sexes: United States-1978. Vital Statistics of the United States, 1978 in Ca-A Cancer Journal for Clinicians, published by the American Cancer Society 32:30, 1982.
77. Wilson RF, Murray C, Antonenko DR: Nonpenetrating thoracic injuries. *Surg Clin North Am* 57:17, 1977.
78. Fagan CJ, Swischuk LE: Traumatic lung and paramediastinal pneumatoceles. *Radiology* 120:11, 1976.
79. Burke JF: Early diagnosis of traumatic rupture of the bronchus. *JAMA* 181:682, 1962.
80. Liedtke AJ, DeMuth WE Jr: Nonpenetating cardiac injuries: A collective review. *Am Heart J* 86:687, 1973.

12

Respiratory Failure

Eliezer Nussbaum, M.D.

Definition

In respiratory failure oxygen delivery and carbon dioxide elimination are severely impaired. Partial pressure of arterial oxygen (Pa_{O_2}) is usually < 60 mm Hg on room air and/or Pa_{CO_2} is > 50 mm Hg.

It is imperative that the prevalent barometric pressure be known when partial pressure of oxygen and carbon dioxide are evaluated. In patients with chronic obstructive pulmonary disease and chronic carbon dioxide retention, changes in partial pressure of arterial carbon dioxide (Pa_{CO_2}) may be more important than baseline values. For example, a rise in $Pa_{CO_2} > 10$ mm Hg per hour may suggest respiratory failure.

Etiology of Respiratory Failure

Respiratory failure[1–3] is not a disease but rather a complication of an underlying syndrome or disease entity such as, status asthmaticus,[4,5] acute epiglottitis, cerebral edema, hyaline membrane disease, pulmonary contusion,[6–8] cystic fibrosis, aspiration of foreign material, etc.

The causes of respiratory failure can be divided into three

Table I

Causes of Respiratory Failure in Children

Central Nervous System (CNS)
Central apnea or primary alveolar hypoventilation
Cerebral edema with rise in intracranial pressure
Intracranial hemorrhage
Meningoencephalitis
Intracranial tumors with autonomic disturbance
Obesity-hypoventilation syndrome
Sedative overdose
Respiratory Tract
Status asthmaticus
Acute epiglottitis
Severe laryngotracheitis
Foreign body aspiration
Pneumothorax
Severe pneumonia (staphylococcal pneumonia, pneumocystis carinii)
Hyaline membrane disease
Adult respiratory distress syndrome
Severe atelectasis
Bronchiolitis
Cystic fibrosis
Pulmonary edema
Diaphragmatic hernia
Cardiovascular Diseases
Congestive heart failure
Severe left to right shunt with pulmonary edema
Cyanotic heart disease with right to left shunt
Severe anemia

major groups: (1) central nervous system; (2) respiratory system; and (3) cardiovascular diseases. (See Table I.)

Pathophysiology

Respiratory failure may result from any of the following: (1) poor ventilation; (2) abnormal diffusion; (3) mismatching between ventilation and pulmonary perfusion; or (4) intrapulmonary shunt.

Although respiratory failure is associated with hypoxemia, the presence of intracardiac shunt or low barometric pressure (high altitudes for example) should be excluded. It is also essential to verify the level of inspired oxygen F_IO_2 so that alveolar-arterial oxygen gradient can be calculated. Normally this gradient is below 15 mm Hg with an increase > 30 mm Hg suggestive of hypoxemia secondary to ventilation-perfusion imbalance, poorly diffused alveoli or intrapulmonary shunting.

Partial pressure of alveolar oxygen can be calculated:

$$P_AO_2 = PiO_2 - \frac{P_ACO_2}{R}$$

$$PiO_2 = F_IO_2 (P_B - PH_2O)$$

PiO_2 is the partial pressure of inspired oxygen, P_ACO_2 is the partial pressure of alveolar carbon dioxide and R represents the ratio of CO_2 production to oxygen consumption. F_IO_2 represents the percentage of inspired oxygen, P_B the barometric pressure and the PH_2O the pressure of water vapor at body temperature (47 mm Hg). For simple calculation R is considered to be 0.8 and P_ACO_2 equals to $PaCO_2$.

The difference between partial pressure of alveolar oxygen and partial pressure of arterial oxygen represents the alveolar-arterial oxygen gradient:

$$P(A\text{-}aDO_2) = P_AO_2 - PaO_2$$

Calculation of $P(A\text{-}aDO_2)$ allows approximation of intrapulmonary shunting.

Types of Respiratory Failure

Respiratory failure[1,2,4,5] can be separated into Type I and Type II respiratory failure.

In Type I respiratory failure ventilation remains acceptable in the face of poor oxygenation. Children in the Type I category have low PaO_2 but normal or even low $PaCO_2$. Alveolar-arterial oxygen gradient is increased and is secondary to respiratory disability such as bronchial asthma, cystic fibrosis, severe atelectasis, etc. Hypoxia, in turn, may result in ventilation/perfusion imbalance leading toward pulmonary vasoconstriction, pulmonary hypertension, increased pulmonary vascular resistance and right-sided failure. In contrast, children with alveolar hypoventilation secondary to CNS causes may not have increased alveolar-arterial oxygen gradient.

Type II respiratory failure represents ventilatory defect with low Pa_{O_2}, rising Pa_{CO_2} and mismatching between alveolar ventilation and pulmonary perfusion. Some children may manifest both Type I and Type II respiratory failure during the course of one disease. For example, in status asthmaticus Pa_{O_2} will be low and Pa_{CO_2} may be originally normal or low (Type I). Subsequently, when status asthmaticus is in a progressive and deteriorating state, some children will manifest Type II respiratory failure with rising Pa_{CO_2} by more than 10 mm Hg per hour or $Pa_{CO_2} > 50$ mm Hg.

In contrast, some children will manifest Type II respiratory failure ($\uparrow Pa_{CO_2} > 50$ mm Hg, $\downarrow Pa_{O_2} < 60$ mm Hg) during the initial course of their disease and may later improve and shift into Type I respiratory failure. For example, a child with barbiturate overdose and severe respiratory depression may show signs of hypoventilation with rising Pa_{CO_2} (CNS) combined with hypoxemia secondary to aspiration and atelectasis. During such course, the patient may recover and regain respiratory drive with subsequent carbon dioxide elimination but persistent hypoxia secondary to remaining atelectasis.

Frequent arterial blood gas determinations are mandatory in patients with respiratory disorders who are in jeopardy of progressing toward respiratory failure.

Clinical Course of Respiratory Failure

The causes of respiratory failure were outlined in Table I. Clinical evaluation of respiratory failure is important but may be insufficient and unreliable. Arterial blood gases are of utmost importance and help in confirming the diagnosis of respiratory failure.[9] In general,[6–8] children in respiratory failure will be tachypneic, dyspneic, tachycardic, occasionally cyanotic (excluded are children who are anemic and therefore cannot demonstrate peripheral cyanosis), exhausted, irritable and lethargic or comatose secondary to carbon dioxide retention. Auscultatory findings reveal diminished breath sounds and occasionally pulsus paradoxus. Any child who is lethargic, restless, dyspneic or confused should have arterial blood gas determinations. Rising $PaCO_2$ may be indicative of primary ventilatory defect. In children who are cyanotic, exhausted, or restless prompt intervention should not be postponed due to unavailability of arterial blood gases. $PaO_2 < 60$ mm Hg (excluding congenital heart disease with intracardiac shunt) and $PaCO_2 > 50$ mm Hg support the diagnosis of respiratory failure.[4,5,9] The importance of serial arterial blood gas determinations is essential.

Therapy

Since all children in respiratory failure are hypoxic, oxygen should be provided regardless of level of carbon dioxide. If the oxygen requirement exceeds 60% therapy should not be withheld for fear of oxygen pulmonary toxicity. Correction of hypoxia and hypoxemia are more critical than oxygen pulmonary toxicity and may prevent lactic acidosis, cytotoxic cerebral edema with rise in intracranial pressure and decrease in cerebral perfusion pressure. Relieving hypoxia may prevent pulmonary hypertension, increased pulmonary vascular resistance and right-side heart failure. It should be remembered that hypoxemia *per se* may result in poor myocardial contractility and pump failure. Oxygen can be given by mask, nasal cannula, hood and tent. A special chapter is devoted to ventilatory support and respiratory care in the pediatric age group. (*See Part III/Chapter 17.*)

Since frequent arterial blood gas monitoring is mandatory in respiratory failure, indwelling percutaneous arterial catheters may be of significant help. Capillary blood gases are not reliable. Other means of monitoring are noninvasive and include ear oxymetry for continuous oxygen saturation monitoring and transcutaneous PO_2 and PCO_2 in children who are spared evidence of circulatory failure. In children with "adult respiratory distress syndrome,"[7,8,10–13] pulmonary artery pressure, pulmonary capillary wedge pressure, partial pressure of oxygen in mixed venous blood, intrapulmonary shunting and cardiac output should be measured by utilizing the Swan-Ganz flow directed balloon-tipped cathe-

Table II

Indications for Intubation and Mechanical Ventilation

- $Paco_2$ rise >10 mm Hg per hour (for example a rise from 40–50 mm Hg) in a child who is exhausted, restless or demonstrates a change in mental status
- $Paco_2$ above 50 mm Hg unresponsive to other modes of therapy
- Poor oxygenation with falling Pao_2 despite oxygen administration (For example, Pao_2 below 60 mm Hg unresponsive to high demands of oxygen supplementation)

ter.[7,8,10,11] Oxygen tissue availability (cardiac output × arterial oxygen content) may be calculated and "best PEEP" may be determined.[11,12] "Best PEEP" is that PEEP at which cardiac output and oxygen tissue availability are optimal.[7,11,12]

The child who is unresponsive to pharmacological therapy should be intubated and supported on the respirator. For example, a child with status asthmaticus and respiratory failure who is unresponsive to isoproterenol intravenous drip[4,5] with continuous rise in $Paco_2$ may require intubation and ventilatory support. Also, children who are exhausted with deteriorating mental status and ineffective ventilation should be ventilated regardless of their arterial blood gases. It is recognized that failure to provide adequate ventilation may result in cerebral edema with rise in intracranial pressure and subsequently poor cerebral perfusion pressure, brain damage and death.

Tables II, III and IV outline the indications for intubation, mechanical ventilation and criteria for weaning a patient off the respirator.

Table III

Indications for Intubation without Mechanical Ventilation

- Life-threatening upper airway obstruction (for example, acute epiglottitis)
- Comatose children with inadequate pulmonary toilet
- Central nervous depression accompanied by fatigue and potential life-threatening aspiration

(In Nussbaum (Ed.): *Pediatric Respiratory Disorders—Clinical Approaches.* Grunne & Stratton [in press].)

Table IV
Indications for Weaning a Child off the Respirator

- $Paco_2$ <50 mm Hg and Pao_2 >80 mm Hg on 40% inspired oxygen
- Negative peak inspiratory pressure > −20 cmH_2O
- Tidal volume more than 5 cc/kg of body weight
- Forced vital capacity more than 15 cc/kg of body weight in a child who can perform the test
- P $(A-aDo_2)$ less than 300 mm Hg on 100% oxygen
- Shunt fraction $(\dot{Q}_S/\dot{Q}_T)$ less than 15% on 100% oxygen
- The ratio of dead space to tidal volume (V_D/V_T) less than 0.55

Children who are candidates for extubation should be able to maintain arterial pH between 7.35 and 7.45, Pao_2 > 80 mm Hg and $Paco_2$ < 50 mm Hg on 40% inspired oxygen, breathe spontaneously, not dyspneic and with adequate cough and gag reflexes. The process of extubation is outlined in *Part III/Chapter 17* dealing with the respiratory care of the pediatric age group.

The use of isoproterenol (Isuprel) in respiratory failure of status asthmaticus is outlined in *Part III/Chapter 14*. The management of the child with adult respiratory distress syndrome is outlined in *Part III/Chapter 15*. The therapy of the child with respiratory failure secondary to acute epiglottitis is outlined in *Part III/Chapter 13*. The management of barbiturate overdose is outlined in *Part IV/Chapter 21*.

References

1. Newth CJL: Recognition and management of respiratory failure. *Pediatr Clin North Am* 26:617, 1979.
2. Martin L: Respiratory failure. *Med Clin North Am* 61:1369, 1977.
3. Wanner A: Conservative management of acute respiratory failure. *Prac Cardio* 5:32, 1978.
4. Simons FER, Pierson WE, Bierman CW: Respiratory failure in childhood status asthmaticus. *Am J Dis Child* 131:1097, 1977.
5. Simpson H, Mitchell I, Inglis JM, et al: Severe ventilatory failure in asthma in children. Experience of 13 episodes over 6 years. *Arch Dis Child* 53:714, 1978.
6. Hopewell PC, Murray JF: The adult respiratory distress syndrome. *Ann Rev Med* 27:343, 1976.

7. Holbrook PR, Taylor G, Pollack MM, et al: Adult respiratory distress syndrome in children. *Pediatr Clin North Am* 27:677, 1980.
8. Lyrene RK, Truog WE: Adult respiratory distress syndrome in a pediatric intensive care unit: Predisposing conditions, clinical course, and outcome. *Pediatrics* 67:790, 1981.
9. Tumalewicz WE: Assessment of arterial blood oxygenation in various states of acute respiratory failure. *Anaesth Resusc Intensive Ther* 3:25, 1975.
10. Peters RM: Lifesaving measures in acute respiratory distress syndrome. *Am J Surg* 138:368, 1979.
11. Gallagher TJ, Civetta JM, Kirby RR: Terminology update: Optimal PEEP. *Crit Care Med* 6:323, 1978.
12. Bone RC: Treatment of adult respiratory distress syndrome with diuretics, dialysis, and positive end-expiratory pressure. *Crit Care Med* 6:136, 1978.
13. Bone RC, Pierce AK, Johnson RL: Controlled oxygen administration in acute respiratory failure in chronic obstructive pulmonary disease. *Am J Med* 65:896, 1978.

13

Acute Epiglottitis and Croup

Christopher J. L. Newth, M.B.

Introduction

In early childhood, inflammation and edema of the laryngeal structures can cause life-threatening upper airway obstruction. Epiglottitis, the more serious type of acute laryngeal obstruction in children, involves the supraglottic laryngeal structures. Croup, the more common and usually less serious disease affects the subglottic area (Fig. 1).

Early distinction between the two diseases is critical, but unnecessary investigation, misdiagnosis and inadequate observation are still common. The general principles of management are now well established, but many physicians and nurses still lack awareness of the implications of upper airway obstruction in a young child, and the result is significant morbidity and even mortality, usually as a result of unrecognized hypoxia.

Incidence

Epiglottitis is a rare disease, although there is a marked regional variation in incidence.[1] In the Panama Canal Zone, epiglottitis is never seen, whereas in Toronto the incidence is 0.07 cases, and in Honolulu 3.1 cases per 1,000 pediatric admissions.[2]

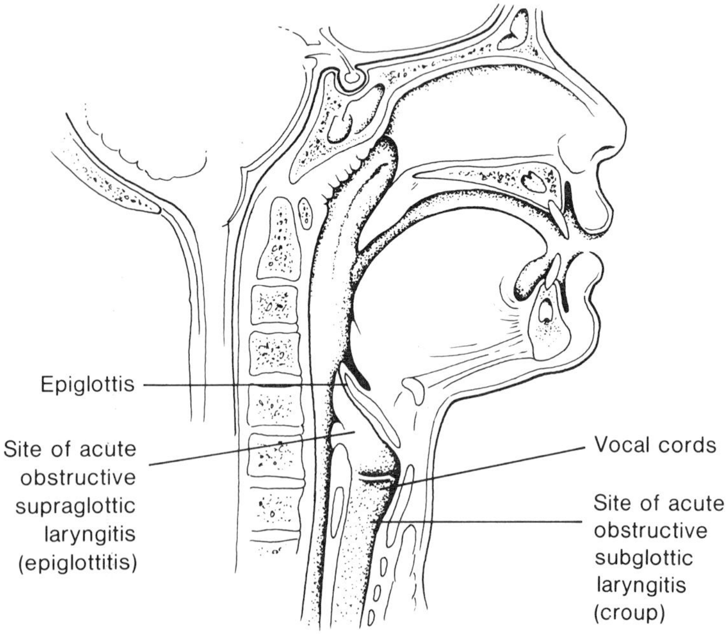

Figure 1. Sagittal section of upper airway showing sites of airway obstruction in croup and epiglottitis.

Croup, on the other hand, is a common disease. The incidence in the community is unknown, but it is probable that less than 10% of cases require admission to hospital.[3] Again, there is considerable geographic variation. In some regions it is almost unrecognized, whereas in Toronto, croup accounts for about 3 per 1,000 pediatric admissions.[2]

Epiglottitis (Supraglottitis)

Acute epiglottitis is defined as acute inflammatory edema and hyperemia involving the epiglottic and aryepiglottic folds. The degree of involvement and swelling of the supraglottic structures may vary, but the pharynx, subglottic region and trachea are never directly affected.

Hemophilus influenzae type B is the infecting organism except in a few cases where beta-hemolytic streptococci are the cause. In addition to local infection of the supraglottic structures, septicemia almost always occurs and is responsible for most of the systemic features of the condition. It is rare for meningitis or septic arthritis to occur as complications.[4] Chest X-ray films show abnormalities in up to 40% of cases and these are usually reported as bronchopneumonia.[4,5] However, these X-ray changes are probably more consistent with atelectasis secondary to airway closure from increased lung water and retention of bronchial secretions.[5]

Clinical Features (See Table I)

The onset is usually quite sudden, although in some children, it is preceded by a minor upper respiratory infection. The parents first usually note that the child seems lethargic, feverish and unwell. These symptoms progress over 2–4 hours, with a sore throat and difficulty in swallowing becoming apparent. The child becomes apprehensive, pale and toxic, and develops a marked tachycardia. As the supraglottic edema accumulates, breathing becomes noisy and the child adopts the characteristic "tripod position," sit-

Table I

Clinical Features of Epiglottitis and Croup

Factor	*Epiglottitis*	*Croup*
Age	Older (3–6 years)	Younger (6 mos–3 yrs)
Sex	Male = Female	Male > Female
Agents	Bacterial (H. influenzae type B + + +) (β-hemolytic strep +)	Viral (Parainfluenza 1 + + +) (RSV, parainfluenza 2, 3, +)
Season	All year	Late Spring and late Fall
Clinical	Sitting Toxic Drooling Stridor } uncommon Sternal recession } uncommon	Lying Nontoxic Not drooling Stridor } common Sternal recession } common
Progression	Rapid	Usually slow
Recurrence	Rare	Fairly common

ting up and leaning forward, with the chin thrust out and drooling saliva. Cough is usually not a prominent symptom and the voice and cry are muffled rather than hoarse. Inspiratory stridor is a late feature and is softer and much lower a pitch than in croup. There is often an intermittent or continuous expiratory snore. Depending on the severity of obstruction there may be suprasternal and sternal retraction, restlessness or cyanosis.

Total airway obstruction with respiratory arrest may occur precipitously at any time without preceding deterioration in clinical signs. This event may be provoked by attempts to visualize the epiglottis using a tongue depressor, forcing the patient to lie flat or by inappropriate investigations such as venipuncture, obtaining arterial blood, or lateral radiographs of the neck. The exact mechanism of this acute obstruction is not clear. The swollen supraglottic structures may be drawn into the glottis plugging the lumen, but in most cases, the epiglottis and aryepiglottic folds are so swollen and rigid that this mechanism is rather unlikely. Alternatively, pain, rigidity and swelling prevent normal swallowing of saliva. Subsequently, the patient aspirates oropharyngeal secretions either spontaneously or secondary to fatigue, septicemia or inappropriate stimulation, and obstructs from laryngeal (vocal cord) spasm.

The diagnosis of acute epiglottitis should be made based upon the history, general appearance of the child and the quality of the stridor. The diagnosis is confirmed by direct visualization of the swollen and inflamed epiglottis, usually during intubation. In the older child, indirect laryngoscopy can be performed quite easily to make a diagnosis. Sometimes, shining a light directly into the pharynx of the *sitting* child reveals the cherry-red, edematous epiglottis. Lateral neck radiographs are generally unnecessary and are potentially dangerous (vide infra).

Blood[6] and laryngotracheal[7] cultures may be positive for H. influenzae type B in up to 90% of the cases. In general, blood cultures are more often positive than pharyngeal and laryngotracheal cultures. Antibiotic treatment should be commenced promptly without waiting for bacteriological proof.

Epiglottitis occurs equally in males and females, and peak incidence is in the three- to six-year-old age group. Epiglottitis is more commonly seen where there are increased hospital admissions for acute respiratory illness and it occurs throughout the year. There can be large seasonal variations between regions, and peaks have been reported in all four seasons.[4,6,8–10]

Croup (Laryngotracheobronchitis)

Laryngotracheobronchitis is the major cause of acute laryngeal obstruction in children and is very commonly seen in pediatric practice. The disease occurs throughout childhood, and occasionally in adults, but the peak incidence is in the second year of life. It is more common in boys than in girls as assessed by hospital admission, and may be recurrent in up to 5% of patients.

Several distinct clinical illnesses have been described in various text books as part of "the croup syndrome," but in my experience there are two illnesses only: spasmodic croup and acute laryngotracheobronchitis.

Spasmodic croup. The child goes to bed well and awakes a few hours later with a classical cough, hoarseness and respiratory stridor, but without coryza or fever. The cause is probably laryngeal edema[11] and, particularly in the older child, vocal cord spasm of unknown origin.[12] It is a short-lived illness, rarely requires upper airway control and is easily managed with mist therapy. It is a relatively *minor* cause of subglottic laryngeal obstruction.

Acute laryngotracheobronchitis. (For clinical features, see Table I.) This is a viral illness and typically the child has coryzal symptoms for one or two days before developing evidence of laryngeal inflammation. The first sign of spread to the larynx is the gradual development of a harsh barking (croupy) cough and hoarse voice. Fever is variable and a mild leukocytosis may be present. The major clinical features are related to inflammatory edema and fibrinous exudate in the subglottic area which narrow the upper airway. This causes inspiratory stridor which initially may be mild and only audible when the child is disturbed and hyperventilates.

In addition, although the inflammation and edema may produce mild changes in the supraglottic area, they commonly extend down the trachea and bronchi producing viscid secretions. There is destruction of the ciliated epithelial surfaces of the trachea and bronchi which adds to the child's difficulty in removing secretions, leading to segmental atelectasis with subsequent mismatch of pulmonary ventilation and capillary perfusion. Involvement of the lower airways, superimposed upon the narrowed subglottic area results in increased respiratory work and hypoxemia. As respiratory effort becomes greater the stridor increases in intensity. As airway obstruction becomes more severe, suprasternal retractions and sternal recession appear, particularly in small infants who have more compliant chest walls. As in other forms of airway obstruction, signs of hypoxemia (restlessness, tachypnea, anxiety, tachycardia) occur before the appearance of cyanosis. Increased work of breathing, hypoxemia (often unrecognized), and lack of fluid and caloric intake will cause fatigue which, if prolonged, will result in hypercapnia and acidosis. Paradoxically, exhaustion may decrease the intensity of the stridor and retractions, and despite a rising heart rate and decreased air entry to the lungs, the inexperienced observer may interpret this as clinical improvement. Ultimately, the patient will collapse and die from hypoxia unless the obstruction of the upper airway is relieved. Fortunately, the vast majority of cases do not follow this pattern and resolve with the appropriate conservative management. Fewer than 2.5% of patients admitted to hospital with croup may require an artificial airway for relief of the obstruction.[3]

Para-influenza virus type 1 is the principal viral agent responsible for acute laryngotracheobronchitis in children.[3,12,13] Para-influenza types 2 and 3, influenza A, respiratory syncytial virus (particularly in children under 12 months of age) and rhinoviruses are next in importance. Measles virus is an infrequent etiological agent, but important if hospital admission is advised.

It has been postulated by Urquhart et al[14] that children with sudden onset "spasmodic" croup have had a prior para-influenza type 3 infection, and develop the disease from a subsequent hypersensitivity reaction to para-influenza type 1 infection.

Primary bacterial infection is now rarely the cause, and secondary bacterial infection is very uncommon although still occasionally reported.[15] However, in the period between 1920 and 1940 (the time demarcated by diphtheria control and the introduction of antibiotics) bacterial and super-infection of what was probably viral croup were commonly seen.[16,17] The usual organisms were Staphylococcus aureus, Streptococcus pneumoniae and Hemophilus influenza. The mortality rate was 10–40% for those hospitalized. Since 1940, this disease entity has almost ceased to exist.

Diphtheria as a cause of croup has rapidly declined with the widespread use of toxoid and is now rare.

Laryngotracheobronchitis occurs throughout the year, but the peak incidence is in the late fall with another smaller peak in the late spring. This pattern is related to the prevalence of para-influenza viruses in the community.[12]

Differential Diagnosis (See Table II)

The diagnosis of acute epiglottitis is rarely difficult, and, in most cases, easy to distinguish from its major differential diagnosis of acute laryngotracheobronchitis on the basis of clinical features. (See Table I.)

A foreign body lodged in the larynx or high in the esophagus can produce stridor and a distressing cough, but unlike croup and epiglottitis the patient is usually unable to vocalize effectively, and is afebrile. There may be a history of a choking episode while eating, or playing with small objects in the mouth. An inhaled laryngeal foreign body should be considered in any case of acute upper airway obstruction even if it can be dismissed immediately on clinical grounds.

Routine roentgenograms of the soft tissues of the neck to confirm an obvious clinical diagnosis are unnecessary. However, croup, epiglottitis, some foreign bodies, and retropharyngeal abscesses have characteristic radiologic appearances and when the diagnosis is truly in doubt, a lateral film of the neck can be invaluable. A person capable of establishing an artificial airway, along with the appropriate equipment, must accompany the child to the Radiology Department.

An inquiry should always be made as to the state of immunization of the patient. Laryngeal diphtheria is now rare, but must be the presumptive diagnosis in an unimmunized child presenting with a membrane on the tonsils. In an immunized child, this membrane is more likely to be from infectious mononucleosis.

Table II

Causes of Acute Upper Airway Obstruction in Decreasing Order of Frequency

Acute laryngotracheobronchitis
Epiglottitis
Laryngeal and upper esophageal foreign bodies
Infectious mononucleosis causing acute tonsillar hypertrophy
Retropharyngeal abscess
Laryngeal diphtheria
Acute angioneurotic edema

Similarly, measles may present with a croup-like prodrome and can cause embarrassment (and danger to an immunocompromised patient) if admitted to an "open" hospital floor.

Angioneurotic edema is a rare but dangerous cause of upper airway obstruction. The obstruction is from the swollen tongue and supraglottic tissues. The diagnosis is often obvious because the lips, cheeks and eyelids are usually involved as well, and urticaria may be present.

Pathophysiology

Croup and epiglottitis are primarily diseases in which there is difficulty *inhaling* air. The airways of a child are large in comparison with those of an adult. However, the absolute diameter of the infant's trachea is small causing a high resistance to airflow. A 1.0 mm increase in the thickness of the mucosa at the subglottic level (secondary to inflammation and edema) may cause a 75% reduction in the cross-sectional area in the neonate, but only a 20% reduction in the adult. Since there is an inverse fourth power relationship of the radius of an airway to resistance, such a decrease in cross-sectional area, as in the case of the neonate, results in a significant increase in airway resistance, and thus respiratory work.

This fixed obstruction should affect inspiration and expiration equally, although in young children, the tracheal cartilages are relatively soft. During inspiration against a fixed obstruction in the extrathoracic airway, large negative intratracheal pressures (relative to the atmospheric pressure around the neck) can be generated immediately below the obstruction by even small infants,[18] with subsequent dynamic narrowing of the extrathoracic trachea[19] which leads to inspiratory stridor (Fig. 2). As a consequence of the increased negative pleural pressure during inspiration, the compliant sternum and rib cage can be deformed with subsequent retraction of suprasternal tissues, sternum and costal cartilages. The opposite occurs during exhalation, with the extrathoracic trachea tending to "balloon". (See Fig. 2.) Thus, the obstruction to airflow is greater during inhalation than exhalation in extrathoracic upper airway obstruction. Figure 3 details these changes in ventilatory mechanics.

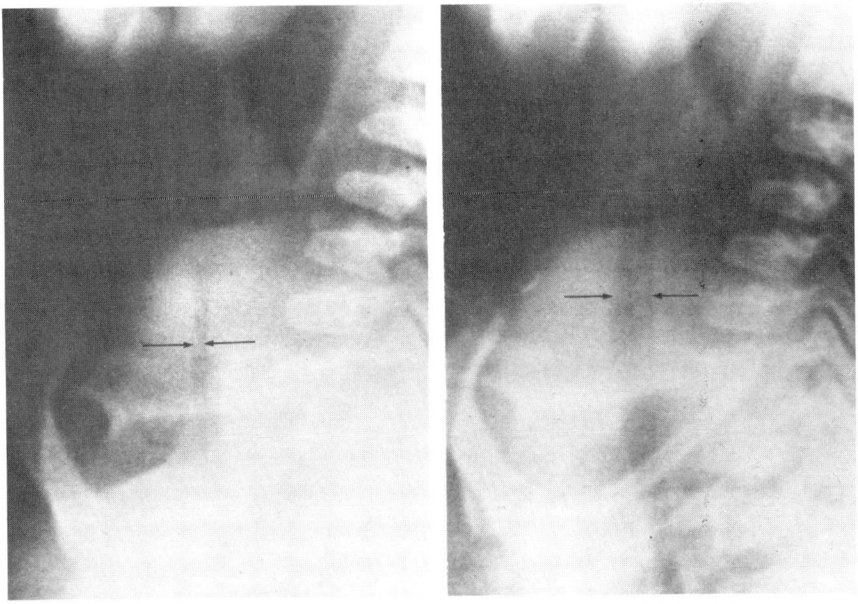

Figure 2. Lateral cineradiograph of the neck of a child with acute laryngotracheobronchitis taken during a single respiratory cycle. On the left is the narrowed extrathoracic trachea (arrows) during inspiration. On the right is the relatively widened extrathoracic trachea (arrows) during exhalation.

Several investigators[20–22] have confirmed that hypoxemia is the earliest important arterial blood gas abnormality in croup and that it is out of all proportion to carbon dioxide retention from alveolar hypoventilation. A recent retrospective study has found the same abnormality in epiglottitis.[5] The most likely cause of this hypoxemia is mismatch of blood and gas in the lung, and several mechanisms may contribute to it either singly or in combination.

First, patients with croup have copious secretions from widespread tracheobronchial inflammation, and the mucociliary "elevator" is lost because of destruction of the ciliated epithelium. In addition, there is an impaired ability to produce an effective cough with which to clear the airways in croup and epiglottitis. Retention

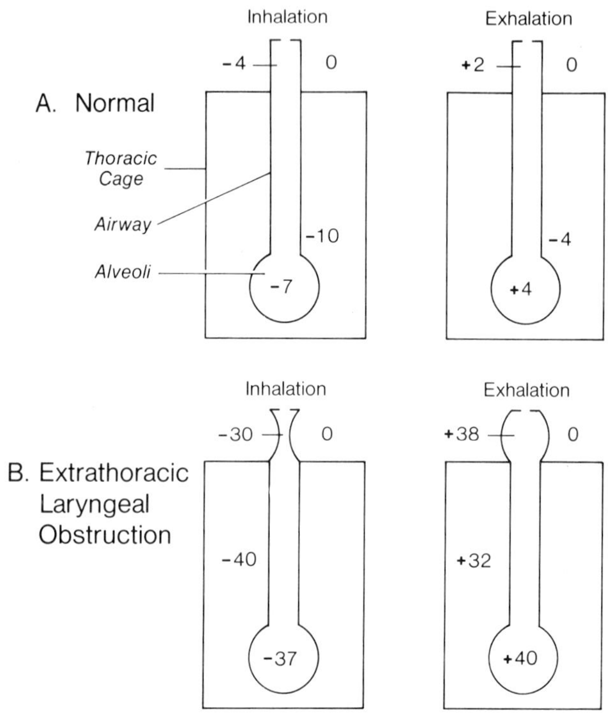

Figure 3. Each of the four diagrams represents the extra- and intrathoracic airways, lungs and thoracic cage. The numbers represent average pressures developed during inhalation and exhalation in (A) a normal child, and (B) a patient with extrathoracic airway obstruction. Dynamic compression causing narrowing of the extrathoracic trachea results both from the large negative pressures generated immediately below the obstruction, and the increased airflow through the narrow segment (Venturi effect).

of these secretions can lead to subclinical plugging of bronchioles and small bronchi and thus ventilation-perfusion mismatch. Occasionally, these secretions may lead to blockage of a larger bronchus and cause overt atelectasis, often of the right middle lobe.[5]

Second, Widdicombe et al[23] have demonstrated in animals that irritation of the larynx and trachea can cause reflex bronchoconstriction of more distal airways. This may happen in croup and epiglottitis patients with subsequent maldistribution of ventilation.

Last, patients with croup and epiglottitis have presented in frank pulmonary edema.[24–26] In less severe cases of both diseases, subclinical increases in lung water may cause small airway closure and flooding of some alveoli with hypoxemia secondary to ventilation-perfusion mismatch, and radiologic evidence of subsegmental atelectasis in any lobe of the lungs.

The reasons for the occurrence of pulmonary edema are uncertain and may differ in croup and epiglottitis. In croup the obstruction may be prolonged and severe. As previously discussed, inspiration through an extrathoracic airway obstruction exaggerates the effects of the normally negative transpulmonary pressure. Transmission of this large negative pressure to the right side of the heart increases venous return and subsequently pulmonary blood flow. At the same time, this pressure is equally applied to the left ventricular (LV) wall and transiently reduces LV output. The net result is an increase in pulmonary blood volume with a consequent increase in transudation of fluid into the peri-bronchial interstitial space. Here, such fluid is normally pumped out of the lungs by the lymphatic system, but the huge negative pressure is also applied transiently to the pulmonary interstitium and may overcome the ability of the lymphatics to remove the fluid, resulting in small airway closure and frank alveolar flooding. This process can cause atelectasis and/or alveolar hypoxia, and thus arterial hypoxemia. A vicious cycle may be established where hypoxia increases cardiac output and hence pulmonary perfusion pressure, causing further accumulation of interstitial fluid with pulmonary edema. As the lung compliance drops, more negative transpulmonary pressures will be needed for ventilation.

In epiglottitis, the same physiologic events occur, but clinical observation indicates that the partial upper airway obstruction is much shorter in time and less severe pre-terminally. Thus, the mean negative transpulmonary pressures are less. Following this reasoning, pulmonary edema (and also hypoxemia and chest roentgenogram film changes) should be a less frequent complication in epiglottitis than in croup, but this is not by experience. Hemophilus influenzae infections of the lungs are associated with pleural effusions in 60–75% of cases. It may be that in epiglottitis the bacteria or (presumed) endotoxins themselves alter pulmonary vascular permeability thus magnifying the effect of the relatively less (c.f. croup) negative intrathoracic pressures and causing increased lung water with all its sequelae.

Therapeutic Measures in Croup

At Home

The majority of infants and children with croup can be managed safely at home by conscientious and reliable parents. A fundamental objective is to prevent unnecessary anxiety and provide minimal disturbance for the child. Water vapour mist seems helpful and can be achieved at home by taking the child into the bathroom and turning on the hot taps. Minor obstruction will usually resolve within the hour. No medications significantly alter the course of mild disease, and sedatives should never be used since they may depress respiration in an already hypoxic child. Restlessness in a child with laryngeal obstruction must be presumed due to hypoxia until proven otherwise and is an indication for hospitalization.

In the Hospital

The management of acute laryngotracheobronchitis is often hindered by the lack of objective but noninvasive measurements which accurately reflect severity of upper airway obstruction and its response to therapy. Clinical scoring systems, assigning a number of points for the presence or absence of each physical sign or symptom, have been proposed by a number of workers;[27–30] all systems seem useful but none appear to have gained universal acceptance. Measurements of total respiratory resistance,[31] cineradiographic changes between inspiratory and expiratory anteroposterior tracheal diameters[30] and arterial blood gases[20–22] have been used in attempts to assess more objectively the severity of upper airway obstruction. These techniques are useful research tools for determining the efficiency of various therapeutic interventions, but in the routine clinical situation have limited application because they often require excessive handling of the child with possible consequent deterioration.

Management

Minimal Disturbance

Any stimulus which provokes anxiety will cause the child to hyperventilate. This will make the inspiratory obstruction worse, thus increasing the work of breathing and oxygen consumption.

Clinical assessments by the attending physicians and nurses should be made frequently, but medical and nursing procedures which disturb the child should be avoided whenever possible. The presence of a parent at the bedside often reduces anxiety, but can also aggravate it on occasion. Occasionally, a younger infant will appear disturbed from hunger, but feeding gives rise to the risk of aspiration of stomach contents either spontaneously or at intubation, should the disease worsen. In such cases, the decision whether to feed or not requires astute clinical judgment. Fever control to reduce oxygen consumption should be achieved through drugs rather than tepid sponging.

A rising respiratory rate correlates well with a falling arterial oxygen tension[21,22] and this may happen quite early in the course of the illness. Most young children have a sleeping respiratory rate of 20–30 per minute, and can easily cope with rates up to 40–50 per minute. Above 50 per minute they may tire very quickly and need relief of airway obstruction. Hypercapnea, however, occurs as a late sign of respiratory failure in croup and it is difficult to detect the classical signs in infants. The indications for airway relief are decreased air entry, increasing (or decreasing) retraction of the chest wall, a rising respiratory rate, and fatigue. If there is any doubt, sampling of arterial blood (with minimal disturbance to the patient) to measure the degree of hypoxemia, hypercapnea and respiratory or metabolic acidosis will be helpful.

Oxygen and Humidification

The hypoxemia in room air which has been demonstrated in hospitalized children with croup results from maldistribution of ventilation and perfusion. The possible mechanisms of (a) diffuse bronchial involvement by the infective viral agent, (b) glottic irritation producing reflex bronchoconstriction, (c) sputum retention causing bronchial obstruction, and (d) pulmonary edema have been discussed in the *Pathophysiology* section. Whatever the mechanism, hypoxemia should be avoided by nursing infants and children in head boxes or oxygen tents supplied with moist nebulized oxygen. Face masks or nasal cannulae are rarely well-tolerated in this age group. An oxygen concentration of more than 30% is rarely required, but the attending physician must be aware of the risks of insidious hypercapnea, having masked the signs of hypoxemia.

Humidification may have a secondary benefit in that animal studies show mist droplets falling on the nasal and supraglottic laryngeal mucosal surfaces reflexly alter the pattern of breathing[32] possibly causing improved respiratory flow rates and less work. This may occur in humans, as well.

Hydration

In most cases of croup this can be accomplished orally by skilled nursing staff. If oral fluids are poorly tolerated, or the child is too ill to drink, intravenous fluids should be substituted. Some very distressed children have a degree of metabolic acidosis which should be corrected.[21]

Racemic Epinephrine

The use of racemic epinephrine in croup is based on its topical vasoconstrictor (alpha) effect when applied to the inflamed, edematous mucosa of the subglottic region. However, its mild bronchodilator (beta) effect may reflexly reduce some laryngospasm or trachealis muscle constriction. Racemic epinephrine is composed of equal parts of the D- and L-isomers of epinephrine. The L-isomer is about 15–20 times more potent than the D- form, and theoretically, a 2.25% solution of racemic epinephrine is equipotent with 1.0% L-epinephrine which could be used instead. Nebulized phenylephrine solution (0.25%) has similar activity.[31]

It is often difficult to compare data from various groups because of the lack of objective measurements of severity of illness and different drug delivery techniques. However, the following conclusions about racemic epinephrine can be accepted:

- Racemic epinephrine delivered by IPPB, intermittent positive pressure breathing, has been associated with a decreased tracheotomy or intubation rate.[33]
- Racemic epinephrine with IPPB provides a relief of upper airway obstruction in croup which is much greater than with either distilled water or normal saline with IPPB.[28,30]
- Despite its popularity in many centers, racemic epinephrine aerosol administered by IPPB is no more effective than that delivered by powered nebulizer and face mask to a spontaneously breathing child.[27]

- Racemic epinephrine appears safe when given as 0.5 ml of 2.25% solution in 3.5 ml water (1:8 dilution). Alternatively, 2 ml of 0.25% phenylephrine solution can be used.[31] These can be given every hour, but if significant obstruction rapidly recurs after three or four one-hourly treatments, an artificial airway should be established.
- Racemic epinephrine does not seem to alter the natural history of acute laryngotracheobronchitis in terms of length of disease, but only in terms of severity.[29] Significant obstruction can recur within a short time of administration with initial complete relief. This is often referred to as a "rebound phenomenon," but is more likely due to worsening disease and rapid metabolism of the drug. Thus, racemic epinephrine should not be used for outpatient therapy.
- Since racemic epinephrine appears to have a beneficial, if short-lived, effect in most cases of croup, its use suggests that the development and trial of longer-acting alpha-agonists should be undertaken.

Other Drugs

Antibiotics. In the vast majority of croup cases, antibiotics have no value because of the viral etiology. The occasional patient will present with evidence of a bacterial infection such as otitis media or tonsillitis. Rarely, nowadays, will a patient with primary viral laryngotracheobronchitis have bacterial superinfection of the tracheal secretions. These patients should be suspected clinically if they have unexpectedly high fever and toxicity, with an elevated absolute band neutrophil count.[15] The tracheal secretions (if obtainable) are grossly purulent and contain many neutrophils, a finding not present in uncomplicated viral infections of the respiratory tract.[34] Cultures of the tracheal secretions reveal a pure or predominant growth of a recognized respiratory tract bacterial pathogen, usually Staphylococcus aureus, Streptococcus pneumoniae or Hemophilus influenzae.

Steroids. The acute anti-inflammatory role of corticosteroids remains highly controversial despite numerous clinical trials,[35–40] largely because of the widely divergent results achieved. The topic was put in perspective by Cherry in 1970,[41] who pointed out that all the studies had been somewhat handicapped by the failure to identify clearly whether the groups being treated had acute laryngotracheobronchitis, spasmodic croup, or, as was most likely, included cases of both. Indeed, future studies on any aspect of croup will require analysis of historic, ecologic, etiologic and clinical features of the cases in order to define the subgroup under investigation.

There is no evidence that a short course of steroid therapy is harmful; neither are there any conclusive data at present that corticosteroids beneficially alter the clinical course of classic viral laryngotracheobronchitis.

Theoretically, steroids may benefit spasmodic croup, where we believe there is no direct infectious involvement of the tracheal epithelium, and obstruction is probably the result of noninflammatory edema within the submucosa of the subglottic trachea. In practice however, steroids will have little apparent effect since this type of croup has a short natural history, and in most cases is easily controlled by mist therapy.

Helium-oxygen Gas Mixtures. Seventy percent helium/thirty percent oxygen mixtures have been used to decrease the work of breathing in supplying oxygen and removing carbon dioxide from the body. The lower density of helium (compared with the nitrogen in air) probably allows better flow through the obstructed segment and conversion of turbulent to laminar flow with a lowering of airway resistance. This technique helps in many cases[42,43] but using a tent or hood requires a lot of relatively expensive gas to maintain an adequate inspired concentration.

Artificial Airway

The technique of upper airway control and the relative safety of nasotracheal intubation versus tracheotomy were the subjects of a recent extensive review.[44] In summary, successful management of the obstructed airway depends upon a team-approach reflecting the skills of its members and the hospital facilities. Either intubation or tracheotomy are safe in some hands, but both can result in serious complications when practiced by inexperienced physicians with inadequate supportive facilities. In a small hospital, without intensive care nursing nor a skilled intubationist readily available, a tracheotomy is probably the technique of choice.

In a hospital with trained personnel and good facilities, such children can be given a general anesthetic (halothane and oxygen with assisted ventilation) safely and when deeply asleep gently intubated via the oral route with an uncuffed polyvinylchloride tube splinted with a stilette. After adequate suctioning of the usually copious tracheobronchial secretions and deepening of the anesthesia, the tube is replaced with a nasal tube. (See Table III for appropriate sizes.) Once the tube is secured, ventilation of both lungs should be checked by auscultation and the position of the tube confirmed by a chest film. Constant nursing supervision and adequate humidification of inspired gases is essential to avoid accidental extubation or blockage, which are the two most serious complications.

The duration of intubation is usually 2–5 days in croup. The child can be extubated when an air-leak develops around the tube, the fever subsides, the tracheobronchial secretions thin and decrease, and any major areas of atelectasis have re-expanded. Following extubation the child should be observed for 1–2 days before discharge.

Therapeutic Measures in Epiglottitis

Once the diagnosis of epiglottitis is made or even strongly suspected, the child should be immediately admitted to hospital. Conservative management is potentially dangerous because of the complication of sudden respiratory arrest and in most cases an artificial airway should be established as soon as possible. In hospital, the child should be accompanied at all times by a physician (with the necessary instruments and other personnel immediately available) who is capable of introducing an artificial airway should respiratory arrest occur.

Table III

Sizes of Endotracheal Tubes for Croup and Epiglottitis

Age of Child	*Size of Tube (I.D.)**
$<$ 6 months	3.0
6 months–2 years	3.5
2 years–5 years	4.0
$>$ 5 years	4.5

*I.D. = Internal Diameter, mm.

Management

Minimal Disturbance and Posture

The risk of sudden laryngeal obstruction is very high in acute epiglottitis, and any event which may precipitate this by causing undue anxiety or physical disturbance to the child must be avoided. This does not exclude continual observation by the attending physician prior to mechanical control of the upper airway. The patient should be nursed in a sitting position propped up with pillows, or allowed to lie on his face. If he is forced to lie flat on his back, he may have difficulty coping with oral secretions, aspiration of which will precipitate laryngeal spasm and complete obstruction.

Oxygen and Humidification

The child should be nursed in an humidified, oxygen enriched (approximately 30% O_2) atmosphere prior to and after control of the airway. Arterial blood gases obtained before intubation add nothing to the management and will unduly disturb the child. Measurements obtained after intubation show no hypercapnea, but sometimes marked hypoxemia.[5]

Hydration

Epiglottitis is an acute illness of only a few hours duration from onset to presentation at hospital. Dehydration is not a problem, and while intravenous fluids and antibiotics are essential after intubation, establishing a route should wait until anesthesia has been administered and an airway secured.

Racemic Epinephrine

There is no place for this drug in the management of acute epiglottitis.

Antibiotics

Appropriate antibiotic therapy rapidly resolves the toxemia and supraglottic edema. The usual causative organism is H. influenzae type B, which is virtually always sensitive to intravenous chloramphenicol 100 mg/kg/day or cefamandole 100–150 mg/kg/day.

Ampicillin 200–400 mg/kg/day intravenously was the antibiotic of choice in the past, but with the large number of resistance H. influenzae organisms (up to 30%) now reported in many centers, it should never be used alone. Similarly, cefamandole should not be used if there is a suspicion of complicating meningitis. Throat swabs and blood cultures should never be taken prior to control of the airway. They can be taken at leisure later, prior to the antibiotic coverage which should be maintained for 5–7 days.

Artificial Airway

A significant mortality (approximately 6%) has been reported with the failure to establish an artificial airway in diagnosed epiglottitis, as opposed to less than 1% in cases with airway control.[45] However, in some centers the incidence of artificial airway control is as low as 70%.[46,47] Children over the age of three years who are not severely obstructed initially can probably be safely managed conservatively in a good intensive care unit provided there are experienced nurses, and physicians immediately available on a 24-hour basis who can quickly intubate a child who deteriorates.

Those who require airway control should be transferred to the operating room and anesthesia induced cautiously using assisted ventilation with halothane and oxygen. No attempt should be made to change the sitting child's position. Provided the epiglottis is lifted well forward with the laryngoscope blade, and a stilette is used in the endotracheal tube, intubation is not usually particularly difficult. Only in rare cases is a person skilled in intubation unable to pass a tube, and then tracheotomy must be performed.

The tube sizes are the same as for croup (see Table III) and the same rules apply for extubation. However, extubation can usually be achieved much earlier, often after 24 hours.[47]

Conclusion

The management of epiglottitis is straightforward once the diagnosis is made. The disease is dangerous only in the failure of physicians to suspect the disease when the child presents at hospital or, having made the diagnosis, time is wasted with various investigations which may be unhelpful, disturbing to the distressed child, and expose him unnecessarily to the risk of respiratory arrest from unrelieved airway obstruction.

In the vast majority of cases, acute laryngotracheobronchitis is not a dangerous disease. However, we lack objective, noninvasive techniques for assessing the severity of this disease and its response to various treatment modalities. The decision when to intubate a child (in the few cases requiring airway relief) depends entirely upon good clinical judgment.

Despite the chest roentgenogram and arterial blood gas data presented here, I do not advocate either investigation in the management of uncomplicated croup or epiglottitis. I have reported these findings merely to emphasize that there is an underlying hypoxemia irrespective of the relief of airway obstruction or the presence of normal chest roentgenograms. This hypoxemia may be severe enough to be life-threatening and these children should be managed always in humidified oxygen.

References

1. Bass JW, Steele RM, Weibe RA: Acute epiglottitis: A surgical emergency. *JAMA* 229:671, 1974.
2. Levison H, Tabachnik E, Newth CJL: Wheezing in Infancy, Croup and Epiglottitis. *In* L. Gluck (ed): *Current Problems in Pediatrics.* Vol. 12, 1982, p. 39–42.
3. Williams HE, Phelan PD: *Respiratory Illness in Children.* Oxford Blackwell Publications, 1975, pp 26–37.
4. Molteni RA: Epiglottitis: Incidence of extraepiglottic infection. *Pediatrics* 58:526, 1976.
5. Costigan DC, Newth CJL: The respiratory status of children with epiglottitis, with and without airway control. *Am J Dis Child,* 1982 (in press).
6. Baxter P, Pashley NRT: Acute epiglottitis—25 years experience in the management. The Montreal Children's Hospital. *J Otolaryngol* 6:473, 1977.
7. Margolis CZ, Ingram DL, Meyer JH: Routine tracheotomy in Haemophilus influenzae type B epiglottitis. *J Pediatr* 81:1150, 1972.
8. Benjamin B, O'Reilly B: Acute epiglottitis in infants and children. *Ann Otolaryngol* 85:565, 1976.
9. Blanc VF, Weber ML, Leduc C, et al: Acute epiglottitis in children: Management of 27 consecutive cases with nasotracheal intubation with special emphasis on anesthetic considerations. *Can Anaesth Soc J* 24:1, 1977.

10. Cohen SR, Chai J: Epiglottitis—20 year study with tracheotomy. *Ann Otolaryngol* 87:461, 1978.
11. Davison FW: Acute laryngeal obstruction in children. *JAMA* 171:1301, 1979.
12. Glezen WP, Loda FA, Clyde WA, et al: Epidemiologic patterns of acute lower respiratory disease of children in a pediatric group practice. *J Pediatr* 78:397, 1971.
13. Horsfall FL, Tamm I: *Viral and Rickettsial Infections of Man.* Fourth Edition, Philadelphia, J.B. Lippincott Co., 1965.
14. Urquhart GED, Kennedy DH, Ariyawansa JP: Croup associated with parainfluenza type 1 virus: Two sub-populations. *Br Med J* 1:1604, 1979.
15. Jones R, Santos JI, Overall JC: Bacterial tracheitis. *JAMA* 242:721, 1979.
16. Brighton GR: Laryngotracheobronchitis. *Ann Otol Rhinol Laryngol* 49:1070, 1940.
17. Orton HB, Smith EL, Bell HO, et al: Acute laryngotracheobronchitis: Analysis of 62 cases with report of autopsies in eight cases. *Arch Otolaryngol* 33:926, 1941.
18. Newton-John H: Pulmonary oedema in upper airway obstruction. *Lancet* 2:510, 1977.
19. Wittenborg MH, Gyepes MT, Crocker D: Tracheal dynamics in infants with respiratory distress, stridor, and collapsing trachea. *Radiology* 88:653, 1967.
20. Wesley AG: Indications for intubation in laryngotracheobronchitis in black children. *South Afr Med J* 49:1126, 1975.
21. Newth CJL, Levison H, Bryan AC: The respiratory status of children with croup. *J Pediatr* 81:1068, 1972.
22. Wesley AG, Bruce R, Holloway R: Arterial blood gases as a guide to management of infective croup. *South Afr Med J* 42:1237, 1968.
23. Widdicombe JG, Sterling GM: The autonomic nervous system and breathing. *Arch Intern Med* 126:311, 1977.
24. Travis KW, Todres ID, Shannon DC: Pulmonary edema associated with croup and epiglottitis. *Pediatrics* 59:695, 1977.
25. Soliman MG, Richer PP: Epiglottitis and pulmonary edema in children. *Can Anaesth Soc J* 25:270, 1978.
26. Galvis AG, Stool SE, Bluestone CD: Pulmonary edema following relief of acute upper airway obstruction. *Ann Otolaryngol* 89:124, 1980.
27. Oh TH, Downes JJ: Comparison of intermittent positive pressure breathing (IPPB) and powered nebulizer to administer racemic epinephrine in croup. New Orleans, *American Society of Anesthesiologists,* Abstracts of Scientific Meetings, 1977, pp 149–150.
28. Westley CR, Cotton EK, Brooks JG: Nebulized racemic epinephrine by IPPB for the treatment of croup. *Am J Dis Child* 132:484, 1978.
29. Taussig LM, Castro O, Beaudry PH, et al: Treatment of laryngotracheobronchitis (croup). Use of intermittent positive-pressure breathing and racemic epinephrine. *Am J Dis Child* 129:790, 1975.
30. Corkey CWB, Barker GA, Edmonds JF, et al: Radiographic tracheal diameter measurements in acute infectious croup—an objective scoring system. *Crit Care Med* 9:587, 1981.

31. Lenney W, Milner AD: Treatment of acute viral croup. *Arch Dis Child* 53:704, 1978.
32. Sasaki CT, Suzuki M: The respiratory mechanism of aerosol inhalation in the treatment of partial airway obstruction. *Pediatrics* 59:689, 1977.
33. Adair JC, Ring WH, Jordan WS, et al: Ten-year experience with IPPB in the treatment of acute laryngotracheobronchitis. *Anaesth Analg* 50:649, 1971.
34. Walsh JJ, Dietlein LF, Low FN, et al: Bronchotracheal response in human influenza. *Arch Intern Med* 108:376, 1961.
35. Turner JA, Morgan EA: Corticotrophic (ACTH) in the treatment of acute
laryngotracheitis. *Am J Dis Child* 83:440, 1952.
36. Vovik A: Corticosteroid treatment of nondiphtheritic croup. *Acta Otolaryngol* 158:163, 1960.
37. Skowron PN, Turner JA, McNaughton GA: The use of corticosteroids in the treatment of acute laryngotracheitis. *Can Med Assoc J* 94:528, 1966.
38. Eden AN, Kaufman A, Yu R: Corticosteroids and croup. *JAMA* 200:133, 1967.
39. James JA: Dexamethasone in croup. *Am J Dis Child* 117:511, 1969.
40. Leipzig B, Oski FA, Cummings CW, et al: A prospective randomized study to determine the efficacy of steroids in treatment of croup. *J Pediatr* 94:194, 1979.
41. Cherry JD: The treatment of croup: Continued controversy due to failure of recognition of historic, ecologic, etiologic and clinical perspectives. *J Pediatr* 94:352, 1979.
42. Kernan JD, Barach AL: Role of helium in cases of obstructive lesions in the trachea and larynx. *Arch Otolaryngol* 26:419, 1937.
43. Duncan PG: Efficacy of helium-oxygen mixtures in the management of severe viral and postintubation croup. *Can Anaesth Soc J* 26:206, 1979.
44. Barker GA: Current management of croup and epiglottitis. *Pediatr Clin North Am* 26:573, 1979.
45. Cantrell RW, Bell RA, Morioka WT: Acute epiglottitis: Intubation versus tracheotomy. *Laryngoscope* 88:994, 1978.
46. Fearon B, Cinnamond M: Tracheotomy in acute supraglottitis (epiglottitis). The treatment of choice. *Laryngoscope* 87:879, 1977.
47. Shann FA, Phelan PD, Stocks JG, et al: Prolonged nasotracheal intubation or tracheostomy in acute laryngotracheobronchitis and epiglottitis? *Aust Pediatr J* 11:212, 1975.

14

The Diagnosis and Therapy of Status Asthmaticus

Stanley P. Galant, M.D.

Introduction

Although the term *status asthmaticus* defies a precise definition, the American Thoracic Society has defined status asthmaticus as an acute asthmatic attack in which the degree of bronchial obstruction is either severe from the beginning or increases in severity and is not relieved by the usual treatment such as epinephrine or aminophylline. Status asthmaticus is a medical emergency requiring expert assessment and management if one is to prevent serious morbidity or death. Several thousand patients (mostly adults) die each year from this condition. The young child particularly less than 5 years is especially susceptible to serious consequences of airway obstruction. It is the purpose of this presentation to provide basic information regarding its pathogenesis, diagnosis and therapy so that the resultant improved patient care will lead to even less morbidity and mortality.

Pathophysiology

Airway Obstruction

Although it is commonly thought that major obstruction frequently occurs at the medium sized bronchi (3 to 5 mm diameter), it has become increasingly clear that obstruction can and does occur in large and small airways (≤ 2 mm). Contributing factors to this obstruction include contraction of bronchial smooth muscle, submucosal edema, hypersecretion of tenacious intraluminal mucus plugs, and extrinsic bronchial compression in the young infant with forceful expiration because of the soft chest wall. The infant and young child would appear to be at increased risk for serious obstruction because of disproportionately narrow small airways, decreased bronchiolar smooth muscle, excessive intraluminal mucus production and decreased static elastic recoil.[1,2]

Biochemical Abnormalities

Hypoxemia. Hypoxemia ($Pa_{O_2} < 95$ torr) is present in almost all cases of status asthmaticus and is usually due to uneven ventilation and perfusion of underventilated alveoli, resulting in right-to-left pulmonary arteriovenous shunting. This is secondary to obstruction of the conducting airways (particularly the small airways). With increased obstruction, hypoventilation becomes an added factor in increasing the hypoxemia.

Hypercapnia. Most patients with status asthmaticus hyperventilate to compensate for hypoxemia as manifested by a low Pa_{CO_2} (25 to 35 torr) on admission. However, with progression of airway obstruction, alveolar ventilation decreases, eventually resulting in hypercapnia ($Pa_{CO_2} > 40$ torr). Hypoventilation is a late, serious manifestation of severe bronchial obstruction. A rising Pa_{CO_2} in the face of worsening clinical pattern is reason for concern, and one should not consider a Pa_{CO_2} of 40 torr to be normal under these circumstances.

Acidosis. Early in the disease process, because of hyperventilation, the patient may have respiratory alkalosis. However, young children frequently develop a metabolic acidosis (a base deficit of ≥ 4 mEq/liter) from tissue hypoxia and the ensuing ketone and organic acid production. Respiratory acidosis (pH under 7.35) is seen as CO_2 retention occurs and indicates alveolar hypoventilation.

Dehydration and Electrolyte Imbalance. The patient with status asthmaticus is frequently thought to be approximately 5% dehydrated due to decreased fluid intake, increased water loss caused by tachypnea (insensible losses), and often the diuretic effect of theophylline. In addition, patients with a history of corticosteroid therapy, particularly within the last six months of admission, should be carefully observed for evidence of adrenal insufficiency (hyponatremia and hyperkalemia).

Assessment of Asthma Severity

The first question facing the clinician with a patient with acute asthma is when to admit the patient to the hospital. Fischl and coworkers[3] found seven parameters useful in predicting which patients require hospitalization: pulse rate; respiratory rate; pulsus paradoxus; peak expiratory flow rate; dyspnea; accessory muscle use; and wheezing. Patients with respiratory distress and poor pulmonary function on admission to the emergency room generally relapsed if sent home instead of being admitted to the hospital.

History

Careful questioning should establish the following: duration of wheezing (mucus plugs take on increasing importance with time); evidence of respiratory infection in patient or family; fluid balance (intake, vomiting, urination); history of allergy to foods and drugs; and dosage and time of medications administered, with particular emphasis on sympathomimetics, methylxanthines, and corticosteroids. A history of previous, severe asthma, especially episodes requiring hospitalization, intensive therapy and corticosteroid use, should signal a high-risk patient.

Physical Examination

Physical examination should include the following: general status of patient (anxiety, alertness, and respiratory distress); height and weight; vital signs including heart and respiratory rate, blood pressure, and pulsus paradoxus;[4] skin and mucous membranes (note state of hydration, pallor, or cyanosis); ears, nose, and throat (examine for infection); chest (note anteroposterior diameter, retractions, and respiratory effort), particularly of sternocleidomastoid muscle (correlates with pulmonary function); air exchange, and adventitious sounds (rhonchi, wheezes, rales); and central nervous system (sensorium and muscle tone). Check for papilledema since its presence means Pa_{CO_2} of about 75 mm Hg. Note that supraclavicular crepitus means pneumomediastinum.

Laboratory Tests

Routine tests include: arterial blood gases (Pa_{O_2}, Pa_{CO_2}, pH, base deficit); serum electrolytes; CBC; urinalysis; and bacterial and viral cultures as clinically indicated. It is our belief that all patients admitted with status asthmaticus should have arterial blood gas determinations on admission; the need for further blood gas tests will depend on the clinical state. Radial and brachial arteries are the best sites for arterial sampling. An indwelling arterial catheter is indicated only in the patient with respiratory failure who will require repeated arterial punctures. The ambient oxygen (F_IO_2) should always be stated when the sample is drawn, to appropriately assess the Pa_{O_2}. Pulmonary function, particularly peak expiratory flow rate (PEFR), can be useful in anyone over 5 years of age. An admission chest film is desirable to rule out pneumonia, atelectasis, pneumomediastinum, and pneumothorax. However, the patient should not be sent to radiology unattended for an extended period of time, since his clinical condition could significantly deteriorate before he reaches the ward.

From these data one should construct a respiratory scoring system or pulmonary index as seen in Table I.

Table I
Pulmonary Scoring System

	0	1	2
PaO_2 (torr)	70–100	≤70 in air	70 in 40% O_2
Cyanosis	none	in air	in 40% O_2
$PaCO_2$ (torr)	<40	40–65	>65
P.P.** (mm Hg)	<10	10–20	>20
Use of accessory muscles	none	moderate	marked
Air exchange	good	fair	poor
Mental status	normal	depressed or agitated	coma

*0 to 4 = no immediate danger; 5–6 = impending respiratory failure; 7 = respiratory failure
**Pulsus Paradoxus

Management of Status Asthmaticus

General Measures

The patient admitted to the hospital with status asthmaticus should be placed in the intensive care unit and have a cardiac monitor.[5] An asthma flow sheet should be made on admission to contain the following data: date and hour of admission; clinical findings and vital signs to include pulsus paradoxus; specific measurements (e.g. blood gases, PEFR, F_IO_2); treatment procedures and medication.

Oxygen. Oxygen administration is mandatory on admission because nearly all patients with status asthmaticus are hypoxemic; 40% humidified oxygen may be delivered quite safely by face mask, tent, or nasal cannula, depending on age of the patient. Continued oxygen administration should be monitored by clinical findings and PaO_2. The latter should be maintained above 60 torr. We do not use mist therapy, since there is no convincing evidence that it helps expectorate mucus; it makes the patient cold and difficult to see, and it may cause increased bronchospasm in some cases.

Intravenous Fluids. Adequate hydration is necessary to loosen and promote expectoration of the thick tenacious mucus plugs. Approximately 1.5 times the usual maintenance 24-hour fluid requirements are recommended to be given intravenously. Caution is advised, however, as too vigorous fluid administration may result in hyponatremia and water intoxication presumably on the basis of increased antidiuretic hormone secretion during the acute phase of status asthmaticus. Furthermore, such therapy might increase fluid in the interstitial spaces around the small airways resulting in increased airway obstruction.

Chest Therapy. Postural drainage and chest percussion can be useful in expectorating mucus plugs, but this procedure should be reserved until patient is over the acute phase and on the way to recovery.

Drug Therapy

Theophylline. A loading dose of 5 to 6 mg/kg *theophylline,* assuming a volume of distribution to be 0.5 liters/kg, will increase the serum theophylline level by approximately 10 mcg/ml. For this reason, if the patient has received theophylline within the previous 12 hours, the loading dose should be reduced by 50%. Following this, the patient should receive theophylline by slow constant infusion. A reasonable maintenance infusion rate would be 0.8 mg/kg/hr for a young child and approximately 0.4 mg/kg/hr for an older child or adult. To assure that the patient is in the therapeutic zone, a serum theophylline level should be drawn on admission and approximately 24 hours after the infusion was started. Before this time the patient may not be in a steady state, making interpretation difficult. Note that children and adult smokers have increased theophylline clearance while patients with congestive heart failure and liver disease have marked decrease in capacity to eliminate theophylline.

Sympathomimetic Drugs. These agents can be useful as an adjunct to theophylline therapy.

Aerosolized agents, either solutions of isoproterenol (0.5%) 0.02 cc/kg or metaproterenol (5%) 0.01 cc/kg (not to exceed 0.30 cc) can be used by diluting them with 2.0 to 3.0 ml of normal saline and giving this mixture by nebulizer or by intermittent positive pressure breathing although some consider the latter contraindicated because of the risk of pneumomediastinum and/or pneumothorax. The frequency of metaproterenol administration is generally every three to four hours, while isoproterenol can be given hourly if several dosages are necessary.

Corticosteroids. Patients who fail to respond to an adequate trial of aminophylline and aerolized sympathomimetic drugs or who have received corticosteroids in the preceding six months are candidates for corticosteroids. The most common errors in using steroids are: (1) not giving a large enough dose during the acute episode; and (2) expecting a rapid response (usual response is within six to eight hours).

Hydrocortisone 125 mg/M^2 every six hours is given as a 10 to 15 minute intravenous infusion or in the six-hour IV bottle. This is continued until the patient is stable and can take steroids by mouth, at which time prednisone 1–2 mg/kg is given until discharge, when steroids are discontinued or reduced to the patient's former schedule. Tapering is not necessary if the total daily steroid course was seven days or less.

Alkalyzing Agents. Sodium bicarbonate is indicated when the pH is less than 7.25 because acidosis of this magnitude impairs systemic, coronary, and pulmonary blood flows. In addition, correction of acidemia is thought to help restore the bronchial smooth muscle response to sympathomimetic drugs.

Several methods are used to arrive at approximate dosage: (1) if base deficit (BD) is present, BD × 0.3 × body weight (kg) = mEq sodium bicarbonate; and (2) if no base deficit exists, 1.5 mg/kg × body weight (kg) = mEq sodium bicarbonate. Note that improved ventilation is most important here, since the acidosis is due primarily to CO_2 retention. However, the increased pulmonary perfusion following bicarbonate therapy often leads to improved CO_2 clearance. The dosage is given over 30 to 60 minutes intravenously. If necessary, this may be repeated once in the first 24 hours without metabolic sequelae. Adverse reactions include metabolic alkalosis and increased load.

Antibiotics. Since most infection-induced exacerbations of asthma are due to viruses, antibiotics should rarely be administered and only if indicated on the basis of cultures or bacterial infection.

Drugs to Avoid. Respiratory depressants such as opiates, propoxyphene, barbiturates, diazepam, and other tranquilizers should be avoided. Whether anticholinergics and antihistamines dry bronchial secretions is controversial, but these drugs are best avoided during the acute phase of status asthmaticus because of this possibility.

Respiratory Failure

Patients with status asthmaticus can develop respiratory failure.[5,6] In one series this occurred in 21% of cases. Wood and Downes[6] have set up a clinical asthma score protocol consisting of such parameters as cyanosis (or PaO_2), nature of breath sounds, use of accessory muscles, degree of expiratory wheezing, cerebral function and $PaCO_2$. Using a 0 to 2 scoring system they categorize patients into pending respiratory failure when clinical score ≥ 5 and $PaCO_2 \geq 55$ torr after conventional therapy and acute respiratory failure for score ≥ 7, $PaCO_2 \geq 65$ torr. (See Table I.) However, a patient may be in impending respiratory failure with a rising $PaCO_2$ which is ≤ 55 torr.

The main *therapeutic modality in the child* is the addition of a constant isoproterenol intravenous infusion. Isoproterenol must be given by a separate intravenous line from that of aminophylline and corticosteroids using a constant infusion pump (IVAC or Harvard). An intraarterial line should be in place for frequent arterial blood gases. The patient must have continuous ECG monitoring and an external defibrillator nearby. Lidocaine (1 mg/kg) may be needed for intravenous infusion.

Isoproterenol is initiated at a dosage of 0.1 mcg/kg/min. The dosage is doubled every 15 minutes until one of the following occurs: (1) $PaCO_2$ falls below 55 torr; (2) heart rate exceeds 200 bpm; (3) an arrhythmia develops (ventricular tachycardia, ventricular fibrillation, frequent ventricular ectopic beats); or (4) a progressive deterioration in clinical state or blood gas status including increasing exhaustion. If this occurs endotracheal intubation and mechanical ventilation should be instituted.

Most cases will respond to a dose of 0.8 to 1.0 mcg/kg/min. If a dose greater than 1.0 mcg/kg/min is required, the increases are made at 20-minute intervals in increments of 0.2 to 0.4 mcg/kg/min. Arterial blood gases and pH are determined every 15 to 20 minutes.

Attempts to decrease the optimal dosage before 12 hours usually lead to exacerbation of airway obstruction. When the $PaCO_2$ remains consistently under 45 torr with a clinical score of ≤ 4, the dosage may be decreased by 0.1 to 0.2 mcg/kg/min at hourly intervals. Isoproterenol must never be stopped abruptly or severe obstruction may recur. This approach has been successful in approximately 70% of children with respiratory failure.

Intravenous salbutamol, because of greater beta-2 adrenergic specificity, has been tried, but remains experimental at this time.[7]

Summary

The time to treate status asthmaticus is before it occurs. Our goal is to keep the patient out of the hospital with excellent allergy care and aggressive pharmacological management.

References

1. Leffert F: The management of acute severe asthma. *J Pediatr* 96:1, 1980.
2. Galant SP: Status asthmaticus in children and adults. *Comprehensive Therapy*. 6:51, 1980.
3. Fischl MA, Pitchenik A, Gardner LB: An index predicting relapse and need for hospitalization in patients with acute bronchial asthma. *N Engl J Med* 305:783, 1981.
4. Galant SP, Groncy CE, Shaw KC: The value of pulsus paradoxus in assessing the child with status asthmaticus. *Pediatrics* 61:46, 1978.
5. Cotton EK, Parry W: Treatment of status asthmaticus and respiratory failure. *Pediatr Clin North Am* 22:163, 1975.
6. Wood DW, Downes JJ, Scheinkopf H, et al: Intravenous isoproterenol in the management of respiratory failure in childhood status asthmaticus. *J Allergy Clin Immunol* 50:75, 1972.
7. Fichett D, McNichol M, Riordan J: Intravenous salbutamol in the management of status asthmaticus. *Br Med J* 1:53, 1975.

15

Adult Respiratory Distress Syndrome in Children

Emily J. Kahlstrom, M.D.

Introduction

The respiratory distress syndrome (RDS) of shock and trauma has been recognized as a disease of adults. The syndrome represents a diffuse systemic capillary leaking of intravascular volume into all tissues of the body with a profound effect on the lung. The lung changes primarily reflect injury to the alveolar capillary membrane with resultant capillary permeability and a defect in surfactant. The pulmonary manifestations include signs of pulmonary insufficiency, impairment in gas exchange, decrease in lung compliance, and diffuse pulmonary infiltrates. The two major determinants of development are shock and major soft tissue injury. Unfortunately, the major descriptions of the subject have been in the adult medical and surgical literature, leaving the pediatrician with the impression that this syndrome occurs only in adult post-trauma patients.

Historical Aspects

The respiratory distress syndrome of shock and trauma was first described by Jenkins, Jones, Wilson and Moyer in 1950.[1] During World War I, major pulmonary problems were attributed to massive pulmonary collapse. Burford and Burbank described the "wet lung" syndrome at the end of World War II.[2] Moon provided the classic description of pathologic pulmonary changes in patients dying of burns and trauma in 1948.[3] Ashbaugh and Petty were first to associate the syndrome with civilian trauma in 1967.[4] Eiseman and Ashbaugh reported the pulmonary effects of nonthoracic trauma, focusing on the magnitude of the problem and significance of the lesion in 1968.[5] Descriptive terms used to describe the pulmonary lesion were "Da Nang Lung," "shock lung," and progressive pulmonary failure. Holbrook, Taylor, Pollack, and Fields reviewed their experience with 18 children in 1980.[6] Their series was collected between 1975 and 1980. Their cases developed the syndrome following nonpulmonary illness or injury. Predisposing causes included septic shock, hypovolemic shock, hypernatremic dehydration, and cardiogenic shock secondary to imipramine poisoning. Five of the 18 patients had sustained cardiopulmonary arrest. Three had significant intracranial hypertension. Lyrene and Truog reviewed their series of pediatric cases of adult respiratory distress syndrome in 1981.[7] Their predisposing causes included smoke inhalation, near-drowning, near-strangulation, dermatomyositis, all diseases that are the primary province of the pediatrician.

Incidence

The incidence of adult respiratory distress syndrome in children is unknown. Lyrene and Truog's pediatric article reports 15 cases collected over a $3\frac{1}{2}$ year period, approximately 1% of medical admissions to their intensive care unit. Pfenninger et al reported a similar incidence in Europe in September, 1982.[8] Holbrook et al did not report the incidence in their unit. Other pediatric centers should be experiencing the same incidence although diagnosed as respiratory insufficiency due to near-drowning, asphyxia, pneumonia, fat embolism, lupus erythematosus, post-traumatic congestive atelectasis, refractory pulmonary edema, pulmonary contusion, and many more.

Mortality and Morbidity

The mortality rate reported by Lyrene and Truog was 60%, comparable to the 25% and 59% in adult populations.[9,10] Blaisdell and Lewis reported a decreasing mortality in trauma cases in their unit from 66% in 1966 to 18% in 1972.[11] They emphasized that decreased mortality can only be achieved through early recognition of patients at risk, early effective respiratory support, and prevention or early treatment of further pulmonary injury such as pneumothorax, pneumonia, and atelectasis. Morbidity of respiratory distress syndrome in children will only be known when it is recognized as a distinct problem and less severe forms are described.

Proposed Etiologic Factors

Nobody knows what causes adult respiratory distress syndrome. A number of factors are probably responsible for the alveolar capillary membrane injury with resultant capillary permeability and defect in surfactant.[9,12–14] The various factors include shock, fluid resuscitation, oxygen therapy, respirator support necessary in treatment, and sepsis. Neurogenic factors also contribute to the development of the syndrome in certain cases.

Fluid overload has had variable prominence as an etiologic cause. Berry described the lung lesion of shock lung in 1963.[15] He felt that fluid overload was a primary factor. Fishman proposed that nonuniform pulmonary perfusion produced high perfusion pressures in certain areas with resultant stretching of pores between endothelial cells and leakage.[16] Crystalloid resuscitation and its effect on plasma oncotic pressure was a concern. The Viet Nam shock unit reported only a slight drop in plasma protein concentration following fluid resuscitation with the most significant drop occurring prior to resuscitation.[17] Moss demonstrated that under experimental circumstances, blood or colloid resuscitation resulted in more lung edema than crystalloid replacement.[18,19] Ashbaugh concluded that massive infusions in the treatment of shock do not cause the syndrome but additional massive infusions will aggravate congestion and edema.[20]

Oxygen toxicity is a known contributing factor.[21] This study also showed that pulmonary changes did not correlate with length of ventilator support. Obviously, respirator therapy may contribute to injury if only through barotrauma. However, the respirator should be primarily viewed as the main method of support while lung healing occurs. This concept is supported by a controlled study in animals demonstrating a decrease in mortality from 19% to 10%.[22]

Sepsis may be followed by respiratory distress syndrome without manifest shock.[23] However, when the syndrome develops within the first 24–48 hours following trauma or nonseptic shock, bacterial infection is unlikely to be an initiating event. Pulmonary insufficiency following primary sepsis or sepsis complicating other causes of respiratory distress syndrome can be related to E. coli endotoxin, live E. coli organisms, and peritonitis induced septicemia experimentally.[24–26] Experimental evidence supports that Gram-negative sepsis causes intravascular coagulation and thereby produces the pulmonary changes of the syndrome.[27,28]

Neurogenic factors also come into play. Several studies show that respiratory insufficiency frequently follows head injury.[29,30] Moss developed an animal model to evaluate the cerebral etiology of shock lung and did produce pulmonary changes which were similar to shock lung. As a result of his studies, he postulated a decrease in hypothalamic perfusion with autonomically mediated increased pulmonary venular resistance and thereby lung changes.[31,32] His studies do serve as an explanation for respiratory distress syndrome in certain patients but not in those who do not develop central nervous system changes.

A multiple of other contributing factors such as the effects of secondary aspiration, atelectasis, pneumothorax, pneumonia, and pulmonary embolism must also be considered. It is important to remember that no single factor explains the entire syndrome.

Clinical Features of Respiratory Distress Syndrome

The syndrome may follow any clinical catastrophe such as major trauma, asphyxia, near-drowning, or sepsis. Less obvious insults such as a partial pneumothorax complicating pneumonia or protracted seizure in an infant with sepsis may herald severe pulmonary disease. The average patient with RDS develops the syndrome within 24–72 hours following the clinical insult. The classical clinical description is a rather sudden onset of dyspnea, labored breathing, tachypnea, tachycardia, fever, hypotension and refractory cyanosis.[33] Infants and small children do not complain of dyspnea. Stiffness of their lungs is clinically reflected by a fast shallow respiratory rate and corresponding decreasing amount of activity. This type of breathing generally does not impress the pediatrician who is used to the labored breathing of the patient with croup or asthma. Cyanosis is difficult to appreciate in infants and children due to their lower hemoglobin levels and tendency to peripheral vasoconstriction. Roentgenographic changes of early "fluffy infiltrates" may be obscured by over-penetrated technique. Initial clinical manifestations, occurring within hours, are limited to tachypnea and tachycardia only. No rales or rhonchi will be heard. Serial blood gas analyses will reveal a concomitant drop in partial pressure of arterial oxygen. Arterial carbon dioxide tensions will be low due to hypoxemic drive unless the pulmonary injury is associated with respiratory center depression. Frequent respiratory rate monitoring will identify the pediatric patient with decreasing pulmonary compliance and permit early therapeutic intervention. Late recognition is a relatively common occurrence in patients with predisposing factors such as sepsis or near-drowning. Here, many hours of generous fluid therapy may have seriously contributed to congestive atelectasis and profound hypoxemia. Clinical manifestations may be delayed after the initial insult until secondary complications including infection, pneumothorax, aspiration, recurrent hypotension, or a profound second hypoxic episode occur. Each subsequent episode should be followed by intensive respiratory monitoring even if apparently minor.

Reported Clinical Course and Complications of RDS

Lyrene and Truog's study reports 60% mortality with mean time of death occurring at six days following the insult and maximal survival to 32 days.[7] Of their nine patients who died, only three died because of refractory hypoxemia. The other six deaths were attributed to irreversible central nervous system damage. These children were described as having inspired oxygen requirements of less than 40%, a decreased need for ventilatory assistance, and improved chest radiographic appearance during the 24 hours prior to death. This would suggest that only 20% of their patients died of the pulmonary involvement, comparable to better statistics reported in the adult respiratory distress syndrome.[9,10] Their most common complication was air leak, occurring in ten of their 15 patients. There was no difference in peak inspiratory pressure and level of positive end-expiratory pressure (PEEP) in those patients who did or did not develop air leak. Secondary infection was suspected in several children but was not confirmed by positive blood cultures. Postmortem lung tissue culture was positive for *Enterococcus* in one patient. Major atelectasis was not mentioned as a complication. Their long-term pulmonary sequelae included only one asymptomatic child with chest radiographic residual linear densities at six months postinjury and another with persistent interstitial infiltrates and obstructive lung disease at nine months posthospitalization. This latter child had a history of prior pulmonary problems (recurrent aspiration pneumonia in early childhood). This represents approximately 30% (two of six) of their survivors. Their neurologic sequelae was the major problem area. Two of six survivors had severe neurologic sequelae while four had none. The sequelae may relate to the initial insult and support prior to initiation of aggressive pulmonary management. Recognition of this syndrome with early monitoring and development of earlier aggressive support might decrease neurological sequelae. A. W. Conn in 1979 described marked improvement in neurologic sequelae of near-drowning patients by early respiratory support and cerebral resuscitative measures.[34]

Pfenninger et al reported 20 cases.[8] Twelve patients survived and eight died. Of the deaths, three had irreversible brain damage and respiratory support was terminated; three died of septicemia; and two had bilateral adrenal hemorrhage with irreversible shock. All of their survivors had normal respiratory function for daily life and only one had a residual motor handicap.

Radiological Features of RDS

Specific radiologic changes for children have not been described. However, changes similar to those seen in adults should be expected. Dyck and Zylak reported the radiographic findings in acute respiratory distress in adults in 1973.[35] Radiographic changes may not be present for 12 hours despite severe pulmonary dysfunction. The early fine reticulonodular changes throughout both lung fields are difficult to note in small children because a standard six-foot film is seldom taken and overpenetration is common. The radiographic changes progress to a virtually confluent pattern over the next 24 hours, correlating with progression of interstitial edema and perivascular cuffing to intra-alveolar edema and hemorrhage.[11] In contrast to the pulmonary edema of cardiac origin, there is often a peculiar sparing of the heart border with more density laterally and at the bases. Also, cardiac size tends to remain normal. The fully developed picture is not dissimilar to that seen in hyaline membrane disease. In contrast, pulmonary contusion generally has an alveolarized pattern localized to the site underlying the thoracic blow. Atelectasis usually is not symmetrical and bilateral. Secondary pneumonia may add local increased radiographic density or may be undetectable because of the primary abnormality. As pulmonary degeneration occurs, pneumatocoeles may develop without secondary bacterial infection.

Pathologic Features of RDS

In 1974, F. W. Blaisdell reported over 200 autopsy results collected, beginning in 1964.[36] In the early cases, death usually occurred within a few hours to days. With the advent of improved respiratory support, the patients in later cases rarely died within the first week of illness. From this autopsy material, Dr. Blaisdell postulated the following sequence of pulmonary microscopic and macroscopic changes that will vary with time, type of support provided, and whether one or more complications have occurred. With repeated insults, new acute changes will be superimposed on chronic changes that have already developed.[36] Microscopic lung sections appear almost normal with thin alveolar walls and minimal congestion. Occasional amorphous masses of granular material containing white cells may be seen in pulmonary arterioles. Between eight and 16 hours, obvious pulmonary microvascular congestion progresses to frank periarterial hemorrhage with interstitial hemorrhage and edema. By 24 hours, widespread intra-alveolar edema and hemorrhage are evident. These changes correlate with the progressive opacification of the roentgenograph. The progression continues with increasing alveolar involvement and associated atelectasis between 48 and 72 hours. By 72 hours, thromboemboli previously present may be diminishing with some evidence of early clearing of edema and hemorrhage. Proteinaceous deposits initially involving alveolar ducts represent hyaline membranes. Macroscopic changes correlate with the microscopic changes. Within hours, petechiae appear over the lung surfaces, lung weights are increasingly heavier, and cut sections appear edematous. By 48 to 72 hours, the lung grossly resembles liver, and inflation does not change the appearance. By one week, inflammatory changes and bronchopneumonia become the dominant lesion. Within the next two weeks, fibroblast proliferation and collagen are much more prominent. The survivor may have a relatively acellular lung replaced by scar tissue, showing widespread degeneration of alveoli, and the appearance of smaller air cysts and even frank pneumatocoeles. The tissue is proportionally avascular with hyaline degeneration of blood vessels. Many of the microscopic and macroscopic changes seen correlate well with the changes of neonatal hyaline membrane disease.[37]

Laboratory Findings of RDS

Decreasing arterial PO_2 values correlate with increasing respiratory rate and progression of disease. Arterial PCO_2 values will remain low or normal until the central nervous system becomes depressed because of severe hypoxia unless the patient has sustained severe central nervous system injury as well. Pulmonary compliance studies are extremely difficult if not impossible in the small child until mechanical intervention has occurred. Effective dynamic compliance may be determined by dividing delivered tidal volume by the difference between peak-inspiratory pressure and end-expiratory pressure measured at the mouth.[4,38]

Differential Diagnosis of RDS

Blaisdell defined nine different explanations for acute respiratory failure following shock and trauma. These include: ARDS, aspiration, simple atelectasis, pulmonary contusion, pulmonary edema, pneumonia, pneumothorax, pulmonary embolism, and fat embolism.[36] ARDS, in addition, may be complicated by all of the above.

Treatment of Respiratory Distress Syndrome

Treatment depends on a clear understanding of predisposing causes, appreciation of clinical course, etiologic factors, complications of the syndrome, and support required during therapy to alter outcome morbidity and mortality. Clearly, respiratory distress syndrome in infants and children may follow trauma such as head injury; massive soft tissue injury; hypovolemic shock as with gastrointestinal bleeding or fluid loss; Gram-negative sepsis with endotoxin damage to the alveolar capillary unit; severe meningitis; intracranial hypertension; and anoxic shock as with near-strangulation or near-drowning. Primarily damaged lungs such as massive aspiration, near-drowning, collagen vascular disease such as lupus erythematosus all share a damaged alveolar-capillary unit, fluid leakage, surfactant decrease, and pulmonary changes in common with respiratory distress syndrome. Here, respiratory distress syndrome may be superimposed on an initial abnormal pulmonary baseline. In addition, any patient with cardiorespiratory arrest should be considered at risk.

All patients described above should have intensive respiratory monitoring every one to two hours for 12–24 hours to alert the physician regarding onset of respiratory distress syndrome. Serial arterial blood gases should correlate with increasing respiratory rate, decreasing lung compliance and severity of disease, as well as the need for therapeutic intervention.

General measures of treatment include elevation of the head and chest which are thought to increase functional residual capacity.[39] Infant seats predispose to body slumping, glossoptosis, and thereby increased inspiratory respiratory effort and possible tendency to aspirate in the infant. Ideally, the head of the bed should be elevated with the infant or child minimally restrained unless respirator dependent. Prone nursing with frequent positional changes may minimize atelectasis. Suctioning may be necessary to clear upper respiratory secretions. Routine postural drainage and percussion have no proven benefit unless lobar atelectasis is present. It should be avoided during the acute phase of illness as it contributes to respiratory fatigue and a potentially earlier need for respiratory intervention.

Volume therapy should include crystalloids necessary for shock resuscitation unless blood loss has been a problem. If the hematocrit drops below 30%, packed red blood cells or whole blood should be combined with crystalloid volume to restore volume to normal. With small infants, patients with severe hypoxemia and patients with pre-existing cardiac compromise, the hematocrit should be maintained at 38–40% to provide an improved oxygen carrying content. Total intravenous and oral fluids should be maintained at one-half to low normal quantities (700–1500cc/kg/24hrs) depending on whether the patient has sustained severe cerebral insult, with potential rise in intracranial pressure. Replacement of all exceptional losses as due to vomiting, diarrhea, gastric suction and urinary losses must be considered.

Diuretics should be used to treat documented or suspected fluid overload, such as may well be present in the fresh water near-drowning patient who required fluid resuscitation for hypotension. Lasix lmg/kg/dose initially may be used to maintain adequate urine output and minimize secondary pulmonary edema. The usual dose interval is six to 12 hours.

Oxygen therapy should be geared to provide an oxygen saturation above 90%. An arterial Po_2 above 60 mm Hg will provide this saturation but not during interruptions of oxygenation as will occur with coughing or suctioning. Ideally, a Pao_2 of greater than 80 mm Hg and less than 150 mm Hg should be maintained. To insure that an adequate oxygen content of 10–13 vol% is maintained, a hemoglobin of 12 gm per dl or higher may be required. If transfusion is required, fresh red blood cells should be used to decrease adverse effects on the oxygen-hemoglobin dissociation curve.[40] High inspired oxygen concentrations may be provided by a ventimask (to 50%), a partial rebreathing mask (>60%), a non-rebreathing mask (>80%), an oxygen tent (40–80%) which is appropriate for the under four-year-old, or an oxyhood (to >80%) in the infant less than four months of age. Remember that oxygen transport represents the product of cardiac output and arterial oxygen content. Therefore, careful monitoring of cardiac output must be maintained.

Corticosteroids have not been shown to be of benefit in ARDS or pulmonary syndromes predisposing to RDS such as near-drowning or aspiration.[41,42] Steroids may be indicated because of associated head injury or cerebral complication of near-drowning.[14]

Antibiotics will be required if sepsis is the precipitating event. If not, careful monitoring for sepsis and pulmonary superinfection should be maintained as they may significantly worsen the pulmonary disease.[43–45] Localized infiltrates, disproportionate temperature, white blood count elevation with shift to the left all suggest secondary infection. Tracheal secretions with evidence of polymorphonuclear cells and bacteria may precede signs of frank infection. Suspected secondary infection should be treated with antibiotics to cover the usual secondary invaders of damaged lungs. Ampicillin will provide coverage for the usual pathogens unless resistant H. influenzae, lactam positive or *Staphylococcus aureus* are suspected. Gram-negative organisms are much more unusual except in the neonate, patient with underlying oncologic problems, or patient who is nutritionally deficient.

Respiratory assistance is the mainstay of therapy for respiratory distress syndrome. Ventilatory criteria have not been established as the syndrome is not uniformly recognized as a pediatric problem. Holbrook's recommendations are reasonable for intervention criteria.[6] The obtunded or hypotonic child should be intubated and ventilated without waiting for laboratory confirmation of respiratory failure. Otherwise a PaO_2 of less than 60 mm Hg on 60% F_IO_2 or $PaCO_2$ of greater than 50–55 mm Hg are criteria for intubation and ventilatory support. For the patient with oxygenation problems only, intubation with continuous positive airways pressure support may suffice. Masks for providing continuous positive airways pressure without intubation are currently being developed. For patients with intracranial hypertension, respiratory intervention should be initiated if the $PaCO_2$ is greater than 40 mm Hg. Here the $PaCO_2$ should be controlled at 25–30 mm Hg. Mechanical ventilation should be provided with a volume-cycled or time-cycled ventilator to provide more uniform volume per breath in patients with very stiff lungs. Delivered tidal volume of 10–15 ml/kg, on an intermittent-mandatory control mode are optimal to avoid significant respiratory acidosis or alkalosis. Pediatric patients may not tolerate low rate intermittent-mandatory-ventilation (IMV) support (lowest normal rate for age), and controlled ventilation with heavy sedation, or paralysis may be required. It is desirable to maintain an end inspiratory pressure of less than

40–50 cc H_2O to decrease the chance of pneumothorax or subcutaneous emphysema. To achieve this goal respirator setting requires higher respiratory rates and a tidal volume of less than 10 ml/kg.

Positive end expiratory pressure (PEEP) increases functional residual capacity, decreases intrapulmonary right to left shunting and improves oxygenation.[46,47] PEEP may be increased by three to five cm of water increments until the F_IO_2 can be decreased to less than 60% to yield a PaO_2 of greater than 80 mm Hg. Lyrene and Truog assessed PEEP response in ten of their 15 patients. These ten patients had a mean increase of 8 ± 6 mm Hg/cm H_2O PEEP with no response noted until at least 10 cm H_2O had been applied. Their average maximum PEEP required was 16 cm H_2O, two-fold greater than reported "optimal PEEP" required in the treatment of hyaline membrane disease.[48] Kirby et al first used high PEEP (>15 cm) to minimize intrapulmonary shunting and improve oxygenation in ARDS.[49] They stress the need for increased fluids and inotropic agents because of the adverse effects of high PEEP on cardiac output. Holbrook et al quote their experience with high PEEP in children stressing the success of high PEEP in selected cases and also the need for a Swan-Ganz flow directed-balloon tipped catheter for measurements of cardiac index, PAP and PCWP.[6] Pulmonary artery catheters should be used whenever high PEEP is considered necessary. Current catheters and introducer systems make pulmonary artery catheterization a bedside procedure in pediatrics.[50] Holbrook recommends increasing PEEP to decrease $\dot{Q}sp/\dot{Q}t$ to approximately 15% while maintaining the cardiac index greater than 3 liters per minute/per/M^2 and av $DO_2 <$ 5 volumes percent with fluids and inotropic agents.[6] $\dot{Q}sp/\dot{Q}t$ is the physiologic intrapulmonary shunt in percent calculated by the following equation:

$$\frac{\dot{Q}sp}{\dot{Q}t} = \frac{CpcO_2 - CaO_2}{CpcO_2 - CmvO_2} \times 100$$

$CpcO_2$, CaO_2, and $CmvO_2$ are the oxygen contents of pulmonary capillary, arterial, and mixed venous blood. As pulmonary capillary blood cannot be directly sampled, alveolar PO_2 (P_AO_2) should be substituted. P_AO_2 may be derived from the following equation:[51]

$$P_AO_2 = F_IO_2 \text{ (P barometric–P } H_2O \text{ vapor)} – PaCO_2/0.8$$

Oxygen content of various samples may be calculated by the following formula:

$$CO_2 = SO_2 \times Hgb \times 1.36 + 0.0031 \times PO_2$$

SO_2 is oxygen saturation. Hgb represent number of grams of hemoglobin. 1.36 is ml O_2 bound to one gram of fully saturated hemoglobin. 0.0031 is the amount of dissolved oxygen per mm Hg PO_2.

With conventional PEEP (15 cm of H_2O or less), central venous and urinary catheter permit monitoring of central venous pressure and urinary output respectively. Arterial catheterization will facilitate blood pressure measurements and blood sampling although conventional blood pressure measurements may suffice. Pulmonary arterial catheterization is not routinely used in patients requiring conventional PEEP.

Conclusion

Adult respiratory distress syndrome represents diffuse systemic capillary leaking of intravascular volume into all tissues of the body with a profound effect on the lung. Historically, the pulmonary process was first identified in adults postshock or trauma with no antecedent pulmonary disease. The syndrome has not been well described in pediatrics and has remarkable similarities to infantile respiratory distress syndrome. The various proposed etiologic factors may affect all children, those with no prior pulmonary problems as well as those with antecedent pulmonary problems. The syndrome should be known as *respiratory distress syndrome* in children. Recognition of the problem and earlier therapeutic intervention in a controlled, systematic way should contribute to decreased morbidity and mortality.

References

1. Jenkins MT, Jones RD, Wilson B, et al: Congestive atelectasis. A complication of the intravenous infusion of fluids. *Ann Surg* 132:327, 1950.
2. Burford TH, Burbank B: Traumatic wet lung: Observations on certain physiologic fundamentals in thoracic trauma. *J Thorac Cardiovasc Surg* 14:415, 1945.

3. Moon VH: The pathology of secondary shock. *Am J Pathol* 24:235, 1948,
4. Ashbaugh DGK, Bigelow DB, Petty TL, et al: Acute respiratory distress in adults. *Lancet* 2:319, 1967.
5. Eiseman B, Ashbaugh DG: Pulmonary effects of nonthoracic trauma. Proceedings of a conference conducted by the committee on trauma, division of medical sciences, national academy of sciences, national research council, Washington, DC, 29 February—2 March, 1968. *J Trauma,* 8 September 1968.
6. Holbrook PR, Taylor G, Pollack MM, et al: Adult respiratory distress syndrome in children. *Pediatr Clin North Am* 26:677, 1980.
7. Lyrene RK, Truog WE: ARDS in Pediatric Intensive Care Unit. *Pediatrics* 676:1981.
8. Pfenninger J, Guber A, Tschäppeler H, et al: Adult respiratory distress syndrome in children. *J Pediatr* 3:352, 1982.
9. Hopewell PC, Murray JF: The adult respiratory distress syndrome. *Ann Rev Med* 27:343, 1976.
10. Amato JJ, Rheinlander HF, Cleveland RJ: Post-traumatic adult respiratory distress syndrome. *Orthop Clinic North Am* 9:693, 1978.
11. Blaisdell FW, Lewis FR: Respiratory distress syndrome of shock and trauma. *Major Problems in Clinical Surgery,* Philadelphia, W. B. Saunders, XXI:8, 1977.
12. Wilson JW, Ratliff NB, and Hackel DB: The lung in hemorrhagic shock. *Am J Pathol* 58:339, 1970.
13. Anderson RR, Holliday RL, Driedger AA, et al: Documentation of pulmonary capillary permeability in adult respiratory distress syndrome accompanying human sepsis. *Am Rev Resp Dis* 119:869, 1979.
14. Petty TL, Reiss OK, Paul GW, et al: Characteristics of Pulmonary surfactant in adult respiratory distress syndrome associated with shock and trauma. *Am Rev Resp Dis* 115:532–536, 1977.
15. Berry RE: Clinical manifestations and treatment of congestive atelectasis. *Arch Surg* 87:153, 1963.
16. Fishman A: Pulmonary edema—The water changing function of the lung. *Circulation* 46:390, 1972.
17. Bredenberg CE: Acute respiratory distress. *Surg Clin North Am* 54:1043, 1974.
18. Moss GS, et al: Hemorrhagic shock in the baboon—circulatory and metabolic effects of dilutional therapy. *J Trauma* 8:837, 1968.
19. Moss GS, et al: The effect of saline solution resuscitation on pulmonary sodium and water distribution. *Surg Gynecol Obstet* 136:934, 1973.
20. Ashbaugh DG et al: Continuous positive pressure breathing in the adult respiratory distress syndrome. *J Thorac Cardiovasc Surg* 57:31, 1969.
21. Nash G, Blennerhasset JB, Pontoppidan H: Pulmonary lesions associated with oxygen toxicity and artificial ventilation. *N Engl J Med* 276:368, 1967.
22. Stallone RJ, Herbst H, Blaisdell FW, et al: Pulmonary changes following ischemia of the lower extremities and their treatment. *Am Rev Resp Dis* 100:813, 1969.

23. Coolins JA: The causes of progressive pulmonary insufficiency in surgical patients. *J Surg Res* 9:685, 1969.
24. Pennington DG, Hyman A, and Jacques, WE: Pulmonary vascular response to endotoxin in intact dogs. *Surgery* 3:246, 1973.
25. Neuhof H, et al: Pathophysiological mechanisms in endotoxin shock and its therapeutic approaches. *In* Bertilli A, Beck N, (eds): *Biochemical, Pharmacological and Clinical Aspects.* New York, Plenum Press 1970.
26. Brown PP, et al: Hemodynamic and respiratory responses of conscious swine to Escherichia coli endotoxin. *J Trauma* 16:184, 1976.
27. Horovitz DL et al: Coagulation changes of septic shock in the subhuman primate. *Ann Surg* 175:417, 1972.
28. Milligan GF et al: Pulmonary and hematologic disturbances following septic shock. *Surg Gynecol Obstet* 138:43, 1974.
29. Froman C: Alterations of respiratory function in patients with severe head injuries. *Chest* 68:736, 1975.
30. Katsurada K, Yamada R, and Sugimoto T: Respiratory insufficiency in patients with severe head injury. *Surgery* 73:191, 1973.
31. Moss G, Staunton C, and Stine AA: Cerebral etiology of the shock lung syndrome. *J Trauma* 12:885, 1972.
32. Motley HL: The influence of short periods of induced acute anoxia on pulmonary artery pressure in man. *Am J Physiol* 150:350, 1947.
33. Jenkins MT, Jones RF, Wilson B, et al: Congestive atelectasis—A complication of the intravenous infusion of fluids. *Ann Surgery* 132:327, 1950.
34. Conn AW, Edmonds JF, Barker GA: Cerebral resuscitation in near-drowning. *Pediatr Clin North Am* 26:691, 1979.
35. Dyck DR, Zylak CJ: Acute respiratory distress in adults. *Radiology* 106:497, 1973.
36. Blaisdell FW: Pathophysiology of the respiratory distress syndrome. *Arch Surg* 108:44, 1974.
37. Spencer H: *Pathology of the Lung.* Volume I, 504. Philadelphia, W. B. Saunders, 1977.
38. Petty TL, Ashbaugh DG: The adult respiratory distress syndrome. *Chest* 60:233, 1971.
39. Hsu HO, Hickey RF: Effect of posture on functional residual capacity post-operatively. *Anesthesiology* 44:520–521, 1976.
40. Woodson RD: Physiological significance of oxygen dissociation curve shifts. *Crit Care Med* 7:368–379, 1979.
41. Calderwood H, Modell J, Ruiz B: The ineffectiveness of steroid therapy for treatment of fresh water near-drowning. *Anesthesiology* 43:642–650, 1975.
42. Wynne JW, Modell JH, et al: Respiratory aspiration of stomach contents. *Ann Intern Med* 87:466–474, 1977.
43. Clowes GHA, Hirsch E, et al: Septic lung and shock lung in man. *Ann Surg* 181:681–692, 1975.
44. Esrig BC, Fulton RL: Sepsis, resuscitated hemorrhagic shock and "shock lung": An experimental correlation. *Ann Surg* 182:218–227, 1975.

45. Walker L, Eiseman B: The changing pattern of post-traumatic respiratory distress syndrome. *Ann Surg* 181:693–697, 1975.
46. Powers SR, Mannal R, Neclerio M, et al: Physiologic consequences of positive end-expiratory pressure (PEEP) ventilation. *Ann Surg* 178:265–272, 1973.
47. Suter PM, Fairley HB, Isenberg MD: Optimum end-expiratory airway pressure in patients with acute pulmonary failure. *N Engl J Med* 292:284–289, 1975.
48. Bonta BW, Uany R, Warshaw JB, et al: Determination of optimal continuous positive airway pressure for the treatment of IRDS by measurement of esophageal pressure. *J Pediatr* 91:449, 1977.
49. Kirby RR, Downs JB, Civetta JM, et al: High level positive end-expiratory pressure (PEEP) in acute respiratory insufficiency. *Chest* 67:156–163, 1975.
50. Pollack MM, Reed TD, Holbrook PR, et al: Bedside pulmonary artery catheterization in pediatrics. *J Pediatr* 96:274–76, 1980.
51. Campbell EJM: The management of acute respiratory failure in chronic bronchitis and emphysema. *Am Rev Resp Dis* 96:626–39, 1967.

16

Pleural Effusion in Children

Robert C. Stern, M.D.

Introduction

Although the lungs are normally immediately adjacent to the internal wall of the thoracic cavity, the two structures are not anatomically joined (except as a result of disease) and a potential space exists between them. Accumulation of fluid within this space is an important manifestation of many intrathoracic diseases as well as some systemic disorders and, in some cases, the compromise of breathing which results becomes the dominant clinical expression of the illness. Thus, the recognition that fluid is present within the pleural space is important from both diagnostic and therapeutic standpoints.

In the human (unlike some of the other mammals, e.g. the dog), the right and left thoracic cavities are completely separated anatomically and, therefore, fluid accumulation which results from unilateral intrathoracic disease usually does not result in bilateral intrapleural fluid accumulation. Systemic diseases also can produce unilateral pleural fluid. The separation of the two thoracic cavities prevents the diagnostic or therapeutic aspiration of fluid from both sides of the chest with a single procedure. Of course, separate right and left thoracic cavities have substantial survival advantages for the normal individual. For example, a penetrating chest injury results in a unilateral pneumothorax as opposed to the bilateral pneumothorax which can occur in a dog after a unilateral penetrating chest injury.

The amount of fluid within the pleural space is determined by a balance among several factors.[2] High pleural capillary hydrostatic pressure and pericapillary colloid osmotic pressure favor the transudation of fluid into the pleural space, whereas high pericapillary hydrostatic pressure and plasma osmotic pressure favor reabsorption of fluid from the pleural space. The net balance in some pleural areas favor transudation of fluid and the net balance in others favor reabsorption so that normally there is a very small amount of intrapleural fluid (from 3–15 ml in the adult) present in health. The lymphatic system, as well as some of the pleural capillaries, is responsible for reabsorption of fluid. The lymphatic system reabsorbs most of the small numbers of large molecules which otherwise would accumulate within the pleural space. Any disturbance in the balance of the relevant pressures or an abnormality in lymphatic drainage can have important clinical implications with regard to the amount and type of pleural fluid which then accumulates.

Pathophysiology

For pleural fluid to accumulate, its rate of formation must exceed its rate of reabsorption. Several basic pathophysiologic mechanisms may be operative, singly or in combination. Two of these result mainly in increased production of fluid. Capillary permeability is increased by a variety of inflammatory situations and the resulting increased volume of fluid production often exceeds the reabsorption rate even if reabsorptive mechanisms are normal. Increased systemic hydrostatic pressure may result in a sufficiently increased fluid production to overwhelm normal reabsorption. One basic mechanism, interference with lymphatic drainage, causes accumulation of pleural fluid mainly by decreased reabsorption.

A few basic abnormalities result in increased production and decreased reabsorption. Intracapillary osmotic pressure decreases in hypoproteinemia. Plasma albumin is the key variable here and severe hypoalbuminemia results in widespread fluid transudation, which includes, but usually is not limited to the pleural space. The ability to reabsorb fluid is also compromised by the low osmotic pressure and, in severe hypoalbuminemia, all reabsorption must be done by the lymphatic system. In patients with congestive heart failure and increased systemic hydrostatic pressure, a pleural effusion is much more likely to occur if the pulmonary venous pressure is also elevated, thus decreasing reabsorption. Finally, with some parenchymal pulmonary diseases, the accentuation of intrathoracic negative pressure generated by the accessory muscles of respiration may be sufficient to decrease pericapillary pressure. A sufficient decrease in pericapillary pressure can result in increased production and decreased reabsorption of fluid.

Clinical Presentation

The major clinical manifestations of pleural effusion relate to the compromise in respiration caused by restriction of the expansion of the lung(s). Dyspnea, tachypnea, retractions, nasal flaring, cyanosis, and orthopnea may be present. When the effusion results from inflammatory diseases, including infection, pleuritic chest pain may precede or accompany the compromised respiration. Occasionally, the chest pain is continuous and dull rather than the typical intermittent and sharp pain accompanying every breath and cough. The signs and symptoms of the pleural effusion may be totally overshadowed by the symptoms of the underlying disease process. In patients with underlying chronic or acute pulmonary disease, the added problems created by effusion may seem to be caused by worsening of the parenchymal disease rather than by the addition of the restrictive effects of pleural fluid, and the diagnosis of a superimposed pleural effusion may be delayed.

Diagnosis

The definitive diagnosis of pleural effusion is made radiologically and confirmed (if appropriate) by thoracentesis. The diagnosis may be strongly suspected clinically, however, on the basis of history and physical findings. Many clinical findings are nonspecific and all vary substantially with the amount of pleural fluid present. The percussion note is dull. Breath sounds are decreased or absent, except in the infant where they may be tubular. A large amount of fluid may cause sufficient shift of the mediastinum to be detected by palpation of the trachea. Fremitus may be decreased. More specific physical findings include a pleural friction rub and a change in physical findings with a shift in position. The pleural friction rub may become louder if the stethoscope is pressed against the chest. Although physical findings may change with a shift in position, a failure to demonstrate such a change does not rule out a pleural effusion, because the amount of fluid may be insufficient or the fluid may be loculated. In adults, a minimum of 300 ml of pleural fluid is believed necessary to produce any of the characteristic symptoms or physical findings. Correspondingly, less fluid would be expected to be detectable clinically in younger patients.

Pleural effusion is often asymptomatic and is discovered when a chest roentgenogram is obtained for another reason. A chest roentgenogram should be obtained when fluid is suspected clinically or when a deterioration of clinical status occurs in an illness which is likely to cause an effusion. Radiologic findings include obliteration of the costophrenic or cardiophrenic angles and a homogeneous density which obscures the underlying parenchyma. (See Fig. 1.) Decubitus and supine films may add additional information by demonstrating a shift in the fluid or by suggesting that the fluid is loculated. (See Fig. 2.) Occasionally, fluid can be suspected when there is widening of the interlobar septae. Usually, plain radiographs are sufficient. In more difficult situations (e.g. determining if a patient with pleural thickening also has an effusion), other radiologic techniques may be useful. Ultrasound can be quite useful to detect very small amounts of loculated fluid, it can be performed at the bedside, is painless and relatively noninvasive, and can usually distinguish fluid from pleural thickening. Computerized axial tomography of the chest, although capable of detecting pleural fluid is usually unnecessary. In some patients the use of ultrasound to pinpoint the optimal site for thoracentesis is extremely important.

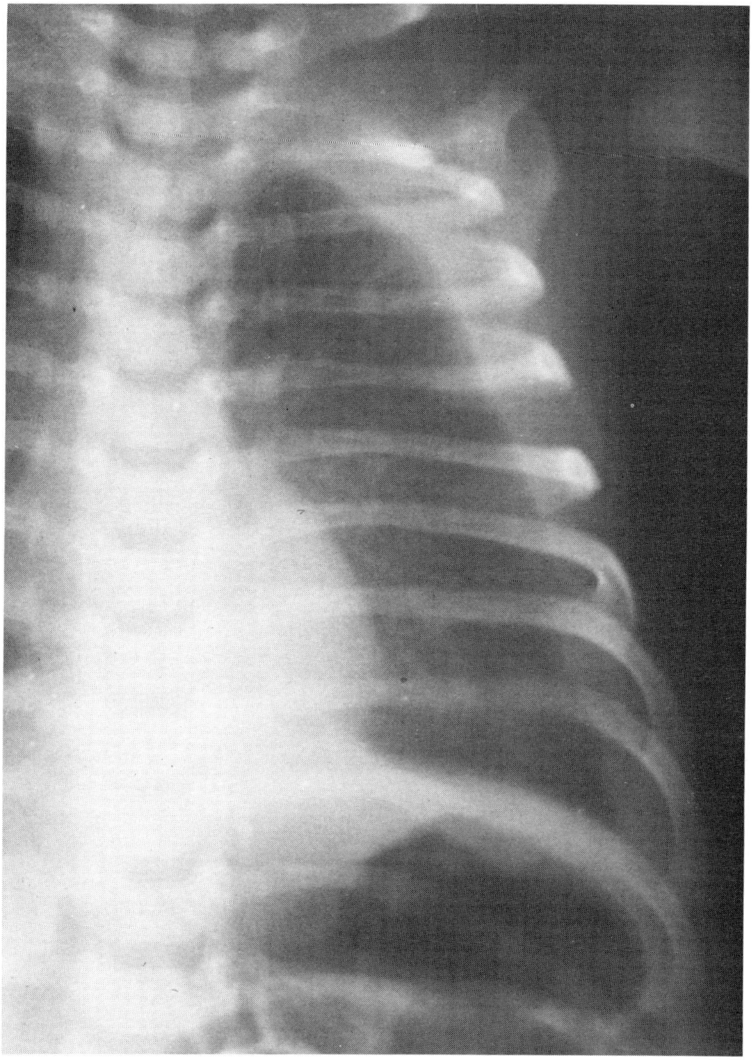

Figure 1. Left pleural effusion in an 18-month-old boy. Note haziness of pulmonary vascular markings caused by the overlying fluid. The fluid can be seen along the left border where it obscures the cardiophrenic angle.

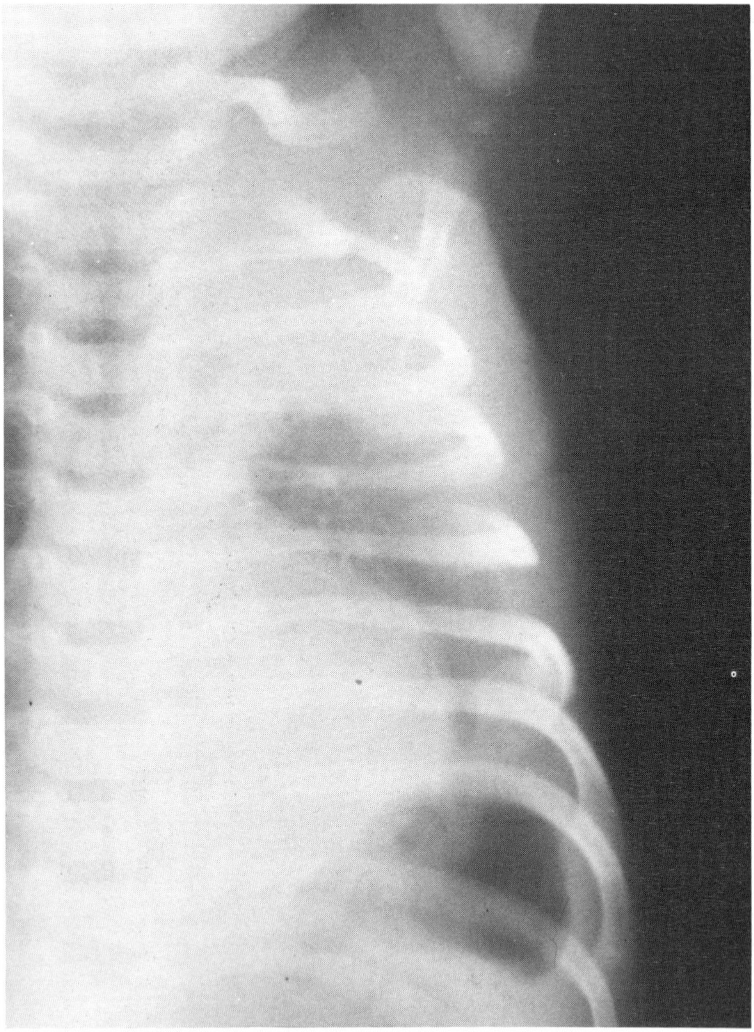

Figure 2. Loculated pleural fluid in an 18-month-old boy. Loculation is clear at the apex where a collection of fluid does not distribute evenly along the lateral border.

Differential Diagnosis

The first step in differential diagnosis, after a space occupying lesion in the pleural space has been demonstrated by chest roentgenogram, is to assign the lesion to one of five general categories: uninfected transudate or exudate (effusion); infected fluid (empyema); blood (hemothorax); chyle (chylothorax); or fibrous tissue (fibrothorax). Fibrothorax may be suspected clinically on the basis of previously diagnosed disease which is known to cause fibrosis and the diagnosis can be confirmed with relative certainty by ultrasound.[4] With rare exception (discussed below), a thoracentesis is needed to differentiate and investigate the other categories of pleural densities.[6]

Relatively few lesions cause massive hemothorax. Trauma is the most common, but local pleural disease (usually a primary or metastatic malignancy) and a dissecting aortic aneurysm are also possible. Similarly, chylothorax almost always results from injury to the thoracic duct. This may be the result of chest trauma or thoracic surgery (particularly for congenital heart lesions in infants). Metastatic malignancy and lymphoma are the other major diagnostic considerations. The thoracic duct normally enters the lower chest on the right side and crosses over to the left before entering the vein in the upper chest. Thus, depending on the location of the injury, either a right or left chylothorax may result.

Empyema is diagnosed when pus is obtained at thoracentesis. The differential diagnosis may be more difficult than with hemothorax or chylothorax, however, in that the source of the infection may not be apparent. Metastatic infection of the pleural space is so rare (if it occurs at all) that, for diagnostic purposes, it is safe to assume that the pleural infection resulted from direct extension. A penetrating chest injury, a surgical incision, or an indwelling catheter or chest tube are obvious sources. Parenchymal pulmonary diseases (e.g. pneumonia and lung abscess) are the most likely possibilities, but subdiaphragmatic abscess or mediastinitis after a perforated esophagus may also have to be considered. Regardless of the clinical impression, any pus should be examined and cultured for all usual pathogens including mycobacteria and fungi. Countercurrent immunoelectrophoresis may be helpful, but is not as high a priority as culture if only a small amount of pus is available for study, because countercurrent immunoelectrophoresis can also be performed on urine.

Nonpurulent uninfected pleural fluid presents an even wider diagnostic spectrum, and a more extensive laboratory investigation is often necessary.[5,7] The overall differential diagnosis is summarized in Table I. Appropriate laboratory examination of pleural fluid is important. The technique of the thoracentesis itself is described under *Therapy*. The handling and analysis of the fluid and the interpretation of the data are discussed here. The precise laboratory tests which should be ordered are determined by the clinical picture and, to some extent, by the amount of fluid available. Every possible test need not be performed on every pleural fluid sample. A small amount of fluid should be cultured on routine media for mycobacteria and, if appropriate, for fungi. If anaerobic infection is a reasonable pre-procedure diagnostic possibility, a portion of the specimen should be cultured anaerobically shortly after its removal. Prior consultation with the microbiology laboratory may be helpful. Other than anaerobic culture considerations, however, this portion of the specimen does not require special handling. Unless there is clear evidence that the effusion is secondary to infection, some fluid should be sent for cell block; this portion of the sample must be treated with an anticoagulant (e.g. heparin) and processed immediately to prevent artifacts which sometimes make an accurate evaluation impossible.

Table I

Major Differential Diagnostic Considerations in Pleural Effusion*

Parenchymal lung infection including pneumonia and tuberculosis
Malignancy
Congestive heart failure
Hepatic cirrhosis
Collagen-vascular disease
Hypoproteinemia
Uremia
Subdiaphragmatic abscess

*These diagnoses account for the vast majority of pleural effusions. Complete differential diagnosis is considered in specialized reviews.[5]

Differentiation between a transudate and an exudate is extremely important and rests on the determinations of serum and pleural fluid protein and lactic acid dehydrogenase[5] (LDH). (Table II.) No special handling of the specimen is necessary for these tests. A pleural fluid-serum protein ratio above 0.5 and/or a pleural fluid-serum LDH ratio above 0.6 and/or a pleural fluid LDH above 200 IU define an exudate. Pleural fluid pH can yield valuable additional information[3] and a sample of fluid should be aspirated into a heparinized syringe and immediately refrigerated or kept on ice for subsequent pH measurement. Most transudates are characterized by a fluid pH above 7.40, while pH measurements below 7.30 usually indicate empyema, malignancy, collagen disease, tuberculosis, and esophageal perforation. Detailed assessment of pleural pH is available in specialized reviews.[7]

Pleural fluid glucose can be particularly low in certain malignancies, tuberculosis, and rheumatoid arthritis. Glucose is also low in empyema fluid. For determination of pleural fluid glucose, a portion of the sample should be treated with sodium fluoride or

Table II

Differentiation Between Major Categories of Pleural Fluid

Characteristic	*Pleural Transudate*	*Pleural Exudate*	*Chyle*
Appearance	Clear	Clear or cloudy	Milky
Cell type	Rare or no cells	Polymorphonuclear leucocytes	Lymphocytes
pH	Above 7.40	Below 7.30	No data
LDH	Below 200 IU/Liter	Above 200 IU/Liter	Below 200 IU/Liter
Pleural fluid/Serum LDH ratio	Below 0.6	Above 0.6	Below 0.6
Pleural fluid/Serum protein	Below 0.5	Above 0.5	No data
Fluid lipid	Low	Low	Very high (Except in unfed newborns)

other appropriate metabolic poison to prevent further glucose metabolism *in vitro*. Although glucose levels can be low in lupus erythematosus, this is not particularly common and the glucose level is often useful in distinguishing lupus from rheumatoid arthritis. In rare patients, an elevated fluid amylase may help in diagnosing pancreatitis. If there is any question of differentiating an effusion from chylothorax, a fluid lipid determination may be useful. In newborn infants, chylothorax may be more difficult to recognize since no lipid will be found in the pleural fluid until after the patient has been started on oral feedings. Pleural biopsy to diagnose malignancy or tuberculosis is rarely necessary in children.

Therapy

Occasional patients with pleural fluid do not need a diagnostic or therapeutic thoracentesis even if pleural effusion has never been present. Three examples will be given: (1) Patients with clear-cut pneumococcal pneumonia (e.g. pneumococcus isolated from blood culture in a patient with lobar pneumonia) already diagnosed prior to onset of effusion. These effusions resolve quickly with antibiotic treatment of the pneumonia and sequelae are rare. (2) Patients with clear-cut congestive heart failure, especially if the onset is acute and can be explained clinically (e.g. a patient with borderline cardiac status is inadvertently given too much IV fluid or blood). Treatment for heart failure can be instituted and the patient reevaluated in several hours. Often the effusion will be rapidly resolved. (3) Afebrile patients with severe hypoproteinemia and anasarca. There are, no doubt, other legitimate situations where thoracentesis can be omitted or at least delayed pending an anticipated rapid response to treatment. Clinical judgment, experience, and common sense are extremely important.

A limited number of therapeutic modalities are available for treatment of symptomatic pleural effusions: simple thoracentesis for removal of sufficient fluid to alleviate respiratory distress; chest tube insertion for prolonged drainage of purulent or rapidly recurrent nonpurulent fluid; and chest tube drainage with chemical pleuradesis to cause adhesion of the lung to the chest wall, thus obliterating the pleural space and totally preventing recurrence of pleural effusion.

Thoracentesis. The site of thoracentesis is chosen high enough to minimize the risk of injury to the lung or abdominal structures, but low enough to ensure that the needle will enter the pleural space below the top of the fluid level with the patient sitting. Usually this site is at the 8th intercostal space at the posterior axillary line. The area of skin overlying the site is infiltrated with local anaesthetic and the needle is advanced slowly. Frequent attempts at aspiration are made while the needle is advanced. If pleural fluid is not obtained, a small amount of an anaesthetic is injected and the needle advanced again. When pleural fluid is obtained, a clamp is placed on the needle at the skin line to mark the depth of the insertion. This needle is then withdrawn slowly while additional local anaesthetic is injected. A larger bore needle is then inserted into the pleural space. This time, a clamp is applied before the needle is inserted to limit the depth of the insertion. This clamp is placed so that the distance from the clamp to the end of the needle is slightly more than the corresponding distance on the needle initially used to inject the local anaesthetic. Once the second (larger) needle is within the pleural space, a plastic catheter is inserted through it and left within the pleural space while the needle is withdrawn. The fluid is then withdrawn slowly. Since the pleural fluid is already out of the vascular space, there is no danger of circulatory collapse if a large amount of fluid is removed. However, a transient failure of expansion of the underlying compressed lung, will result in a potentially undesirable shift of the mediastinum toward the side of the thoracentesis. Thus, the patient should be observed carefully during the procedure and the withdrawal of fluid temporarily stopped if dyspnea, chest pain or repetitive coughing occurs. A repeat chest film should be obtained after the procedure; the pulmonary parenchyma will be easier to evaluate without the overlying fluid and the film will allow assessment of the success of the procedure.

Chest Tube Drainage. The most common indication for chest tube drainage is a parapneumonic exudate, especially if the pleural fluid pH is low. The duration of chest tube drainage is dictated by the patient's fever curve, the amount of continuing drainage and the appearance of the chest roentgenogram.

Chest Tube Drainage with Chemical Pleuradesis. Occasional patients with inoperable malignancies have rapidly recurring pleural effusion. If these patients become substantially less dyspneic after each thoracentesis, chemical pleuradesis should be considered.[1] The chest tube is inserted and as much fluid as possible is drained. For malignant effusion, talc and tetracycline are the most commonly used sclerosing agents. Quinacrine is also effective, but is difficult to obtain in the United States. Tetracycline is usually well tolerated and successful. Tetracycline (500 to 1000 mg for a teenager and graded lesser amounts for smaller patients) is inserted through the chest tube which is then clamped. The patient is then rotated through several positions and held in each for a few minutes to allow contact with all areas of the pleura. For example, the patient is placed head down and then turned on the right side, back, left side and face down; the procedure is then repeated with the bed level and then with the head up. This treatment may be repeated daily for two or three days unless prior fever or chest pain indicate that sufficient pleural inflammation has already occurred. Pre-treatment with narcotic and/or preliminary insertion of local anaesthetic into the pleural space via the chest tube may be desirable, since the introduction of the therapeutic agent, e.g. tetracycline, may be quite painful.

Prognosis

The overall prognosis is totally dependent upon the underlying disease. A pneumococcal pneumonia with a pleural effusion will totally resolve with antibiotic treatment and leave no sequelae. Patients with inoperable malignancy obviously have a dismal prognosis regardless of the specific therapy employed for the pleural effusion. The immediate prognosis, i.e. the probability that breathing will be improved by thoracentesis and removal of fluid, is excellent.

Prevention

Prevention is rarely an issue in pleural effusion. In patients with inoperable intrapleural malignancy, chemical pleuradesis could be considered before actual effusion has occurred. However, this lesion often presents with effusion and the opportunity to use pleuradesis preventively is rare.

References

1. Bayly TC, Kisner DL, Sybert A, et al: Tetracycline and quinacrine in the control of malignant pleural effusions. *Cancer* 1978; 41:1188–1192.
2. Black LF: Pleural Disease. Basics of Respiratory Disease 1978; 6:1–6.
3. Good JT Jr, Taryle DA, Maulitz RM, et al: The diagnostic value of pleural fluid pH. *Chest* 1980; 78:55–59.
4. Gryminski J, Krakowka P, Lypacewicz D: The diagnosis of pleural effusion by ultrasonic and radiologic techniques. *Chest* 1976; 70:33–37.
5. Hirsch A, Ruffie P, Nebut M, et al: Pleural effusion: laboratory tests in 300 cases. *Thorax* 1979; 34:106–112.
6. Light RW, Girard WM, Jenkinson SG, et al: Parapneumonic effusions. *Am J Med* 1980; 69:507–512.
7. Sahn SA: Pleural manifestations of pulmonary disease. *Hosp Prac* 1981; 16:73–89.

17

Respiratory Care of the Pediatric Patient

Martha I. Ellington, RRT

Introduction

Over the years much experience has been gained in respiratory care for the premature infant as well as for the adult patient. Many clinical studies have been conducted on these two age groups. This has resulted in a clearer understanding and a greater standardization of procedures in the care of these patients. Unfortunately, the same is not true for the pediatric patient. Respiratory care of this middle age range, between one month and eighteen years, still remains a mystery to many in the health care field.

In the past, respiratory care of the pediatric patient fell to those with experience in adult pulmonary medicine or to pediatricians unfamiliar with modern respiratory care techniques. This, fortunately, is changing. The pediatric patient is recognized as a distinct entity and not just as a "little adult." The patient is seen to have a different spectrum of pulmonary disease problems requiring different approaches.

In researching this chapter, it was truly a disappointment to see that little concrete information is available (in comparison to other age groups). This, too, is changing, and we, as clinicians, will benefit but most importantly, so will the children.

Supplemental Oxygen Administration

The indications for the administration of supplemental oxygen are the same for every patient: (1) to relieve hypoxemia and improve availability of oxygen to tissues; (2) to decrease the work of breathing; and (3) to decrease myocardial work.[33]

Most devices for adult use have been scaled down for use in children. In addition, there are devices adapted for the specific need of the pediatric patient. The success of any device will depend largely on the child's acceptance of it. Reassurance and patience will aid in this acceptance.

Humidifiers and Aerosol Units

A humidifier is a device designed to deliver a maximum amount of water vapor without producing particulate water (mist).[3,33] To accomplish this the source gas is passed over or bubbled through the sterile water in the humidifier. Humidifiers are used with most oxygen delivery equipment to increase the water content of the dry source gas. The water may be at room temperature or heated. Small bore oxygen tubing is used to link the actual delivery device and the humidifier. Examples of the devices used with humidifiers are: nasal cannulae; oxygen hoods; simple, venturi and non-rebreathing masks.

An aerosol unit will provide the patient with water in particulate form (mist).[3,33] The formation of the mist is accomplished by the insertion of a hollow tube into the sterile water reservoir. A high pressure gas flow over this tube will cause the water to be drawn upward. At this point the water is dispersed into small particles by the high pressure gas flow or it is "smashed" against a baffle to break it up into particles. The water can be heated to increase particles and help thin secretions, or it can be left cool to help soothe airways and decrease laryngeal edema. Large bore tubing with a condensation collection bag incorporated is used to link the actual delivery device and the aerosol unit. Examples of devices used with aerosol units include aerosol masks, tracheostomy collars, and T-bars.

Nasal Cannulae

Nasal cannulae have two prongs, each which fit just inside the opening of the nares. They are fairly well tolerated and will provide continuous oxygen even while the child is eating. If the prongs are too large for the child, they can be trimmed or cut out completely leaving only open holes which are then positioned just outside the nares.[13]

The fraction of inspired oxygen (F_IO_2) cannulae deliver is highly variable. F_IO_2 has been estimated at 0.22–0.50 depending on the child's ventilatory pattern. Cannulae can be run at an oxygen flow rate of 0.5 liters per minute (LPM) to 6 LPM.[3,26,33] An increase above 6 LPM may prove uncomfortable since it will dry out the nasal passages and may cause gastric distention.

The F_IO_2 delivered will not be affected by mouth breathers, since the nasopharynx acts as a reservoir for nose and mouth breathers. A change in the child's tidal volume, respiratory rate, or inspiratory flow rates will alter the F_IO_2.[25,33]

Nasal catheters consist of a single catheter which is inserted nasally to a point just above the uvula. They are managed the same way as cannulas. Catheters can be very uncomfortable, and it is rare that a child will accept this device.[3,7,25,33]

Masks

Simple Mask. These are cone shaped and made to cover the nose and mouth with the remaining area inside the mask acting as a reservoir. These masks should not be run at less than 6 LPM; 6–8 LPM is optimal. This is recommended so that there will be enough flow available to flush the mask of exhaled gas. In this way the possibility of CO_2 rebreathing is eliminated. Flows above 8 LPM may cause a build-up of pressure within the mask and thus may impede exhalation. The F_IO_2 provided is estimated at 0.35–0.45.

Venturi Mask. These masks are fitted with a venturi device which entrains room air by use of the Bernoulli principle to create known and stable oxygen concentrations. These masks come with adapters to provide various oxygen concentrations, the most common are F_IO_2s of 0.24, 0.28, 0.31, 0.35, 0.40, and 0.50.

Due to the entrainment of room air, the total liter flow of gas provided to the child is higher than with a simple mask. Because of this, they are more comfortable to wear and more easily tolerated by the air hungry patient. The venturi mask is considered a high flow oxygen system.[33]

Non-rebreathing Mask. This device incorporates a reservoir bag with a one-way valve going from bag to mask. A one-way valve is also situated on either side of the mask over each exhalation port which prevents room air entrainment during inspiration. The mask should fit snugly and the reservoir bag must remain inflated during use with only partial collapse during inspiration. Minimum allowable flow rate is 8–10 LPM. With a proper fit and the use of an oxygen blender, any F_IO_2 from 0.22–1.0 can be delivered.

Aerosol Masks and Tracheostomy Collars. These devices are used to deliver oxygen and particulate water. The aerosol mask is a cone shaped device which fits over the patients nose and mouth. It has two large open ports at either side to allow for the escape of excess mist. Provided a good seal is obtained and the flow rate used is high enough to meet the child's minute volume, the F_IO_2 delivered can be as high as 100% source gas.

Tracheostomy collars are also cone shaped but are much smaller and made to fit over a tracheostomy tube. Their fit is much looser and they can only deliver an F_IO_2 up to 0.5, approximately, when an oxygen flowrate of 6–15 LPM is used. Both the aerosol mask and tracheostomy collar are used with an aerosol unit.

Tents. Tents are not the optimal device to use when precise oxygen concentrations are required. Their efficiency is directly related to how well the canopy has been sealed and how often it must be opened for patient care. Oxygen concentrations vary widely. Under optimal conditions, an F_IO_2 of approximately 0.3–0.35 can be obtained. Unfortunately, it is not a steady and stable F_IO_2 due to the problems already listed.[35]

Although the newer model tents no longer require ice in order to cool, they can still be cumbersome and require frequent monitoring. Source gas should be delivered at 12–15 LPM to ensure proper circulation of air and diffusion of exhaled CO_2. The temperature inside the tent must be maintained 6°–8°F below room temperature to ensure patient comfort and cooling.[26] If supplemental oxygen is not required, compressed air can be used.

Mist tents have been found to be fairly well tolerated by small infants but they can be difficult to maintain with active toddlers.

Hoods. Hoods[3,7,26,35] are made in a variety of styles and sizes.

Typically, they are made of clear plastic. They provide a controlled environment of oxygen, humidity, and temperature for small infants (generally less than 5 kg body weight). To deliver the oxygen, a heated passover humidifier is preferred to an aerosol unit. This is because the dense mist of an aerosol unit may hinder the clinician's visibility of the child and the rain-out will increase the undesirable cooling effect on the infant's head. To insure that the infant is not cooled needlessly, care must be taken that the gas entering the hood does not strike the infant's head directly. The hood may already be designed to do this or it can be accomplished by putting a T-bar on the end of the large bore tubing which enters the hood.

The semicircular opening for the infant's head must not be so snug that it will not allow exhaled CO_2 to escape around the infant's neck. Gas flow must be set at a minimum of 7 LPM; enough to flush exhaled CO_2 from the hood. F_IO_2 of 0.22–1.0 can be obtained with proper application. Ideally, the F_IO_2 should be analyzed continuously, and monitored at least every 1–2 hours, or more often if necessary.

T-bars. T-bars are T-shaped adaptors used to deliver humidity and particulate water to patients with endotracheal or tracheostomy tubes. A heated nebulizer is used with large bore tubing which is connected to the T-bar. A short length of large bore tubing is added to the distal end of the T-bar to act as a reservoir and prevent room air entrainment. Flows must be high enough to meet the child's minute volume. In order to accomplish this, set the flow rate high enough that mist is visible at the distal end of the reservoir tubing even during inspiration, allowing the child to receive 100% source gas.

A water condensation collection bag should be placed inline to prevent excess condensation from occluding the tubing.

Incubators and Isolettes. These can be used to deliver low to moderate concentrations of oxygen.[3,25] Depending upon oxygen liter flow, an F_IO_2 of approximately 0.4 or lower can be obtained. If higher concentrations are needed, an oxygen hood should be used.

Maintaining a stable F_IO_2 within the isolette can be very difficult due to frequent opening of the ports for patient care. Flexible sleeves in place at each port will help to prevent this but fluctuations may still occur. This is not the device of choice when a stable F_IO_2 is necessary.[7]

Hazards and Complications of Oxygen Administration

Oxygen is a drug and can be very dangerous. Its administration must be closely monitored. Damage to the retinal capillaries in the form of retrolental fibroplasia can occur as a result of an excessive PaO_2. Children exposed to high concentrations of oxygen for more than 24–48 hours have shown evidence of pulmonary oxygen toxicity. This toxicity is manifested by a decrease in surface-active substances (surfactant), impairment of mucociliary activity, and atelectasis with ensuing ventilation/perfusion abnormalities.[25] Lung congestion, alveolar exudation, and hemorrhage have also been reported.[9]

Serial blood gas analysis is imperative during oxygen therapy so that the F_IO_2 can be lowered without delay as the condition of the child's lungs improves.

When using a hood, tent, isolette, or T-bar, analyze the F_IO_2 at *least* every two hours. Be sure the analyzer is calibrated daily on room air and 100% oxygen. Keep in mind that there are children as well as adults who are CO_2 retainers. Extra care must be taken when administering oxygen to these children since they too can have their ventilatory drive impaired by an excess PaO_2.

Administration of Aerosolized Medication

There is an extensive list of medications which can be effectively applied to the respiratory tract. They include bronchodilators, mucolytics, and antibiotics. It was once felt that the best way to deliver these medications was by the use of Intermittent Positive Pressure Breathing (IPPB). Although there has been much controversy surrounding IPPB, it does have its place in the treatment of atelectasis, CO_2 retention or pulmonary edema. Its use, however, is contraindicated in some situations, i.e. untreated pneumothorax, and bullous disease.

IPPB is not the ideal way to deliver aerosolized medications to the pediatric patient, as it can be a very frightening experience. More often than not, the child will be too young or too frightened to cooperate with a mouthpiece treatment. This will necessitate the use of a face mask, adding greatly to the child's anxiety. It may also necessitate the use of force, which is not very desirable. The net effect of this experience is often a worsening of the child's condition and a very frustrating experience for the therapist.

A more effective method of administering aerosolized medications is with the use of a hand-held nebulizer. The nebulizer can be connected to an aerosol mask or mouthpiece depending on the child's age and ability. The gas flow to the nebulizer can be adjusted to regulate the amount of mist being produced. There is no positive pressure to frighten and confuse the child. If the patient should cry, he will not adversely affect the treatment and may enhance it by the deep breaths taken.

Chest Physiotherapy (CPT)

At first glance this mode of therapy[3,26,35] may seem very simplistic and unsophisticated. In reality it can be most effective in helping the respiratory impaired child to clear secretions and improve ventilation/perfusion abnormalities. The total regimen consists of five parts: postural drainage, percussion, vibration, segmental breathing and coughing. It may not be feasible to use all modalities on the same child at one time; however, benefits can still be obtained.

Care must be taken to prepare the child for the CPT session. This should be turned into "fun and play time" for the child. Although the preparation may take extra time for the therapists, it is time well spent since the child will be better able to cooperate and will tolerate the session better with less anxiety and fear.

Postural Drainage. This technique utilizes the basic principle that gravity will help to drain lung segments. A working knowledge of the pulmonary anatomy of pediatric patients of different age groups is essential.

The child with diffuse chronic lung disease will probably require drainage of a majority of segments. Positioning children with localized disease will be determined by the chest X-ray and by auscultation. The number of sessions per day will depend on the child's condition and his level of toleration. Postural drainage may be done therapeutically or prophylactically (on the child with chronic disease). Depending on the child's age, size and condition, he may be positioned on the bed, padded tilt board, isolette (limited), or the therapist's lap.

Percussion. This technique is accomplished by lightly clapping the child's chest with a cupped hand. The cupped hand forms a cushion of air that softens the blow and is transmitted into the chest. There are devices on the market which can be used in place of a cupped hand, and they are especially useful for smaller children.

Percussion is done when the child is in each postural drainage position. Care must be taken to regulate the force of the clapping according to the child's size and tolerance of the procedure.

Vibration. This technique can be very helpful when combined with percussion to further mobilize secretions towards the larger airways. It is done during the patient's exhalation and is accomplished by using the hands or fingers, depending on the child's size. The therapist stiffens the upper arms and gently shakes the hands or fingers on the child's chest in a vibrating manner.

Segmental Breathing. This is a technique which can be very helpful to the older child and adolescent. It has to be learned and mastered by the patient and, therefore, is of little value in the infant and small child. What the adolescent attempts to do is inhale while actively expanding predominantly one lung or portion of one lung. This is accomplished by having the therapist place his hands firmly over the area the patient is to expand. The patient then inhales and attempts to expand the chest directly under the therapist's hands. Light but constant pressure is applied by the therapist throughout this maneuver.[7,33]

Coughing. Once CPT has been accomplished, it is vitally important that the loosened and drained secretions be removed. The child must be encouraged to cough and if unable, should be instructed to breath deeply then exhale quickly in the hopes that this will elicit a cough. If an effective cough cannot be obtained because the child cannot cough, is uncooperative or too young, then naso-orotracheal suctioning should be performed.[9,33]

Intubation

Intubation refers to the placement of an artificial airway into the respiratory tract. It is best undertaken in a controlled setting, although most often this is not possible. In the acute situation, an oral route should be attempted since technically the procedure is easier. The tube can later be changed to the nasal route for greater stability or if longer term ventilation is anticipated.

The primary indications for intubation are: (1) apnea, and other indications for ventilatory support or CPAP; (2) upper airway obstruction; (3) prevention of aspiration; (4) control of ventilation; and (5) neuromuscular disorders (i.e. Guillain–Barré).

The endotracheal tubes used should meet the following requirements: (1) They must be of a uniform diameter. One of the first tubes available was the Cole tube.[7] They were designed with a tappered end about 1.5 cm from the end. The purpose of this was to prevent accidental intubation into a main stem bronchus. It is generally felt that the physical presence of this shoulder on the epiglottis may produce trauma and inflammation. (2) They should be implant-tested to ensure bio-compatibility. (3) They should be flexible while retaining their integrity. (4) They must be radiopaque.[7]

Prior to the intubation procedure, all necessary equipment should be assembled and ready at hand. This equipment includes: (1) A laryngoscope and several blades with functioning light. A straight blade should be used on infants less than 2 years of age due to the sometimes large floppy epiglottis which must be lifted out of the way. (2) Orotracheal tubes in several sizes. Uncuffed tubes are used in infants and small children to decrease the chance of tracheal wall pressure damage. The narrow cricoid cartilage of these small children usually provides an adequate seal. See Table I for approximate orotracheal tube sizes for children of different ages. (3) Suction equipment. (4) Resuscitation bag, mask and oxygen. (5) Oral airway or bite block. (6) ETT securement equipment.

The actual intubation should be carried out by the person most qualified. The child's head should be placed in the "sniffing" position[11] (hyperextension will close the airway). The laryngoscope should be held in the left hand and the orotracheal tube in the right. The tube should be passed as atraumatically as possible.

Close monitoring of the child during the procedure is essential. Each intubation attempt should last no more than 30 seconds. Hyperoxygenation and ventilation with bag and mask should be done between attempts.[3]

Once the tube has been passed, the breath sounds must be

Table I
Orotracheal Tube Sizes

Age	*I.D. (Internal Diameter)*
Newborn (less than 1.0 Kg bw)	2.5 mm
Newborn (greater than 1.0 Kg bw)	3.0 mm
1–6 months	3.5 mm
6–12 months	4.0 mm
12–18 months	4.5 mm
18–36 months	5.0 mm
3–4 years	5.5 mm
5–6 years	6.0 mm
6–7 years	6.5 mm
8–9 years	7.0 mm
10–11 years	7.5 mm
12–14 years	8.0 mm

evaluated for equality. The tube should be temporarily secured and a chest X-ray taken. Once the tube is found to be in optimal position it can be better secured.

Mechanical Ventilation

The criteria for initiating artificial ventilatory support in children are basically the same as those for adults. These criteria include the mechanical failure of breathing whether it be pulmonary or nonpulmonary in origin (apnea); ventilatory insufficiency as evidenced by hypercapnea associated with acidosis; and hypoxemia and chest wall instability secondary to surgery and/or trauma. Children who will undergo therapeutic coma for the treatment of head injuries are also candidates for mechanical ventilation. In this way assisted ventilation is used deliberately to keep $PaCO_2$ low to promote cerebral vascular constriction and to aid in reducing cerebral edema. Impending ventilatory failure, as evidenced by fatigue and deteriorating lab values, should certainly be included in this list.

It is to the child's benefit if intubation and commitment to mechanical ventilation are carried out in a controlled and non-acute situation.

Expert clinical judgment is necessary to evaluate a child's need for mechanical ventilation. Laboratory data that are abnormal for one child, may be well tolerated by another.

Ventilators

Since the care of the pediatric patient was recognized as separate in many respects, a wide variety of ventilators have been developed that are specific to pediatrics.[1] The ultimate choice of a pediatric ventilator rests with each individual respiratory therapy department. That choice may be based on such things as the average age and weight of children requiring mechanical ventilation at that hospital, the most common disease entities treated at that hospital, and the ventilator's versatility and cost.

Adult Ventilators in Pediatrics. With the help of certain modifications, adult ventilators have been used on the pediatric patient. Modifications include the use of a humidification system with a smaller compressible volume, and patient tubing that has a smaller diameter and a lower compliance factor.

Although this has been shown to work, it is not optimal. For the most part, these ventilators were never intended for use in pediatrics. They are usually volume-cycled ventilators whose capacity at the low end of the volume scale is not adequate. Some have been known to deliver a volume of gas even while set on a tidal volume of zero. Also, the response time to initated breaths may not be what is desired for the tachypneic child.

Since there are a wide variety of ventilators available,[1,7,23,25] it is helpful to know some desired characteristics of a versatile and reliable ventilator for pediatrics. (See Table II.)

Modes. In the *control* mode the ventilator takes over completely in providing the child with a total minute volume.[31] Sedation alone or in conjunction with a paralyzing agent is often necessary in order to fully control the child's ventilation. A true control mode indicates that even without sedation or paralyzation, the child is prevented from triggering the ventilator to initiate a breath. For this reason, a true control mode is rarely used. We may control a child's ventilation, but when the sedation or paralyzing effects begin to lessen, the ventilator must be able to respond to the child's inspiratory efforts. High levels of anxiety as evidenced

Table II

Characteristics of Pediatric Ventilators

- Accurate delivery of preset tidal volume (especially at low volumes).
- Ability to deliver gas at rapid rates.
- Flexible ventilation modes: assist/control, Intermittent Mandatory Ventilation (IMV) or Synchronized Intermittent Mandatory Ventilation (SIMV), spontaneous breathing.
- Ability to deliver Positive End Expiratory Pressure (PEEP) and Continuous Positive Airway Pressure (CPAP).
- A humidification system with a low compressible volume.
- Accurate measurement of proximal airway pressure.
- Variable inspiratory and expiratory times.
- Accurate oxygen blender.
- Alarm system sensitive to high pressure, low pressure (disconnect) and ventilator malfunction.
- Adjustable pop-off system. This will vent excessive pressure to the atmosphere in the event of increased pressure build-up in the patient circuit. This can be due to such things as kinked tubing, obstruction, or system malfunction.
- Variable gas flow rates.
- Adjustable ventilation wave form.
- Inspiratory pause.
- Compatible patient circuit with a low compliance factor (less than 1.5 ml/cm H_2O and less than 1.0 ml/cm H_2O for children less than 10 kg body weight).[23]

by increased heart rate and blood pressure have been noted when an apparently sedated and/or paralyzed child attempts to inspire and receives nothing from the ventilator.

The *assist* mode indicates that all breaths delivered are initiated by the child. This means that when the child generates negative pressure (below zero or PEEP level set), the ventilator will deliver a preset volume or pressure. However, there are definite disadvantages to the assist mode. A minimal back-up rate is not employed, therefore, a dangerous situation will arise if for some reason the child stops assisting or if the machine does not sense small amounts of negative pressure generated by the child.

A combination of assist and control will alleviate many of the problems associated with using either mode alone. This is termed *assist/control.* The child will receive a preset number of breaths at a preset volume or pressure. Intermittently, he may initiate further breaths at the same preset volume or pressure. A problem which may occur is overventilation with resultant respiratory alkalosis. Another problem may be asynchronous breathing, especially in the anxious and tachypneic child.

When a ventilator has a free flow of gas which the child can draw from between mandatory ventilator breaths, we have an *IMV system* (Intermittent Mandatory Ventilation).[11] The child's spontaneous breaths are at his own rate and volume. The mandatory breaths are delivered at specific time intervals at a preset volume or pressure. The ventilator does not take into account what phase of respiration the child is in before delivering a breath, which can result in a breath being delivered during the child's expiratory phase. The IMV mode has proven to be well tolerated and its use has been successful in synchronizing a child's breathing to the ventilator. It is a valuable tool during weaning although it is not exclusively used for weaning.[24,39] IMV using high mandatory breath rates has been tolerated well by children who are difficult to synchronize with the ventilator and who are not yet ready to wean.

SIMV (Synchronized Intermittent Mandatory Ventilation) differs from IMV only in that the mandatory breaths are synchronized with the child's own breathing.[14] When a mandatory breath is due, the ventilator will delay delivery of the breath until the child begins an inspiratory effort. If the child does not initiate a breath within a certain time frame, the ventilator will then deliver a breath. SIMV is said to be superior to simple IMV because it synchronizes ventilation with the patient. However, results of studies have not supported this theory.

PEEP (Positive End Expiratory Pressure) is a technique used to increase and maintain airway and alveolar pressures above atmospheric. PEEP has been shown clinically and experimentally to be one of the most effective ventilatory techniques in the treatment of hypoxemia associated with reduced functional residual capacity (FRC), such as in Respiratory Distress Syndrome.[27] It has also been used for internal splinting of the chest wall in cases of chest trauma with flail chest.

PEEP has been used to help stabilize and expand fluid-filled alveoli. Due to the increased distention of the alveoli, the fluid no longer fills the entire alveolus but now forms a flattened layer through which oxygen is permeable.

Because FRC is increased by PEEP, an improvement in lung

compliance and a decrease in work of breathing is achieved. Alveoli are recruited and kept above their critical closing volumes. This increases lung volume and decreases the ventilatory pressures necessary to reexpand the lungs with each breath. Ventilation occurs at the steeper more compliant portions of the pressure volume curve of the lungs.

If the PEEP level becomes excessive a decrease in compliance will be seen. This is due to overdistended alveoli because now ventilation occurs at a higher, "flatter" portion of the pressure volume curve.[18]

The epiglottis of a spontaneously breathing child creates back pressure to the alveoli keeping them partially distended and so decreasing the work of breathing. This effect is bypassed with an endotracheal or tracheostomy tube in place. Routinely, a PEEP of 2 cm H_2O is added to our intubated pediatric patients in an attempt to restore this phenomena.

PEEP levels in the range of 4–15 cm H_2O are not uncommon in pediatrics. Levels above 15 cm H_2O are occasionally necessary in the child with severe RDS. Clinical studies have proven that the early institution of PEEP can be very desirable in the treatment of RDS. It is much easier to maintain alveoli open than to open alveoli that have already collapsed.

Contraindications and Complications.[18] There are a number of relative contraindications to the use of PEEP. A major one occurs in those diseases in which the FRC is already at a level above normal (air trapping), i.e. bronchopulmonary dysplasia, asthma, emphysema and cystic fibrosis. Unilateral lung disease, i.e. segmental pneumonia, is also a contraindication since the PEEP level applied may take the path of least resistance and thus cause overdistention to unaffected "normal" portions of the lungs.

Untreated pneumothorax is a contraindication for PEEP. Also, if a child has intracranial hypertension, PEEP should be used very judiciously. This is because the increased intrathoracic pressure may cause a decrease in venous return from the cerebrum thus causing pooling of blood in the brain and potentially accentuating cerebral edema.[25]

Complications of PEEP include barotrauma as evidenced by pneumothorax, pneumomediastinum and subcutaneous emphysema. Decreased cardiac output can occur due to decreased venous return or a decrease in left ventricular volume with septal shift. The decrease in venous return is caused by pressure exerted on the heart and great vessels and by the lack of negative intrathoracic pressure during inspiration. This negative pressure helps to pull venous blood back to the heart thus further compromising the hypovolemic child.[8]

CPAP (Continuous Positive Airway Pressure) is the same as PEEP except that it is applied to the spontaneously breathing patient. In order to apply CPAP effectively, it is necessary for the patient to be able to adequately ventilate spontaneously. Indications for its use include refractory hypoxemia without excessive elevation in $PaCO_2$ and the decreasing of the work of breathing. Apnea in the premature infant has also been treated successfully with low levels (less than 5 cm H_2O) of CPAP.

It has been over ten years since CPAP was first described by Gregory[19] et al. Since then its uses and methods of application have increased. CPAP has been shown to retard the progress of disease, improve oxygenation, and reduce the need for high toxic levels of oxygen, decrease surfactant consumption, and improve the pattern and regularity of the patient's breathing.[12,20]

A variety of methods can be used to apply CPAP. Most are considered forms of threshold resistors. Upon exhalation, the patient must exceed the threshold pressure which is constantly applied by the CPAP valve system. Such devices include the underwater seal and Emerson PEEP valve.

Another way to create CPAP is with the use of a variable orifice causing a fixed resistance to exhalation. The amount of gas flow through the system will also influence the amount of CPAP. The Baby Bird PEEP valve, Carden valve and the Gregory system are all variable orifice CPAP systems.[3]

These methods have been shown to be effective but they can be cumbersome to set up and maintain. Provided that one is available, a much simpler method is the use of a continuous flow or demand flow ventilator. In this way the pressure manometer, humidification and alarm system of the ventilator are utilized without the need for further adaptations.

There are various airways which can be used to deliver CPAP to the pediatric patient. The easiest to maintain and most well tolerated is the endotracheal tube (nasal or oral) or tracheostomy tube (cuffed or uncuffed depending on age and size). CPAP by way of a tightly sealed mask has been used successfully on the adult population.[36] Children, on the other hand, do not tolerate this technique at all. An effective seal is extremely difficult to maintain, pressure damage has been noted on the eye area, and significant gastric distention has been noted.

The Gregory hood is a pressurized box which totally encloses the infant's head. Due to its association with intracranial hemorrhage and pressure necrosis of the infant's neck, this device is no longer used.

Nasal prongs have been used in neonates to administer a CPAP of up to 12 cm H_2O. This method is not effective in most pediatric patients because they are no longer obligatory "nose breathers," and therefore, the pressure applied cannot be adequately maintained. Studies have demonstrated that the use of nasal prong CPAP can increase the infant's work of breathing by as much as 94%. For this reason it cannot be recommended.[17]

Contraindications and Complications. Contraindications and complications are generally the same as those which apply to PEEP, namely, barotrauma and impedence of venous return with impaired cardiac output.

High Frequency Ventilation (HFV). Although it is not new, HFV[6,10,15] has recently been receiving publicity as the "new" technique of mechanical ventilation. Ventilation with a respiratory rate of less than 60 per minute is not considered high frequency. HFV is measured in cycles per minute where 60 cycles/min is equal to one Hertz (Hz). HFV refers to two different methods of ventilation. One uses a jet with substantial air entrainment at 1–2 Hz. The second uses an oscillator or a jet without air entrainment at frequencies of 4 Hz or more. It has been established that excellent gas exchange can be maintained using volume as low or even lower than dead space volume. The HFV increases molecular kinetic energy and so facilitates diffusion of gas within small airways and alveoli even at low volumes. It has been shown that both animals and humans become apneic while receiving HFV. In the future this may prove very useful.

The usage of HFV is still experimental. No standards have been set regarding optimal ventilator or circuit set-ups. We do know that a ventilator with very rapid response times and a patient circuit with a very low compressible volume are required. Optimal monitoring of the patient receiving high frequency ventilation is also not yet known. Certainly, mean airway pressure plays a significant role.

The choice of patients who would benefit from HFV is also not clear. What is clear, however, is that a lot more research needs to be done before this method can be widely adopted.

Care and Monitoring of the Child Receiving Assisted Ventilation

Once a child has been intubated it is imperative that a chest x-ray be obtained. Not only should the lung fields be examined but also the position of the endotracheal tube. It is very important that the child's head be kept in a neutral position during the x-ray.[29] This is because extension or flexion of the neck can alter endotracheal tube (ETT) placement. Optimal position of the tube tip is one to two centimeters above the carina. Serial chest x-rays will be required to further evaluate the child's lung fields on a day-to-day basis.

Once the ETT is found to be in optimal position, it must be adequately secured so as to prevent accidental extubation. An oral airway should be in place if the child has a tendency to bite down on the oral ETT. Oral endotracheal tubes can be secured in a variety of ways. One that works very well for small infants is the "mustache" method. A piece of elastoplast is placed above the infant's upper lip (resembling a mustache) with the aid of tincture of benzoin to improve adhesiveness. A narrow (1 cm) length of cloth tape is then wound around the endotracheal tube at the approximate level where the tube will meet the infant's lips. Sutures are then drawn through the tape around the ETT and the elastoplast on the infant. These sutures are tied together to secure the tube. Care is taken not to pierce the ETT or the infant when suturing.

On an older child the oral endotracheal tube is best secured with a length of cloth tape whose center portion is double backed (so as not to adhere to the back of the child's neck). Approximately 3–4 cm of the tape is allowed to adhere to the child's cheeks on either side before the tape is wound around the ETT. A nasotracheal tube can also be secured in this fashion with the addition of a piece of cloth tape that is wound around the tube and secured to the superior portion of the child's nose. This will prevent the tube from slipping down or out. Depending on the child's size and level of activity, the tape does not need to encircle the child's head.

Tracheostomy tubes are best secured using a padded neck strap that can be individually adjusted using Velcro. Conventional trach ties can also be used. In both instances care must be taken to ensure that the ties are neither too loose nor too tight.

Humidification

Since heat and moisture loss via the respiratory tract of infants can be critical, all gases delivered to the intubated or tracheotomized child should be adequately humidified and warmed.

Not only will heat and moisture loss be minimized, but secretions will also be kept thin and easier to manage. The airways of a child have a much smaller diameter than those of an adult and are more easily obstructed by thick, tenacious, dehydrated secretions.

Suctioning

This procedure[3,28,34] is necessary to aid the intubated or tracheotomized patient in the removal of secretions. A sterile technique must be used to avoid introducing pathogens to the lower airways. A suction catheter no more than half the diameter of the endotracheal tube or tracheostomy tube should be used. In this way the spontaneously breathing child can still breathe around the catheter.

The catheter should be advanced without suction to a point of resistance (carina), pulled back a bit, and then intermittent suction can be applied while the catheter is removed in a rotating fashion. In this way, trauma to the bronchial mucosa can be minimized. A small amount of normal saline (0.25–0.5 cc) may be helpful in clearing thick secretions.

Each suction attempt should last no more than 10 seconds.[3] A resuscitation bag delivering an F_IO_2 approximately 0.1 higher than the child is already receiving should be ready for use between suction attempts. One of the first signs that indicates a child may not be tolerating the suctioning procedure is a decrease in heart rate. Therefore, the ECG should be closely monitored.

Blood Gas Analysis

Blood gas monitoring[3] is an integral part of oxygen therapy and ventilator management. No child should be placed on oxygen or ventilatory support without the availability of quick and accurate blood gas analysis. It is clear that the way a child appears clinically may be very different from what is actually going on metabolically.

As in the adult, the child offers several sites from which to obtain an arterial sample for analysis. The preferred site is the radial artery due to its accessibility and presence of ulnar artery collateral circulation. An Allen test should be performed to ensure that this collateral circulation is present. Brachial arteries should be reserved as a last resort due to the absence of collateral circulation and the high danger of hematoma and embolus formation.

Obtaining an accurate and safe arterial blood sample from a child can take a lot of patience and expertise. Most children are not cooperative during the procedure and their blood gas values may be altered due to their anxiety and apprehension. An arterial catheter is ideal in situations where multiple samples will be required and continuous blood pressure monitoring is desirable. Samples can be obtained without disturbing the child. Occasionally, one or both radial arteries are by-passed for the first few punctures if they are being "saved" for the impending placement of an arterial catheter.

Although arterial punctures and catheters bring with them certain hazards and complications, they are the ideal methods for sampling blood gases. In the event that neither is possible, capillary blood samples can be obtained. The primary puncture site is the lateral or posterior side of the heel. The big toe, thumb or fingertip, ear lobe and lateral side of the palm can also be used.

The capillary bed must be arterialized for at least 5 minutes prior to each puncture. This is accomplished by wrapping the area with a warm moist washcloth or rubber glove loosely filled with warm water. The washcloth or glove should be covered with a dry washcloth or disposable diaper to retain the heat. Care must be taken not to apply excessive heat since burn injuries can occur. Only trained and experienced personnel should attempt the capillary stick since the blood gas values can be greatly altered by faulty technique.

A capillary blood gas sample obtained under optimal conditions will correlate with the arterial values fairly well in regard to

$PaCO_2$, pH and bicarbonate. The correlation with PaO_2 is not as accurate and should be viewed as limited. PcO_2 can, however, be very successfully used for trending.

Blood gas analysis should be done 20–30 minutes after the child is placed on any form of assisted ventilation or oxygen. Follow-up blood gases should be obtained once the child has stabilized and after each ventilator and/or oxygen setting change. Blood gases should also be obtained whenever the child's condition dictates.

Compliance Studies[4,5,7]

Pressure-volume measurements are simple, noninvasive ways of assessing physiologic defects of the airways or lung parenchyma. These measurements are performed on patients who are intubated and mechanically ventilated on volume ventilators that do not have continuous flow. In conjunction with other clinical and radiologic data, pressure-volume measurements may help distinguish abnormalities associated with changes in lung recoil (i.e. pulmonary edema, atelectasis, pneumonia and other parenchymal pulmonary pathologies), from abnormalities associated with increased airway resistance (i.e. retained secretions, bronchospasm and other primary airway disorders).

Pressure volume measurements involve plotting the static and dynamic compliance at several tidal volumes, usually not to exceed the sigh volume. The static and dynamic compliance curves reflect the static-elastic properties of the lungs and chest wall. In addition, the dynamic compliance curve reflects the flow resistive properties of the airways. Static compliance is the ratio of volume change (Δ V) to associated pressure change (Δ P) during interruption of air flow (plateau pressure after transient occlusion of the expiratory flow). Dynamic compliance is the ratio of volume change (Δ V) to associated pressure change (Δ P) between points of zero flow just prior to tidal volume delivery, and at peak tidal volume delivery.

When there is a parallel shift to the right of both curves it indicates diseases characterized physiologically by an increase in elastic recoil of the lungs or chest wall. If only the dynamic compliance curve is shifted to the right, it indicates diseases associated with increased airway resistance. Often a shift in the curve(s) will occur before there is significant deterioration of the patient's blood gases, clinical or radiologic status.

Serial determinations are much more useful than isolated measurements. Studies should be done at least every eight hours and whenever the patient's condition changes. New baseline measurements should be done after each alteration in mechanical ventilator settings. For accurate determinations the child should be relaxed and breathing in cooperation with the ventilator. If not, small amounts of sedation may be used. Keep in mind that these measurements uncover functional disturbances but do not make a diagnosis.

Optimal PEEP Determinations

Optimal PEEP[4,16,30] has been described as that level which provides the highest static compliance, smallest arterial/venous saturation difference, and the highest possible Pa_{O_2} while causing the least reduction in cardiac output. Optimal PEEP does not necessarily mean the highest Pa_{O_2} will be obtained.

A simple and noninvasive way of estimating optimal PEEP on a patient receiving mechanical ventilation is by plotting a static compliance curve. The patient receives the same tidal volume while static compliance measurements are done on zero PEEP up to 10 or 12 cm H_2O (possibly higher) in increments of 2 cm H_2O. That level which produces the highest static compliance while not causing a deterioration in the patient's condition (as evidenced by changes in blood pressure, heart rate and agitation) is the PEEP level on which the patient is placed. Blood gas determinations are done 20 minutes following to evaluate Pa_{O_2}. Accuracy of the static compliance measurements will greatly depend on whether the patient is relaxed and breathing in cooperation with the ventilator. Sedation or even a paralyzing agent may be required during the determinations.

If the patient has a functional Swan-Ganz flow directed balloon tipped catheter in place, intrapulmonary shunt determinations can be done to calculate optimal PEEP level.[23] The intrapulmonary shunt is made of two parts: the normally occurring anatomical shunt caused by the draining of the thebesian and bronchial veins into the left side of the heart (normally 2–5% of the total cardiac output), and any pathologically occurring physiological shunt caused by nonventilated alveoli (for whatever reason) which remain perfused. Bed-side intrapulmonary shunt determinations include anatomical and physiological shunt fractions. True physiological shunt units have a ventilation/perfusion ratio of zero. They do not respond to oxygen administration and account for the clinical necessity of positive end expiratory pressure.

Bed-side intrapulmonary shunt determinations are accomplished by drawing simultaneous arterial and mixed venous (from pulmonary artery) blood samples for blood gas analysis. These samples are drawn on various levels of PEEP ranging from zero to 10 or 12 cm H_2O (possibly higher), usually in increments of 3 or 4 cm H_2O. A cardiac output determination should also be done at each PEEP level. The formula used to calculate the intrapulmonary shunt is as follows:

$$\dot{Q}_s/\dot{Q}_T = \frac{Cc{o_2} - Ca{o_2}}{Cc{o_2} - C\bar{v}{o_2}}$$

$\dot{Q}_T$ = total cardiac output
$\dot{Q}_s$ = that portion of the cardiac output that does not exchange with alveolar air
$Cc{o_2}$ = pulmonary capillary oxygen content
$Ca{o_2}$ = arterial oxygen content
$C\bar{v}{o_2}$ = mixed venous oxygen content[38]

The optimal PEEP level is that which yields the least shunt value while only minimally compromising the cardiac output (if at all) and provides the highest $P\bar{v}{o_2}$ possible to ensure the best possible tissue oxygenation. Intrapulmonary shunt determinations should be done at least every 24 hours, preferably every eight hours when the patient's condition warrants it.

Capnography

A capnograph[3] is a device used to continuously monitor exhaled CO_2. It can be used on mechanically ventilated or spontaneously breathing patients.

If the patient has normal ventilation/perfusion ratios, the peak exhaled CO_2 will correlate well with arterial CO_2. If the patient is suffering from shock, pulmonary hypertension, pulmonary embolus, broncho-pulmonary dysplasia or other situations where there is ventilation in excess of perfusion, the capnograph can still be used successfully to trend end tidal CO_2 ($P_{ET}CO_2$) with $PaCO_2$.

For use on a spontaneously breathing child, the sampling tube should be taped so that the tip is just inside the child's nares. Appropriate adapters are used for inline monitoring of the mechanically ventilated child. A simultaneous blood gas should be obtained for correlation.

To ensure accuracy, care must be taken to keep the sampling line free of moisture and mucus. A two point calibration procedure with a known high and low CO_2 concentration should be done approximately every eight hours.

Transcutaneous PO_2/PCO_2[3]

This technique allows for continuous monitoring of the patient's oxygenation or ventilatory state. Two separate electrodes are used for measuring PO_2 or PCO_2. They contain a modified Clark or Severinghaus electrode which includes a heating element and are attached to the patient's skin using a double sided adhesive ring.

Either electrode can be used alone or they can be used simultaneously on the same patient. Good capillary perfusion and blood pressure should be present for optimal correlation. Also, the electrodes should not be placed over areas with increased subcutaneous fat deposits, increased skin thickness, or directly over areas where large blood vessels are present. The upper chest is a good site on most infants. The abdomen and inner thigh are acceptable on neonates.

A two point calibration should be done prior to placing the electrode on the patient. Once the electrode is placed, it should be allowed to stabilize for approximately 20 minutes before readings are taken. At that time, the reading should be correlated with simultaneous blood gas analysis.

The position of either electrode must be changed frequently. Time intervals will depend on the patient's condition and the heating temperature used. The range is usually from 2–6 hours. At least a one point calibration should be done prior to replacing the electrode. Recorrelation with blood gas analysis should be done each time the electrode is repositioned.

When either electrode is in place, pressure over it should be avoided since this will cause a decrease in capillary blood flow and may also increase the possibility of a thermal skin injury.

Ear Oximetry

This is a noninvasive method of acquiring data on the ratio of oxygen content to the total oxygen capacity. This ratio is the oxygen saturation. This instrument operates by passing light through living tissue (pinna or earlobe). By determining the amount of light absorbed, oxygen saturation data can be determined. Hemoglobin saturation is very closely related to PaO_2. Once a correlation is established with blood gas analysis, the device is very reliable for continuous monitoring. New smaller models have been developed that make the application to pediatrics even better.

The Weaning Process[2,11,12,21,22,25,32,37,39]

A great deal of information has been compiled and many guidelines have been established about when the initiation of mechanical ventilation is necessary. Unfortunately the same is not yet true regarding the optimal time to take a patient off mechanical ventilation.

Due to all of its inherent problems and complications, mechanical ventilation must be discontinued at the earliest possible time consistent with patient safety. This does not mean that weaning attempts should be made without rational decision making since this will usually result in unnecessary cardiopulmonary stress that may lead to a longer ventilator course.

A significant point that must be stressed when a child is committed to a ventilator is the establishment of a working diagnosis i.e. identification of the underlying disease which caused the need for mechanical support of ventilation. The major guidelines for discontinuing ventilator care are evidence of improvement or reversal of that disease process and its inherent complications. Pulmonary and cardiovascular measurements provide objective criteria used in making the clinical judgement that the underlying disease process is sufficiently reversed.

Although the dictionary definition of wean is "to withdraw," the common connotation of the term is "to gradually ease away." There are still some institutions which continue to employ an *all or nothing* method of weaning. The patient is alternately completely dependent on the ventilator and then he must breathe entirely on his own for varying lengths of time. This method may be physiologically and psychologically unsound as evidenced by the anxiety, tachypnea and increased oxygen requirements caused by the abrupt discontinuation of all ventilatory support. Considered a more physiologically sound method is the progression from assist/control to IMV or SIMV.

One of the first things that should be done prior to beginning the weaning process is the discontinuation of all sedatives and paralyzing drugs. Whenever possible, serious weaning should be attempted early in the day and not late at night when the child is likely to be tired. This is especially true for the older child and adolescent.

There are several parameters that should be evaluated at the outset: (1) spontaneous tidal volume should be greater than 5 cc/Kg body weight (bw); (2) forced vital capacity of at least 10–15 cc/Kg bw (can be measured in a cooperative child); and (3) negative inspiratory force (NIF) of greater than -25 to -35 cm H_2O. NIF measures general muscular strength and degree of large airways obstruction. This is most useful in evaluating the ability of the child to tolerate increased work of breathing demands that may be imposed as ventilatory support is decreased.

If possible the following measurements can also be done. Dead space/tidal volume (V_D/V_T) ratio which should be less than 0.55 to 0.6. Normal V_D/V_T of a spontaneously breathing patient is 0.2 to 0.4. A normal patient on a ventilator has a V_D/V_T of less than 0.5. Intrapulmonary shunt fraction ($\dot{Q}_s/\dot{Q}_T$) should be less than 15%.

Other parameters that should be monitored include the F_IO_2 which should be at 0.4 or below. PEEP level can be minimal although this is not absolutely necessary since CPAP can be continued after mechanical ventilation is discontinued. Vital signs including blood pressure must be stable and not excessive (especially respiratory rate and effort). Respiratory and metabolic acid base status must be stabilized and under control according to the child's normal status. The same is true for other blood gas parameters. The child who is receiving pharmacologic agents for blood pressure elevation or positive inotropic drugs must be carefully evaluated to ensure that any potential blood gas abnormalities will not aggravate an already compromised situation.

Once all the necessary measurements have been made and evaluated and the child is found in a satisfactory status, the weaning process can continue. Whenever possible, psychological preparation should be given to the child according to his developmental level. If the parents are at the bedside, the procedure should also be explained to them. Lower the F_IO_2, IMV rate or PEEP in accordance with the clinical picture and blood gases. Ideally only one parameter should be changed at a time so that any problems encountered may be easily identified. The child should be kept on at least 2 cm H_2O PEEP in conjunction with IMV. This will aid the child in tolerating the resistive properties of the endotracheal/tracheostomy tube.

Once the child is doing well on a low IMV rate (generally less than or equal to 5 breaths/min), with stable F_IO_2 requirements of 0.4 or less, with a satisfactory metabolic and cardiopulmonary status, the decision to extubate may be entertained. At times a trial on a T-tube or CPAP set-up with supplemental oxygen may be desirable to further evaluate spontaneous breathing capability without increase in work of breathing.

Extubation and Decannulation

Prior to extubation/decannulation,[25] weaning from mechanical ventilation as well as other criteria must be completed. (See Table III.) The child must be able to maintain adequate blood gas values while on minimal IMV parameters or while breathing spontaneously on a T-tube or CPAP set-up. The indications for the artificial airway must be resolved.

The volume and consistency of the child's secretions should be evaluated. The child should be able to mobilize his secretions adequately. If not, extubation may not be timely. Gag reflex should also be intact to prevent possible aspiration. Airway obstruction is a contraindication to extubation or decannulation. The cardiovascular status should be stable and any amount of supportive phar-

Table III

Criteria to Be Met Prior to Extubation or Decannulation

Successful weaning from mechanical ventilation
Adequate blood gases while on minimal IMV or T-tube
Indications for the airway must be resolved
Able to mobilize own secretions
Intact gag reflex
Stable cardiovascular status
No problem with infection

macology should also be considered. Infection should not be a problem.

It has been recommended that the child be kept NPO for approximately six hours prior to extubation. The stomach can be emptied via a nasogastric tube if time does not permit. This is done to minimize the risk of aspiration. If possible the procedure should be explained to the child to the degree he is capable of comprehending. Whenever possible extubation or decannulation should take place early in the day when the child is more likely to be the most alert and when hospital staffing is usually at its optimum.

All necessary equipment must be at hand for the extubation procedure i.e. suction, oxygen delivery system for use post-extubation, resuscitation bag and mask and reintubation equipment. To avoid any transient hypoxemia during the procedure the child should be preoxygenated with a higher F_IO_2 for approximately five minutes. The child should be in a semi- or high-fowlers position if possible. Suction should be very thorough; endotracheally, orally, and nasally. If the endotracheal or tracheostomy tube is cuffed, all air must be removed from the cuff and pilot balloon. A sterile suction catheter is placed in the airway and the child is asked or stimulated to cough so that the tube is removed during the peak cough effort. Suction is applied during the removal.

In instances of prolonged intubation, swelling or stridor, aerosolized racemic epinephrine may be given as indicated. The child should then be placed on a replacement O_2 delivery system at an F_IO_2 0.10 higher than before.

A tracheostomy tube is always removed in an anatomical configuration consistent with the shape of the tube. The stoma is covered with Vaseline gauze reinforced with a 4 × 4 gauze folded in half and taped air-tight to permit effective coughing and talking.

Post-Extubation/Decannulation Monitoring

The newly extubated/decannulated child must be closely monitored for signs of airway obstruction i.e. stridor or other breathing difficulties. The cardiopulmonary status must be evaluated for any signs of decompensation i.e. tachycardia, hypertension, tachypnea with increased work of breathing. Blood gas analysis should be done 30 minutes post-extubation and again as the child's condition warrants and for the purpose of tapering the supplemental oxygen. A chest X-ray should also be done to evaluate any developing post-extubation atelectasis. Above all, the child should be encouraged to cough and take deep breaths and should be kept as calm as possible. Reintubation equipment should be readily available.

Summary

The techniques of care and modes of therapy described are, by no means, all that are involved in the respiratory care of the pediatric patient. This chapter attempts to gather and outline those areas that are most pertinent to children. Additional knowledge and expertise is gained daily in this once uncharted field of medicine. Interested clinicians must do their part to enhance this process by researching and becoming familiar with new knowledge gained in this area of respiratory care.

References

1. Abrahams N, Fisk GDC, Vonwiller JB: Evaluation of infant ventilators. *Anaesth Intensive Care* 3(1):6–11, 1975.
2. Belani KG, Gilmour IJ, McComb RC, et al: Preextubation ventilatory measurements in newborn and infants. *Anesth Analg* 59(7):467–72, 1980.
3. Blodgett D: *Manual of Pediatric Respiratory Care Procedures.* Philadelphia, JB Lippincott, 1982.
4. Bone RC: How to select the best PEEP for ARDS mechanical ventilation: Maximizing therapeutic value. *J Resp Dis* 3(2):87–95, 1982.

5. Bone RC, Jantten D, Heithold R: Utilization of pressure–volume curves in the pediatric patient. *J Pediatr Surg* 13(2):157–62, 1978.
6. Boros SJ, Campbell K: A comparison of the effects of high frequency–low tidal volume and low frequency–high tidal volume mechanical ventilation. *J Pediatr* 97(1):108–12, 1980.
7. Burton G, Gee G, Hodgkin J: *Respiratory care, A Guide to Clinical Practice.* Philadelphia, JB Lippincott, 1977.
8. Cassidy SS, Gaffney FA, Johnson RL Jr: A perspective on PEEP. *N Eng J Med* 304:421–2, 1981.
9. Cox JMF: Prolonged pediatric ventilatory assistance and related problems. *Crit Care Med* 1(3):158–67, 1973.
10. DeLemos RA, Merdith KS: High frequency ventilation: Panacea or problem? *Pediatrics* 69(2):240, 1982.
11. Douglas ME: Intermittent mandatory ventilation: Why the controversy? *Crit Care Med* 9(8):622–3, 1981.
12. Felley TW: Problems in weaning patients from ventilators. *Resident and Staff Physician* 51–9, 1976.
13. Fuchs PL: Getting the best out of oxygen delivery systems. *Nursing* 10(12):34–43, 1980.
14. Fuchs PL: Understanding continuous mechanical ventilation. *Nursing* 9(12):26–33, 1979.
15. Gallagher TJ: High frequency ventilation: A passing fancy? *Chest* 80:659–60, 1981.
16. Gallagher TJ, Civetta JM, Kirby RR: Terminology update: Optimal PEEP. *Crit Care Med* 6(5):323–6, 1978.
17. Goldman SL, Brady JP, Dumpit FM: Increased work of breathing associated with nasal prongs. *Pediatrics* 64(2):160–4, 1979.
18. Gong Jr H: Positive-pressure ventilation in the adult respiratory distress syndrome. *Clin Chest Med* 3(1):69–88, 1982.
19. Gregory GA, Kitterman JA, Phibbs RH, et al: Treatment of the idiopathic respiratory distress syndrome with continuous positive airway pressure. *N Engl J Med* 284:1333–1340, 1971.
20. Hegyi T, Hiatt IM: The effect of continuous positive airway pressure on the course of respiratory distress syndrome: The benefits of early initiation. *Crit Care Med* 9(1):38–41, 1981.
21. Hodgkin JE: Ventilatory assistance *Am J Surg* 138:374–78, 1979.
22. Hodgkin JE, Bowser MA, Burton G: Respiratory weaning. *Crit Care Med* 2(2):96–102, 1974.
23. Holbrook PR: Taylor G, Pollack MM, et al: Adult respiratory distress syndrome in children. *Pediatr Clin North Am* 27(3):677–85, 1980.
24. Hollinger IB: Postoperative management: Ventilation. *Int Anesthesiol Clin* 18(1):205–16, 1980.
25. Levin, Morriss, Moore: *A Practical guide to Pediatric Intensive Care.* CV Mosby Co, 1979.
26. Lough MD, Doershuck CF, Stern RC: *Pediatric Respiratory Therapy.* Chicago, Year Book Medical Publishers, 1974.
27. Lyrene RK, Truog WE: Adult respiratory distress syndrome in a pediatric intensive care unit: Predisposing conditions, clinical course, and outcome. *Pediatrics* 67(6):790–5, 1981.

28. McFadden R: Decreasing respiratory compromise during infant suctioning. *Am J Nurs* 81(12):2158–61, 1981.
29. Oaks AR: *Critical Care Nursing of Children and Adolescents.* Philadelphia, W.B. Saunders Co., 1981.
30. Reines HD, Civetta JM: The inaccuracy of using 100% oxygen to determine intrapulmonary shunts in spite of PEEP. *Crit Care Med* 7(7):301–3, 1979.
31. Rose DK, Froese AB: Changes in respiratory pattern affect dead space/tidal volume ratio during spontaneous but not during controlled ventilation: A study in pediatric patients. *Anesth Analg* 59(5):341–9, 1980.
32. Scoggin CH: Weaning respiratory patients from mechanical support. *J Resp Dis* 13–23, 1980.
33. Shapiro BA, Harrison RA, Trout C: *Clinical Application of Respiratory Care.* Chicago, Yearbook Medical Publishers, 1975.
34. Sinbruner G, Coradello H, Fodor M, et al: Effects of tracheal suction on oxygenation, circulation, and lung mechanics in newborn infants. *Arch Dis Child* 56(5):326–30, 1981.
35. Slonim NB, Schneider SN, Weng TR, et al: *Pediatric Respiratory Therapy, An Introductory Text.* New York, Glenn Educational Medical Service Inc. 1974.
36. Smith RA, Kirby RR, Gooding JM, et al: Continuous positive airway pressure (CPAP) by face mask. *Crit Care Med* 8(9):483–5, 1980.
37. Vidyasagar D, Wai W: Respiratory weaning of the newborn: Some practical considerations. *Crit Care Med* 3(1):16–22, 1975.
38. West JB: Respiratory Physiology—The Essentials. Baltimore, Williams and Wilkins Co., 1974.
39. Williams JMH: IMV and weaning. *Chest* 78(6):804, 1980.

Part IV

Trauma, Acute Poisoning and Bleeding Disorders in Children

Part IV covers the aspect of traumatic injuries in children including spinal cord injuries and burns. A chapter on poisoning has been included in this part because of its frequent occurrence in children. Bleeding and clotting disorders related to trauma and burn injuries as well as the importance of disseminated intravascular coagulation (DIC) are discussed in the concluding chapter.

18

Traumatic Injuries in Children

Morris J. Asch, M.D.
Neil J. Sherman, M.D.

Traumatic injury has long been recognized as the leading cause of death in children one through 15 years of age. It accounts for approximately 50% of deaths in children in the United States and other industrialized nations and this percentage does not seem to vary from year to year (Table I).[1] In a compilation of statistics in 1974 the automobile was the leading cause of death followed in order of frequency by burns, drowning, fatal injuries caused by firearms, and deaths due to poison ingestion.[2] There is no reason to believe that these statistics have changed significantly in the ensuing years. What has changed, is an appreciation of the magnitude and importance of trauma as a disease process in the pediatric age group. Public awareness through media attention, education, and legislation has been the thrust of a major emphasis in accident prevention. Examples of this are the elimination of lead based paint, the Flammable Clothing Act, and the First Ride, Safe Ride Program in California sponsored by the American Academy of Pediatrics, stressing automobile restraints and safety for children.

In the last decade, the dramatic improvement in transport systems including helicopter and fixed wing evacuation, along with the emergence of regional trauma centers have provided a vastly superior capability in the early care of the injured child. With these specialized facilities, many people feel that the accident victim who

Table I

Causes of Death in Children in the United States in 1975[1]

Cause of Death	*Percent of Total Deaths*
Trauma	48
Infections	14
Cancer	11
Congenital malformations	11
All others	16

reaches the emergency room alive should not die in the emergency room. As greater attention has been focused on traumatic injuries in children, the compilation of data and evaluation of results have followed, resulting in the establishment of a children's trauma registry, regionally and nationally. As information emerges from these centers vital data are being accumulated and correlated such as time lag between injury and arrival to the hospital, location and distribution of regional centers, appropriate level of training of personnel, and the performance of the trauma team in specific injuries. When one considers that almost all pediatric accident victims have been previously healthy and further considers the prolonged rehabilitation and lifetime loss of work potential, then all of these efforts in education, prevention and improvement in care are clearly worthwhile.

The trauma team should be well organized, experienced and led by an emergency room physician or trauma surgeon. A separate pediatric area for ease of patient flow and facility in finding pediatric equipment is advisable. Radio transport systems will usually allow the emergency room team to be prepared for the specific injuries before a patient arrives.

Following severe injury there is a clear list of priorities of evaluation and treatment which should be followed. The most immediate and potentially life-threatening problems are respiratory impairment with failure of oxygenation and ventilation following head and neck, maxillofacial or thoracic injuries. Clearing of the airway followed by mask ventilation using an oxygen reservoir and finally endotracheal intubation are used to establish adequate ventilation. The possibility of cervical spine injury should always be considered. Longitudinal traction on the head should be maintained while securing ventilation to prevent spinal cord injury. Arterial blood gases should be obtained to measure the efficiency of treatment. While ventilation is being secured adequacy of circulation is assessed by measuring blood pressure using the proper size blood pressure cuff for the large and smaller child to prevent spurious values.

Obvious areas of external hemorrhage can be temporarily controlled by direct pressure or tourniquet application. Profusely bleeding scalp laceration can be controlled by slight elevation of the head and neck and direct pressure. Deeper scalp wounds with associated intracranial bleeding cannot be controlled in this fashion. Rapid insertion of an intravenous cannula percutaneously or by cutdown is necessary for fluid and blood administration. Scalp vein needles should be avoided if at all possible. If the injury is primarily thoracic and/or upper body, then lower extremity intravenous portals are preferable; whereas if the injury seems to be primarily abdominal and/or lower extremity, then upper extremity and/or head and neck portals are more desirable. Treatment of circulatory insufficiency manifested by shock is performed by immediate intravenous administration of 20 cc per kilogram of Ringers lactate solution followed by 10–20 ml per kilogram of whole blood if necessary.

Once the immediate life-threatening areas of establishing adequacy of respiratory and circulatory function have been established, the next priority should be the evaluation of intraperitoneal and retroperitoneal injury. Insertion of a Foley catheter, and immediate urine analysis should be done looking for hematuria. Abdominal examination in the conscious child will usually allow for reasonable assessment of the presence of intraperitoneal injury. Chest and abdominal X-rays as well as X-rays of the skull and involved areas of possible fracture should be obtained. Some centers recommend the use of peritoneal aspiration and lavage in all cases of suspected abdominal injury. The authors prefer to reserve this for comatose or semicomatose children and prefer repeated abdominal examination. This will be dealt with in further detail below. Injuries to the brain and spinal cord are the next order of priorities since they do not threaten death as rapidly as the injuries mentioned above. Open cranial wounds should be cleansed and debrided and neurosurgical evaluation obtained.

Further down the list of priorities, which are usually not immediately life-threatening, are thermal injuries, extensive soft tissue injuries, peripheral vascular injuries without hemorrhage, peripheral nerve injuries and fractures. A complete physical examination and evaluation accompanied by appropriate laboratory and x-ray examinations will obviously lead to the diagnosis of these injuries. Wounds with suspected fractures or dislocations should be temporarily immobilized prior to obtaining an x-ray of the appropriate area. After this order of priorities has been exercised and stabilization achieved, then the patient is admitted either to an intensive care unit or general floor care depending upon the extent of the injury.

Specific Injuries

Thoracic Injuries

Thoracic injuries are much less common than abdominal injuries in children. The incidence of associated abdominal injuries in most series is 20–25%. The majority of thoracic injuries are due to blunt trauma related to vehicular accidents. The percentage of penetrating injuries is higher in thoracic injury than in abdominal trauma, and lower in children than in adults because children are less prone to gunshot and knife wounds. Although physical examination is important, a good upright anterior/posterior roentgenogram of the chest remains the hallmark of diagnosis. Thoracic injuries can be divided into pulmonary or mediastinal with the former being subdivided into hemopneumothorax and contusions and the latter subdivided into injuries to the tracheobronchial tree, esophagus, heart and great vessels.

Hemothorax and *pneumothorax* separately or in combination account for about 50% of thoracic injuries. Blunt injuries more often cause pneumothorax while penetrating injuries are associated with a higher incidence of hemothorax. After the suspected diagnosis is confirmed by chest x-ray and the necessity for immediate ventilatory support assessed then tube thoracostomy is usually the first procedure required. This procedure is easily performed at the bedside under local anesthesia. The pleural cavity is best entered in the 5th or 6th intercostal space in the anterior axillary line. If the problem is primarily pneumothorax then the tube can be angled superiorly for better removal of air. Blood is better drained by leaving the tube lower in the pleural cavity and using a larger chest tube. An incision is made on top of the rib and the thoracic cavity entered with either a trochar or large clamp. Prior to entering the thoracic cavity all connections should be checked so that immediate attachment of the tube to underwater drainage and 15–20 cm of negative pressure can be accomplished. Chest tube placement will usually result in rapid lung expansion and removal of blood with clinical improvement. Persistent significant air leak or bleeding should alert one to the possibility of injury to the tracheobronchial tree or great vessels. Occasionally thoracotomy is necessary to control bleeding particularly after penetrating injuries. Concern regarding great vessel injury should be even greater if there is mediastinal widening, first or second rib fracture, or fracture of the scapula or clavicle. After stabilization, angiography should be performed if great vessel injury is suspected.

Pulmonary contusion is a less common but usually a more serious problem caused by severe blunt or crushing trauma. Tachypnea and hypoxia as determined by arterial blood gases are usually present at the outset. Initial chest X-ray may be normal followed in several hours by fluffy infiltrates progressing to complete whiteout in severe injuries. Edema and bronchospasm are the main pathophysiological components and early ventilatory support is often required. There is a high mortality associated with severe pulmonary contusion with the only hope for improved survival resting with the use of extracorporeal membrane oxygenator support.

Mediastinal injuries are much less common than pulmonary injuries. Trauma to the trachea, or main bronchi is usually life-threatening and requires rapid selective intubation of the noninjured bronchus via tracheostomy followed by surgical repair after exact anatomic diagnosis has been made by endoscopy. Injuries to the heart and great vessels are fortunately rare in children. They usually cause life-threatening hemorrhage and require immediate surgical intervention with the capability of using cardiopulmonary bypass.

Esophageal injuries can be caused by blunt or penetrating trauma. The diagnosis is suspected by the presence of pneumomediastinum and confirmed by contrast esophagram and esophagoscopy. Treatment consists of broad-spectrum antibiotics, thoracotomy and repair using postoperative tube thoracostomy drainage.

Abdominal Injuries

Traumatic injury to the abdomen is the most common type of injury seen in the pediatric age group. The vast majority of injuries, about 90% in most series as reported by Welch,[3] are due to blunt trauma. Penetrating injuries are more common in reports that include more, and older, teenagers where knife and gunshot wounds become more prevalent. The two main causes of injury reported by Velcek et al[4] are vehicular accidents in 41%, and falls in 27%.[4] This holds true for most series. Other causes include accidents related to play, penetrating object injuries, and assault. The spleen is injured much more frequently than any other organ, followed in order of frequency by renal and hepatic injuries (Table II).[5–9] Major associated injuries, most often fractures and head injuries, occurred in 61% of the patients in one series, underscoring the severity of the trauma.[8]

The child presenting with abdominal trauma is usually in the 6–10 year age range, frightened and somewhat difficult to evaluate. If the child is conscious and the physician patient and gentle, a reliable abdominal examination can usually be obtained. Unless the child is in shock the initial examination should be performed prior to obtaining blood tests or starting intravenous fluids. Gentle stethoscope palpation and percussion should be used before direct palpation. Repeated abdominal examination is often helpful. Initial laboratory tests should include complete blood count, amylase, and urinalysis. Supine and upright abdominal roentgenograms should be obtained as well as chest and pelvic x-rays if indicated. If the child is stable and the evaluation has failed to reveal abnormalities by physical or laboratory examination, one must determine whether hospitalization or observation by the parents at home is advisable. This depends somewhat on the reliability of the parents and one should always err on the side of being conservative. If specific injuries are suspected then intravenous fluids are started, blood for type and cross-match sent and appropriate x-ray examination obtained.

Table II

Organs Injured Following Blunt Abdominal Trauma in Children[5–9]

Organs Injured	*Tank*[5]	*Levy, Linder*[6]	*Richardson*[7]	*Sinclair, Moore*[8]	*Hood, Smyth*[9]	*Total Number Injured Each Organ*
Spleen	30	23	17	43	29	142
Kidney	18	20	6	20	48	112
Liver	8	5	11	22	33	79
Retroperitoneal hematoma	—	10	3	—	29	42
Stomach	1	2	—	—	5	8
Duodenum	5	—	1	4	6	16
Pancreas	5	—	—	7	1	13
Small bowel	8	2	5	3	8	26
Large bowel	3	1	—	—	8	12
Bladder	3	1	2	5	10	21
Diaphragm	—	2	—	—	3	5
Others	1	—	3	17	21	42
Total Injuries						518

Evaluation for abdominal injury in the neurologically impaired child is more difficult and often requires ancillary techniques such as peritoneal lavage. Some authorities feel that diagnostic peritoneal lavage as first described by Root et al[10] should be performed on all patients with suspected abdominal injury. Most experience has been reported in adults where there is a small percentage of false positive and negative results as well as complications. The trend in children has been away from performing routine diagnostic peritoneal lavage. The authors agree with this approach since the complication rate seems to be a little higher in children and further physical examination is usually masked. We have reserved diagnostic peritoneal lavage for the patient with suspected intra-abdominal injury where neurological impairment makes evaluation by physical examination difficult or unreliable. An incision is made in the midline below the umbilicus under local anesthesia after emptying the bladder with a Foley catheter. In children under six, a 14-gauge intracath with extra holes is inserted into the peritoneal cavity and used for the lavage. A pediatric peritoneal dialysis catheter is used in children over six after actual dissection with good light and retractors is carried out down to the peritoneum so that controlled entry into the peritoneal cavity can be achieved between mosquito clamps. Fifteen ml/kg of Ringers lactate is instilled rapidly and drained as completely as possible. Quantitative measurement of red blood cells, white blood cells and amylase is obtained with a positive test considered to be greater than 100,000 RBC's per ml. Rapid evaluation by seeing if one can read newsprint through a bottle of the return fluid has been considered reliable in most centers.

Other criteria for a positive peritoneal lavage are more than 500 WBC/mm^3, amylase greater than 100 Somogy units and the presence of bile or bacteria.

In summary, initial evaluation and management of the pediatric trauma patient involves first establishing the adequacy of airway and ventilation followed by assessment of intravascular volume. After these immediate life-threatening areas have been evaluated a general complete examination looking for abdominal injury, fractures, neurological injury or other problems is carried out. This is followed by specific organ system evaluation as described below and appropriate consultation as indicated.

Splenic Injury

As stated earlier the spleen is the most common organ injured following abdominal trauma. A history of a fall or upper abdominal trauma, which may be relatively minor is usually given. Upper abdominal pain and tenderness are almost always present. Any rib fractures on the left side and an X-ray demonstration of same should heighten one's suspicions. Left shoulder pain referred from diaphragmatic irritation is often present. The initial complete blood count usually shows a normal hemoglobin and hematocrit but there is often an immediate rise in white blood count to greater than 15,000/mm^3. Abdominal X-rays are seldom helpful although occasionally one can see an increase in the splenic shadow or medial displacement of the stomach. If splenic injury is suspected it should be confirmed as soon as possible by radionuclide scan of the spleen using Technetium-99 sulfur colloid. An area of decreased isotope uptake indicating decreased blood supply in the area of injury can be seen on the scan as an actual laceration or transection (Fig. 1A), or in small injuries as a subcapsular defect. Once the diagnosis has been established then one must determine if this is an isolated problem, as is usually the case, or whether there are injuries to other intra-abdominal organs. If laparotomy is not indicated for other reasons then a conservative surgical approach using splenic repair or a completely nonoperative approach has become increasingly prevalent. The predominant feeling of trying to preserve the spleen followed Singer's review in 1973 which showed that when splenectomy was performed for trauma the incidence of postsplenectomy sepsis is 58 times that found in the general population.[11] Sherman and Asch were among many surgeons who demonstrated that splenic repair rather than splenectomy was quite feasible and safe.[12] Douglas and Simpson were among the first to report a series of children with documented splenic injury managed without surgery.[13] More recently Welch reported a series of 12 consecutive patients with proven splenic injuries managed without surgery.[3] A specific policy was described including the use of transfusion. The authors have used this nonoperative approach successfully on many occasions if surgery was not required for other reasons. Careful observation in an intensive care unit by an experienced surgeon is necessary with serial measurement of hemoglobin and hematocrit. If the patient is unstable or abdominal findings worsen then exploration should be considered. In the stable patient hemoglobin and hematocrit levels equilibrate in about 48 hours with improvement in the abdominal findings shortly thereafter. After tolerating diet most patients can be discharged in less than a week. True delayed splenic rupture is rare and does not preclude the above approach. Vigorous activity is prohibited for six weeks and contact sports for three months. This approach is illustrated by the case of an 11-year-old girl seen in the emergency room with left upper quadrant tenderness after falling off a horse. A large splenic laceration was noted on Technetium-99 sulfur colloid scan of the liver and spleen. (See Fig. 1A.) No other injuries were apparent and she was managed nonoperatively and discharged on the sixth hospital day. A repeat liver spleen scan six weeks following the injury showed complete healing (Fig. 1B).

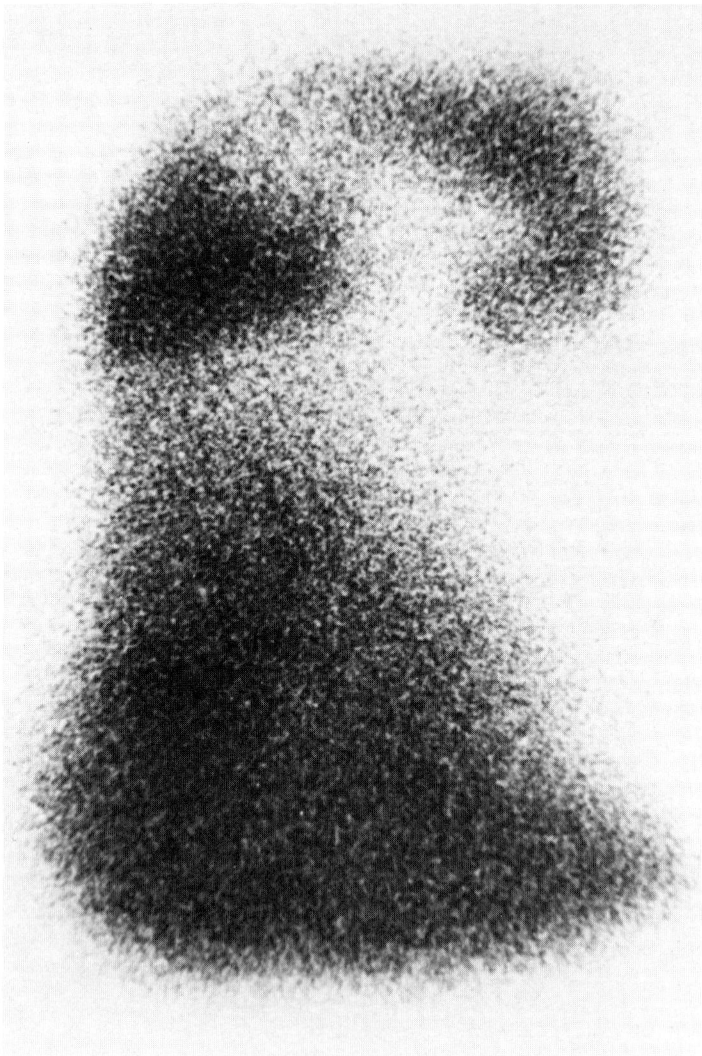

Figure 1A. Radionuclide liver/spleen scan, anterior/posterior view demonstrating large splenic laceration.

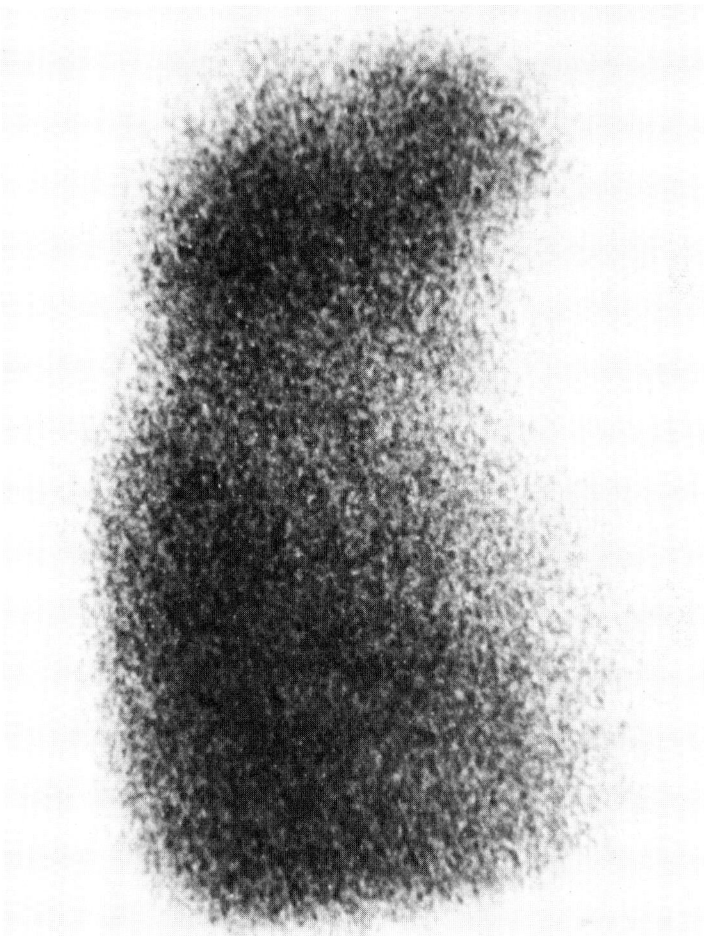

Figure 1B. Radionuclide liver/spleen scan, six weeks after patient was treated non-operatively, demonstrating good healing.

Kidney Injuries

The kidney is the second most common organ injured following blunt abdominal trauma. The anatomical position of the kidneys in children make them more prone to injury than adults. Children have less perirenal tissue and fat and the kidneys occupy a more intraperitoneal position. Relatively minor trauma may cause significant kidney injury in patients with renal abnormalities such as horseshoe kidney, hydronephrosis or renal tumors. There are associated injuries of the central nervous system, intraperitoneal injuries or fractures in 30–40% of children with renal injuries.

Abdominal or flank pain and hematuria are the usual presenting symptoms of kidney injury. Some patients present in shock due to severe retroperitoneal or intraperitoneal hemorrhage. If there is major bleeding into the collecting system, bladder clots occasionally cause inability to void or bladder spasm. Physical findings include abdominal tenderness and/or rigidity. A paralytic ileus is often seen secondary to retroperitoneal or intraperitoneal blood.

The diagnosis of kidney injury is confirmed when microscopic or gross hematuria is present. If the patient with significant trauma does not void shortly after entering the emergency room catheterization of the urinary bladder should be performed. Uson and Lattimer have divided renal injuries into injuries of the kidney proper and those of the kidney appendages such as renal vascular pedicle, perineal fat and ureter.[14] They further divide injuries of the kidney proper into five types: simple contusions with integrity of the renal capsule and pelvis; superficial laceration with associated tear of the cortex; deep laceration with concomitant rupture of the capsule and calices; rupture of the pelvis; and "shattered" kidney. Once the diagnosis of renal injury is suspected there is a fairly standardized way to proceed diagnostically although there is some difference of opinion about treatment. An intravenous pyelogram is obtained and if it is normal, or shows delayed visualization or minor extravasation then conservative management with bedrest is prescribed. If there is major extravasation, or nonvisualization then transfemoral arteriography is immediately performed looking for an injury to the renal vascular pedicle. A stable retroperitoneal renal hematoma should be treated nonoperatively, if possible, because exploration and untamponading of the hematoma may result in uncontrollable bleeding and the loss of an otherwise salvageable kidney. Evidence of damage to the renal vascular pedicle on arteriography dictates immediate laparotomy to try and save the kidney. A long midline incision with exposure and control of both renal vascular pedicles prior to opening Gerota's fascia allows for optimum control. Further operative details are beyond the scope of this chapter. Major extravasation with an intact renal vascular pedicle would be treated nonoperatively by most authorities including the authors. Patients treated nonoperatively may have a persistent ileus, develop fever or a retroperitoneal urine collection causing a mass or "urinoma." Most of these problems resolve with time although occasionally "urinomas" require drainage. Late complications include hypertension, stone formation and caliectasis. All patients with significant renal injury managed nonoperatively should have follow-up intravenous pyelograms and blood pressure measurement at six weeks, three and six months following injury. Although there is some controversy in managing renal injuries the trend in recent years has been to be as conservative as possible since this has led to the greatest degree of kidney preservation.

Liver Injuries

Hepatic injuries follow closely behind renal injuries in order of frequency of organs injured in children with abdominal trauma (Table II). Major liver injury causes the highest mortality rate among abdominal organs injured. A great many patients with significant juxtahepatic vascular injury and hemorrhage die before reaching the hospital and many more die in the operating room due to uncontrollable hemorrhage. Mikeskey et al reported a 40% mortality in the first decade of life following blunt abdominal trauma causing liver injury.[15]

Patients with liver injuries present with abdominal pain and are frequently in shock. The normotensive patient who has upper abdominal pain and tenderness and does not have hematuria is suspected of having an injury to the spleen or liver. After obtaining blood for type and cross-match and starting a large intravenous cannula in the upper extremity a radionuclide liver/spleen scan should be performed if plain and upright roentgenograms of the abdomen are normal. There is a high correlation between arteriography and radionuclide scan of the liver and some cases of hepatic injury can be managed without operation. Richie and Fonkalsrud reported four patients with subcapsular hematomas of the liver who were followed with serial hepatic scans to healing without surgical intervention.[16]

The child presenting in shock without hematuria most likely has a significant hepatic or splenic laceration causing major hemorrhage. If blood pressure stabilization can be obtained by an infusion of Ringers lactate and 5% albumin solution through large bore intravenous cannulas in both upper extremities then consideration should be given to obtaining a radionuclide scan of the liver and spleen or celiac arteriography while making preparations for laparotomy. Recurring or persistent hypotension demands immediate laparotomy. Monitoring of blood pH and correction of acidosis is extremely important in these patients and should be followed on a serial basis. Moderate hypothermia[33–34] should be prepared for both before and during surgery since it has been shown to minimize necrosis and increase tolerance to hepatic vascular inflow occlusion often required in surgery for control of hemorrhage. Details of surgical management will not be elaborated upon here except to say that despite wide exposure through laparotomy and thoracotomy incisions, hepatic vascular inflow occlusion, packing and internal venous bypass shunting there remains a very high mortality with hepatic rupture and/or juxtahepatic vascular injury. In recent years, a more conservative surgical approach of hepatic artery ligation coagulation and packing, trying to avoid hepatic resection if possible, has been recommended. Unfortunately there remains a great deal of room for improvement in the results of management in patients with major hepatic injuries.

Injuries to the extrahepatic biliary tree are uncommon but do occur and should be carefully searched for during any laparotomy for trauma. Penetrating injuries occasionally cause laceration of the gall bladder and there are numerous reported cases of tears and disruption of the hepatic and common bile ducts following blunt trauma. If these injuries are diagnosed at laparotomy successful repair with T-tube drainage as indicated can usually be achieved. Broad-spectrum antibiotic coverage following hepatic or bile duct injury is recommended to minimize hepatic necrosis and cholangitis.

Intestinal Injuries

Injuries to the intestinal tract, although not as common as injuries to the spleen, kidney and liver, do comprise a significant number of injuries following abdominal trauma, and most of them require surgical intervention. Perforations are more common in children than in adults because the relatively thinner abdominal wall in children provides less protection. This allows, for instance, a relatively minor blow to the abdomen to cause perforation in a child who has just eaten. It also maximizes the contrecoup effect after trauma and deceleration in the proximal jejunum and distal ileum where these injuries are most common. Signs and symptoms of intestinal injury vary with the severity of injury from mild abdominal tenderness with a small mesenteric hematoma to abdominal rigidity with a free perforation. The initial plain and upright roentgenograms of the abdomen frequently do not show free intraperitoneal air in children with intestinal perforations. One must base the decision to perform laparotomy upon abdominal physical findings or pursue diagnosis with the use of a contrast upper gastrointestinal series using water soluble contrast material. Recently computerized axial tomography examination of the abdomen has been helpful in diagnosing duodenal and pancreatic injuries.

Gastric injuries are relatively uncommon and often occur following blunt trauma in the child with a full stomach resulting in perforation. The children usually present with peritoneal signs or total abdominal rigidity, and are often diaphorectic and hypotensive. Free intraperitoneal air is usually seen on an upright roentgenogram of the abdomen following a gastric perforation. Laparotomy is performed after starting intravenous fluids and antibiotics. Most gastric perforations are on the anterior wall of the stomach and are easily sutured with the main problem being cleansing of the intraperitoneal contamination. Survival should be excellent without other associated life-threatening injuries.

Duodenal injuries are more common than gastric injuries and can be divided into perforation and intramural hematoma with the latter being more common. Because of its retroperitoneal location perforations of the duodenum cause less symptoms and are more difficult to diagnose than other gastrointestinal perforations.

There is usually some epigastric or right upper quadrant tenderness and there may be an elevation of the serum amylase. Upper gastrointestinal roentgenograms using water soluble contrast will usually lead to the diagnosis. Laparotomy is performed after starting antibiotics and making sure that intravascular volume is satisfactory. Wide exposure of the duodenum and pancreas using a Kocher manuever is necessary for complete evaluation since there may be an associated pancreatic injury. Direct suture of the perforation with reinforcement by a patch of omentum or an intestinal serosal patch usually results in a satisfactory closure. Postoperative nasogastric tube decompression and antibiotics are required. Results of the repair of duodenal perforations have been good with excellent survival in the absence of other life-threatening injuries.

The more common injury to the duodenum is intramural hematoma resulting from contusion, usually of the second portion of the duodenum. The patient usually has very little abdominal pain or tenderness but demonstrates persistent vomiting or high output through the nasogastric tube. The vomiting is caused by obstruction of the duodenal lumen by the intramural hematoma and the associated edema. An upper gastrointestinal series will confirm the suspicion of duodenal obstruction with the intramural hematoma causing diagnostic x-ray findings. There is some disagreement in treatment recommendations for duodenal hematoma although in recent years most authors have recommended surgery. The intramural hematoma will slowly resorb and the duodenal obstruction will usually resolve in two to three weeks. Many patients have been treated successfully without surgery using nasogastric suction and intravenous fluids with parenteral nutrition waiting for the duodenal lumen to open up. If surgery is performed shortly after the diagnosis is made, morbidity can be decreased and hospitalization shortened by one or two weeks. At the time of surgery the intramural clot is evacuated and meticulous hemostasis obtained by electrocautery. The patient can usually begin feedings several days after surgery and can go home several days later.

Pancreatic injury has been included with intestinal injury because of its close proximity to the intestine and the frequency with which pancreatic and intestinal injuries coexist. Traumatic pancreatitis may occur following a relatively minor injury. The head and body of the pancreas join just anterior to the vertebral column and even a mild blow from a bicycle handlebar can cause the pancreas to be pushed against the spine. Patients usually complain of upper abdominal pain and often have persistent vomiting. Measurement of serum amylase on a daily basis will usually confirm the diagnosis of pancreatic injury although the combination of measuring serum and urine amylase has been shown to be much more accurate in making the diagnosis of pancreatitis. This is because urinary amylase stays elevated longer than serum amylase. The extent of the injury varies from mild contusion of the pancreas to complete transection with disruption of the head from the body and tail of the pancreas. Milder injuries usually resolve without surgery following treatment with nasogastric decompression and intravenous fluids. Total parenteral nutrition may be required in cases of prolonged elevation of the serum amylase and protracted ileus. In more severe cases of pancreatic injury with or without ductal disruption, pancreatic fluid extravasates retroperitoneally and occasionally intraperitoneally. This causes increasing peritoneal signs and "third space" fluid loss into the peritoneal cavity. Progressive abdominal findings correlated with the clinical course may indicate the necessity for laparotomy. At the time of surgery, debridement of necrotic pancreatic tissue and drainage are carried out, or if there is severe disruption of the body and tail of the pancreas distal pancreatectomy with drainage may be required. The most complex problem seen is a combination of injury to the head of the pancreas and duodenum. Various types of resection and drainage including pancreaticoduodenectomy have been used in treatment. Fortunately this injury is quite rare. Total parenteral nutrition is often helpful in the postoperative management of these patients since prolonged ileus and delay in return of gastrointestinal function are common. Pancreatic injury and necrosis will sometimes result in the formation of a pancreatic pseudocyst. These can be seen as early as one week following injury and manifest themselves by increasing abdominal distention and tenderness with persistent elevation of the serum or urine amylase. The diagnosis can be confirmed by ultrasound or computerized axial tomography and the size of the cyst can be followed on a serial basis by these modalities. Many of these pseudocysts will require internal drainage into the stomach or jejunum. The danger of an enlarging pseudocyst is that it may bleed or rupture into the free peritoneal cavity. Internal drainage of a pseudocyst is not recommended before two and a half to three weeks following injury because prior to this the cyst wall is not thick enough to allow suturing to the intestinal tract. As can be appreciated from the above description the types of pancreatic injury are quite varied and manifest themselves in different ways. Careful serial examination and laboratory evaluation is required to achieve optimal results.

Jejunoileal injuries usually occur in the first 10–20 cm of jejunum or last 10–20 cm of ileum. This is because of the transition from retroperitoneal or fixed intestine to intestine on a free mesentery both at the ligament of Trietz and at the ileocecal junction. The jejunum just distal and the ileum just proximal to these fixed areas suffer a maximal shearing force, the so-called *contrecoup effect,* after a relatively minor blow or automobile deceleration injury. Children with these injuries usually present with abdominal pain and tenderness. It is remarkable that in many cases initial supine and upright roentgenograms of the abdomen fail to show free intraperitoneal air. The decision to perform surgery is usually made on the basis of increasing abdominal findings or a subsequent roentgenogram showing free intraperitoneal air. A contrast upper gastrointestinal series or peritoneal lavage revealing bacteria or bile may also be helpful in leading to the diagnosis. At the time of surgery perforations are usually found on the antimesenteric surface and are easily sutured. Occasionally there is a complete disruption of the bowel and debridement of the ends with limited resection and primary anastomosis is required. It is remarkable that some of these perforations are discovered during routine examination of the bowel when laparotomy is performed for other indications. This underscores the importance of checking all viscera at the time of laparotomy for trauma including examination of the entire gastrointestinal tract. The results of repair of an isolated small bowel injury are usually excellent with the occasional complication of a postoperative subphrenic or intraperitoneal abscess because of contamination. Antibiotics are started prior to surgery to minimize this problem.

Colonic injuries are relatively uncommon and are caused in almost equal frequency by blunt and penetrating trauma. As one might expect injuries due to blunt trauma are most common in the younger child and are often associated with pelvic injuries while penetrating injuries become more common in teen-aged children. The usual signs and symptoms are lower abdominal pain and tenderness with increasing peritoneal signs as peritoneal contamination increases. In a major pelvic crush injury these signs and symptoms may be difficult to distinguish from other aspects of the injury such as bladder contusion, pelvic fracture or retroperitoneal hematoma. A supine and upright roentgenogram of the abdomen may reveal free intraperitoneal air in the presence of a colon perforation. A rectal perforation may not cause free intraperitoneal air and after careful rectal examination a water soluble contrast enema should be done if there is any suspicion of a rectal or lower colonic perforation. Treatment of colonic perforations consists of exteriorization of the injury as a colostomy if possible. Lower colonic and rectal injuries should be repaired and protected by a proximal diverting colostomy which can be closed in four to six weeks depending on the patient's condition. There has been some enthusiasm for primary closure of small isolated colonic perforations due to knife or gunshot wounds without performing a colostomy. The results in the series reported have been good especially if it is an isolated injury. As with any intestinal perforation the most common complication is postoperative pelvic or subphrenic abscess. The use of broad-spectrum antibiotics will minimize this problem.

Pelvic Injury

Injury to the lower abdomen and pelvis usually results from blunt or crushing trauma. In younger children it is not uncommon for a parent to unknowingly roll over the child with the wheels of an automobile while backing out of the driveway. Physical examination may disclose areas of pelvic bony tenderness or instability. Aside from skull fractures, fracture of the pelvis is the most common bony injury in traffic accidents. After patient stabilization and pelvic bone X-rays the presence of retroperitoneal hemorrhage with or without associated vascular injury should be assessed. Retroperitoneal hemorrhage may be severe and is occasionally life-threatening. In the absence of other indications for surgery retroperitoneal hemorrhage is not in itself an indication for laparotomy. In fact, it is the majority opinion that at the time of laparotomy nonenlarging retroperitoneal hematomas should not be opened or evacuated for fear of releasing the tamponade and causing uncontrollable hemorrhage. Vascular injury to the iliac or femoral vessels may occur with pelvic injury. If there is any abnormality of the pulse or Doppler flow measurement then arteriography should be done to define the vascular anatomy.

Genitourinary injuries are quite common following pelvic trauma. In the presence of a pelvic fracture a urethrogram should be performed prior to inserting a Foley catheter to prevent conversion of a urethral tear into a disruption. The urethrogram is done by inserting a syringe into the urethral meatus and injecting 5 cc of contrast material. A cystogram should be done to detect bladder injury. A good washout view of the bladder may detect a small amount of extravasation of contrast due to a small bladder tear.

Urethral injuries are treated by splinting with a Foley catheter which may have to be inserted via a cystotomy guide. Bladder perforations can usually be closed easily with the closure being protected by bladder drainage with a Foley catheter for 7–10 days postoperatively.

Because of the multiple aspects of pelvic injury it is crucial to use a stepwise methodical approach in evaluation and treatment in order to achieve optimum results.

Summary

A perspective on the magnitude of trauma as cause of injury and death has been given. Our greatest hope for decreasing the incidence of this disease lies in the area of public education and accident prevention. Better transport mechanisms and regionalization of trauma facilities have allowed the injured child to obtain more rapid and expert initial evaluation. Despite this the mortality for major head and thoracic and abdominal injuries remains significant.

A detailed discussion of the initial approach to the childhood trauma victim is given, including priorities of evaluation and treatment. Specific recommendations in the approach to thoracic and abdominal injuries are reviewed. Since this has been written from the perspective of the pediatric intensive care unit, details of operative management have been omitted.

References

1. Haller JA Jr: An overview of pediatric trauma. *Current Concepts in Trauma Care.* Nov:16–20, 1977.
2. Garfinkel J, Chabot JJ, Pratt MW: *Infant, Maternal and Childhood Mortality in the U.S.* DHEW publication no. (HSA) 75-5013 (Rockville, Md. Health Services Administration, 1968–1973.)
3. Welch KJ: Abdominal injuries. *Pediatric Surgery.* Third Edition, Vol. 1, pp. 125–149.
4. Velcek FT, et al: Traumatic death in urban children. Presented at the Annual Meeting, *American Academy of Pediatrics,* Chicago, October 18, 1976.
5. Tank ES, Eraklis AJ, Gross RE: Blunt abdominal trauma in infancy and childhood, *J Trauma,* 8:439, 1968.
6. Levy JL, Linder LH: Major abdominal trauma in children. *Am J Surg,* 1970.
7. Richardson JD, Belin RP, Griffen WO: Blunt abdominal trauma in children. *Ann Surg,* 1972.
8. Sinclair MC, Moore TC: Major surgery for abdominal and thoracic trauma in childhood and adolescence. *J Pediatr Surg* 9:155, 1974.
9. Hood JM, Smythe BT: Nonpenetrating intraabdominal injuries in children. *J Pediatr Surg* 9:69, 1974.
10. Root HD, et al: Diagnostic peritoneal lavage. *Surgery* 57:633, 1965.
11. Singer DB: Post-splenectomy sepsis. *In* Rosenberg HS, Bolander RP (eds): *Perspectives in Pediatric Pathology.* Chicago, Year Book Medical Publishers, 1973, pp. 285–305.
12. Sherman NJ, Asch MJ: Conservative surgery for splenic injuries. *Pediatrics* 61:267–271, 1978.
13. Douglas GT, Simpson JS: Conservative management of splenic trauma. *J Pediatr Surg* 6:565, 1971.
14. Uson AC, Lattimer JK: Genitourinary tract injuries. *Pediatric Surgery.* Third Edition, Vol. 1, pp. 162–176.
15. Mikeskey WE, Howard JM, DeBakey ME: Collective review: Injuries of the liver in 300 consecutive patients. *Surg Gynecol Obstet* 103:323, 1956.
16. Richie JP, Fonkalsrud EW: Subcapsular hematoma of the liver. *Arch Surg* 104:781, 1972.

19

Spinal Cord Injury in Infants and Children

Barry B. Ceverha, M.D.

Introduction

Pediatric spinal cord injury may best be managed by understanding differences of anatomical and biomechanical factors unique to the spine of young children. Injury associated with the pliable spine of the neonate differs dramatically from the mature spine of the older child. Consequently, dependent upon the development of the neural tissue and mechanism of injury, the child presents with varying clinical features. Treatment, directed towards managing and preventing further injury, is influenced by such factors.

Epidemiology

It is generally accepted that spinal cord injuries in children are an uncommon phenomenon. Most authors estimate the actual frequency of admissions to spinal cord rehabilitation centers to be approximately 2–4%. By contrast in the adult, over 10,000 new cases of cervical spinal cord injury alone are reported each year and account for the majority of admissions to these centers.

Figure 1 illustrates a high correlation of frequency of spinal cord injury with increasing age. This may be related to certain anatomical features of the infant spinal column, as well as the exposure to certain mechanisms of injury that occur only as one gets older.

The majority of spinal cord injuries occurring in children less than one year of age may be attributed to obstetrical complications occurring with breech delivery. Maekawa has reported a quite unusual case of tetraplegia in a newborn delivered by Caesarean section. X-rays a few days before birth demonstrate marked hyperextension of the cervical spine.

The majority of injuries in a toddler or school age child are related to motor vehicle accidents or falls from playground equipment. Table I demonstrates the etiology of these injuries as reported by Anderson[1] in a series of 156 cases treated at the Mayo Clinic. Sports related injuries increase in frequency as the child enters the competitive arena. Football is frequently indicted as a major causative factor. Water related injuries such as diving and water skiing account for 6%.

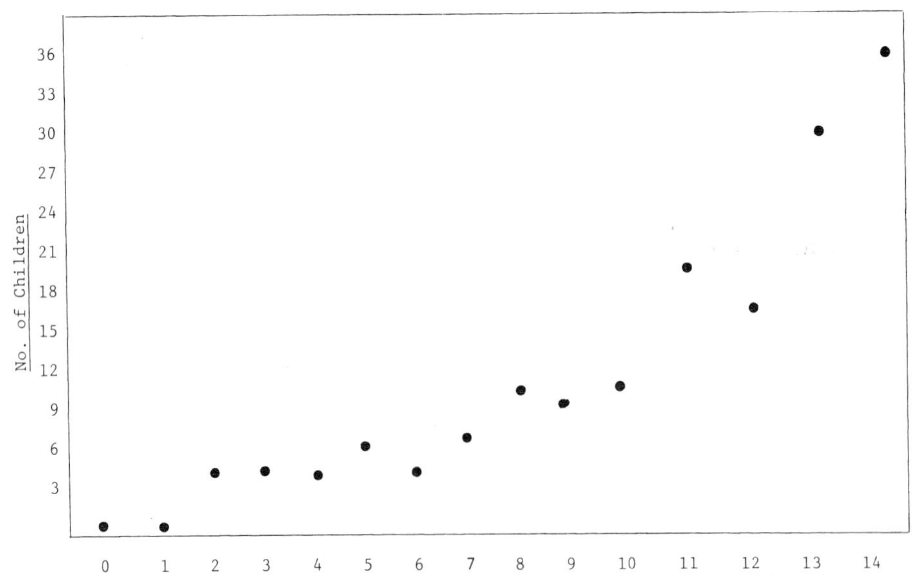

Figure 1. Increasing frequency of spinal injury with age.

Table I
Cause of Spinal Injury (156 Cases)

Mode	*Number*	*Percent*
Automobile accidents	33	21
Fall	28	18
Sports	16	10
Farm-related accidents	11	7
Winter activities	10	6
Water activities	9	6
Playground activities	8	5
Bicycle accidents	7	4
Pedestrian-auto accidents	6	4
Other motorized vehicle accidents	5	3
Horseback riding	5	3
Corticosteroid therapy	5	3
Gunshot or knife wound	3	2
Not stated	10	6

Violent injuries such as gunshot wounds and stabbings account for only 2% of injuries reported. Burke[3] reports a surprisingly high incidence of this type of injury in the southern California area; 18% of admissions to the Pediatric Regional Spinal Cord Center are related to violence.

The most common sites of fracture are in the cervical and thoracic regions. Anderson[1] analyzes the fracture sites, and groups them into six locations (Table II). The most common sites of fractures are the cervical spine above C4 (25%) and the thoracic area from T6 to T12 (27%). The incidence of fracture at other vertebral levels ranged from 6–17%. Fractures that are most common in adults are much less frequent in the infant and child. True fractures of the odontoid process in these patients under the age of three are regarded as rare. Ewald[6] reviews only four previously reported cases of odontoid fracture in this age group. Hangman's fracture, a fracture-dislocation of C2-C3, and a relatively common fracture in adults, are also considered rare in the pediatric age group. Weiss[15] reports a single case of a 12-month-old with this injury and describes only one other case in the world literature.

Table II

Site of Injury to Spinal Nervous System (156 Cases)

	Fracture	
Level	*Number*	*Percent*
Above C4	39	25
C4 to C7	22	14
T1 to T5	15	10
T6 to T12	42	27
L1 to L4	27	17
L5 to Sacrum	9	6

Radiological Findings

Radiological signs of vertebral injury are not apparent in more than one-half of the injuries reported below age ten. The younger the patient is, the less likely X-ray evidence will confirm fracture. In Melzak's series,[12] no fracture could be detected in 16 to 29 patients with traumatic paraplegia. Slight wedging may be observed, but flattening of the normal convex end-plates of the vertebral body are frequently the only signs of recent trauma. Hachems[8] radiologic findings in 18 pediatric spinal cord injuries are listed in Table III. True fracture lines are very uncommon in the young child, and prior to puberty, totally avulsed vertebral corners are an exception. Because of these difficulties, spinal cord injury may remain unrecognized, especially in the comatose child.

Table III

Radiological Signs of Vertebral Lesion (18 Cases)

	0–10 Years	*10–15 Years*
No evidence of lesion	5 cases	3 cases
Slight compression (squaring)	2	2
Fracture-dislocation	1	2
Multiple fragments	1	2

With severe ligamentous and muscular injury, one can, at times, demonstrate pathological cervical hypermobility by doing *careful* extension and flexion lateral views of the neck to identify the involved level. This procedure should be performed only in the presence of experienced personnel. Extreme caution must be exercised to prevent rapid or exaggerated movements of the head which would promote further injury. Tomography and computerized tomography of the spine are techniques that also may prove useful in demonstrating subtle bony abnormalities in the acute setting.

Biomechanical Factors

Cervical Spine

There are marked anatomical and physiological differences in the infant spinal column compared with the older child and adolescent. The infantile vertebral bodies are elastic cartilages surrounded by connective tissue. In autopsy specimens, it can be shown that the bony column can stretch at least two inches, but the spinal cord accommodates to a much lesser degree. Breig[2] has noted that the spinal cord adapts to changes in canal length by a mechanism of plastic deformity. There is some elongation of the spinal cord in flexion and shortening of the cord in extension. There may be as much as 25% change of length in cord. But the cord does not freely move up and down the spinal canal, and is restricted by extrinsic factors such as nerve roots and dentate ligaments, as well as intrinsic factors such as the pia and axons themselves. In flexion then, the cord is "stretched" to its limit. Any existing pathological changes in the canal such as disc protrusion, dislocation or bony ridges will indent the anterior aspect of the cord, causing further injury.

Spinal cord damage without demonstrable skeletal injury may result from a variety of circumstances. Temporary dislocation in hyperextension can occur with rupture of the anterior longitudinal ligament. The ligamentum flavum may bulge forward during forcible hyperextension, as in motor vehicle accidents when the head is held immobile and the body is thrown forward. Greatest bulging of the ligamentum has been shown to occur between C3 and C6—the region where most cervical pathology is located.

Glasauer[7] constructs the mechanism of injury to the cervical spinal cord in vehicular accidents as follows: upon impact, acceleration with hyperextension of the head and neck occurs, followed by forcible flexion of the proportionate large head causing traction and actual stretching, possible impingement or even compression of the spinal cord resulting in damage. This mechanism resembles that of birth injury in which traction on the body applied during delivery of the head in breech presentation may result in tearing of the cord.

These mechanical factors are also complicated by the immature and tenuous vascular supply of the spinal cord. The blood supply is marginal under normal conditions, because of inadequate collateral circulation and vascular anastomotic channels. The areas of the cord in which the circulation is most tenuous is the T4 and L1 segments. These regions are felt to be "watershed" regions and are particularly susceptible to perfusion changes. It is not uncommon to note a fracture-dislocation at C5–C6, but the patient will demonstrate clinically or at necropsy, T4 segment necrosis. In addition, vascular spasm and cord edema may further compromise the already reduced tissue blood flow and further damage the spinal cord.

As the child gets older and the spine matures, the muscular, ligamentous, and bony structures are firmer and less amenable to stretch forces. Hyperextension, flexion and rotatory forces are more likely to produce actual tissue damage and fracture with direct pressure applied to the cord and its vascular supply. Stretching of the cord plays a much less significant role. Radiographic evidence of spinal column injury is apparent as actual fractures and ligamentous tears are more likely to occur.

Thoracolumbar Fractures

Injuries to the thoracic or lumbar spine are caused by either a closed mechanism or by penetrating wounds, such as gunshot or stabbing. The mechanisms of closed injury to this region are basically the same as elsewhere in the spine: flexion, extension, rotation and compression. Bony and ligamentous injury determines the end result rather than stretching or elastic properties of the spinal cord. Because of the heavy and well-formed spinal column, it takes much more force to disrupt and injure the thoracolumbar spine. The injuries are more extensive and by this fact are more apparent on x-ray.

Closed injuries are usually flexion caused by acceleration or deceleration with the fixed part of the body acting as a fulcrum, allowing the unrestrained portion to flex acutely on the fixed portion of the body. Compression fractures may occur by themselves or with flexion and/or rotatory forces. Axial compression such as landing on the feet or buttocks from height will cause this type of injury. When a injury does occur at this level, there is apt to be more neural injury than at other parts of the spine. The spinal cord occupies a greater proportion of the spinal canal in the thoracic region and is thus more susceptible to processes that narrow the canal. The vascular supply of the thoracic cord is more tenuous than other regions, making ischemia more likely. It takes tremendous force to produce fracture, and greater destruction results to the neural elements and surrounding structures.

Clinical Features

Early recognition of spinal injuries is critical if one is to aggressively treat the existing injury, or to prevent further damage from an unsuspected fracture. In the newborn and infant, it is at times difficult to recognize neurologic deficit from spinal cord injury. The standard method of pinching extremities and watching movement patterns may in some cases identify gross complete injury, but may not identify subtle motor and sensory abnormalities. Attention to respiratory patterns, noting intercostal muscle movement, abdominal breathing patterns, and unexplained cyanosis and hyperpnea may point toward neurologic dysfunction. Absence of sweating below the physiological level of dysfunction is another subtle but useful diagnostic sign of spinal cord injury. Distended bladder or recurrent urinary tract infections, priapism, patulous anus, absence of Moro's reflex, and general hypotonia may provide useful information in diagnosing spinal cord dysfunction in this age group.

Several clinical syndromes have been reported by Crothers[4] in those infants surviving spinal cord injury: (1) unilateral or bilateral brachial plexus palsies and/or cranial nerve deficit; (2) permanent flaccidity and anesthesia below the level of physiologic or anatomic cord transection; and (3) initial flaccidity and anesthesia (spinal shock) but followed by the development of hyperreflexivity.

As the age of the patient increases, so does the ability and ease of the physician to diagnose spinal cord injury. This is presumably due, at least in part, to the patient's ability to speak and localize discomfort. Hubbard[10] evaluated the presentation of 42 spinal injured children and his findings are noted in Table IV. Stable and unstable fractures presented somewhat differently and this is noted. Pain and tenderness were the most common findings. The pain may be localized to the fracture area, referred to another site, or as with cervical fractures, presented as acute torticollis. Neurologic symptoms, such as numbness, tingling, or dysesthesias and/or an abnormal neurologic exam were present only in the unstable fracture category.

Special consideration must be given to those patients presenting with possible spinal injury whose level of consciousness is seriously impaired. For the patient who can talk and/or follow commands, a more complete neurological evaluation is possible. A detailed reflex and sensory examination will usually allow the physician to localize the general physiologic or anatomical level of injury. If a patient is unconscious, however, an accurate neurologic

Table IV

Signs and Symptoms of Spinal Injuries in Children (42 Cases)

	Percentage of Cases	
Signs and Symptoms	*Stable*	*Unstable*
Pain (spine, abdomen)	86.2	92.8
Tenderness (spine, abdomen)	89.2	92.8
Tingling, numbness, weakness	3.5	57.1
Radiation of pain	0.0	7.1
Inability to walk	3.5	42.8
Muscle spasm	3.5	42.8
Abnormal neurologic exam	0.0	57.1

examination is not possible, making localization or indication of spinal cord injury difficult.

Table V lists general helpful signs that may be apparent in a comatose patient suggesting spinal cord injury. Flaccid areflexia, as well as flaccid rectal tone, strongly suggests spinal cord dysfunction. Therefore, when first evaluating any severely injured patient, the examiner should immediately perform a rectal exam noting presence or absence of bulbocavernous reflex or rectal sphincter tone.

When the injury is in the high cervical area, respiratory paralysis will occur. Diaphragmatic breathing is another valuable sign suggesting cervical or high thoracic cord dysfunction.

Due to the sympathectomy effect from spinal cord injury, hypotension is a very common problem in cervical and thoracic cord injury. One must always consider other causes of hypotension in the spinal injury patient as well. Intrathoracic and intra-abdominal hemorrhage occur commonly in the mulitple trauma patient and must be considered. Chest X-ray and peritoneal lavage are mandatory in the hypotensive trauma victim with known or suspected spinal cord injury.

Treatment

There are three goals in the management of the patient with spinal cord injury. The first and foremost is to protect the patient

Table V

Spinal Injury Signs in the Comatose Patient

- Flaccid areflexia, especially with flaccid rectal sphincter
- Diaphragmatic breathing
- Patient can flex forearms but not extend them
- Facial grimaces to pain above clavicle but not below
- Hypotension without other evidence of shock (i.e., hypotensive with warm extremities)
- Priapism is an uncommon but characteristic sign
- Gibbus or obvious spinal deformity
- Loss of bulbocavernous reflex

from any additional damage to either ligamentous, bony, or neural structures. The second is to treat the neurological injury. The third is to realign the spine and insure stability.

First Aid and Transportation

The most important approach for care of any patient with spinal cord injury is to prevent further deformity by spinal immobilization. Every unconscious patient should be treated as if they have a spinal cord injury. The patient should never be picked up or transported in the sitting or reclining position. Whenever possible, he must be rolled into the supine position on a flat surface. The basic principle is to maintain the body in a strictly neutral position at all times. This may be accomplished by specially designed extraction boards currently being utilized by paramedical personnel to provide traction and support on head and feet while others support the chest and pelvis. These concepts must be followed even in the emergency room where the patient must be transferred to a bed or x-ray table.

Immobilization and Traction

Once a fracture has been identified, steps must be taken to avoid further deformation of the injury. With cervical fractures, head traction must be applied in order to immobilize and eventually reduce the fracture site. Skeletal traction is the best method.

Gardner-Wells skull fixation tongs are currently being used in emergency departments because of their ease in application. They cannot be used, however, in infants because of the soft nature of the skull. Wide cranial burr holes with wire traction has been advocated by Hoen[9] for use in infants and small children, but carries some risk of hemorrhage and infection. Halter traction, by means of cloth straps under the chin and occiput, is a temporary available method. The disadvantage to this approach occurs when the patient requires reduction with the use of heavy weights. Pressure areas may develop on the chin and occiput.

Once the proper means of immobilization has been decided upon, weight must be applied to prevent movement of the head (usually 2–5 lbs), and to attempt reduction of the fracture-dislocation. This should be performed slowly and cautiously. Generally, small increments of weight are added under fluoroscopic monitoring to prevent severe distraction and to recognize when reduction occurs. Once the reduction is accomplished, weight may be removed to maintain alignment.

Symptomatic Treatment

Respiratory Problems

Disturbances in respiratory function occur to some degree in every patient with cervical or high thoracic spinal cord injury. Lesions above the C4 level, produce diaphragmatic and intercostal paralysis with resultant apnea. Preservation of diaphragmatic breathing may reduce vital capacity from 50–60% of predicted values. In addition, the ability to cough is markedly impaired. Failure to remove secretions may add to the patient's respiratory embarrassment by adding atelectasis and pneumonia to the already severely compromised patient.

For these reasons, steps must be taken to assist respiration, coughing, and expectoration. In the acute phase of the injury, serial measurement of vital capacity is mandatory to provide information of failing respiratory effort. Deep breathing exercises, I.P.P.B. and frequent suctioning will aid respiratory effort and must be provided. If respiratory efforts are failing, intubation and early tracheostomy are essential.

Cardiovascular Problems

As mentioned previously, loss of vasomotor tone from spinal cord injury will produce hypotension and, at times, bradycardia. No specific treatment is required for this as long as oxygenation is adequate and perfusion to the kidneys is sufficient as evidenced by adequate urine output. Fluid challenge and/or sympathomimetic agents are recommended to bolster blood pressure and pulse if needed.

In acute spinal cord injury, there is a very high incidence of deep vein thrombosis and subsequent pulmonary embolism. Immobilization of the patient, muscular paralysis, and vasomotor paralysis associated with decreased pulmonary ventilation and venous return, are all factors which retard venous blood flow. For these reasons, prophylactic anticoagulation is begun immediately.

Thermoregulatory Control

Normal sympathetic pathways between the midbrain and the lateral sympathetic plexi are frequently disrupted with lesions of the cervical spinal cord. Consequently, there is loss of sweating below the level of injury, altering normal dispersal of heat. This is further aggravated by a reduction of heat loss because of diminished pulmonary ventilation. Hyperthermia then results. It is necessary to cool the patient by reduction of the external temperature. This can be accomplished by the application of ice packs, but is more efficiently achieved through the use of electric fans or air conditioning units.

Surgical Intervention in Spinal Cord Injury

The surgical management of spinal cord injury is controversial. Attention has been directed towards decompression of neural elements, reduction of bony abnormalities, and fusion and stabilization of the unstable spine. Decompressive laminectomy provides inspection of the spinal canal with identification of gross pathology and removal of compressive forces from the spinal cord and involved nerve roots. It can, however, also provide further bony instability and adversely interfere with the vascular supply of the cord. In addition, it has been argued that one cannot decompress violent forces which have already been expended and that removal of these forces is of little or no value. One must consider that the full extent of damage to the cord has been brought about immediately or soon after the insult, and that removal of compressive factors is of no apparent value. An exception is the patient who has preservation of some neurologic function and subsequently demonstrates deterioration. Decompressive laminectomy may be of value in this situation to arrest the progression.

Surgical reduction with simultaneous fusion of spinal fractures promotes early mobilization of the patient and facilitates entry into rehabilitation programs. These procedures should be delayed, if possible, until seven to ten days postinjury. This significantly reduces postoperative morbidity, particularly with reference to pulmonary complications.

Bladder and Gastrointestinal Tract Considerations

With any spinal cord injury, one must expect and then treat the neurogenic bladder. This should be managed acutely by indwelling bladder catheterization when hourly urine quantification is important. In the subacute phase, intermittent catheterization is preferred because of the lower risk of infection as well as the ability to begin initial aspects of the bladder training.

Gastrointestinal disturbances such as intestinal ileus are also common with spinal cord injury. Gastric intubation is mandatory in the acute phase of the injury to prevent aspiration of stomach contents in the immobile patient. Prophylactic antacids or gastric acid inhibiting agents are recommended to reduce the possibility of stress ulceration.

Pharmacologic Treatment of Spinal Cord Injury

The pathologic processes that occur following spinal cord injury are various and extensive, making pharmacologic treatment difficult and ineffective. Edema, contusion, and hemorrhage of the gray matter promote cord swelling and vascular compromise. As this progresses, edema extends into the adjacent white matter. Further vascular compromise occurs secondary to liberation of vasoactive amines, which results in ischemia in the already severely compromised cord.

Various pharmacological treatment approaches have been advocated in patients with both complete and incomplete myelopathies secondary to trauma. High potency glucocorticoids, loop and osmotic diuretics, hypothermia, barbiturates, and biogenic amine blockade have been utilized in experimental models with varying degrees of success. To date, however, no carefully constructed double-blind study exists evaluating these agents in human subjects.

Despite no proven effectiveness in the clinical state, glucocorticoids are frequently utilized in the treatment of edema associated with spinal cord injury. Osmotic agents such as mannitol and urea have been recommended for the same purpose. Spinal injury centers are currently evaluating these agents in an objective fashion to determine their usefulness and will, it is hoped, provide guidelines for their use.

Conclusion

Spinal cord injury is an uncommon entity in the pediatric age group and accounts for only 2–4% of all admissions to spinal cord rehabilitation centers.

Radiological findings are not apparent in more than one-half of the injuries reported below the age of ten. Careful tomography of the suspected region or flexionextension lateral cervical x-rays may disclose subtle changes not apparent with conventional studies.

Anatomical and biomechanical differences in the infant spinal column as compared with the older child account for varying degrees of spinal cord injury. Infant spinal cord injury tends to occur from stretching forces as in hyperextension or flexion. Actual tissue damage due to fracture produces the majority of injuries in the older child.

Clinical features, which facilitate early recognition of spinal injury, may be affected by age of the child and level of consciousness. The examiner must focus on subtle changes of nervous system function, such as altered respiratory patterns and absent rectal sphincter tone, as well as obvious motor and sensory dysfunction.

Goals in the management of the patient with spinal cord injury include prevention of further injury, treatment of neural tissue damage and stabilization of the spinal column. Prevention of further injury is attempted by cautious immobilization and traction of the spine in addition to treatment of system dysfunction related to nervous system interruption.

Although controversial in its effectiveness, various pharmacological approaches may be utilized to retard the pathological processes which occur following injury. Surgical intervention is limited to decompression of neural tissue and stabilization by fusion of the spinal column.

References

1. Anderson M, Schutt A: Spinal injury in children: A review of 156 cases seen from 1950 through 1979. *Mayo Clin Proc* 55:499–504, 1980.
2. Breig A: *Biomechanics of the Central Nervous System.* Stockholm, Almqvist & Wiksell, 1960.
3. Burke DC: Traumatic spinal paralysis in children. *Paraplegia,* 11:268–276, 1974.
4. Crothers B: Paralysis due to injury of the spinal cord. *Practice of Pediatrics.* Fourth Edition, Lippincott, Philadelphia, 1959, p. 13.
5. De Souza SW, Davis JA: Spinal cord damage in a newborn infant. *Arch Dis Childhood* 49:70–71, 1974.
6. Ewald F: Fracture of the odontoid process in a seventeen-month-old infant treated with a halo. *Bone and Joint Surg* 8:1636–1640, 1971.
7. Glasauer F, Cares H: Biomechanical features of traumatic paraplegia in infancy. *J Trauma,* 2:166–170, 1973.
8. Hachem HJ: Spinal cord injury in children and adolescents: Diagnostic pitfalls and therapeutic considerations in the acute stage. *Paraplegia* 15:55–64, 1977–1978.
9. Hoen TI: A method of skeletal traction for treatment of fracture-dislocation of cervical vertebrae. *Arch Neurol* (Chicago) 36:158, 1936.
10. Hubbard DD: Injuries of the spine in children and adolescents. *Clin Orthop Relat Res* 100:56–66, 1974.
11. Kahn GA, Crosby EC, Schneider RC, et al: Correlative Neurosurgery. Second Edition. Springfield, Illinois, Charles C. Thomas, 1969.
12. Melzak J: Paraplegia among children. *Lancet* 2:45–48, 1969.
13. Pang D, Wilberger J: Spinal cord injury without radiologic abnormalities in children. *J Neurosurg* 57:114–129, 1982.
14. Schulman ST, Madden J, Esterly J, et al: Transection of spinal cord: A rare obstetrical complication of cephalic delivery. *Arch Dis Childhood* 46:291, 1971.
15. Weiss MH, Kaufman B: Hangman's fracture in an infant. *Am J Dis Child,* 1926:268–269, 1973.

20

Burns in Children

Morris J. Asch, M.D.
William Dean Davies, M.D.

Traumatic injury is the leading cause of death in children 1 to 15 years of age, and, following vehicular accidents, burns are the second most common cause of death in this age group. Among the 300,000 people hospitalized due to burns in the United States each year 20% of them are children.[1] Most burn injuries in children occur in the home and are presumably preventable; however, despite an active prevention program by the American Burn Association and other groups the number of home accidents has not decreased. Scald injuries are the most common cause of burns in children older than three. The typical injury that one sees is the result of a toddler pulling boiling coffee or water onto himself producing a scald burn of the face and neck, chest and arms. These are usually less than 10% body surface burns and not life-threatening in nature. One of the first decisions that the physician, seeing a burn in the emergency room, must make is whether the patient requires hospitalization, and if so, is the injury severe enough to warrant transfer to a hospital with a formal burn service or unit.

Initial Evaluation

The turmoil caused by a screaming child after an accidental injury, often accompanied by guilty parents, may lead to a less than thorough examination and disposition. A careful, methodical initial evaluation is essential to decide on inpatient versus outpatient treatment and to prevent the needless transfer of patients with small burns to hospitals with specialized burn facilities.

As in any trauma victim an established order of priorities is followed and respiratory problems must be dealt with first. Most burn victims do not have immediate respiratory problems unless they have an inhalation injury or carbon monoxide poisoning. Obtaining a history of closed space injury or carbon monoxide contact is important. Physical examination following inhalation injury may reveal singed nasal vibrissae, pharyngeal edema or carbonaceous sputum. Carbon monoxide combines with hemoglobin producing carboxyhemoglobin, thus preventing adequate tissue oxygenation. The patient may complain of headache or dizziness and physical examination reveals the classical cherry red skin and mucous membranes accompanied by tachypnea and tachycardia. Immediate treatment should be started in a patient showing confusion and lethargy, since carbon monoxide levels may not be readily available. This consists of humidified high concentration oxygen administration by mask followed by endotracheal intubation and ventilatory support as indicated by respiratory failure and arterial blood gas determination.

After a thorough examination, attention should then be directed to the burn wound itself. Chemical burns should be copiously irrigated with warm saline solution. Patients who have had cold or icewater applied to their burns prior to arriving at the hospital, should have an immediate core body temperature measurement. Significant hypothermia often follows this treatment in burns greater than 15% of the body, particularly in infants and young children.

When examining the burn, careful evaluation should be made as to the possibility of child abuse. Documented child abuse accounts for 15–20% of pediatric burn admissions, with most of them occurring in the toddler age group. The pattern of a burn usually leads one to suspect child abuse, particularly a scald burn without splash marks. A good review of child abuse through burning, including suggestive burn patterns and a physician suspicion index, has recently been completed by Deitch and Staats.[2]

Estimation of burn size is the next priority as this will determine necessity for and level of hospitalization, and guide intravenous fluid administration. Over-estimation of burn size is the most frequent error made, often leading to unnecessary hospitalization or transfer to a burn unit. The well established rule of nines, assigning 9% or a multiple thereof to various areas of the body, provides a good estimate of total body surface burn in children over 14 years of age. This method assigns 9% for the head, 18% for the anterior trunk and posterior trunk, 9% for each upper extremity and 18% for each lower extremity. The significantly higher percentage of body surface accounted for by the head and neck in children under 14 years of age requires a mapping out of the burn on the Lund-Browder diagram,[3] or some modification thereof (Fig. 1) and is essential for an accurate estimate of burn size in children.

Diagnosing the depth of burn is important for early treatment and prognostication. First degree burns are painful and erythematous without vesicle formation, and are thus easy to distinguish from second and third degree burns. A sunburn is the most common type of first degree burn. Unless first degree burns cover a large surface area they can be symptomatically treated for pain and fever and do not require hospitalization. Second degree, or partial thickness burns are usually caused by hot or scalding water or flashes of flame. They are painful and on examination vesicle formation is seen. Partial thickness burns appear pink or mottled and sensation to touch can be elicited. Third degree or full thickness burns are usually caused by flame, scald immersions, scald spills in small infants and electrical injury. They usually appear white and dry and are anesthetic to touch. Experienced observers often have difficulty differentiating between deep partial and full thickness burn injuries and it is best to inform the parents that this distinction may not be clear in some areas of the burn for 5–10 days or even longer.

Following evaluation of burn size and depth one must decide if the patient should be hospitalized and if the facilities of a specialized burn care unit are required. Guidelines are given below but individual assessment as to injury and responsibility of the parents should be made when deciding on inpatient or outpatient treatment. In general, second degree burns greater than 10% body surface (5% in children under 2 years of age) require hospitalization. Smaller burns with a significant third degree component or involving the face, hands, feet or perineum may require inpatient care. Evacuation to a hospital with special burn treatment facilities should be considered in burns greater than 20% of total body surface or with a greater than 10% third degree component, electrical injuries and burns complicated by associated injuries or fractures.

Early Management

After initial appraisal has led to a decision to hospitalize, a logical sequence of therapy should follow. As mentioned above early respiratory problems are unusual but occasionally do occur after inhalation injury or carbon monoxide poisoning. Oxygen by mask is administered for mild respiratory distress. Further respiratory support should be guided by arterial blood gas analysis. Carbon monoxide poisoning can be detected by measurement of carboxyhemoglobin saturation. Increased carboxyhemoglobin is not significant after 72 hours. Levels of carboxyhemoglobin greater than 50% are associated with a high mortality.[4] The main therapy for carbon monoxide poisoning is high flow oxygen administration. Other early treatments for inhalation injury include humidification and frequent suctioning. Frequent blood gas measurement should be done to evaluate the need for respiratory support. Airway edema may lead to complete airway obstruction in the first 12–24 hours post-burn and an endotracheal tube may need to be placed for a progressive rise in arterial P_{CO_2}. Complete airway obstruction may occur rapidly and suddenly in the smaller child with inhalation injury, and prophylactic endotracheal intubation should be considered in such patients to avoid sudden respiratory arrest. Ventilator support is carried out as in any other patient, guided by arterial blood gas analysis. Frequent suctioning is necessary and airway clearance can sometimes be improved by suction bronchoscopy. The use of systemic corticosteroids for inhalation injury is somewhat controversial and their use is not recommended in most centers.[5] Tracheostomy should be avoided if at all possible. Endotracheal tubes can be left in place safely for 3–5 days before considering tracheostomy.

The use of intravenous fluid administration is necessary in all major burns. Burns less than 10% of the body can usually be managed solely by oral fluids with careful monitoring of intake and urine output. Some burns between 10–20% can be managed with oral fluids only but many, particularly those in younger children, will require intravenous fluids. An intravenous cannula inserted aseptically in an unburned area should be started as soon as possible.

Physiological Principles of Fluid Resuscitation

Thermal injury is followed by loss of capillary integrity and an increase in capillary permeability. This loss creates a change in the functional fluid volume resulting in fluid exudation and protein leakage from the intravascular into the extravascular space. In burns greater than 25–30% of surface area, free exchange between the intravascular and extravascular spaces is seen not only in the burn wound but also in unburned areas of the body. In addition to the loss of capillary integrity, microtechnique measurements of membrane potential have shown a significant decrease in potential across the cell membrane in skeletal muscle in both burned and non-burned areas.[6] This loss of transmembrane potential renders the sodium pump less effective, allowing for an influx of sodium ion into the cell. The loss of capillary permeability and decrease in cell membrane potential account for the tremendous fluid and sodium requirement necessary for resuscitation of burn shock in the first 48 hours following injury. In larger burns (>30%) these physiological changes are also seen in the non-burned parts of the body resulting in generalized edema. Due to the loss of capillary integrity colloidal elements freely move from the intravascular to the extravascular space. It has been shown in several studies that the use of colloid containing solutions in the first 24 hours post-burn does not increase plasma volume.[7] Capillary integrity recovers somewhere between 20–30 hours following a burn, and intravenous administration of colloid can effectively increase plasma volume after that time. Another major physiological abnormality noted following large burns is a depression of cardiac output, due at least in part to the decrease in intravascular volume. Cardiac output has been measured following burns and studies have shown that immediately following burn injury there is a de-

AREA	0–1	1–4	5–9	10–15	Adlt.	% 2°	% 3°	% Total
Head	19	17	13	10	7			
Neck	2	2	2	2	2			
Ant Trunk	13	13	13	13	13			
Post Trunk	13	13	13	13	13			
R. Buttock	2½	2½	2½	2½	2½			
L. Buttock	2½	2½	2½	2½	2½			
Genitalia	1	1	1	1	1			
R.U. Arm	4	4	4	4	4			
L.U. Arm	4	4	4	4	4			
R.L. Arm	3	3	3	3	3			
L.L. Arm	3	3	3	3	3			
R. Hand	2½	2½	2½	2½	2½			
L. Hand	2½	2½	2½	2½	2½			
R. Thigh	5½	6½	8	8½	9½			
L. Thigh	5½	6½	8	8½	9½			
R. Leg	5	5	5½	6	7			
L. Leg	5	5	5½	6	7			
R. Foot	3½	3½	3½	3½	3½			
L. Foot	3½	3½	3½	3½	3½			
				TOTAL				

A.

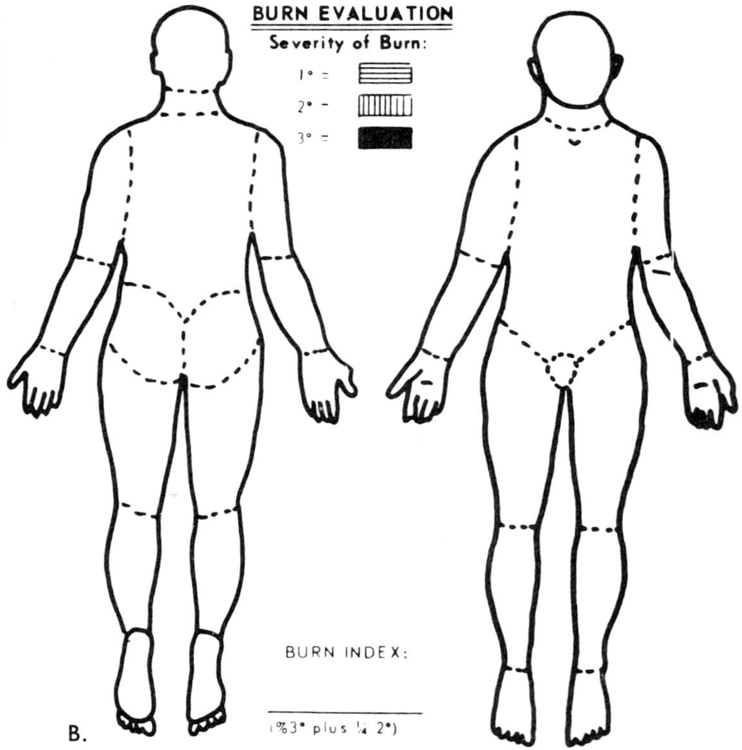

B.

Figure 1 A. and B. Represents burn index charts, and *C.* shows patient's medical history. (From Burn Service, Torrance Memorial Hospital Medical Center.)

C.

ADMITTED BURN CENTER AM
DATE ______________ HOUR: ______________ PM
AGE ______ SEX ______________ RACE ______________
DATE AND TIME BURNED ______________________________
CIRCUMSTANCE OF BURN ______________________________
____
____
____

ETIOLOGY OF BURN FLAME INDOORS-OUTDOORS FLASH
(CIRCLE) HOT LIQUID IMMERSION-SPLASH
CONTACT CHEMICAL-ELECTRICAL

______________ GOOD FAIR POOR
INFORMANT RELIABILITY (CIRCLE)

TREATMENT PRIOR TO ARRIVAL
BURN CENTER: AM
PM
____
DATE TIME
____
NATURE OF RX
____
____
____

WEIGHT (KG) ______________ % BURN ______________

ALLERGIES ______________________________

ANTICIPATED BLOOD NEEDS:
____
____

ANTICIPATED 1ST SURGERY
DATE ______________________________

Figure 1C.

crease in cardiac output to 50–75% of normal depending on the size of the burn.[8] This gradually returns to normal by 24–36 hours post-burn but remains below normal in the first 24 hours following injury despite apparently adequate intravenous fluid resuscitation. Following return of cardiac output to normal, a hyperdynamic state occurs and cardiac output levels of 2–3 times baseline are not unusual. The release of vasoactive substances and the isolation of a burn toxin, which is a myocardial depressant, have been cited as the reasons for the early loss of capillary permeability and the immediate drop in cardiac output described above.[9] With this brief background in burn shock physiology one can better approach and manage fluid resuscitation.

Resuscitation Formulas

In 1952, Evans measured red blood cell and plasma volume loss in burned animals, empirically doubled this volume and came forth with the first formula for replacement therapy in burns.[10] (See Fig. 1.) After using this formula for a number of years a statistical evaluation of the actual amount and type of fluid required and the rate of administration was done at the Brooke Army Burn Unit. From these data the Brooke formula[11] was devised (see Fig. 1) and used successfully for many years. One of the important facts pointed out in the Brooke formula was that the largest loss of fluid seemed to occur in the first several hours post-burn. The Brooke formula, and the Parkland formula described below, advocated giving 50% of the calculated fluid in the first eight hours post-burn and the remaining 50% in the next 16 hours. The Parkland formula (Fig. 1) introduced by Baxter, utilized the growing appreciation of the importance of the sodium ion in burn resuscitation coupled with the knowledge that colloid solution administered in the first 24 hours post-burn does not remain in the intravascular space.[12] Hypertonic sodium solution resuscitation should be mentioned since it is used with good results in a number of burn centers. Sodium chloride is added to Ringers lactate and distilled water so that a solution containing 300 mEq of sodium/liter is achieved.[13]

Table I
Formula Guides to Fluid Resuscitation

		First 24 Hours	*Second 24 Hours*
Evans formula	Colloid solution (blood, plasma)	1.0 ml/kg/% burn	0.5 ml/kg/% burn
	Electrolyte solution (Lactated Ringers)	1.0 ml/kg/% burn	0.5 ml/kg/% burn
	Glucose water	Maintenance (2000 ml in adult)	Maintenance (2000 ml in adult)
Brooke formula	Colloid solution (blood, plasma)	0.5 ml/kg/% burn	.25 ml/kg/% burn
	Electrolyte solution (Lactated Ringers)	1.5 ml/kg/% burn	.75 ml/kg/% burn
	Glucose water	Maintenance (2000 ml in adult)	Maintenance (2000 ml in adult)
Parkland formula	Colloid solution (5% albumin)	None	As indicated to maintain urine volume (500–2000 cc)
	Electrolyte solution (Lactated Ringers)	4 ml/kg/% burn	½–⅔ first day needs
	Glucose water	None	None

The solution is administered at a rate to produce 30 ml of urine per hour in adults and proportionately less, on a weight basis, in children.

All of these formulas when used properly will be successful in the resuscitation of burn shock. The Parkland Formula is the one most widely used today since it seems to encompass current physiological concepts and is relatively easy to use, although there are many respected burn specialists who advocate using more concentrated salt solutions. An example of the calculations derived from the Parkland Formula in a 20 kilogram child incurring a 30% burn is shown in Table II.

Table II

Fluid Calculations Using Parkland Formula in 20 Kg Child with 30% Burn

	First 24 Hours	*Second 24 Hours*
Electrolyte solution (Lactated Ringers)	2400 cc (50% in first 8 hours) (50% in next 16 hours)	½ to ¾ first day amount
Colloid (5% Albumin solution)	None	As indicated by urine output (300–600 cc)

Monitoring Fluid Resuscitation

The goal of successful resuscitation is to provide enough intravascular volume so that adequate perfusion of the heart, kidney, brain and other vital organs is achieved while minimizing the total fluid and sodium load. There is good evidence that post-traumatic pulmonary insufficiency and burn edema can be lessened if total fluid and sodium load are minimized. It should be emphasized that the formulas described are an initial guide to starting fluid resuscitation but should be constantly evaluated and changed according to the patient's response. These formulas are reasonably accurate in predicting the amount of fluid required in small to medium size burns but, as pointed out by Reckler and Mason, frequently fall far short in burns over 50% of the body.[14] Monitoring patient response consists, for the most part, in following the basic clinical parameters of pulse, blood pressure and urine output, with the last being most crucial. Insertion of a Foley catheter into the bladder is essential for the constant monitoring of urine output in patients with burns greater than 20% of the body. A urine output of one ml/Kg/hr should be produced in an infant or small child to ensure adequate renal perfusion. In children, over 30 kilograms a urine volume greater than 30 ml/hr is sufficient. If the urine volume is below 1 ml/Kg/hr the intravenous fluid rate is increased by at least 20%. Conversely, if urine output is greater than 2 ml/kg/hr the intravenous fluid rate is decreased. Frequently, a slight fall in blood pressure will precede a drop in urine output. Arterial blood gas analysis is useful in patients with large burns. A mild metabolic acidosis is not unusual in the first 24 hours post-burn but a base excess of greater than minus ten almost always indicates inadequate resuscitation. Invasive monitoring using a central venous pressure or a Swan-Ganz catheter can be helpful in larger burns. This is particularly true if a greater volume of intravenous fluid than expected is being replaced followed by an inadequate urine output. In this situation the use of a diuretic, such as Lasix, can be considered, but only after all other modalities have been exhausted. Because of the danger of sepsis when central venous lines are used these lines should be discontinued after 48–72 hours. As in most situtations there is no substitute for clinical experience as a guide to the successful manipulation of intravenous fluids in the resuscitation of burn shock.

Other Early Considerations

Nasogastric decompression of the stomach should be used in patients with burns greater than 25% of the body because of the associated ileus. The nasogastric tube should be passed in the emergency room to prevent vomiting and aspiration during transfer to the intensive care unit. The ileus usually lasts for two days after which time the nasogastric tube can be discontinued.

After the patient's respiratory status is secure and fluid resuscitation is well underway attention should be directed to early wound care. The burn is gently cleansed with warm saline solution preferably in the hydrotherapy bath. The authors prefer debridement and removal of blisters in large burns. Hair, in and around the burned area, should be shaved. Small amounts of an antiseptic solution, such as hexachlorophene soap or Povidone-iodine 10% solution should be used during this initial cleansing. Immersion in hexachlorophene-containing solutions should be avoided since there have been reports of seizures due to hexachlorophene absorption. Analgesia prior to the initial debridement and subsequent hydrotherapy treatments is advisable but general anesthesia is not indicated. After initial debridement topical antibiotics are applied and this will be discussed in further detail below.

During fluid administration significant edema occurs in deep partial thickness and full thickness burns. This edema may cause constriction at the elbow, wrist, knee or ankle in circumferential burns of the extremity leading to circulatory compromise of the fingers or toes. Elevation of the extremity with active massage may decrease the edema but relief of the constriction may be required by incising the eschar, or escharotomy. This procedure involves incision of the skin and subcutaneous tissue along the medial and lateral aspect of the extremity taking care to include constricting joint surfaces. Incision of the fascia, or fasciotomy, is not necessary. Immediate spread of the tissue with rapid improvement in circulation is usually apparent. Although a decrease in sensation may indicate circulatory compromise, an objective method of evaluating the adequacy of circulation includes serial measurement of digital blood flow by the Doppler ultrasonic flowmeter. Escharotomy is not a difficult procedure and is usually associated with minimal bleeding but should be done by an experienced burn surgeon.

A tetanus toxoid booster should be given to patients who have had a complete immunization series. In patients not previously immunized human tetanus immune globulin should be administered along with tetanus toxoid, and the immunization course completed.

Further Management Considerations

After the early acute problems have been evaluated and dealt with long-range management considerations must be addressed. The primary goals of therapy must always be kept in mind: survival and achievement of an optimal functional and cosmetic result with a minimum of morbidity and hospitalization. Burn patients manifest a spectrum of problems which require the expertise of multiple medical specialists. In addition to physicians, involvement of other health care professionals such as burn nurse specialists, physical therapists, nutritionists and social workers has become essential in the total care of the burn patient. The best direction and coordination of the care of the burned child is done by a surgeon experienced in burns, preferably a pediatric surgeon.

Late Fluid and Nutritional Management

Following the initial large sodium and fluid requirements there is a return to normal functional fluid space dynamics. Capillary membrane integrity and cell membrane potential return to normal and the intravascular volume stabilizes. A large diuresis and natriuresis is usually observed after the first 48–72 hours. It is important not to replace the large fluid volume lost in the urine at this point but instead switch to a program of fluid maintenance. The usual fluid maintenance requirements based on weight or surface areas can be used.

There are two additional special problems in burn patients which must be taken into account: increased evaporative water loss and increased potassium loss. Because of the loss of the burned skin as an effective regulator of evaporative water loss there is an increased amount of evaporative water loss which is directly proportional to the size of the burn. Multiple studies of evaporative water loss using metabolic bed scales have been done and the amount of fluid lost is usually between 1–2 ml/kg/% burn/24 hours.[15] The 20 kg patient with a 30% burn would lose somewhere between 300–600 cc per day. The fluid lost is mostly salt free and should be replaced by D5W or D5¼ normal saline solution, using daily weight, serum sodium, serum and urine osmolality as a guide. As time progresses the patient can take fluid orally or via a nasogastric tube feeding.

There is a larger than normal potassium loss in burn patients because of tissue breakdown and the ongoing catabolic process. Increased amounts of intravenous potassium are usually required, carefully monitored by serum potassium levels and ECG.

The combination of the catabolic process associated with burn injury and the prolonged hypermetabolic state places the burn patient at a severe nutritional disadvantage. Before the importance of aggressive nutritional support was recognized it was not uncommon for patients with burns greater than 30% total body surface to lose 20% of their lean body mass in the first 3–4 weeks following injury. It has been shown that this depleted nutritional state is associated with impaired neutrophil function and an increased rate of sepsis and mortality.[16] Nutritional support should be started after completion of fluid resuscitation, usually 48–72 hours following injury. This is best provided by normal feeding with careful calorie counts. Many children will not eat well due to a combination of the injury, hospital environment and unfamiliar food. Constant drip feedings through a small nasogastric tube should be started early. A variety of elemental diets are available for tube feeding and manipulation may be necessary if diarrhea is encountered. Intravenous nutrition can be used as a supplement or for brief periods as the main source of caloric support. Enteral feeding is most preferable because of the dangers of sepsis associated with intravenous nutrition, particularly if central venous hyperalimentation is used. The goal of nutritional support is to provide 80–100 calories/kilogram/day guided by daily weights, and bi-weekly serum albumin measurements. This vigorous approach to nutrition should be pursued until the burn wound is almost completely healed or grafted.

The Burn Wound

After the evolution of fluid resuscitation programs all but prevented mortality from renal shutdown the next great problem to be solved was sepsis due to the burn wound. It had been appreciated for many years that fatal sepsis occurred with burn wound infection. Teplitz described the actual process of burn wound sepsis, quantitating the number of bacteria in eschar and subeschar tissue and the histological features which were associated with lethal bacterial invasion of the burn wound.[17] Topical antibacterial agents applied to the burn wound markedly decrease the volume of bacteria but do not sterilize the wound. This allows the body's host defense mechanisms to control the microbial population decreasing the incidence of subeschar bacterial invasion with marked decrease in the incidence of lethal burn wound sepsis. Silver nitrate, used as a 0.5% solution in bulky dressings, was the first topical antibacterial agent used on the burn wound. This has been replaced by several sulfa based creams which seem to be more effective and have fewer complications. The first of these creams described was 10% Mafenide. Bruck, Asch and Pruitt reported a series of 412 burns in children, comparing results prior to and after the use of Mafenide topical antibacterial therapy. The decreased incidence of death due to sepsis was striking, changing from 34.1% in the non-Mafenide treated group to 4.4% in the Mafenide treated group.[18] Similar results have been reported in a number of other series. Because Mafenide causes inhibition of carbonic anhydrase, and is painful when applied to partial thickness burns, its use has been mostly supplanted by another agent, silver sulfadiazine. These agents are applied to the burn wound twice a day, with reinforcement as necessary. The topical antibacterial creams are applied directly to the open burn wound which may be left open, or covered with a light gauze dressing. Although the authors prefer the open method, small children frequently rub the cream off and dressings are necessary. Daily cleansing and debridement with evaluation of the burn wound is done in a hydrotherapy bath.

Aside from the topical antibacterial agents antibiotics are used only when indicated for specific infections. Routine penicillin G administration for the first 5–7 days post-burn was recommended in the past to prevent streptococcal sepsis. There is no good evidence that this use of penicillin G is beneficial and most centers have abandoned this practice. The majority of burn patients, however, do receive antibiotics at some time during their hospital stay with pulmonary infections being the most common reason for antibiotic usage.

The *sine qua non* for recovery of the burn patient is closure of the burn wound. This should be done as soon as possible with maximum preservation of function. Partial thickness burns, with proper therapy, as previously described, will usually heal in 10–20 days. Full thickness burns require grafting, which may be done early by excising the eschar or later by allowing the eschar to separate. Eschar separation usually occurs between 3–4 weeks post-burn and is aided by daily hydrotherapy and debridement. Skin grafting is performed either early or after eschar separation, frequently testing the wound as a recipient site with human allograft skin or another biological dressing.

Temporary biological dressings are used in partial and full thickness burns throughout the course of the burn wound. The most frequently used biological dressing is electron beam sterilized, refrigerated porcine xenograft although a number of other artificial coverings have recently become available. Biological dressings promote healing in partial thickness burns, increase comfort, and decrease evaporative fluid loss. Their use in full thickness burns aids in preparation for grafting and also provides temporary wound coverage. Skin grafting of burns requires experience, judgement, and skill. In children there are the added difficulties of working with thin skin, and in larger burns limited availability of donor sites. Sheets or large strips of autograft provide the best cosmetic and functional results following skin grafting. Meshed autograft is used very frequently to increase coverage and in areas of mixed partial and full thickness burn to allow for fluid drainage through the interstices.

Early tangential excision of full thickness and deep partial thickness burns has gained increasingly widespread usage.[19] The advantages of early tangential excision are: early wound coverage of full thickness injury thus decreasing the possibility of sepsis in very large burns; achievement of better function and cosmesis in deep partial thickness burns particularly of the hands and face; and a markedly shortened hospital stay. Bleeding during burn excision is minimized by tourniquet application or infiltration with xylocaine with dilute epinephrine in excisions involving the trunk. Excisional therapy can be started when the patient is stable following fluid resuscitation, usually by the third to fifth day. In patients with inhalational injury, excision may need to be delayed further until the pulmonary situation stabilizes.

Donor sites require special attention in children. One can easily create a full thickness loss while taking skin because of the thinness of a child's skin. Donor sites are also a potential source of sepsis and should be left exposed if possible and checked repeatedly. There are many other details of wound coverage and skin grafting which are beyond the scope of this chapter. Following wound coverage most of the burn team's energy is directed toward physical therapy and long-term rehabilitation. Prevention of contractures, assisting in social adjustment and many other things allow the burned child to re-enter his world in a normal fashion.

Summary

Burns are the second leading cause of death due to trauma in children. The majority occur in the home and are preventable. Initial evaluation and treatment should follow the priorities established for any trauma patient, dealing first with respiratory problems and shock and then ruling out associated injuries. The size of the burn wound is accurately assessed and the need for and level of hospitalization ascertained. Intravenous fluid resuscitation is then started using one of the currently recognized burn shock formulas as a guide. Fluid requirements are continuously re-evaluated according to the patients physiological responses, mainly urine output. After initial fluid resuscitation a maintenance program allowing for evaporative water loss and strong nutritional support is pursued. The burn wound after initial debridement is managed with topical antibacterial agents to prevent sepsis. Partial thickness burns are allowed to heal whereas full thickness burns may be excised and grafted early or are allowed to separate and are grafted later. Successful management of the burned child is best achieved by using a team approach.

References

1. Berman W, et al: Childhood burn injuries and deaths. *Pediatrics* 51:1069, 1973.
2. Deitch EA, Staats M: Child abuse through burning. *J Burn Care* 3:2, 1982.
3. Lund, CC, Browder NC: The estimation of areas of burns. *Surg Gynecol Obstet* 79:352, 1944.
4. Artz C, Moncrief J, Pruitt B: *Burns a Team Approach.* Philadelphia, W.B. Saunders Co., 1979, pg. 42.
5. Artz C, Moncrief J, Pruitt B: *Burns a Team Approach.* Philadelphia, W.B. Saunders Co., 1979, pg. 101.
6. Baxter CR: The response to initial fluid and electrolyte therapy of burn shock. *In* Lynch JB, Lewis SR, (eds.): *Symposium on the Treatment of Burns.* Vol. 5. St. Louis, C.V. Mosby Co., 1973, p. 42.
7. Baxter CR: Fluid volume and electrolyte changes in the early postburn period. *Clin Plast Surg* 1:693, 1974.
8. Asch MJ, et al: Systemic and pulmonary hemodynamic changes accompanying thermal injury. *Ann Surg* 178:218, 1973.
9. Baxter CR, Cook WA, Shires GT: Serum myocardial depressant factor of burn shock. *Surg Forum* 17:1, 1966.
10. Evans EI, Purnell OJ, Robinett PW, et al: Fluid and electrolyte requirements in severe burns. *Ann Surg* 135:804, 1952.
11. Moncrief JA: Effect of various fluid regimens and pharmacologic agents on the circulatory hemodynamics of the immediate postburn period. *Ann Surg* 164:723, 1966.
12. Baxter CR: Crystalloid resuscitation of burn shock. *In* Stone H, Polk

HA, (eds): *Contemporary Burn Management.* Boston, Little, Brown and Co., 1971.
13. Monafo WW: The treatment of burn shock by the intravenous and oral administration of hypertonic lactated saline solution. *J Trauma* 10:575, 1970.
14. Reckler JM, Mason AD Jr: A critical evaluation of fluid resuscitation in the burned patient. *Ann Surg* 174:15, 1971.
15. O'Neil J: *Burns, Pediatric Surgery.* Vol. 1, Third Edition, Chapter 11, p. 195.
16. Lennard ES, et al: An immunologic and nutritional evaluation of burn neutrophil function. *J Surg Res* 16:286, 1974.
17. Teplitz, C: Pathogenesis of Pseudomonas vasculitis and septic lesions. *Arch Pathol* 80:297, 1965.
18. Bruck H, Asch M, Pruitt B: Burns in children: A 10-year experience with 412 patients. *J Trauma* 10:8, 1970.
19. Monafo W, Aulenbacher C, Pappalardo C: Early tangential excision of the eschars of major burns. *Arch Surg* 104:503, 1972.

21

Pediatric Poisonings

Hugo L. Folli, PHARM.D.

Introduction

Accidental poisonings in children are a major health problem in this country. A poisoning is considered *accidental* in children under five years of age; whereas poisonings after the age of five should be considered self-induced and appropriate psychological evaluation should be provided.

Accidental poisonings may occur as early as six months of age but become prevalent at two to three years. The agents most commonly involved are shown in Table I.[1]

The number of fatal poisonings has steadily decreased over the last 15 years probably due to widespread use of pediatric intensive care units, improvements in supportive care, new developments in the identification and quantification of poisons, and newer means to promote clearance or removal of poisons from the body. The Poison Prevention Packaging Act enacted in 1970 has significantly contributed to the reduction of accidental ingestions in children under five years of age.[2] Government efforts to require child-resistant containers began late in 1972 with aspirin-containing products being the first to be regulated. It is estimated that over 190,000 hospital emergency room visits for ingestions were prevented during the five-year period from 1973 to 1978.[2] The number of ingestions of all regulated products declined by 45% in

Table I[1]

Common Serious Poisons that Affect Children

Drugs	*Others*
Acetaminophen	Alcohol
Acetylsalicylic acid	Camphor
Antiarrhythmics	Caustics
Anticonvulsants	Corrosives
Antidepressants	Insecticides
Antihistaminics	Heavy metals
Antihypertensives	Herbicides
Barbiturates	Organophosphate pesticides
Bronchodilators	Petroleum products
Digoxin	
Iron salts	
Narcotics	
Phenothiazines	

the same time period. The number of deaths associated with accidental ingestions has steadily declined from 2.1 per 100,000 children in 1964 to approximately 0.5 per 100,000 children in 1978.[2]

Early intervention in most poisonings will prevent serious sequelae. The general approach to management of an acute poisoning includes: (1) respiratory and cardiovascular support; (2) diagnosis and identification of the poison; (3) evacuation of the poison from the stomach (unless specifically contraindicated); (4) administration of an antidote or gastrointestinal decontaminant, if available; and most important of all, (5) intensive supportive care when needed.

Diagnosis

Pediatric poisonings often result in emotional stress for the family, and the reliability of an admission history may be questionable. More than 50% of such histories may overestimate or underestimate the quantity or variety of drugs or poisons taken.[3] Fortunately, in many pediatric poisonings the substances (or containers) involved in the event are often found near the child.

In those instances when the nature of the substance ingested is unknown, a list of common signs and symptoms associated with toxic ingestions may be of value in identifying a particular class of poison (Table II).[4]

If the poison is known, evaluation of potential toxicity should be made to determine if any treatment is required. The initial history should include the amount that was ingested. A swallow of liquid has been approximated as 0.21 ml/kg body weight, or about 4–5 ml in a three-year-old.[5,6] The amount ingested in milligram-per-kilogram body weight can also be approximated from the number of missing pills or capsules. If in doubt about the amount, one should err toward the largest estimated quantity ingested in

Table II[4]

Signs and Symptoms Caused by Some Drugs in Toxic Ingestions

Drug	*Clinical Manifestations*
Amphetamines	Argumentative, tremors, tachycardia, hypertension, mydriasis, dry mouth, hallucinations, convulsions, coma
Atropine-like (atropine, scopolamine)	Agitation, hallucinations, ataxia, mydriasis, thirst, tachycardia, muscle spasms, convulsions, coma
Barbiturates and tranquilizers	Slurred speech, nystagmus, pallor cyanosis, ataxia, respirator paralysis, shock, coma
Opiates	Euphoria, miosis, ataxia, respiratory paralysis, coma
Organic phosphates or some mushrooms	Salivation, lacrimation, urination, defecation, miosis, pulmonary congestion, convulsions
Phenothiazines	Tetanic rigidity, oculogyric crisis, hypotension, ataxia, blindness
Salicylates	Headaches, tinnitus, blindness, vomiting, hypotension, tachycardia, shock, hyperpnea, fever, coma
Tricyclic antidepressants	Blurred vision, tachycardia, arrhythmias, hallucinations, convulsions, coma

determining therapy. Toxicity ratings of some products may be correlated to the amount ingested (Table III).[7]

Substances which have been ingested and generally have not produced significant toxicity except in large doses are listed in Table IV.[8]

In cases where an unknown substance is ingested, laboratory identification is of the utmost importance.[1,9]

Recent advances in toxicologic methodology have made possible the identification and quantification of hundreds of chemicals in blood, urine, and other body fluids or tissues. Most large teaching institutions and many metropolitan areas have laboratories which can provide these services within a short period of time.

The importance of laboratory analysis is threefold: (1) while most poisonings are handled with supportive care alone, some may respond better to specific therapy (e.g. acetaminophen); (2) documentation of the poisoning for the patient's and institution's welfare, should any legal proceeding result in the future, as in the case of a battered child; and (3) a negative screen can aid in the differential diagnosis of intoxication versus neurological or psychological etiologies as a cause of the patient's symptoms.

Selective use of screening tests for groups of drugs known to elicit the patient's symptoms (Table V[4]) can provide valuable information promptly and economically. Several available drug screens are listed in Table VI.

A drugs-of-abuse screen will detect those drugs most often encountered in drug abusers. Confirmation of a positive result is

Table III[7]

How Much Is How Toxic in Humans

	If Probable Oral Lethal Dose Is:	
Toxicity Rating	*Dose (mg/Kg)*	*For 70-kg Person Equivalent to*
6 super toxic	5	7 drops
5 extremely toxic	5–50	between 7 drops and 1 tsp
4 very toxic	50–500	between 1 tsp and 1 oz
3 moderately toxic	500–5000	between 1 oz and 1 pt or 1 lb
2 slightly toxic	5000 to 15,000	between 1 pt and 1 qt
1 practically nontoxic	>15,000	>1 qt

Table IV[8]

Nontoxic Ingestions

Abrasives
Antacids
Antibiotics

Baby product cosmetics
Ballpoint pen inks
Bathtub floating toys
Body conditioners

Calamine lotion
Candles (beeswax or paraffin)
Carboxymethyl cellulose
Chalk (calcium carbonate)
Clay (modeling)
Corticosteroids
Cosmetics
Crayons (marked A.P., C.P.)

Dehumidifying packets (silica or charcoal)
Deodorants
Deodorizers (spray and refrigerator)

Elmer's glue®
Etch-A-Sketch®
Eye makeup

Fish bowl additives

Glues and pastes
Glycerol
Golf ball (core may cause mechanical injury)
Greases
Gums

Hair products (dyes, sprays, tonics)
Hand lotions and creams

Indelible markers
Ink (black, blue)

Kaolin

Linoleic acid
Linseed oil
Lipstick
Lubricant
Lubricating oils

Magic markers
Magnesium silicate
Makeup (eye, liquid facial)
Motor oil

Newspaper

Paint—indoor or Latex
Paraffin
Pencil (lead-graphite, coloring)
Petroleum jelly (Vaseline)
Play-Doh®
Polaroid® picture coating fluid
Porous-tip ink marking pens
Prussian blue (fericyanide)®
Putty (less than 2 oz.)

Rouge

Sachets (essential oils, powder)
Sesame oil
Shoe polish (most do not contain aniline dyes)
Silica
Silly Putty® (90% silicones)
Spackles
Suntan preparations
Sweetening agents (saccharin, cyclamate)

Teething rings
Thermometers (mercury)
Titanium oxide
Tooth paste (without fluoride)

Vaseline®

Water colors

Zinc oxide
Zirconium oxide

Table V[4]

Emergency Symptoms and Signs which may be Encountered in a Poisoning

Ataxia
- Alcohol
- Barbiturates
- Bromides
- Carbon monoxide
- Hallucinogens
- Heavy metals
- Organic solvents
- Phenytoin
- Tranquilizers

Convulsions and Muscle Twitching
- Alcohol
- Amphetamines
- Antihistamines
- Boric acid
- Camphor
- Chlorinated hydrocarbon insecticides (DDT)
- Cyanide
- Lead
- Organic phosphate insecticides

(Continues)

Convulsions and Muscle Twitching
- Plants (lily-of-the-valley, azalea, iris, water hemlock)
- Salicylates
- Strychnine
- Withdrawal from barbiturates, benzodiazepine (Valium, Librium), meprobamate

Coma and Drowsiness
- Alcohol—ethyl
- Antihistamines
- Barbiturates and other hypnotics
- Carbon monoxide
- Narcotic depressants (opiates)
- Salicylates
- Tranquilizers

Paralysis
- Botulism
- Heavy metals
- Plants (coniine in poison hemlock)
- Triorthocresyl phosphate

Pupils

Pinpoint
- Mushrooms (muscarine type)
- Narcotic depressants (opiates)
- Organic phosphate insecticides

Nystagmus on Lateral Gaze
- Barbiturates
- Minor tranquilizers (meprobamate, benzodiazepine)

Dilated
- Amphetamines
- Antihistamines
- Atropine
- Barbiturates (coma)
- Cocaine
- Ephedrine
- LSD
- Methanol
- Withdrawal-narcotic depressants

Pulse Rate

Slow
- Digitalis
- Lily-of-the-valley
- Narcotic depressants

Rapid
- Alcohol
- Amphetamines
- Atropine
- Ephedrine

Respiratory Alterations

Rapid
- Amphetamines
- Barbiturates (early)
- Carbon monoxide

Slow or Depressed
- Alcohol
- Barbiturates (late)
- Narcotic depressants (opiates)

Table V

Emergency Symptoms and Signs which may be Encountered in a Poisoning *(Continued)*

Methanol
Petroleum distillates
Salicylates

Tranquilizers

Wheezing and Pulmonary Edema
Mushrooms (muscarine type)
Narcotic depressants (opiates)
Organic phosphate insecticides
Petroleum distillates

Paralysis
Organic phosphate insecticides
Botulism

Mouth

Salivation
Arsenic
Corrosive
Mercury
Mushrooms
Organic phosphate insecticides
Thallium

Dryness
Atropine
Amphetamines
Antihistamines
Narcotic depressants

Breath Odor

Acetone: acetone, alcohol (methyl, isopropyl, phenol, salicylates)
Alcohol: alcohol (ethyl)
Bitter almonds: cyanide
Coal gas: carbon monoxide
Garlic: arsenic, phosphorus, organic phosphate insecticides, thallium
Oil of wintergreen: methyl salicylate
Petroleum: petroleum distillates
Violets: turpentine

Skin Color

Jaundice (hepatic or hemolytic)	Cyanosis	Red Flush
Aniline	Aniline dyes	Alcohol
Arsenic	Carbon monoxide	Antihistamines
Carbon tetrachloride	Cyanide	Atropine
Castor bean	Nitrites	Boric acid
Fava bean	Strychnine	Carbon monoxide
Mushroom		Nitrites
Naphthalene		
Yellow phosphorus		

Violet Emesis often with Hematemesis

Aminophylline
Bacterial food poisoning
Boric acid
Corrosives
Fluoride
Heavy metals
Phenol
Salicylates

Abdominal Colic

Black widow spider bite
Heavy metals
Narcotic depressant withdrawal

Table VI
Laboratory Analysis in Drug Ingestions*

DRUG	SCREEN TYPE: Drugs of Abuse	SCREEN TYPE: Alkaloids/ Bases	SCREEN TYPE: Coma Panel	SCREEN TYPE: Hypnotics/ Tranquilizers	FLUID SAMPLE: Blood	FLUID SAMPLE: Urine	FLUID SAMPLE: Gastric	RESULTS: Qualitative	RESULTS: Quantitative**
Alcohols			+		+				+
Amphetamines	+	+				+		+	
Antihistamines		+				+		+	
Atropine		+				+		+	
Barbiturates	+		+	+	+	+		+	+
Benzodiazepines		+	+	+	+	+		+	+
Cocaine		+				+		+	
Opiates	+	+				+		+	
Pentazocine		+				+		+	
Phencyclidine	+	+				+	+	+	
Phenothiazines	+					+		+	
Propoxyphene	+		+		+	+		+	+
Salicylates			+		+				+
Tranquilizers		+		+	+	+		+	+
Tricyclic Anti-depressants		+				+	+	+	+

*The laboratory should be contacted for specific drugs in each category.
**Quantitative results can be obtained from blood samples only.

desirable, especially if there are legal consequences. The alkaloids and other organic-bases screens will detect antihistamines, analgesics, narcotics, benzodiazepines, and tricyclic antidepressant drugs which are often encountered in many pediatric poisonings. These are drugs which are, in many cases, rapidly removed from the blood. The coma panel offers valuable information especially in cases of coma of unknown etiology. This panel will identify 90% or more of the agents responsible for toxic coma in drug-poisoned patients.[10] The sedative hypnotics and tranquilizers screen include most drugs found in suicidal or accidental severe poisonings.

The fluid samples most often submitted for toxic analysis include urine, serum, and gastric aspirate. On occasion, cerebrospinal fluid may also be used. The best samples to obtain depend on the situation at hand, as well as the most likely fluid where the agent may be detected. It is important to consult the toxicology laboratory early so that the correct samples can be obtained in the appropriate volumes and containers. Urine and gastric contents samples provide only qualitative information. In cases where actual measurement of the toxin is needed, a serum sample must be obtained.

Interpretation of the results must be done with caution and should be correlated with the clinical status of the patient. The laboratory should be consulted regarding their "normal" values which may be different from published figures.[11] Some problems

Table VII

Problems Encountered in Associating Reported Levels with Clinical Status

Effects of co-ingested drugs
- Additive effects (diazepam and chlordiazepoxide)
- Antagonistic effects (barbiturates and amphetamines)
- Synergistic effects (alcohol and diazepam)

Simultaneous measurement of drug and inactive metabolites

Interpatient variation of drug tolerance
- Genetic variation
- Tolerance (habitual user)
- Altered disposition (e.g., renal failure)

encountered in associating reported levels with clinical status are shown in Table VII.

The pharmacokinetics of drugs taken in an overdose are often assumed to be similar to those observed after therapeutic doses, but in reality may differ considerably.[12] An understanding of these differences should contribute to a rational medical management of these situations.

An overdose may result in dose-dependent (nonlinear) kinetics processes which affect absorption, bioavailability, distribution and elimination of the drug. Pathophysiologic changes may also result from a drug overdose. Gastrointestinal motility may be decreased resulting in decreased rate and increased amount of drug absorbed.[12] Decreased cardiovascular and pulmonary function may lead to higher than expected blood concentrations and decreased drug clearance.[12] Changes in urine pH may significantly affect the renal elimination of weak acids or bases. Drug-induced renal or hepatic damage may severely alter drug elimination. Hypothermia, a common complication of drug overdose, might retard distribution and also reduce drug clearance.[12]

In most ingestions, qualitative detection of a particular drug is all that is necessary. There are some instances, encountered especially in pediatric poisonings, where actual quantification in the serum is of the utmost importance because of the frequency of serious sequelae and the need for crucial therapeutic maneuvers (Table VIII).[13]

Table VIII

Common Types of Poisoning for which Toxicologic Measurements Are Most Likely To Be Important

Salicylate	Nitrates–Methemoglobin
Barbiturates–comatose patient	Organophosphates–pseudo–cholinesterase
Acetaminophen	Heavy metals
Iron products	Tricyclic antidepressant
Methanol	Theophylline
Acute arsenic	Anticonvulsants
Carbon monoxide–carboxyhemoglobin	

Treatment: General Measures

Supportive Therapy

Initial assessment of the patient will determine the general treatment measures required. Cardiopulmonary support, assisted ventilation, continous positive airway pressure, and supplemental oxygen may be required. Continuous electrocardiographic (ECG) monitoring is essential.[1] Appropriate antiarrhythmic therapy should be instituted if indicated. These drugs should be used with extreme care especially in the presence of cardiotoxic poisons. (The reader is referred to *Chapter 9* on cardiopulmonary resuscitation for appropriate dosages.)

The treatment of shock will be determined by its etiology. Hypotension should be managed with fluids, albumin or plasma, and if necessary, with appropriate vasopressor agents. (*See Chapter 9.*) Fluid and electrolyte disturbances should be managed using the principles for similar clinical situations.

Coma, if present, should initially be managed in the appropriate manner regardless of the suspected cause. The severity of coma can be evaluated using the following scale:[14]

Level 0–Asleep but can be aroused and can answer questions.
Level 1–Comatose; does withdraw from painful stimuli; reflexes intact.
Level 2–Comatose; does NOT withdraw from painful stimuli; most reflexes intact; no respiratory or circulatory depression.
Level 3–Comatose; most or all reflexes are absent but without depression of respiration or circulation.
Level 4–Comatose; reflexes absent; respiratory depression with cyanosis, circulatory failure or shock.

In all cases of coma of unknown etiology, naloxone (Narcan®) should be administered in a dose of 10 mcg/kg/dose. Larger doses may be repeated if there is little or no response to the initial dose. Convulsions can be treated with the appropriate medications. (See *Chapter 5* on seizure disorders.) The potential for additive or synergistic CNS depressant effects of certain drugs with anticonvulsants should be kept in mind, especially in the patient without an artificial airway.

Prevention of Absorption

Gastric removal of ingested poison remains the mainstay of early treatment in the majority of poisonings. Decontamination can be achieved by induced emesis or gastric lavage and aspiration. Mechanically-induced emesis by stimulation of the posterior pharynx has been shown to be largely ineffective in recovering stomach contents.[15] Chemically-induced emesis has been tried with a variety of agents. Most of these have been proven not only unpredictable in efficacy, but also extremely dangerous, and their use should be condemned. Hypertonic saline solution, for example, has caused fatalities in children.[16] Concentrated copper sulfate solutions, a local irritant, have produced deep gastrointestinal ulcerations, liver necrosis, and renal damage in some patients.[17] The use of liquid dishwashing detergents has also been suggested to induce emesis.[18] Although their use appears safe, confusion at the time of the poisoning may lead one to use the toxic laundry or electric dishwashing detergents with disastrous results. Thus, the use of these agents should be reserved only for those circumstances where emesis is necessary and syrup of ipecac is unavailable, an unlikely situation in the hospital setting.

Pharmacologically-induced emesis can be accomplished by the use of syrup of ipecac or apomorphine. Syrup of ipecac, derived from the dried root of *Cephaelis ipecacuanha* is the emetic of choice. It has maintained an extraordinary record for safety over the last ten years with only four reports of toxicity documented.[19] Administration of the *extract* (14 times more potent than the syrup) should not occur, since it has been removed from the market.

Ipecac acts by a local and central effect. The effect is seen within 20 minutes in over 90% of patients.[19–22] Administration with milk can increase this time to about 30 minutes.[21] Concurrent administration with carbonated beverages may cause abdominal distention but does not affect efficacy.[23] If these fluids are used, it is recommended that clear beverages (e.g. 7-UP®) be used rather than the fruit- or cola-flavored drinks so as not to mask the color of the emesis and complicate identification of the ingested substance.[23] The efficacy of syrup of ipecac in antiemetic ingestions (e.g. phenothiazines) has been proven in adults and children.[24] The time to successful emesis may be slightly prolonged to 30 minutes. The success rate is 81% after one dose and 95% after two doses.[24] The recommended doses of syrup of ipecac are given in the chart below.[19]

Age	*Dose*	*Concurrent Fluids*
Less than 6 months	Not recommended	—
6–8 months	5 ml	60–120 ml
9–11 months	10 ml	60–120 ml
1–12 years	15 ml	120–240 ml
Over 12 years	30 ml	240–480 ml

The maximum single dose is 30 ml. A second dose may be given if no emesis occurs within 30 minutes of the first dose. In many cases, stimulation of the posterior pharynx with a soft tooth-brush 15 to 20 minutes after ipecac administration will induce the emetic process. If no emesis occurs following two doses of ipecac, a charcoal slurry should be given and lavage may be performed if indicated. Children given ipecac may become drowsy following the emesis.[19] Emesis may continue for up to two hours. Vomiting may be effectively stopped by restricting fluids for one hour following the last emesis.

Apomorphine, a narcotic derivative, acts by stimulation of the chemoreceptor trigger zone.[21] Its action is within five minutes and response rate is above 90%.[20,21,25] The removal of stomach contents, approximately 30%, is no better than with ipecac.[25] The more rapid effects of apomorphine are outweighed by the fact that preparation of the drug requires dissolution and filter sterilization of apomorphine tablets prior to use, a process which requires up to 15 minutes to complete. At the recommended dose of 0.07 mg/kg, given subcutaneously or intramuscularly, it caused central nervous system depression in up to 60% of children.[20] Naloxone can be used to reverse this effect.

Although both apomorphine and syrup of ipecac have been shown to be equally effective, the use of the former should be limited to well-equipped and well-staffed medical units.[1,21,22] The ease of administration, documented efficacy and safety of syrup of ipecac make it the drug of choice for the induction of emesis in most clinical situations.

Contraindications to any form of emesis include:[1,5] (1) ingestion of strong bases or acids; (2) loss of gag reflex; (3) drowsy, unconscious, or seizing patient; and (4) corrosive ingestion.

Gastric lavage is the alternative to pharmacological evacuation of the stomach. It should only be performed under close medical supervision. The efficacy of lavage is often overshadowed by the delay in instituting the procedure following the poisoning. A study comparing lavage versus syrup of ipecac found an average delay of 91 minutes from the time of poisoning to the initiation of lavage procedures compared to 17–82 minutes for ipecac-induced emesis.[26] In certain poisonings, ipecac-induced emesis may be superior to gastric lavage in removing gastric contents.[27] The percentage of stomach contents removed by lavage declines to 26% and 8% at 30 and 60 minutes respectively, following gastric instillation of barium sulfate suspension.[21,28] Lavage is indicated when a potentially serious poisoning has occurred and emesis is contraindicated or ineffective. Lavage is contraindicated with corrosive or caustic agents. Its use in petroleum distillate ingestions remains controversial. In the comatose patient, lavage should be performed following protection of the airway by a cuffed endotracheal tube.[5,6] The largest catheter possible should be used (8–26 F or larger[6,22,29,30]). In infants and younger children, the oral passage is the easier route and less traumatic. For older children the nasal route is preferred.[30] Passage of the tube may be easier if it is immersed in cold water and lubricated with a water-soluble gel. The patient should be placed on the left side with the head hanging over the edge of the bed and face down.[30] Stomach contents should be aspirated prior to instilling the lavage solution. Contents may be sent for analysis if necessary. The lavage fluid should be instilled in small aliquots 10–12 times or until clear. Small amounts should minimize the chance of stomach content passage into the small intestine.[6,30] The solutions preferred for pediatric lavage are normal or half-normal saline. Tap water may cause water intoxication in a small child.[30] Once the lavage is completed, the tube may be used to administer an antidote or to instill activated charcoal. Complications of gastric lavage, although rare, include aspiration of gastric contents, laryngeal spasm, esophageal and gastric perforation, and cardiac arrest.[21,26]

Another method of decreasing gastrointestinal absorption of ingested poison is by the administration of activated charcoal powder. Activated charcoal is the residue of destructive distillation of organic materials. Activity as an adsorbent depends on its small particle size, large surface area, and low content of adsorbed substances which are removed by the activation process. Activated charcoal powder, N.F., should not be confused with the Universal Antidote, a mixture of activated charcoal, magnesium oxide and tannic acid. This combination has been proven to be considerably less effective than activated charcoal alone and should not be used.[31]

Activated charcoal tablets, even if crushed, are not as effective as the powder.[21] Activated charcoal, N.F., is available from different manufacturers under their trade names. Three products known to be equally effective are Activated Charcoal, N.F., (Merck and Co.), Nuchar C® (West Virginia Pulp and Paper Co.), and Norit A® (American Norti Co.).[32] A large number of compounds are adsorbed by activated charcoal powder (Table IX[31,33–38]).

The greatest effect on decreased systemic adsorption of toxin is obtained when activated charcoal is administered within 30 minutes of ingestion.[39] If syrup of ipecac has been given, one must wait for emesis to occur before activated charcoal is given, as it may bind the ipecac and prevent emesis.[39]

Activated charcoal can be effective in preventing absorption when administered several hours postingestion if the ingested agent has low gastrointestinal solubility, if it decreases gastric motility (e.g. opiates, anticholinergics), or is a delayed-release preparation.[21,39,40] Compounds which undergo enterohepatic circulation (e.g. tricyclic antidepressants, phencyclidine) may be effectively removed by repeated doses of activated charcoal.[37,40]

Activated charcoal should be administered in a minimum dose of 30-50 gm.[21,39] Doses up to 120 gm have been recommended.[39] It should be given in a water slurry or mixed with 50–150 ml of 70% sorbitol. Sorbitol will increase palatability, as well as promote gastrointestinal passage of the charcoal-drug mixture with no loss of efficacy.[39,41] Activated charcoal is nontoxic but if administered too rapidly, especially following ipecac-induced emesis, it may produce further vomiting.[21] Aspiration of the charcoal and gastric contents resulting in acute airway obstruction and severe bronchospasm has been reported.[42]

The use of cathartics to speed up gastrointestinal transit of the unabsorbed toxin has been advocated for many years. There

Table IX
Adsorption of Chemicals by Activated Charcoal*

Good Adsorption	*Fair/Poor Adsorption*	*Minimal/No Adsorption*
	Medicinals	
Acetaminophen	Barbital sodium	Alcohol Ethyl
Aspirin	Chlorpromazine	Boric acid
Atropine	Glutethimide	Water-insoluble compounds
Barbital	Hexobarbital sodium	
Chloroquine	Isoniazid	
Chlorpheniramine	Methylsalicylate	
Chlorpromazine	Phenobarbital sodium	
Cocaine	Prochlorperazine	
Colchicine	Promazine	
Dextroamphetamine	Promethazine	
Digitalis	Propoxyphene	
Ethchlorvynol	Quinacrine	
Glutethimide	Quinidine	
Hexachlorophene	Quinine	
Imipramine	Salicyclic acid	
Iodine	Thioridazine	
Ipecac		
Meprobamate		
Morphine		
Narcotics (synthetic)		
Nicotine		
Nortriptyline		
Opium		
Penicillin		
Pentobarbital		
Phenobarbital		
Phenolphthalein		
Phenytoin		
Potassium permanganate		
Primiquine phosphate		
Propantheline		
Propoxyphene		
Salicylamide		
Secobarbital		
Sulfanilamide		
Tricyclics		

*Adapted[31,33–38]

Table IX

Adsorption of Chemicals by Activated Charcoal *(Continued)*

Good Adsorption	*Fair/Poor Adsorption*	*Minimal/No Adsorption*
	Industrial Products	
Antimony	Lead	Acids, Minerals
Bichloride mercury	Phenol	-hydrochloric
Camphor	2-4 D (2-4	-nitric
Gasoline	dichlorophenoxy-	-sulfuric
Kerosene	acetic acid)	etc.
Mercuric chloride	Malathion	
Methylene blue		Alkali, strong
Oxalates		-potassium
Parathione		hydroxide
Phenol		-sodium
Phosphorus		hydroxide
Potassium permanganate		etc.
Selenium		Alcohol methyl
Silver nitrate		Cupric copper
Strychnine		Cyanide
Thallium		DDT
Tin		Ferrous iron
		Ferrous sulfate
		Malathion
		N-methylcarbamate
		Sodium
		metasalicylate
	Plants or Plant Products	
Aconite		
Cantharides		
Delphinium		
Hemlock		
Muscarine		

are no clinical studies to confirm the efficacy of this form of therapy. Cathartics may be useful in reducing the absorption of drugs which are incompletely or slowly absorbed and in pediatric patients with a comparatively short intestinal tract.[43] Different types of cathartics are available (Table X[43]). In most cases, a saline cathartic, such as magnesium citrate, sulfate or sodium sulfate, can be used. Sorbitol and mannitol can also be used. Disodium phosphate so-

Table X[43]
Cathartics Used in Poisonings

Agent	*Dose*	*Contents*
Disodium phosphate solution (Fleets®)	0.5 ml/kg (10–24% solution) Maximum 100 ml	Na^{+} = 1607 mEq/liter $PO_4^{=}$ = 4147 mEq/liter
Magnesium sulfate	250 mg/kg (10% solution)	Mg^{++} = 8.3 mEq/gm
Magnesium citrate	0.5 ml/kg Maximum 240 ml	Mg^{++} = 16 mEq/gm
Sodium sulfate	250 mg/kg (10% solution)	Na^{+} = 14 mEq/gm
Sorbitol	50–150 ml (70% solution)	
Mannitol	50–100 ml (10–20% solution)	

lutions (Fleets® enema) have also been used but carry a higher potential for severe fluid and electrolyte imbalance due to their high sodium and phosphate concentration.

Toxicity with saline cathartics can be avoided if fluid and electrolyte losses are measured and properly replaced. Magnesium cathartics should be avoided in patients with renal dysfunction. Disodium phosphate solutions can cause severe calcium and phosphate imbalances and should be administered with proper monitoring of the patient. Oil cathartics should never be used due to the danger of aspiration.

A roentgenological flat plate of the abdomen can detect any unabsorbed and unremoved drug which may be radiopaque. Most enteric-coated tablets appear to be radiopaque.[44]

Hastening Removal from the Body

Forced Diuresis. Increased urine output (3–6 ml/kg/hr) by administration of large amounts of fluid is seldom of significant use in poisonings as a means to increase toxin excretion.[1,5,14] In some instances, renal excretion can be enhanced by alkaline or acid diuresis. Alkalinization of the urine (pH 7–8) with sodium bicarbonate (2–3 mEq/kg/4–6 hrs) will promote removal of weak

bicarbonate (2–3 mEq/kg/4–6 hrs) will promote removal of weak acids, such as long-acting barbiturates, salicylates, and isoniazid.[1,14] Acid-forced diuresis (pH 4.5–5.5) with ammonium chloride (75 mg/kg/6 hrs) may enhance the excretion of weak bases, such as amphetamines, strychnine, and phencyclidine.[14] The use of such techniques should not take the place of good supportive management. The benefits of such methods rarely exceed the potential complications of fluid overload and electrolyte imbalance, especially in young patients.[1,5,14,40]

Dialysis. The usefulness of peritoneal dialysis or hemodialysis procedures in acute poisonings is limited. The number of drugs effectively removed by either method is small. The efficiency of dialysis depends upon: (1) the permeability of the dialysis membrane to the toxin; (2) the apparent volume of distribution of the toxin; drugs with extensive distribution in body tissues will not be easily dialyzable (e.g., tricyclic antidepressants); (3) the relative amount of toxin cleared from the body compared to the normal biological pathways of elimination must be significant; and (4) the degree of serum protein binding; highly bound toxins are not easily dialyzable.

Dialysis should not be a routine procedure in the management of severe poisonings. It should be reserved for those cases of stage 3 or 4 coma caused by dialyzable drugs which cannot be treated by conservative means.[14] In the pediatric patient, dialysis may be of greatest use in correcting fluid, electrolyte and acid-base disturbances that do not respond to standard therapy.[14] For those poisons which are dialyzable (Table XI), peritoneal dialysis is less effective than hemodialysis,[45] but peritoneal dialysis may be easier to perform in the small patient.[14]

Hemoperfusion. Hemoperfusion has become increasingly more popular in recent years as an adjunct to the treatment of the poisoned patient. In this procedure, blood is pumped from the patient through a column of adsorbent material (activated charcoal, ionic or nonionic exchange resins) and recirculated back to the patient. Hemoperfusion is less expensive and much simpler than hemodialysis.[46] This procedure is most efficacious for toxins with low intrinsic body clearance and relatively small volume of distribution (Table XII).[47]

Lipid-soluble drugs and highly protein-bound drugs which are inefficiently removed by hemodialysis may be removed more efficiently by hemoperfusion.[45] Rapid technological advances in this

Table XI

Dialyzable Drugs*

Alcohols (methanol, ethanol, isopropanol)
Ammonia
Amphetamines
Boric acid
Calcium
Chloral hydrate
Chlorates
Digoxin
Ethylene glycol
Halides (bromide, chloride, fluoride, iodide)
Heavy metals
Lithium
Methotrexate
Paraldehyde
Phenobarbital
Potassium
Quinidine
Quinine
Salicylates
Strychnine

*Adapted[1,14,46]

Table XII

Drugs Removed by Hemoperfusion*

Ammanita phalloides
Barbiturates† (short and intermediate acting)
Digoxin
Ethchlorvynol†
Glutethimide†
Methaqualone
Methyprylon
Paraquat
Phenobarbital
Phenytoin
Salicylate (dialysis preferred)
Theophylline
Tricyclic antidepressants

*Adapted[46,47]

†Rebound increase in blood concentration with possible clinical deterioration may occur after hemoperfusion is complete, so repeated hemoperfusions may be necessary.

field will undoubtedly provide adsorbing materials of greater efficiency and specificity.

As with dialysis, hemoperfusion should be reserved for those patients in stage 4 coma who are unresponsive to other supportive treatment.[1,46] The potential complications of hemoperfusion include embolization of adsorbed particles, depletion of blood cells (notably platelets), hypocalcemia, hypophosphatemia, hypoglycemia, and hypothermia.[47] The risks of embolization and thrombocytopenic effects have been reduced with newer techniques. Electrolyte abnormalities are usually minor and easily treatable.[46,47] Body temperature may fall by one or two degrees due to cooling of the blood as it passes through the resin. This effect is rarely significant.[47]

The decision to use dialysis or hemoperfusion as an adjunct to supportive treatment is a difficult one. In their review of the subject, Winchester, et al[45] suggest some criteria which may be used to arrive at a decision: (1) severe clinical intoxication with abnormal vital signs (i.e. hypotension unresponsive to standard treatment, apnea, severe hypothemia); (2) ingestion and probable absorption of a potentially lethal dose; (3) blood levels in the potentially lethal range; (4) a degree of intoxication that impairs the normal route of excretion of the drug or an underlying disease which impairs the normal pathways of elimination; (5) toxins which are metabolized to more noxious metabolites (e.g., methanol to formaldehyde); (6) progressive clinical deterioration despite proper supportive treatment; (7) poisonings with agents known to produce delayed toxicity (e.g. pagaquat, amanita phalloides, acetaminophen); and (8) development of complications of coma, such as pneumonia or septicemia (Table XI[1,14,46] and Table XII[46,47]).

Antidotes

The number of useful antidotes is limited. Antidotes, if available, should be used in conjunction with the appropriate supportive care. The ideal antidote should have at least four properties:[48] (1) either reverses or neutralizes the effect of the offending agent; (2) has no action of its own; (3) is easy to administer; and (4) is free of unwanted side effects.

Many existing standard texts confuse antidotes with drugs used for the treatment of poisonings. In many cases, some contain old antidotes which may cause more harm to the patient or are useless (Table XIII[48]). In cases for which a specific antidote can be used, it is important to follow the route, dose and monitoring parameters very closely.[48,49] Many of these agents can cause severe toxicity. Table XIV[48] lists the current available antidotes.

Poisoning Information Resources

To provide safe, effective and timely treatment of poisoned patients, the information used must be readily accessible and current. Many sources of information currently available are often outdated and, in many cases, contain incorrect recommendations. This is particularly true for some manufacturers' labels.

There are a number of periodically updated poison information resources currently in use. POISINDEX®, a system of microfiche which is reviewed and updated quarterly, is far superior to other systems.[50] It contains information on over 300,000 commercial products, plants and poisonous snakes. Compared to other

Table XIII[48]

Antidotes No Longer or Seldom Used

Old Antidote	*Was Used For*	*Now Preferred*
Ammonia water	Formaldehyde	Protein
Barbiturates	Seizures	Diazepam
Caffeine with sodium benzoate	CNS depression	Supportive care
Chloral hydrate	Seizures	Diazepam
Cysteamine	Acetaminophen	Acetylcysteine
Ephedrine	CNS depression	Supportive care
Hydrochloric acid	Various bases	Dilution with water
Levallorphan	Narcotics	Naloxone
Levarterenol	Depression	Supportive care
Methionine	Acetaminophen	Acetylcysteine
Nikethamide	CNS depression	Supportive care
Paraldehyde	Seizures	Diazepam
Pentylenetrazol	CNS depression	Supportive care
Picrotoxin	CNS depression	Supportive care
Tannic acid	Alkaloids	Activated charcoal
Universal antidote	Many	Activated charcoal

similar systems, it is superior in the frequency of finding entries of substances involved in pediatric poisonings, management information, and time required to obtain the information.[50] In conjunction with this system, consultation with one of the Regional Poison Control Centers can provide the most accurate and timely information on poisoning management. A current list of existing regional centers is published yearly by the National Clearinghouse for Poison Control Centers, Rockville, Maryland, 20857.

Specific poisoning treatments are purposely omitted, as it is superfluous to attempt consolidation of the vast amount of updated treatment modalities. The information presented in this chapter is designed to aid in the initial management of the poisoned child. Further treatment should be implemented following consultation with one of the aforementioned resources.

Future Trends in Treatment

Recent developments in immunotherapy of digitalis toxicity represent a new and important advance in the treatment of pediatric poisonings.[51,52] Continued research in this area should result in safer and more effective means to treat other drug intoxications. Thus, the importance of updated poisoning information cannot be overstated.

(See following page for Table XIV: Selection and Use of Antidotes.)

[1](Used with kind permission from Kilham HA: Hospital management of severe poisoning. *Pediatr Clin North Am* 27:603, 1980.)
[4](Used with kind permission from Mofenson HC, Greensher, J: The unknown poison. *Pediatrics* 54:336, 1974. Copyright American Academy of Pediatrics 1974.)
[8](Used with kind permission from Rumack BH: *Poisindex Management of Nontoxic Ingestion.* Poisindex Co., 1981.)
[48](Used with permisson from Spoerke DG: Guide to the acquisition, storage, and use of antidotes. *Am J Hosp Pharm* 38:498, 1981.)

Table XIV[48]
Selection and Use of Antidotes

Antidote Name	Indications for Use	Dose
Acetylcysteine	Acetaminophen >7.5 g or 120 μg/ml at 4 hr after ingestion	Orally, 140 mg/kg initially and 70 mg/kg maintenance for 14 doses
Activated charcoal	Adsorbant for many poisons	Ten times dose ingested or 50 g for adults and 25 g for children
Alcohol (ethyl)	Methanol, ethylene glycol	Loading dose, 1 ml/kg; maintenance (est), 7–10 ml/hr
Aluminum hydroxide gel	As a neutralizer, delays absorption	Child, 5–30 ml; adult, 15–60 ml
Amyl nitrite	Cyanide poisoning	Inhaled for 30 sec every 2 min until i.v. started. I.v. dose is based on hemoglobin. A normal child (12 kg) would receive 10 mg/kg
Atropine sulfate	Cholinergic poisonings especially caused by organophosphates or carbamates	0.015–0.05 mg/kg Adult, 2–12 mg in first 2 hr Child, 1–2 mg in first 2 hr
Botulism antitoxin	Botulism	10,000 units injected i.v. every 4 hr
Calcium disodium edetate (EDTA)	Lead	75 mg/kg/24 hr in 3–6 divided doses for 5 days. A second course may be given in 2 days. No more than 500 mg/kg/course
Calcium gluconate	Hydrofluoric acid or fluoride	External, no limit. Injection, small volumes at site of burn
Castor oil	Phenols	30–60 ml
Cyanide kit	Cyanide	See individual agents (amyl nitrite, sodium nitrite, thiosulfate)
Deferoxamine	Iron	15 mg/kg/hr i.v.; 90 mg/kg up to max of 1 g dose every 8 hr, i.m.
Dimercaprol (BAL)	Heavy metals except iron	Lead, 4 mg/kg every 4 hr × 5 days. Others, 2.5–5 mg/kg every 4 hr × 2 days
Diphenhydramine	Phenothiazine dystonias	1–5 mg/kg to max of 50 mg over 2 min
Lactrodectus mactans antivenin	Black widow spider bite	1 ampul

Table XIV[48]
Selection and Use of Antidotes *(Continued)*

Route	Special Information Relating to Administration, Dose, or Legal Questions	Precautions or Hazards	Systemic or Local
p.o.	Is mixed in liquid and administered. This is not yet fully FDA approved. Rocky Mountain Poison Center has an IND	Vomiting is a common side effect. Therapy is not useful >12 hr after ingestion	Systemic
oral	Mixed with water and administered as a slurry.	Will absorb and inactivate ipecac if the two are given together	Local
oral or i.v.	There is little data on childhood alcohol toxicity; care must be taken in giving drug		Systemic
oral or external			Local
inhaled, i.v.		Should not be given while Na nitrite is given i.v.	Systemic
i.m., i.v.			Systemic
i.v.	Skin test required for serum sickness. Temp >37 °C will destroy antitoxin. Dose should be discussed with Centers for Disease Control, Atlanta; 404-329-3644	Temp >37 °C may form toxic substances	Systemic
i.m. deep, i.v. slow		Kidney tubular necrosis	Systemic
oral, external	Use of injected calcium salts for HF is questionable but still accepted in many places	Bradycardia, local necrosis when injected	Local/systemic
oral	Unusual case where oil will retard rather than promote absorption	Contraindicated in phosporous poison or chlorinated hydrocarbons; may increase absorption	Local
inhalation, i.v.			Systemic
i.v., i.m.	Urine may turn red when using this antidote. I.v. dosing is preferable, but i.m. may be used if the patient is not in shock		Systemic
i.m.			Systemic
i.v.			Systemic
i.v.		Beware of sensitivity reactions	Systemic

Table XIV[48]
Selection and Use of Antidotes *(Continued)*

Antidote Name	Indications for Use	Dose
Magnesium hydroxide gel	Acids, sodium fluoride	30–60 ml
Magnesium sulfate	Arium salts	2–5% solution in lavage or 30 g p.o.
Methylene blue	Methemoglobin-causing agents such as nitrites	0.1–0.2 ml/kg of 1% solution (1–2 mg/kg)
Naloxone	Narcotic poisoning	1-ml ampul (0.4 mg) given when necessary to prevent respiratory depression. Several ampuls may be needed, depending on situation
Neostigmine	Tubocurarine	0.5 to 2 mg
Nicotinamide	Vacor	Adult, initially 500 mg i.m., i.v., followed by 200–300 mg every 4 hr for 48 hr. Child, half adult dose
Oxygen	Carbon monoxide	100% oxygen
Penicillamine	Heavy metals—Cu, Pb, Hg, As	100 mg/kg/day for up to 5 days
Physostigmine	Tricyclic, anticholinergic poisoning like atropine, jimson weed, etc.	Child, 0.5 (max of 2 mg); adult, 1–2 mg as needed
Phytonadione	Warfarin	Child, 1–5 mg; adult, 10 mg
Potassium permanganate	Alkaloids	1:5,000 or 1:10,000 solution
Pralidoxime	Organophosphate	Adult, 1 g i.v. at 0.5 g/min; child, 25–50 mg/kg. May repeat ×3 at 8–12 hr intervals
Protein	Tannins, formaldehyde	Meat, soup, bread in significant amounts
Snake bite antivenin *Crotalidae* *Micrurus*	Rattlesnake Coralsnake	3–10 5-ml vials in 500 ml over 1 hr; 3–20 vials may be used in first 6 hr
Sodium bicarbonate	Iron	Child, ca. 50 ml of 5% sodium bicarbonate
Sodium sulfate	Barium	2–5% solution in lavage, 10 ml of 10% solution i.v. slowly
Sodium nitrite	Cyanide poisoning	Child, 6.6–11.6 mg/kg depending on Hb; adult, 300 mg (in 10 ml)
Sodium thiosulfate	Cyanide poisoning	Child, 1.1–1.95 mg/kg depending on Hb; adults, 12.5 g in 50 ml
Starch	Iodine	As much as can be tolerated, 3–10% solution
Zinc DTPA	Radioisotopes, plutonium	1 g (30 μmol/kg) over 1 hr, immediately and daily

Table XIV[48]
Selection and Use of Antidotes *(Continued)*

Route	Special Information Relating to Administration, Dose, or Legal Questions	Precautions or Hazards	Systemic or Local
topical/oral	First irrigation on acids is water. Do not wait to find a neutralizing gel		Local
oral			Local
i.v.	Treatment is unnecessary unless methemoglobin is >30%	Saliva or other fluids may turn blue	Systemic
i.v.	Drug has short duration. Repeat administration may be necessary	Administration of naloxone to addict may cause withdrawal symptoms	Systemic
i.v., slowly	No more than 5 mg should be given		Systemic
i.v., i.m.	Most of experience is with animals. Data are sketchy for humans	Treatment initiated 3–4 days after ingestion showed no improvement	Systemic
inhalation	Half-life of CO in 100% O_2 is about 40 min		Systemic
oral	Long-term therapy should not exceed 40 mg/kg/day		Systemic
i.v.	Is metabolized in 30–60 min. May need repeat dosing	Should be test dose of 0.5 mg in child and 1–2 mg in adult before using. Do not use as a drip	Systemic
i.v., i.m.			Systemic
lavage	Rarely used	Safety is marginal	Local
i.v.	Is of little use if given >36 hr after exposure. Is an adjunct to atropine		Systemic
oral	Provides alternate substance to human tissue for toxin reactions		Local
i.v. (if i.v. impossible, i.m. in buttocks)		Always do skin test first because of possible allergic reaction. Never inject in finger, toe or at bite site	Systemic
oral/lavage			Local/systen
oral, i.v.	i.v. only in severe poisonings		Local
i.v.	If symptoms persist >30 min a second dose, half of original, may be given	Excessive amounts of this antidote may result in fatal methemoglobinemia	Systemic
i.v.	Should be given over a 10-min period		Systemic
oral	Provides alternate substrate to human tissue for toxin reactions. Flour, bread, milk may be used if starch not available		Local
i.v. (may be given sub q) i.m. (painful on inhalation)	Is investigational. The Ca salt is more toxic than the Zn salt	Not recommended for pregnant women or children. Is toxic to fetus, kidney and liver	Systemic

References

1. Kilham HA: Hospital management of severe poisoning. *Pediatr Clin North Am* 27:603, 1980.
2. Walton WW: An evaluation of the poison prevention packaging act. *Pediatrics* 69:363, 1982.
3. Wright N: An assessment of the unreliability of the history given by self-poisoned patients. *Clin Toxicol* 16:381, 1980.
4. Mofenson HC, Greensher J: The unknown poison. *Pediatrics* 54:336, 1974.
5. Pagliaro LA, Levin RH: *Problems in Pediatric Drug Therapy.* Illinois, Drug Intelligence Publications, Inc., 1979.
6. Graef JW, Cone TE: *Manual of Pediatric Therapeutics.* Second Edition, Boston, Little, Brown and Co., 1980.
7. Gosselin RE, Hodge HC, Smith RP, et al: *Clinical Toxicology of Commercial Products.* Fourth Edition, Baltimore, Williams & Wilkins Co., 1976.
8. Rumach BH: *Poisindex Management of Nontoxic Ingestion.* Poisindex Co., 1981.
9. Flanagan RJ, et al: Value of toxicological investigation in the diagnosis of acute drug poisoning in children. *Lancet* II:682, 1981.
10. Scherz RG: The differential diagnosis of coma due to poisoning and exogenous toxins. *Pediatrician* 6:190, 1977.
11. Done AK: The toxic emergency—in the blood. *Emerg Med* 7:193, 1975.
12. Rosenberg J, et al: Pharmacokinetics of drug overdose. *Clin Pharmacokinet* 6:161, 1981.
13. Done AK: The toxic emergency—asking for lab backup. *Emerg Med* 9:91, 1977.
14. Rumach BH: *Poisindex Management of General or Unknown Poison Management.* Poisindex Co., 1981.
15. Dabbons IA, et al: The ineffectiveness of mechanically induced vomiting. *J Pediatr* 66:952, 1965.
16. Barer J, et al: Fatal poisoning from salt used as an emetic. *Am J Dis Child* 125:889, 1973.
17. Chuttain HK, et al: Acute copper sulfate poisoning. *Am J Med* 39:849, 1965.
18. Gieseker DR, Troutman WG: Emergency induction of emesis using liquid detergent products: A report of 15 cases. *Clin Toxicol* 18:277, 1981.
19. King WD: Syrup of ipecac: A drug review. *Clin Toxicol* 17:353, 1980.
20. Lovejoy FH: Priorities in poisonings. *Emerg Med* 11:265, 1979.
21. Easom JM, Lovejoy FH: Efficacy and safety of gastrointestinal decontamination in the treatment of oral poisoning. *Pediatr Clin North Am* 26:827, 1979.
22. Keller EL: Poisoning in children—an approach for the primary physician. *Postgrad Med* 65:177, 1979.

23. Uden DL, et al: The effect of carbonated beverages on ipecac-induced emesis. *Ann Emerg Med* 10:79, 1981.
24. Manoguerra AS, Krenzelok EP: Rapid emesis from high-dose ipecac syrup in adults and children intoxicated with antiemetic or other drugs. *Am J Hosp Pharm* 35:1360, 1978.
25. Corby DG, et al: Clinical comparison of pharmacologic emetics in children. *Pediatrics* 42:361, 1968.
26. Reid DHS: Treatment of the poisoned child. *Arch Dis Child* 45:428, 1970.
27. Boxer L, et al: Comparison of ipecac-induced emesis with gastric lavage in the treatment of acute salicylate ingestion. *J Pediatr* 74:800, 1969.
28. Abdallah AH, Tye A: A comparison of the efficacy of emetic drugs and stomach lavage. *Am J Dis Child* 113:571, 1967.
29. Weir MR, Patterson HS: Tube size, lavage, and emesis. *Pediatrics* 69:388, 1982.
30. Arena JM: Poisoning—treatment and prevention—Part I–III, *JAMA* 232:1272, 233:358, 233:900, 1975.
31. Picchioni AL, et al: Activated charcoal vs. universal antidote as an antidote for poisons. *Toxicol Appl Pharmacol* 8:447, 1966.
32. Picchioni AL, et al: Activated charcoal preparations—relative antidotal efficacy. *Clin Toxicol* 7:97, 1974.
33. Chin L, et al: The action of activated charcoal on poisons in the digestive tract. *Toxicol Appl Pharmacol* 16:786, 1970.
34. Holt LE, Holz PH: The black bottle. A consideration of the role of charcoal in the treatment of poisoning in children. *J Pediatr* 63:306, 1963.
35. Picchioni AL: Activated charcoal—a neglected antidote. *Pediatr Clin North Am* 17:535, 1970.
36. Rauws AG, Van Noorwijk J: Activated charcoal in tricyclic antidepressant overdose. *Br Med J* 4:298, 1972.
37. Decker WJ, et al: Adsorption of drugs and poisons by activated charcoal. *Toxicol Appl Pharmacol* 13:454, 1968.
38. Dawlings S, et al: Effect of delayed administration of activated charcoal on nortriptyline absorption. *Eur J Clin Pharmacol* 14:445, 1978.
39. Greensher J, et al: Activated charcoal updated. *JACEP* 8:261, 1979.
40. Black JA, et al: *Pediatric Emergencies.* Chap. 8, London, Butterworths Co., 1979.
41. Cooney DO: Palatability of sucrose-, sorbitol-, and saccharin-sweetened activated charcoal formulations. *Am J Hosp Pharm* 37:237, 1980.
42. Pollack MM, et al: Aspiration of activated charcoal and gastric contents. *Ann Emerg Med* 10:528, 1981.
43. Riegel JM, Becker CE: Use of cathartics in toxic ingestions. *Ann Emerg Med* 10:254, 1981.
44. Handy CA: Radiopacity of oral nonliquid medications. *Radiology* 98:525, 1971.
45. Winchester JF, et al: Dialysis and hemoperfusion of poisons and drugs—Update. *Trans Am Soc Artif Intern Organs* 23:762, 1977.

46. Done AK: The toxic emergency—What's with hemoperfusion? *Emerg Med* 13:199, 1981.
47. Pond S, et al: Pharmacokinetics of haemoperfusion for drug overdose. *Clin Pharmacokinet* 4:329, 1979.
48. Spoerke DG: Guide to the acquisition, storage, and use of antidotes. *Am J Hosp Pharm* 38:498, 1981.
49. Rumach BH: Poisindex Management—Drugs Used in Toxicology. Poisindex Co., 1981.
50. Yokel RA, et al: A comparison of four toxicology resources in respect to rates of retrieval and time required. *J Pediatr* 92:145, 1978.
51. Zucker AR, et al: Fab fragments of digoxin-specific antibodies used to reverse ventricular fibrillation induced by digoxin ingestion in a child. *Pediatrics* 70:468, 1982.
52. Murphy DJ, et al: Massive digoxin poisoning treated with Fab fragments of digoxin-specific antibodies. *Pediatrics* 70:472, 1982.

22

Bleeding and Clotting Disorders

Jerry Z. Finklestein, M.D.
James A. Baker, M.D.

Introduction

The child who presents to the Pediatric Emergency Room or Intensive Care Unit with a bleeding problem should be evaluated for both a congenital and an acquired hemostatic abnormality. While the pediatrician often focuses upon the hereditary bleeding disorder, the majority of hemorrhagic problems seen in a Pediatric Intensive Care Unit are acquired.

Bleeding disorders may be associated with a blood dyscrasia such as leukemia, congenital heart disease, liver problems, and renal disease. Platelet disorders are often acquired. A bleeding problem may be secondary to marked thrombocytopenia either due to an immune phenomenon, bone marrow production defect or secondary to an underlying collagen vascular disorder. The child with sepsis harbors the risk of developing disseminated intravascular coagulation or thrombocytopenia secondary to circulating immune complexes. The management of bleeding in the sick neonate will not be included in this review.

Pathophysiology

Hemostatis involves a series of interactions. Blood vessels, platelets and plasma factors are active in this process which results in the formation of a firm clot. When a vessel is broken, platelets adhere to the subendothelial layer, aggregate and form a temporary plug capable of arresting bleeding. Vasoconstriction occurs in the venules and arterioles but its role in arresting bleeding at the level of these small vessels is probably not significant. A fibrin clot forms in intimate association with the platelets to form a firm plug. The loss of the endothelial cell at this site of damage, in addition to exposing the basement membrane and connective tissue, removes an important source of inhibitors of hemostasis. These cells release a potent inhibitor of platelet aggregation, PGI_2, and appear to be involved in the activation of several inhibitors of clotting.[1,2,3] Figure 1 illustrates the major components of hemostasis. A discussion of several additional points of interest follows.

The term *contact phase* includes a negatively charged surface (which can be basement membrane, connective tissue or in the laboratory glass), prekallikrein (Fletcher Factor), high molecular weight kininogen (Fitzgerald Factor), and factor XII, all of which can cause abnormal clotting tests but none of which cause bleeding in patients. Thrombin, in addition to splitting off the small polypeptide from the ends of fibrinogen to form fibrin, activates factor XIII which, in turn, acts on fibrin to form the firm covalently bound clot.

Plasmin is rapidly destroyed by a very potent inhibitor, called alpha-2-antiplasmin. When plasmin is infused into the blood stream it lasts for only fractions of a second. This antiplasmin does not affect plasminogen or plasmin bound to a clot, thus localizing fibrinolysis. The chief activator of plasminogen is a substance from the endothelial cell.

Platelets are made in the marrow from megakaryocyte cytoplasm; platelets circulate as discs but readily form long pseudopods. A number of factors have been attributed to platelets, and assigned arabic numbers. The most commonly utilized term is *platelet factor 3* which is a phospholipid substance from their wall necessary in the intrinsic and common pathway of the coagulation scheme. Several clotting factors including fibrinogen and Factor V are intimately bound to platelets and participate in clotting at the platelet surface.

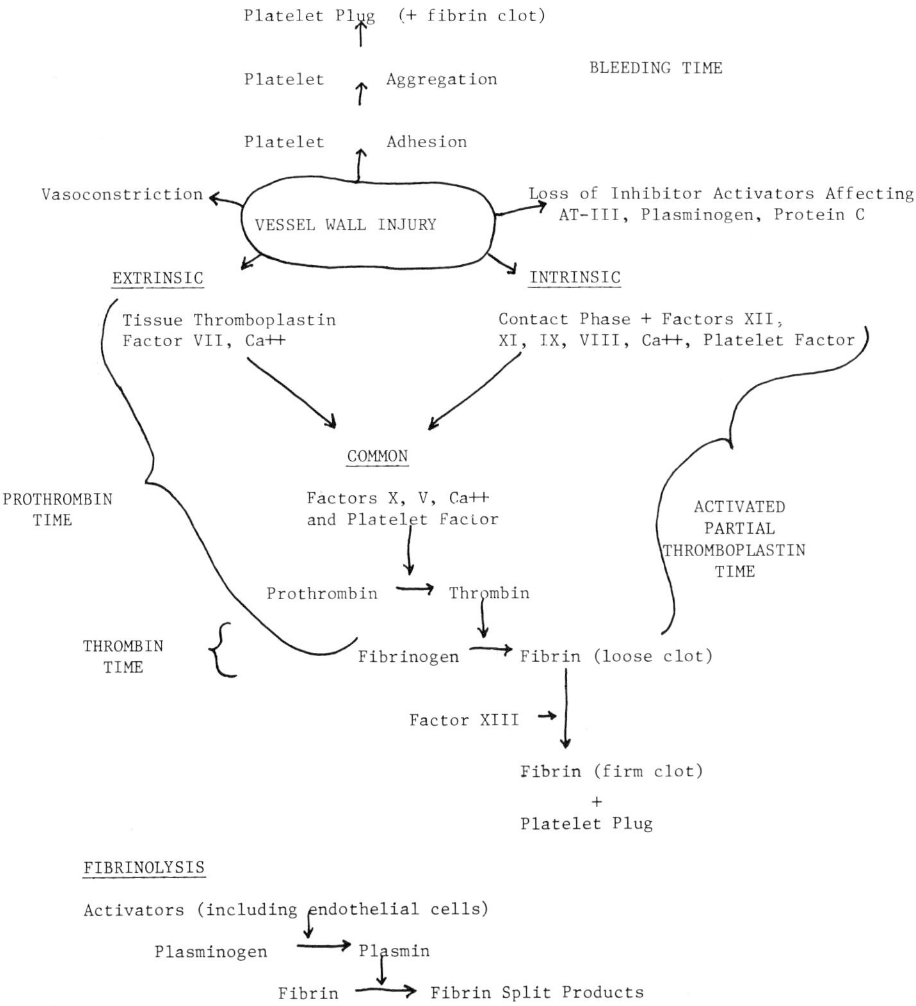

Figure 1. Simplified scheme of hemostasis.

Clinical Presentation

The importance of a family history cannot be over-emphasized. While most children presenting to an Intensive Care Unit with a bleeding problem will have an acquired disorder, hereditary disorders are often identified by a simple family history. This is especially important in pediatrics where the child's life span is often too short to permit him to manifest a bleeding problem. Surgery is an excellent test of hemostasis. Thus, a question about prior surgery is important but should be followed by asking specifically about T&A, the removal of teeth and circumcision. Routine immunization or other intramuscular injections followed by a hematoma should be noted. The normal child who is the first offspring may show bruises that are considered to be excessive by neophyte parents while subsequent children will be termed as normal. A recent change or the presence of several bruises not on the shins and not related to trauma may be significant. The formation of hemarthrosis, large soft tissue hemorrhages and hematuria are definitely abnormal. Gross gastrointestinal bleeding is very rare in children and requires investigation. Hyperextensible joints may be a clue to the bleeding disorder in Ehlers-Danlos syndrome but is often difficult to assess in children. While epistaxis usually is of uncertain significance, it can be a clue to a problem. As a general rule, disorders of platelets lead to skin and mucous membrane bleeding, and disorders of clotting factors lead to deep hemorrhage or hemarthrosis, yet exceptions are often seen.

Malignancies, cardiovascular shock, giant hemangioma, hemolytic transfusion reactions, trauma, burns, heatstroke, viral or bacterial diseases, or damage to endothelial cells may result in thromboplastic material being released and lead to disseminated intravascular coagulation (DIC) and a consumptive coagulopathy. A child who bleeds and in whom thrombocytopenia is identified almost always has one of the following: a blood dyscrasia, immune thrombocytopenia, a drug-induced thrombocytopenia or DIC. Bleeding secondary to an inhibitor or antibody against clotting factors is very rare in children. The most common inhibitor is probably the lupus type which causes a prolonged activated partial thromboplastin time, and multiple abnormal factor assays, but no bleeding problems; it is most often not associated with lupus erythematosis.

While external blood loss is readily determined, internal bleeding may be more difficult to identify. Once it is confirmed that a patient is bleeding, a series of laboratory aids may be necessary in deciding if this is related to a hemostatic defect. (Table I.)

Table I
Diagnostic Considerations

Presenting Problem of Bleeding Appears to be Associated With:	*Physicians Should Consider the following Etiologic Factors:*
1. Family history of hemophilia	Prolonged PTT-assay VIII and IX
2. Sepsis, trauma, malignancy	DIC (see Table II)
3. Liver disease	Depressed clotting factors including vitamin K factors, excessive fibrinolysis, thrombocytopenia, DIC
4. Kidney disease	Thrombocytopenia or platelet function defect
5. Surgery	Operative technique, DIC, massive or incompatible blood transfusions
6. Mucocutaneous bleeding	Thrombocytopenia, platelet function disorder, von Willebrand's disease

Bleeding and the Surgeon

Many patients present to the Intensive Care Unit with bleeding associated with surgery. Realizing that surgery is a major challenge of the hemostatic mechanism, physicians must consider that any surgical patient is at risk to develop a serious bleeding problem related to an even mild underlying defect. A careful history and screening tests of hemostasis together will almost always indicate the possibility of a disorder; a firm specific diagnosis should be established prior to surgery. It is no longer acceptable for a child to go to surgery without an evaluation of hemostasis unless there is an emergency situation without sufficient time.

A patient who experiences bleeding which increases during surgery, generally has an acquired disorder related to the surgical procedure.[4] The differential diagnosis includes operative techniques, disseminated intravascular coagulation, the fibrinolysis syndrome, acquired thrombocytopenia or an incompatible blood transfusion. Primary fibrinolysis is rare; fibrinolysis is usually secondary to DIC. Thrombocytopenia may occur as part of the disseminated intravascular coagulation syndrome and as a result of massive or incompatible blood transfusions. The child who undergoes cardiac surgery with a cardiac bypass may develop severe bleeding diathesis. This is often due to a platelet function defect. However, it has been proposed that primary fibrinolysis may be an etiological factor.

Post-operative hemorrhage is most often due to a mechanical problem related to primary surgical hemostasis. Conditions similar to those described as occurring during surgery may present following the completion of the surgical procedure. For example, a massively swollen neck after head and neck surgery may be a clue to an underlying hemophilia and can be rapidly fatal.

Disseminated Intravascular Coagulation

Disseminated intravascular coagulation (DIC) is an acquired consumptive coagulopathy. It can be produced by either generalized activation of the clotting mechanism or localized activation. It may be sudden or gradual in onset, acute or chronic in duration. Corrigan[5,6] has indicated that a number of pediatric equivalents can be hypothesized as acting in a manner similar to experimental triggering agents in the causation of this phenomenon. Table II is from Corrigan's work and indicates that infections, bacterial septic shock, viral or protozoal disease may result in the release of thromboplastic material.[6] This may also be the mechanism in cases where DIC occurs with certain malignancies, e.g., acute stem cell leukemia.[7]

Patients with DIC have reduction in clotting factors II, V, VIII and fibrinogen. The activated partial thromboplastin time is often prolonged and the prothrombin time is almost always prolonged. Thrombocytopenia, hypofibrinogenemia and elevation of fibrin split products are usually present. The identification of a significant number of fragmented red blood cells on a blood smear may indicate DIC. Corrigan has listed a comparison of screening tests and specific tests to differentiate between DIC and entities confused with DIC such as liver disease, vitamin K deficiency and changes associated with massive volume replacement (Table III).[6] Specifically, the child in an Intensive Care Unit setting may present

Table II

Disseminated Intravascular Coagulation and Consumption Coagulopathy: Triggering Mechanisms

Experimental Agent	*Possible Clinical Equivalent*
Bacterial products (i.e., endotoxin)	Gram-negative septicemia
Thromboplastic material (tissue juices)	Shock Endothelial damage (virus, bacterial, rickettsia, heat stroke) Trauma/burns Malignancies Hemolytic transfusion reaction
Antigen-antibody complexes	Immune disease (purpura fulminans?) Anaphylactic shock
Blood stasis	Generalized: shock Localized: giant hemangioma
Particulate matter	Hemolytic transfusion

(Modified from Corrigans)

with problems requiring differentiation between DIC and liver disease. Factor VIII activity is helpful since it is normal or elevated in liver disease and usually low in severe DIC. Platelets are usually low in DIC and normal in liver disease.

The Child with Liver Disease

It has been estimated that up to 85% of patients with liver disease have abnormal hemostasis and yet less than 25% bleed.[8] Clotting disorders associated with hepatocellular disease must be considered in children. Prothrombin time can be prolonged in obstructive jaundice (due to vitamin K deficiency only). All clotting factors except for VIII may be reduced in patients with liver disease. Similarly, anti-thrombin III and plasminogen may be low. Thrombocytopenia can also be found in liver disease. This may be

Table III

Comparison of Screening Tests and Specific Tests between DIC and Entities Confused with DICA* (from Corrigan)

Tests	*DIC*	*Liver Disease*	*Vitamin K Deficiency*	*Dilutional Changes Associated with Massive Volume Replacement*
Screening tests				
PTT	P	P	P	P
PT	P	P	P	P
FSPs	+	+/O	O	O
Fibrinogen level	R	R	N	R
Specific tests				
Factor II	R	R	R	R
Factor V	R	R	N	R
Factor VIII	R	N-E	N	R
Platelet count	R	N-R	N	R
"Soluble fibrin"	+	O	O	O

*Key: PTT = partial thromboplastin time; PT = prothrombin time; P = prolonged; N = normal; R = reduced; + = present; O = absent; E = elevated

due to an enlarged spleen with splenic sequestration, but occasionally liver disease alone appears to cause low platelets. Table III will aid the clinician in differentiating between liver disease and disseminated intravascular coagulation.

DIC has also been described in individuals with advanced liver disease. The treatment of the coagulation defect associated with liver disease is replacement of clotting factors; fresh frozen plasma is usually the treatment of choice.[9] Prothrombin complex concentrates may halt the bleeding; since these concentrates can produce DIC or thrombosis, heparin may be added. Platelet transfusions may be necessary in specific situation. (When liver disease is mild, the deficiency in vitamin K dependent factors may be helped with the administration of vitamin K.)

Renal Problems and Hemostasis

Children with chronic renal disease with renal failure and uremia appear to have a plasma compound that inhibits platelet function and/or platelet production.[10] Patients with chronic renal disease without uremia may have defects in the hemostatic mechanism secondary to endothelial cell injury or defects secondary to the loss of the clotting factors associated with proteinuria. In addition, other studies have revealed that these children may have elevations in fibrinogen degradation products with an activation of the plasma fibrinolytic system.[11] Thus, with abnormalities noted in platelets, clotting factors and fibrinolysis, it is apparent that sophisticated evaluations will be necessary in order to delineate which, if any, therapy is necessary.[12] On occasion, therapy may be clotting factor replacement or platelet transfusion but usually platelet function defects can only be corrected by dialysis since transfused platelets acquire the defect from the plasma. Rarely, anti-thrombotic therapy or fibrinolytic therapy is needed.

Cyanotic Congenital Heart Disease and Bleeding

Individuals with cyanotic congenital heart disease may have thrombocytopenia, prolonged thrombin times, prolonged partial thromboplastin times, hypofibrinogenemia, abnormal platelet function, defective clot retraction, and accelerated fibrinolysis.[13] These abnormalities do not occur in any consistent manner and vary in frequency and severity and may or may not be related to the degree of hypoxemia and polycythemia seen in children with this abnormality. While in some cases clotting factor changes are related to the inability of the liver to synthesize these factors or to scavenge the fibrin degradation products from the circulation, it is difficult to interpret the multitude of results reported.[14,15] Other reports have been published regarding platelet survival and platelet function in children with cyanotic congenital heart disease.[16] The aim of therapy must be directed at the replacement of depleted clotting factors and/or platelets. This can be accomplished with fresh frozen plasma and with platelet concentrates if required.

There have been some cases in which intravascular coagulation is described and heparinization suggested.

Immune Thrombocytopenic Purpura (ITP)

Immune thrombocytopenic purpura is a benign disease in children which becomes chronic in 10–20% of cases but rarely is life-threatening. Yet, intracranial hemorrhage is described in approximately 1% of patients with this disorder, and thus is a prime consideration in a child who presents with thrombocytopenia and cerebral bleeding. While the diagnosis can be established with a bone marrow aspiration and identification of platelet antibodies, controversy exists regarding management for this disorder. The majority of children with ITP remit spontaneously, and yet most physicians utilize corticosteroids for the general treatment of this disorder. It is the child who arrives in the Intensive Care Unit that must be considered, and for these individuals the diagnosis should be confirmed. Treatment should include corticosteroids at high doses (prednisone, 2 mg/kg/day or the equivalent for approximately four weeks). Platelets as an emergency transfusion and splenectomy may be indicated for children with a CNS bleed. More recently, infusion of IgG has been used to block the reticuloendothelial system and provide temporary therapy for thrombocytopenia.

Von Willebrand's Disease

This is the most common congenital bleeding disorder and may present as a mild defect which first manifests itself with major surgery or trauma; hence it warrants particular discussion. The bleeding defect is usually related to the platelet problem and hence is of a mucocutaneous nature; in rare cases the factor VIII clotting activity is extremely low causing a hemophilia-type problem.

The classic tests for its detection have included a long bleeding time and a low factor VIII coagulant activity with a long APTT. These tests are, however, abnormal in only approximately 70% of cases and hence other tests are often necessary to exclude this possibility. The best single test is the factor VIII related antigen whereby the level of the von Willebrand's factor is measured by an antibody. This is low in the vast majority of von Willebrand's patients and is normal in hemophilia. Probably of equal sensitivity but somewhat more difficult to perform is the ristocetin co-factor assay. This is based on the observation that the antibiotic ristocetin causes aggregation of platelets in the presence of the von Willebrand's factor.

In the treatment of this disorder it is important to realize that the defect lies in a large multimeric plasma factor, sometimes called von Willebrand's factor, which is necessary for platelets to adhese to surfaces such as collagen. The platelets themselves are functionally normal. Hence, cryoprecipitate rather than platelet transfusions are indicated.

Massive Blood Loss

Following massive blood loss with multiple transfusions, a bleeding defect often occurs. In the case of an adult this does not occur until after approximately 15 units of blood in a 5-hour period. (This translates into approximately one and a half total blood volumes.) At this time the primary defect is a thrombocytopenia but may also include a functional platelet defect. With platelet counts below 70,000 in major surgery and trauma, bleeding problems may develop. To prevent this in an adult, it is suggested that approximately 8 units of platelets be infused after each 10 units of banked blood or if platelets are readily available, one may wait until the platelet count falls below 100,000/cu mm. Two units of fresh frozen plasma are also often given with each 10 units of banked blood to replace any possible clotting factor defect, although the need for this is debatable in patients transfused with whole banked blood. In a child the blood volume is approximately 70 to 80 cc per Kg. Thus, any child requiring 100 cc/Kgm of blood in a 5-hour period should be considered as having received "massive" transfusions which may lead to a bleeding defect. Platelet and fresh frozen plasma replacement therapy are considerations in these situations.

The Laboratory

Simple guidelines should be followed by the physician in selecting the appropriate tests of hemostasis.[17] Sample collection with young children requires patience and understanding as a free flow of blood is important in order to assure accurate test results. The standard screening tests are: (1) complete blood count including platelet count; (2) prothrombin time; (3) activated partial thromboplastin time; and (4) template bleeding time.

The complete blood count will determine whether the child is anemic or thrombocytopenic. Mild clotting factor deficiencies, moderate fibrinogen deficiency, a mild DIC, and very rare defects such as factor XIII and alpha-2-antiplasmin deficiency, even if severe, would not be identified by these screening tests.

For the collection of blood sample, many laboratories insist upon a two syringe technique. Free blood flow is important. If a clot is formed in the test tube, no matter how small, the test results are not valid. If the sample is obtained with difficulty, it is quite likely that the test result will not be valid. Samples collected from a vein superior to an IV site can give a picture similar to DIC but without fibrin split products. Polycythemic blood or poor filling of tubes may give erroneous results. Samples that stand for long periods of time will suffer depletion of certain factors and alter test results. Specimens should be centrifuged and the plasma separated and frozen at −30°C or below for delayed testing. The choice of sodium citrate anticoagulant in siliconized tubes is important, and the ratio of anticoagulant to the blood sample is crucial. Children with cyanotic congenital heart disease and hematocrits greater than 50% will need lesser amounts of sodium citrate to assure an appropriate ratio.

The ordering of laboratory tests should be carried out with a differential diagnosis in mind. A summary of the common tests[17] follows.

Prothrombin Time (PT)

The prothrombin time measures the time required for plasma to clot after tissue thromboplastin and calcium have been added.

It requires prothrombin (factor II), factor V, factor VII, factor X and fibrinogen.

The usual normal range is 11–12.5 seconds. It is more sensitive to mild factor deficiencies than the activated partial thromboplastin time in detecting factors below the 50% level. For this reason, mild prolongations of the PT are not as important as are mild prolongations of the APTT which is less sensitive. Patients with vitamin K deficiency, liver disease, malabsorption problems and children exposed to anticoagulants may have a prolongation of the prothrombin time. Patients who have deficiencies in any of the above factors may have a prolonged prothrombin time. A simple procedure in a patient with a long protime for no apparent reason is to give I.M. or I.V. vitamin K and repeat the protime 8 hours later.

Activated Partial Thromboplastin Time (APTT)

The activated PTT measures the intrinsic system. An activator and a substitute for platelet factor 3 is added. Normal values for APTTs vary from laboratory to laboratory but are usually less than 47 seconds. Term infants may range between 50–84 seconds. Factors may be reduced to as low as 25% of normal, and still show a normal APTT. Thus, the sensitivity of the test barely detects minor deficiencies. For this reason, only slight prolongations above normal cannot be ignored as they may reflect, for example, a factor VIII level of 20% which could cause severe bleeding with major surgery. It is essential that each lab determine an accurate upper limit of normal for each batch of reagent. Reporting results as a control plus the patient without a normal range is not adequate. Fibrinogen when it is markedly reduced, e.g., less than 80 mg/dl, may result in a prolonged activated partial thromboplastin time. This test then measures deficiencies of fibrinogen, prothrombin, factors V, VIII, IX, X, XI, XII as well as the contact phase factors known as Fletcher Factor (Prekallikrein) and Fitzgerald Factor (high molecular weight kininogen). Warfarin therapy, liver disease, circulating anticoagulants, and fibrin degradation products may all prolong the APTT. In cases where the APTT is long and the PT normal, diagnostic possibilities include deficiencies in factors VIII,

IX, XI, XII, contact factors or anticoagulants. Inhibitors, e.g., factor VIII inhibitors, may similarly affect the APTT. Before embarking on an expensive work up in a patient with a long APTT, it is wise to repeat the test. Many centers use the APTT to monitor the administration of heparin.

Thrombin Time

The thrombin time measures the ability of fibrinogen to generate fibrin and is affected by fibrin split products, heparin and the concentration of fibrinogen. A normal thrombin time is within 3 seconds of the control. Any disorder lowering fibrinogen, (e.g., DIC) causing abnormal fibrinogens (such as dysfibrinogenemias in liver disease) or inhibitors such as fibrin split products, may prolong the thrombin time. Heparin used to keep intravenous lines clear may cause an abnormal thrombin time. Correction of the long thrombin time by adding toluidine blue will confirm the presence of heparin in the specimen.

Fibrinogen

Quantitation of plasma fibrinogen can be done in most hospital laboratories. Decreased levels are documented in hereditary disorders as well as acquired disorders such as disseminated intravascular coagulation, severe liver disease or in cases with fibrinolysis. The usual value for children is 150–400 mg/dl depending upon the technique utilized.

Platelet Count

An estimate of platelet numbers can always be made by examining a well prepared peripheral blood smear. The direct counting method utilizing an electronic particle counter or a phase microscope is preferable. The normal platelet count for a child ranges between 150,000–450,000/mm^3.

Bleeding Time

To test platelet function and the integrity of small vessels, a template bleeding time is done. This procedure is standardized and requires a technician who is competent in the procedure. The patient's arm should be under steady support, the blood pressure cuff maintained at 40 mm of mercury, the device should be standardized, the flow and blotting must be uniform, and ideally normal values obtained for each laboratory for children of various ages. Usually the template bleeding time, e.g., Simplate or Mielke, is less than 8 minutes. The test is prolonged in thrombocytopenia (below 100,000/mm^3), many platelet function disorders, some children with von Willebrand's disease, and occasionally in individuals with vascular abnormalities. When prolonged in the face of a normal platelet count, platelet function studies may clarify. However, a careful drug history is essential before using this expensive testing.

The Coagulation Laboratory

Institutions who care for the critically ill child should have access to a laboratory which can provide more than routine screening tests. The laboratory should be able to perform platelet function tests, clotting factor assays, quantitation of factor VIII related antigen, a solubility test for factor XIII, ristocetin co-factor assay, a test for anti-thrombin III, tests for fibrinolysis, and procedures for indicating inhibitors such as the lupus type and against factor VIII.

Differential Diagnosis

A complete history and physical examination will usually suggest to the clinician the correct diagnosis; laboratory tests confirm or clarify this impression. Abnormalities of hemostasis to be considered are shown in Table IV.

Table IV
Abnormalities of Hemostasis

A. Disorders of Clotting Factors

Prolongation of activated partial thromboplastin time
- Factor VIII deficiency:
  - hemophilia A
  - von Willebrand's disease
  - associated with disseminated intravascular coagulation
- Factor IX deficiency:
  - inherited (Christmas disease)
  - associated with liver disease
  - induced by Coumarin
  - Vitamin K deficiency
- Factor XI deficiency:
  - inherited
- Factor XII deficiency:
  - laboratory phenomenon
- Inhibitors:
  - lupus type
  - against Factor VIII

Prolongation of prothrombin time
- Factor II, VII, X deficiency:
  - inherited
  - acquired in liver disease
  - Coumarin compound induced
  - Vitamin K deficiency
- Factor V deficiency:
  - inherited
  - acquired in liver disease
  - associated with a malignancy
  - seen in DIC

Prolongation of thrombin time
- Fibrinogen deficiency:
  - an inherited disorder
  - the result of severe liver disease
  - the result of DIC
- Presence of heparin
- Presence of fibrin split products

B. Platelet Disorders

C. Blood Vessels

D. Thrombosis

Platelet Disorders

Thrombocytopenia. Patients may present with low platelet counts in immune thrombocytopenic purpura, or thrombocytopenia associated with hemangiomas, cyanotic congenital heart disease, or the Wiskott-Aldrich syndrome, collagen vascular diseases, in thrombotic thrombocytopenia purpura, purpura fulminans or the hemolytic uremic syndrome. In these cases there are generally at least adequate numbers of megakaryocytes in the bone marrow. Thrombocytopenia secondary to decreased megakaryocytes is usually associated with loss of other marrow elements such as in aplastic anemia or in marrow replacement as with tumor or leukemia. The rare primary defect of megakaryocytes alone is sometimes associated with absent radii.

Thrombocytopathy. Patients who bleed and have normal platelet counts may have abnormal platelet function either congenital or acquired or secondary to drug ingestion.

Blood Vessels

Disorders of blood vessels are rare in children. The Ehlers-Danlos syndrome, anaphylactoid purpura, the metabolic disorder of scurvy, and prolonged corticosteroid therapy may produce this problem. Since there are no good tests for this problem, the primary reliance is on the history and physical and the absence of detectable defects in hemostasis.

Thrombosis

Children who present with venous thrombosis or pulmonary embolism should be considered for anticoagulant therapy. Heparinization and coumadin are effective. Low dose heparin does protect against deep vein thrombosis in selected post-operative patients. Long-term prevention may require the use of a non-steroid anti-inflammatory drug such as aspirin. Aspirin inhibits platelet release reactions and may lead to a prolongation of the bleeding time.

A common cause for post-operative thromboembolism is venous stasis. However, when repeated thrombotic problems occur in a young person, underlying conditions such as diabetes, obesity, the nephrotic syndrome, smoking, AT-III deficiencies, plasminogen abnormalities, protein C deficiency, and dysfibrinogenemia should be considered.

Although a number of inhibitors of coagulation have been identified, recent investigations have suggested that anti-thrombin III plays an important role in the balancing of the clotting process *in vivo*.[18] It was realized that there are a number of activities in plasma that seem to interfere with the function of thrombin. One of these, anti-thrombin III, is a serine protease inhibitor. Since many activated clotting factors are serine proteases, AT-III blocks many factors in addition to thrombin. AT-III is apparently the sole means of action of heparin. Heparin greatly increases the action of AT-III, and in the absence of AT-III, does not inhibit clotting, even in large doses. AT-III deficiency should be considered in the differential diagnosis of an individual who presents with a hypercoagulable state.

Therapeutic Considerations

The therapy for children who have bleeding and clotting disorders depends on accurate identification of the pathogenesis and etiology of the disorder. The following products are available for treatment.

Platelets

In most countries, platelets can be readily obtained and may be used to control or improve hemostasis in children who have thrombocytopenia associated with acute leukemia, bone marrow failure, or chemotherapy. Volume considerations are important in the child.

Spontaneous bleeding problems do not usually occur until a platelet level falls below 30,000. Thus, there is no indication for platelets in cases in which the platelet count is above that level and in which there is no frank bleeding. Platelet transfusions are not usually indicated for individuals with immune thrombocytopenic purpura unless they have severe life-threatening bleeding in which case the transfusion is given in conjunction with other therapeutic approaches. In individuals who have thrombocytopenia secondary to infection, platelet transfusions usually are not helpful until the infection is controlled. One unit of platelets will raise an adult's platelet count by 10,000 cells/mm^3, when measured 1 hour post-transfusion. The *in vivo* half-life is about four days for platelets stored for less than 72 hours at room temperature. A practical approach is to administer platelets on a volume of 10 cc/kg in over one hour.

Plasma Factors

There are a large number of plasma products available for the treatment of bleeding due to hereditary and acquired disorders. Table V outlines some of the therapies that are proposed for hemostatic defects due to clotting abnormalities. For factor VIII, doses are given utilizing either cryoprecipitate, or commercial concentrate. Similar therapies, when appropriate, are listed for factor IX deficiency and deficiencies of other clotting factors as well as von Willebrand's disease. Commercial products are packaged in vials which are labeled with exact number of units of replacement factor in the reconstituted product. The merits of these products include ease of reconsitiution, small volume and rapid attainment of the desired hemostatic level. The disadvantages include the risk of hepatitis and the recently described acquired immune deficiency syndrome, isoimmune hemolytic anemia with factor VIII concentrates and risk of generalized thrombosis with prothrombin concentrates. For factor VIII deficient patients with infrequent need for therapy, cryoprecipitate is preferable to concentrate because of the exposure to fewer donors. The table suggests guidelines for repetition of treatment. The half-life of factor VIII is about 12 hours; whereas the half-life for factor V is 36 hours, the half-life for factor VII is only five hours. This must be considered in terms of frequency of replacement therapy.

Table V
Replacement Factors

Factor	*Preferred Preparation*	*Half-Life Hours†*	*Increase in Plasma After I.U./Kg(x)*	*Hemostatic Level: Minor Trauma*	*Hemostatic Level: Major Trauma or Surgery*	*Level for Maintenance Hemostatis*
VIII	Fresh frozen plasma, Cryoprecipitate, concentrate (Commercial)	12–15	2%*	20–30%	50%	10%
IX	Fresh frozen plasma, Commercial concentrate Prothrombin complex	18–24	1%	15%	25%	5–10%
W? disease	Cryoprecipitate, fresh frozen plasma	24–48	3%	20–30%	50%	10%
XI	Fresh frozen plasma	24–48	2%	10–15%	20%	10%
VII	Fresh frozen plasma, Commercial concentrate (Prothrombin complex)	5	1%	5–10%	10%	5%
V	Fresh frozen plasma	12–36	1.5%	10%	25%	5%
X	Fresh frozen plasma, Commercial concentrate (Prothrombin complex)	24–60	1%	10%	15%	5%
II	Fresh frozen plasma, Commercial concentrate (Prothrombin complex)	72	1%	15%	25%	10%
I	Cryoprecipitate	80	1–1.5 mg/100 ml	150 mg/100 ml	200 mg/100 ml	100 mg/100 ml

(X) One unit is the amount of clotting factor of normal fresh pooled citrated plasma.
*Example: A 20 kgm child will require 500 units to raise his factor VIII level to 50%. This can be accomplished with commercial product or approximately seven bags of cryoprecipitate when one bag contains 70–75 units of factor VIII. Volume restrictions on a child limit a plasma infusion to 10 to 15 cc/Kgm repeated every 6 to 8 hours or as necessary.
†Half life refers to second and subsequent infusions.

Heparin

When an individual presents with DIC, the treatment must be directed to the underlying disease. Rarely does one have to treat the hemostatic abnormality. However, when this is necessary, the depleted clotting factors should be replaced, and in occasional specific cases heparin may be necessary. Most clinicians no longer utilize heparin in patients with DIC; replacement therapy along with treatment of the primary disease is the preferred treatment. On occasions where it is felt that specific organ damage may be occurring due to clotting, it may be elected to interrupt the DIC with heparinization. In these cases, fibrinogen concentration can be utilized as a guide for the effectiveness of the therapy and heparinization can be carried out, preferably on a continuous IV basis (600 units/kg per 24 hours). Heparin may be neutralized by protamine sulfate administered intravenously as 1 mg for each 100 units of heparin.

Prognosis

The prognosis of the child who presents to the Intensive Care Unit with a bleeding or clotting disorder will usually depend on the prognosis of his underlying disease since most of these disorders are acquired or are a secondary phenomenon. Thus, therapy must be directed to the underlying disease; the treatment of the hemostatic abnormality is usually secondary to the primary treatment. Patients presenting to the Intensive Care Unit with a congenital hereditary abnormality will have a prognosis dependent on the underlying abnormality, the clinical presentation, the organs involved, bleeding diathesis, and the skill of the therapist.

References

1. Feinstein DI, Rapaport SI: Acquired inhibitors of blood coagulation. *In* Spaet TH, (ed): *Progress in Hemostasis and Thrombosis.* New York, Grune & Stratton, Inc., 1972, p 75.
2. Teger-Nilsson A: Antithrombin in infancy and childhood. *Acta Paediatr Scand* 64:624, 1975.
3. Prevention of Thrombosis *Lancet,* 127, January 15, 1977.

4. Bowie EJW, Owen Jr CA, Hagedorn AB: The diagnosis and management of unusual bleeding in the surgical patient. *Surg Clin of North Am* 49:1161, 1969.
5. Corrigan Jr JJ: Disseminated intravascular coagulation: Pathogenesis, diagnosis and management. *In* Lusher JM, Barnhart MI, (eds): *Acquired Bleeding Disorders in Children.* New York, Masson Publishing Inc., 1981, p 27.
6. Corrigan JJ Jr: Heparin therapy in bacterial septicemia. *J Pediatr* 91:695, 1977.
7. Edson JR, Krivit W, White JG, et al: Intravascular coagulation in acute stem cell leukemia successfully treated with heparin. *J Pediatr* 71:342, 1967.
8. Owen CA Jr: Coagulation disorders associated with hepatocellular disease. *In* Lusher JM, Barnhart MI, (eds): *Acquired Bleeding Disorders in Children.* New York, Masson Publishing, Inc, 1981. p 41.
9. Spector I, Corn M, Ticktin HE: Effect of plasma transfusions on the prothrombin time and clotting factors in liver disease. *N Engl J Med* 275:1032, 1966.
10. Lazerson J: Hemostatic defects associated with renal failure. *In* Lusher JM, Barnhart MI, (Eds): *Acquired Bleeding Disorders in Children.* New York, Masson Publishing Inc, 1981. p 83.
11. Frumin AM: Platelet function, coagulation, and fibrinolysis. *In* Jepson JH, (ed): *Hematologic Problems in Renal Disease.* Reading, MA, Addison-Wesley Publishing, 1979. p 193.
12. Green D, Arruda H, Honig G, et al: Urinary loss of clotting factors due to hereditary membranous glomerulopathy. *Am J Clin Pathol* 65:376, 1976.
13. Warrier AI: The hemorrhagic diathesis associated with cyanotic congenital heart disease. *In* Lusher JM, Barnhart MI, (eds): *Acquired Bleeding Disorders in Children.* New York, Masson Publishing Inc, 1981. p 91.
14. Ekert H, Gilchrist GS, Stanton R, et al: Hemostasis in cyanotic congenital heart disease. *J Pediatr* 76:221, 1970.
15. Komp DM, Sparrow AW: Polycythemia in cyanotic heart disease. A study of altered coagulation. *J Pediatr* 76:231, 1970.
16. Waldman JD, Czapeck EE, Paul MH, et al: Shortened platelet survival in cyanotic heart disease. *J Pediatr* 87:77, 1975.
17. Hillman C, Lushner JM: Tests of blood coagulation: Technical points of clinical relevance. *In* Lusher JM, Barnhart MI, (eds): *Acquired Bleeding Disorders in Children.* New York, Masson Publishing Inc, 1981, p 107.
18. Marciniak E: Antithrombin III: Its role as a coagulation inhibitor. *In* Lusher JM, Barnhart MI, (eds): *Acquired Bleeding Disorders in Children.* New York, Masson Publishing Inc, 1981, p 115.

Part V

Intensive Care of Children with Infections

Systemic or local infections are potential complications of any child admitted to a pediatric intensive care unit. Some children are admitted because of primary infectious disorders while the course of others is complicated by a secondary, life-threatening infection. Acute infection in children is one of the most common entities in pediatric intensive care and, therefore, the entire part has been devoted to this topic.

23

Intensive Care of Children with Infections

Gerald R. Greene, M.D.

Acute Infections in Children

General Considerations

Acute infections in infants and children are common and are caused by a variety of microorganisms including bacteria, viruses, rickettsiae, protozoans, fungi, chlamydia, mycoplasma, and mycobacteria. Infections in children that are severe enough to require intensive care are far less common and will be the focus of this chapter. Certain potentially overwhelming infections will be discussed. Aside from the infection itself, complications such as shock, renal failure, disseminated intravascular coagulation, and cerebral edema can be life-threatening. These complications require rapid identification and prompt institution of appropriate supportive care. If the infectious agent cannot be treated primarily, supportive care is all that can be offered to the patient. The severity of a given infection and the likelihood of complications are dependent upon a complex interaction of patient attributes, host-parasite relationships, and the characteristics of the infectious agent. Infants and children may acquire potentially life-threatening infections from the community or from hospitalization. Certain patients such as prematures, neonates, immunosuppressed and debilitated children are most likely to suffer infection with unusual opportunistic organisms or have a severe illness when infected by a common pathogen.

The physician should be aware of the presenting signs and symptoms of infection in infants and children and the common treatable pathogens in his geographic area. He should be able to obtain a careful, focused medical history, physical examination and laboratory analysis of a possible infection. Symptoms of infection may be general or localized and may be obvious or cryptic. Usually, the younger the child the less specific are the signs and symptoms of a given infection. Also, young infants and immunosuppressed children tend to localize infections poorly and may have several sites involved, generalized septicemia or more than one infection simultaneously.

A history of previous infections and their severity should be obtained as well as records of previous hospitalizations. Recent exposure to ill persons or an illness in the family is useful information. A history of travel or of visitors may imply exposure to pathogens not ordinarily found where the patient lives. Visitors from other locations may harbor nonindigenous organisms. A recent history of camping or swimming may suggest other infections. The consumption of nonpasteurized dairy products may be a clue to an infectious etiology. A history of exposure to farm animals, exotic pets and birds should be obtained. The physician should be aware of infections currently prevalent in the community. A history of allergies, particularly those due to antibiotics, should also be documented for any child suspected of infection.

Although not always present, a fever is usually considered suggestive of an infection. Infants and prematures may manifest hypothermia as an indication of infection. Conditions such as heat stroke, collagen-vascular disease, central nervous system injury, and malignancy may also cause fever in children. A recent review of the initial management of febrile children is available.[1] The height of the fever, and other physical and historical findings, as well as the age and general appearance of the child suggest the need for laboratory investigation and urgency in the initial management of the patient. However, the physician cannot always depend upon his first assessment of the severity of an infection.[2] Specific physical findings may be present to indicate a localized infection, and this is ordinarily the case with children beyond infancy. Such findings might include tachypnea and rales associated with pneumonia, lethargy, and meningismus associated with meningitis, cellulitis, pseudoparalysis of a limb due to osteomyelitis, an enlarged tender liver and jaundice with hepatitis or petechiae due to meningococcemia. Physical findings related to infections may be either confusing or inapparent. For example, persistent emesis may be the only manifestation of urinary tract infection in neonates.

The type and extent of an initial laboratory investigation for possible infection is determined by the history and physical examination and may be directed by specific information. The initial tests usually include a complete blood count with differential and a urinalysis. Other laboratory tests which might be useful at this stage are a chest roentgenogram, sputum culture, urine culture, blood culture, lumbar puncture, stool culture, tests of hepatic function, and specific roentgenograms. In addition, the severity of the patient's illness might indicate the need for more sophisticated tests, such as computerized axial tomography, radionucleotide scan, ultrasound scan, and tests such as counterimmunoelectrophoresis and latex agglutination for the presence of bacterial antigens in body fluids.[3–5] Tests for acute phase reactants such as erythrocyte sedimentation rate or C-reactive protein may help delineate a bacterial process. Serological evaluation for the development of antibodies to a wide variety of infectious agents may be considered, and in obscure cases a clotted tube of blood drawn initially in the hospital course and saved may later be useful for serological evaluation. Skin tests for various pathogens may be applied. Cultures for viruses, chlamydia, fungi, mycobacteria, anaerobic bacteria, and mycoplasma may be indicated.

It is sometimes necessary to start antibiotic therapy prior to the availability of culture and antibiotic susceptibility results. It is certainly not always necessary to start antibiotics in children with suspected infection. Many infections in children are viral and self-limited, and the physician must avoid the temptation to use antibiotics in all children who present with a fever. There are certain situations, however, such as fever in neonates, immunosuppressed children or those with malignancies, in which it may be life-saving to use antibiotics rapidly. There are patients whose presenting signs and symptoms point to an overwhelming bacterial infection, such as purulent spinal fluid, consolidated pneumonia with high fever, or characteristic findings of septic shock in which it is also necessary to utilize antibiotics before culture data are available. Before antibiotics are prescribed in such a patient, appropriate cultures and stains should be obtained in order that therapy be evaluated and changed in case of antibiotic failure. A gram stain of sputum, spinal fluid, urine, pus or empyema fluid may indicate a likely pathogen and should be performed at the time of admission. In young infants and immunosuppressed children where Gram-negative enteric bacteria as well as staphylococci and streptococci are likely pathogens, empiric antibiotic therapy usually consists of a penicillin and an aminoglycoside. An antibiotic appropriate for anaerobic bacteria may be used if there is a ruptured viscus or deep tissue abscess. In children beyond infancy, the antibiotics which are prescribed before culture information becomes available depend upon the site of infection and likely pathogens.

Infections Acquired in the Hospital

Introduction

Hospitalized infants and children are at risk in acquiring infections. Infection rates range from less than 1% in the normal newborn nursery to approximately 4–6% on the general pediatric ward and up to 25% in the neonatal intensive care unit.[6,7] The likelihood of a hospital-acquired *nosocomial* infection is related to the severity of the patient's illness, the patient's location in the hospital, and any underlying conditions which predispose to infection. Infections acquired on the general pediatric ward and in the nursery tend to be respiratory and viral in etiology and may be severe.[8] Immunosuppressed patients and patients that are in neonatal or pediatric intensive care units can develop bacterial or fungal infections which may be life-threatening.[9] Ventilatory support, indwelling vascular lines, urinary catheters, and other invasive life-saving procedures and devices increase the likelihood of nosocomial infection. Broad-spectrum antibiotics suppress the normal flora and allow colonization and possibly infection with organisms indigenous to the hospital that are resistant to commonly used antibiotics. Pediatric patients who develop a fever in the hospital present the physician with a dilemma.[10,11] Such infections are often difficult to evaluate and yet because they can be life-threatening, require rapid identification and treatment.

Pathophysiology

Hospital infections may be caused by microorganisms already resident in or on the patient *endogenous* or those acquired from other persons in the hospital or the hospital environment *exogenous.* Endogenous infections tend to occur in children who have illnesses which result in impairment of defense mechanisms such as malignancies or those who are taking immunosuppressive medication. A breach of the body's natural barriers with devices such as indwelling intravascular lines, central nervous system shunts, and urinary catheters can also lead to nosocomial infections caused by the patient's endogenous flora. Infections due to exogenous microorganisms may be acquired from hospital personnel usually by the respiratory route, but also by contact or fomites and reflect patterns of infection in the community or adjacent patients.[12] The most likely source of exogenous flora, however, is hospital personnel who do not adhere to hand-washing and isolation procedures. Exogenous flora may also be introduced as a consequence of a wide variety of procedures performed in the hospital.

A hospital-acquired infection is initiated when a microorganism, either endogenous or exogenous, finds itself in a hospitable environment for multiplication in a patient. Depending upon that patient's ability to respond, there may be no apparent infection, a mild or localized infection, or a disseminated infection. Bacteria and fungi may multiply in tracheostomy tubes, indwelling catheters and neurosurgical shunts and be relatively free of the body's defense mechanisms. Multiple-resistant hospital pathogens may colonize and infect pediatric patients whose normal flora and/or defenses have been suppressed by medication.

Clinical Presentation

The clinical presentation of a hospital-acquired infection depends upon the type of organism, the location, and the underlying status of the patient. Hospital-acquired viral upper respiratory tract infection may be manifested by low-grade fever, rhinorrhea, cough, sputum production, and pharyngitis; whereas hospital acquired Gram-negative septicemia may present as chills, confusion, lethargy and sudden shock. In neonates and prematures, hospital-acquired infection may be manifested by very nonspecific signs and symptoms. An infant that had been previously thermostabile may suddenly manifest temperature swings. The infant may change its feeding habits, become lethargic, irritable, or develop abdominal distension. Often the earliest clue to an acquired infection in an infant or premature is an uneasy feeling on the part of the physician or nurse that the baby is not well. More obvious manifestations of neonatal hospital-acquired infection include jaundice, emesis, diarrhea, shock, convulsion, or coma. In older children, fever may be the only sign of a hospital-acquired infection, and if the patient has a malignancy or is taking immunosuppressant medications, the development of fever in the hospital requires immediate attention and antibiosis. Some hospital-acquired infections may be obvious, such as phlebitis at an intravenous site or infected surgical wound. Noninfectious processes which may cause fever in hospitalized children include drug fevers, transfusion reactions, postsurgical atelectasis, and malignancies.

Diagnosis

The diagnosis of a hospital-acquired infection may be apparent or may require extensive laboratory and radiological investigation. Blood and urine cultures are usually performed in hospitalized children that develop fever. Tachypnea and/or rales heard in auscultation suggest the need for a chest X-ray. A bulging fontanel, lethargy, irritability, and meningismus indicate the need for a lumbar puncture. Stool culture and stool assay for viral pathogens may be indicated if diarrhea is present. If initial laboratory testing fails to reveal the diagnosis and etiology of a hospital-acquired infection, more extensive investigation may be necessary such as radionucleotide scans, specialized radiological procedures, bone marrow aspiration, skin testing, sophisticated culture techniques, biopsies, and serological testing.

Therapy

Therapy of a hospital-acquired infection depends upon the type of infection and the etiology. The acquisition of fever in prematures and immunosuppressed children is an indication for a rapid investigation and the initiation of antibiotics appropriate for potential pathogens. The development of chills, confusion and shock also suggest the need for blood cultures, fluid replacement, and antibiotics directed at the likely causes of septic shock. In many instances no specific therapy is needed or available as in the case of viral upper respiratory infections. Antiviral chemotherapy, if available, may be considered in overwhelming hospital-acquired viral infections. Surgery may be necessary to drain postoperative or wound abscesses or to excise infected veins. Infected indwelling catheters should be removed and replaced. Replacing life lines and neurosurgical shunts may pose a therapeutic dilemma if no other access sites are available. In general, however, antibiotics will not eradicate microorganisms from these devices. Candida may infect patients on broad-spectrum antibiotics, and antifungal therapy may be necessary.

Prognosis

Prognosis in hospital-acquired infections varies from excellent, in respiratory viral infections, to very poor, in hospital-acquired septic shock, and neonatal sepsis which may have up to an 80% mortality. Prognosis can be improved by rapid detection and identification of hospital-acquired infections with the rapid institution of appropriate therapy.

Prevention

Hospital-acquired infections cannot be totally prevented. The proximity of sick children to each other, the likelihood that personnel working in the hospital may acquire infections in the community and bring them into the hospital, and the need for invasive procedures along with the use of antibiotics in patients with infections mean that nosocomial infections will probably always be with us; however, the incidence of such infections can be reduced by proper management of medical equipment, by adherence to isolation and hand-washing techniques, avoiding crowding of patients by replacing urinary and vascular catheters at appropriate intervals, and by a heightened awareness of the situations in which such infections occur and their potential lethality.[13]

Neonatal Sepsis Syndrome

Introduction

The neonatal sepsis syndrome encompasses a constellation of signs and symptoms, rather than a specific entity, suggestive of infection. Case fatality rates range from 20–75%.[14] Due to immature defense mechanisms and lack of immunological experience, the neonate, in particular the premature infant, has a higher incidence of infection than older children, ranging from 1 to 10 per thousand live births.[14,15] Also, infections in neonates are more likely to disseminate. Because of a limited repertoire of responses, the manifestations of infection in the neonate are often subtle and usually do not indicate the organ system involved. Non-infectious processes can lead to a similar symptom complex. Because infection in neonates may disseminate rapidly, it is necessary to obtain appropriate laboratory studies and cultures and initiate broad-spectrum antibiosis as soon as an infection is suspected. Less than half of such investigations yield a pathogen. Only 5–15% of blood cultures obtained as part of an investigation for suspected neonatal sepsis are positive.

Young infants have immature metabolic pathways which prolong the detoxification of antibiotics.[16] In most instances, the usual dose of an antibiotic in these patients is lower and administered less frequently than in older individuals.[16] Certain antibiotics have very specific toxicity for neonates as well. It is sometimes feasible to stop antibiotic therapy when cultures have been negative for 72 hours if the infant has improved rapidly. In other instances, the clinical course or the identification of a specific infection dictates the duration of antibiotic therapy.

Pathophysiology

Several factors contribute to the increased incidence of infections in prematures and neonates. The common bacterial pathogens are acquired from maternal vaginal and fecal flora as well as the nursery environment.[16] Complications of pregnancy such as prolonged rupture of membranes, amnionitis, maternal fever, prematurity, or the use of forceps increase the likelihood of neonatal bacterial infection.[15,16] Any invasive procedures in the hospital such as indwelling urinary or intravascular catheters and ventilatory support increase the likelihood that pathogens will breach natural barriers to infection.[15] Other factors which may increase the likelihood of infection in newborns include the degree of crowding in the nursery, the attention to isolation and hand-washing procedures by hospital personnel, the presence in the nursery of an infected hospital staff person, or inadequate ventilation systems.[7]

Immaturity of the premature and newborn infant's defenses contributes to the likelihood that colonizing organisms will gain access to ordinarily sterile areas and cause localized or disseminated infection. The natural barriers such as the skin and mucous membranes may not be as efficient as in older children and adults.[17] Bowel wall anoxia may allow gastrointestinal flora to invade. Neonates lack specific secretory IgA antibodies which coat the mucous membrane barrier.[18] The umbilicus is a potential avenue from the skin to the circulation. Transplacental maternal IgG provides only partial humoral antibody protection.[15] Some fractions of IgG (particularly IgG 2) and maternal IgM, do not readily pass the placenta.[15] The infant is passively protected against only those pathogens to which the mother has made IgG antibodies. Premature infants may receive only a fraction of the usual transplacental maternal antibodies. The newborn has reduced circulating levels of most components of complement.[15,19] There is recent experimental information suggesting that cord blood contains an excess of suppressor lymphocytes which may be necessary for the fetus to survive *in utero* but may prevent a normal lymphocytic response to infection postnatally.[20] Neonatal T-lymphocytes and macrophages are apparently less able to process antigens for identification by B-lymphocytes and subsequent antibody production.

Phagocytic cells from prematures and neonates are less able to transmigrate vascular walls and are less efficient killers as measured by chemiluminescence.[15,16,21,22] The neutrophil storage pool in neonates dying of sepsis was found to be depleted in one study, implying a limited reserve.[23] These immature defense mechanisms increase the likelihood that infection will occur and, once established, will disseminate rapidly.

The bacteria that cause neonatal septicemia are different from those commonly infecting older children and are acquired during birth or in the nursery. Currently, the most commonly identified neonatal pathogen is the Group B streptococcus *S. agalactae.*[14] Early onset Group B streptococcal septicemia is manifested by an overwhelming systemic infection including pneumonia which mimics the respiratory distress syndrome.[24] This entity is usually seen within the first 48 hours after birth and may be rapidly fatal in spite of the institution of appropriate antibiotic therapy. Early onset Group B streptococcal septicemia has a significant mortality rate. This rate may be declining because the organism may be becoming less virulent, or infection is being recognized and treated earlier.[25] Infants infected later in the postnatal period usually have a localized process such as meningitis, pneumonia, cellulitis or osteomyelitis. The Group B streptococcus is usually susceptible to penicillin or ampicillin. An aminoglycoside may provide a synergistic effect.

The second most common cause of severe infections in neonates is *E. coli.* Serotype K1 is most commonly responsible for life-threatening infections. In one study 80% of *E. coli* meningitis and 40% of *E. coli* septicemia in neonates were caused by the K1 organism.[26] *E. coli* are usually susceptible to an aminoglycoside; however, specific antibiotic sensitivities should dictate the appropriate medication to be used.

Staphylococcus aureus also causes neonatal infections. This organism is usually acquired from nursery personnel. Infection may occur in the spectrum from cutaneous bullae to life-threatening meningitis or sepsis. Other organisms which can cause infections in neonates include *Listeria monocytogenes,*[27] and other streptococci (enterococcus) and Gram-negative enteric bacteria such as klebsiella and pseudomonas.

Clinical Presentation

Nonspecific signs and symptoms herald the neonatal sepsis syndrome. There may only be an uneasy feeling on the part of the nurse or physician that the baby is not well.[16] An infant that was previously thermostabile may demonstrate temperature swings manifested by frequent adjustments of the isolette temperature. The baby may become weak, lethargic, feed poorly, develop apnea, and/or bradycardia spells, or have a change in coloration. More serious signs of neonatal sepsis include abdominal distension, jaundice, shock, convulsion, and coma. Not all infants with these symptoms are infected. Other possible causes include intracranial hemorrhaging, electrolyte imbalances, and pulmonary or cardiac insufficiency. The symptoms usually do not suggest the involved organ system. An infant with tachypnea may have meningitis rather than pneumonia. Convulsions may indicate a urinary tract infection or septicemia rather than a central nervous system infection.

Due to the nonspecificity of signs and symptoms and since bacterial infections may disseminate early, an infant suspected of sepsis should have a rapid investigation including laboratory evaluation of all common sites of infection, and then a broad-spectrum antibiosis should be instituted.[15] Only a fraction of investigations for sepsis yield positive cultures, and many infants are treated for sepsis on clinical grounds.

The diagnostic investigation for suspected neonatal sepsis is a broad one and includes a careful review of maternal history and any maternal cultures; a thorough physical examination; a complete blood count with differential; a blood culture; a urinalysis and urine culture (suprapubic aspiration if possible); a chest roentgenogram and a lumbar puncture. If pneumonia is suspected, a tracheal aspirate may be appropriate. Surface and upper respiratory cultures are not usually helpful. Other roentgenograms and laboratory tests may be suggested by the infant's clinical condition. Certain nonspecific tests for inflammation may help in differentiating a bacterial infection from other conditions causing the signs and symptoms of the neonatal sepsis syndrome. Such tests include c-reactive protein, sedimentation rate, nitroblue tetrazolium test and leukocyte alkaline phosphatase level. Although a positive test is suggestive of a bacterial process, none of these tests have been proven to be specific.[15] Perhaps the most useful laboratory tests include the absolute neutrophil count, absolute band count, immature to total neutrophil ratio and platelet count.[15,28] In one study, neonates surviving septicemia had significant elevated neutrophil counts and band counts, and those who died had neutropenia and thrombocytopenia.[29] Tests for the presence of bacterial antigens in body fluids may also be used in the neonatal sepsis investigation and are diagnostic if positive.[14,30]

Therapy

Antibiotic therapy for neonates suspected of sepsis usually includes a penicillin and an aminoglycoside, most commonly ampicillin and gentamicin.[15] If a staphylococcal infection is suspected, a beta-lactamase resistant penicillin, such as nafcillin or methicillin, may be added or substituted in the antibiotic regimen. Depending upon culture results and sensitivity testing, other antibiotics may be indicated in the treatment of neonatal infections, and rarely an antiviral or antifungal agent may be indicated. Newer penicillins and cephalosporins hold promise in resistant infections.[31] In these latter instances, consultation with an infectious disease expert is suggested. Because of immature metabolic pathways, dosages of antibiotics are reduced in neonates and administered less frequently.[16] Antibiotic serum levels, if available, should be monitored.[16] Treatment for neonatal septicemia is usually administered for at least ten days and may last three weeks or more. If the infant recovers rapidly, antibiotics may be discontinued after 72 hours of therapy if the cultures are negative and no specific infection is identified or if another etiology of the symptoms becomes apparent.

Several adjunctive therapeutic modalities have been suggested as possibly useful in the neonatal sepsis syndrome. These include exchange transfusion, neutrophil transfusion, fresh frozen plasma and pooled immune serum globulin. None of these therapies have been firmly established but may be useful in specific cases.[15] The physician should be aware of complications of neonatal infection such as disseminated intravascular coagulation shock, renal failure and respiratory failure. Prompt recognition of such complications may result in timely institution of life-saving supportive measures.

Certain antibiotics have unique toxic effects in the neonate. The sulfonamides displace bilirubin from albumin binding sites and result in an increased level of free bilirubin.[16] Chloramphenicol administered in usual adult doses results in toxic levels in the neonate and may result in fatal shock (gray baby syndrome).[16] Antibiotic dosages in neonates are adjusted with advancing age.[16] The physician or pharmacist should have access to current pharmacological data when prescribing antibiotics for newborns.

Prognosis

Prognosis in the neonatal sepsis syndrome depends upon the age at onset; the causative organism; the location of the infection; the susceptibility of the organism to antibiotics; and any underlying metabolic, structural or immunological abnormalities of the infant. In general, neonatal sepsis has a 10–20% mortality. The more rapidly subtle signs of neonatal infection are recognized and investigated, and antibiotics started, the more likely there will be a favorable outcome to therapy. However, in some instances, the institution of antibiosis has no effect on the inexorable course of the illness.

Prevention

Although neonatal sepsis cannot be prevented entirely, the incidence can be reduced by avoiding crowding, observing isolation procedures, properly maintaining equipment, and attending to hand-washing.

Septic Shock Syndrome

Introduction

The septic shock syndrome occurs when homeostatic mechanisms are abnormally triggered and unbalanced. The process is usually initiated by infection with a Gram-negative bacteria. Occasionally Gram-positive bacteria, fungi, viruses, and rickettsia may cause the syndrome.[32] Although not fully understood, a combination of bacterial components and toxins causes intravascular activation of the clottting, fibrinolytic, complement and kallikrein systems.[33,34] Activated polymorphonuclear cells release damaging oxidants and enzymes.[35] The net result is peripheral vascular dilation and loss of intravascular fluid into the tissues. Circulatory failure, disseminated intravascular coagulation and multiple organ system failure may ensue.[33,34] Septic shock syndrome usually occurs in those individuals who are susceptible to opportunistic infections. Severely ill patients hospitalized for other reasons are at high risk, particularly those who are neutropenic.[34] Meningococcemia may rapidly progress in a similar fashion.[36,37] Toxic shock syndrome, recently described, also has many features in common with septic shock.[38,39] These two potentially fatal illnesses tend to occur in young and otherwise healthy individuals. Noninfectious causes of shock due to circulatory maldistribution include anaphylaxis, head injury and drugs.[32]

Approximately one in one-hundred hospitalized patients will develop the septic shock syndrome.[34] There is a 20–50% mortality rate.[34] When fully developed, multiple organ system and circulatory failure occur simultaneously, requiring therapy best performed in a sophisticated intensive care unit. Awareness of those factors, which predispose patients to septic shock, as well as the early warning signs of the syndrome will lead to prevention or more rapid diagnosis and earlier treatment.

Pathophysiology

The candidate endotoxin is the lipid A portion of the outer cell layer of Gram-negative bacteria.[33,34] Lipid A when injected into animals causes many but not all of the changes seen in septic shock.[33,34] However, since Gram-positive bacteria and other microorganisms can occasionally cause septic shock, other cellular components or toxins may also have a causative role.

Circulating endotoxin causes intravascular activation of Hageman factor (XII) which in turn initiates the coagulation and fibrinolytic cascades with the consumption of clotting factors resulting in disseminated intravascular coagulation (DIC).[40] Abnormal bleeding may occur. In addition, the complement cascade is activated resulting in the release of chemotactic factors, neutrophil activating factors and mediators of inflammation which cause vascular dilation and leak of intravascular fluid into the interstitium.[34,35] The activated neutrophils aggregate in the microvasculature causing obstruction to blood flow and additional vascular damage.[41] Activated neutrophils release oxidants and enzymes that further damage tissues and vascular endothelium.[35] Damaged endothelium results in platelet aggregation and contributes to disseminated intravascular coagulation. Thrombocytopenia is often an early sign of DIC.[40] Activated Hageman factor also triggers the kallikrein-kinin system resulting in the release of bradykinin which causes peripheral vasodilation, peripheral vascular pooling, and vascular damage with loss of intravascular fluid into the tissues.[34]

Initially, in the course of septic shock, the patient manifests an increased heart rate and peripheral vasodilation without an actual drop in blood pressure. This stage is called compensated or "warm shock."[32,33,34,42] Later, as peripheral vasodilation increases and fluid is lost into the tissues, there is impairment of blood return to the heart. The patient becomes hypotensive. There is peripheral vasoconstriction, and the patient appears to be cold and cyanotic. This stage is called uncompensated or "cold shock." It is far more difficult to treat and may be irreversible.[32,33,34,42] Hypoxic, undercirculated tissues, particularly striated muscle, initiate anaerobic metabolism with lactate as an end product resulting in metabolic acidosis.[32,34,42] Endotoxin or anoxia may also have a suppressant effect on the myocardium so that the overall picture is one of peripheral vascular pooling, loss of intravascular fluid into the interstitium, acidosis and decreased blood return to a possibly inefficient heart.

There is the potential for multiple organ system involvement.[32,33,34] Aggregates of platelets and activated neutrophils in the pulmonary microvasculature lead to diminished pulmonary blood flow, vascular damage, and leak of intravascular fluid into the alveoli and intraalveolar spaces resulting in pulmonary edema (adult respiratory distress syndrome or shock lung).[43] Diminished oxygenation because of pulmonary edema results in even further reduction in delivery of oxygen to tissues. Respiratory failure may result. Hypovolemia may lead to pre-renal azotemia. Shock may lead to acute tubular necrosis and renal failure.[32,34] Hepatic function may be affected, possibly due to a direct effect endotoxin or undercirculation with hepatocellular damage.[44] Acidosis and hypoxemia may affect central nervous system functioning. Cerebral edema may be present.[44]

In meningococcemia, there is vascular damage due to microseptic emboli causing bleeding into the skin and other sites. These areas are extended as further embolization takes place and disseminated intravascular coagulation occurs.[36] Meningitis may accompany meningococcemia.[36] In addition, there may be bleeding into the adrenal glands (Waterhouse-Friderichsen Syndrome) resulting in fatal shock.[36] The toxic shock syndrome is quite similar to septic shock but is due to a toxin produced by *Staphylococcus aureus*.[45,46] There may be hypotension and multiple organ system failure.[38,39]

Clinical Presentation

The patient with septic shock syndrome is often already hospitalized for other reasons.[34] Underlying conditions which predispose children to Gram-negative bacterial septicemia and shock include immunodeficiency syndromes, immunosuppressive medication, malignancies, prematurity, structural defects, asplenia, neutropenia, burns, indwelling catheters and surgery. Although fever is a usual concomitant of endotoxemia, some patients, particularly neonates, become hypothermic.[33,34] Bed-shaking chills are described as a premonitory sign of Gram-negative septic shock. The child may act scared or confused or become agitated. Neonates may display abdominal distension, decreased feeding and apnea-bradycardia spells. Older children may have tachycardia, tachypnea, mild hypotension, neutropenia, thrombocytopenia, and mild acidosis.[34] These rather soft signs should alert the physician to an impending septic shock syndrome. The patient may have a "toxic appearance" with a blank apathetic facies, relative inactivity, and inattention to his surroundings. Children with meningococcemia may have petechiae on the skin, conjunctivae and mucus membranes.[36] A febrile, toxic appearing child should be totally undressed for examination of all areas of skin. Patients with the toxic shock syndrome may have a diffuse erythematous flush as well as a toxic appearance and hypotension.[38,39] Fainting or dizziness may herald the toxic shock syndrome.

Diagnosis

The diagnosis of early septic shock syndrome is based upon clinical presentation. Symptoms such as hypothermia, confusion, tachycardia, and tachypnea in patients with high-risk underlying conditions should be enough to suggest that early intervention is necessary. Since the process may be rapidly fatal, therapy must be initiated before the etiologic agent is known; however, appropriate cultures should be obtained prior to the institution of specific antibiotic therapy. Two to three blood cultures, if possible, should be obtained quickly when septic shock is suspected. The following initial laboratory tests are usually appropriate: urinalysis and urine culture, chest roentgenogram, culture of other sites, abdominal scans and lumbar puncture. A gram stain of urine or spinal fluid may reveal the causative organism. In meningococcemia, the organisms may be seen in smears from petechiae which have been scraped with a surgical blade so that serum exudes. A glass slide is then touched to the serum, allowed to dry and either stained with methylene blue or gram stain. The small diplococci will be found in inflammatory cells. Rapid diagnostic techniques may identify some pathogens before cultures are available.[4,5] The bacteriology laboratory should be asked to save causative organisms for possible determination of minimal bactericidal and inhibitory titers to various antibiotics. In postpubescent women who present with an erythematous flush and hypotension, a vaginal culture should also be obtained along with a menstrual history, and a history of the use of vaginal tampons.[39] Toxic shock syndrome can also occur in children and males although less frequently.[38,47] Staphylococci causing toxic shock may be submitted to a reference laboratory for assay for toxin production. A gallium scan may reveal an obscure focus of inflammation in patients with no obvious source for septicemia. Special attention should be directed to any organ system which has an anomalous structure.

Treatment

Treatment should be instituted as soon as septic shock is suspected. Rapid decisive therapy may prevent progression to irreversible shock and death.[34,44] Treatment and supportive measures for diminished function of many organ systems may be necessary simultaneously.[34,44] Such patients are appropriately monitored and cared for in an intensive care unit.[44] Frequent measurement of vital signs and electronic monitoring of cardiac and respiratory function as well as accurate tabulation of intake and output are necessary. Intervals between measurements can be increased as the patient improves. Most patients with septic shock syndrome also require an indwelling arterial catheter for blood gas determinations and either a central venous pressure or Swan-Ganz catheter in order to direct fluid replacement therapy and monitor cardiac and pulmonary function.[33,34,44] An indwelling urinary catheter to follow output and response to medications may also be indicated.[44] The frequency of various laboratory tests is dependent upon the severity of the patient's illness.

All organ systems which can be potentially involved in the toxic shock syndrome should be evaluated for normal functioning at appropriate intervals. Urinalysis as well as creatinine and blood urea nitrogen determinations should be followed to determine adequate renal functioning. Pre-renal azotemia should be differentiated from that due to acute tubular necrosis. It may be necessary to measure serum and urine osmolalities. Tests of clotting mechanism status such as the prothrombin time, partial thromboplastin time, fibrin degradation products, and platelet counts will help to determine the presence and degree of intravascular coagulation. Blood gases, preferably arterial in origin, should be measured to indicate the presence of acidosis and hypoxemia and as an indication of pulmonary function. Frequent determinations of serum electrolytes such as sodium and potassium will allow appropriate monitoring of fluid replacement therapy. It may also be necessary to measure calcium and phosphorus and magnesium as these ions can be deficient in septic shock syndrome. Tests of liver function may be necessary at intervals. If possible, the patient should be weighed daily. Indwelling catheters, vascular and urinary, as well as prostheses made of plastic or metal, and neurological shunts should be suspected as a possible cause of septicemia and should be cultured and probably removed if found to be infected.

Antibiotic therapy appropriate for suspected bacterial pathogens should be started after the initial cultures and laboratory tests. Physicians should be aware of the more common hospital "flora" and those organisms which are prevalent in their community.[34] This information will aid in the initial choice of antibiotics. In most instances, septic shock syndrome is due to Gram-negative enteric organisms for which an aminoglycoside or a newer penicillin or cephalosporin is indicated. If staphylococcus is suspected as in the toxic shock syndrome, an anti-staphylococcal penicillin should be included in the initial therapy. The meningococcus is susceptible to penicillin and ampicillin. When sepsis arises from either pelvic or gastrointestinal sources, anaerobic bacteria may be responsible and chloramphenicol, clindamycin or cefoxitin, which have broad antianaerobic spectra may be indicated. Usually in patients who do not have an obvious source for sepsis, an aminoglycoside and a penicillin are used until antibiotic susceptibilities are available to more specifically direct therapy.

The objective of fluid replacement therapy for septic shock is restoration of the functional intravascular volume.[34,44] Ordinarily, this is done with either central venous or Swan-Ganz pressure monitoring. A series of fluid challenges is administered intravenously depending upon the degree of shock, renal function, and cerebral edema. Each challenge usually is 10–20 cc per kilogram and is administered over one to two hours.[44] Response to intravenous fluid replacement is measured by affect on blood pressure, central venous pressure and urinary output. The goal of fluid therapy is to restore intravascular volume and resolve hypotension without fluid overload and cardiac failure.[44] The patient's maintenance fluid requirements should not be overlooked. The presence of cerebral edema, renal failure, pulmonary edema or cardiac failure affects fluid replacement therapy and may necessitate the use of diuretics and peripheral vasoconstrictive drugs.

Depending upon the degree of shock and "vascular leak," initial intravenous fluid replacement therapy may be either colloid or crystalloid. If a crystalloid solution is used, it should be isotonic.[44] Hypotonic solutions will not be useful in the treatment of septic shock. Since there may be hepatic dysfunction impairing the metabolism of lactate, it is probably more appropriate to use sodium chloride rather than sodium lactate in the initial fluid management.[44] If the patient is anemic, fresh whole blood is indicated and also may supply needed clotting factors. Albumin, usually a 5% solution, or fresh frozen plasma which also contains clotting factors may be used as a colloid source to reconstitute functional intravascular volume. If there is a significant loss of protein from the vascular space, continued use of albumin intravenously may contribute to the accumulation of edema fluid. Usually colloid and crystalloid solutions are utilized during fluid replacement therapy. It may take several days to several weeks for fluid lost into the interstitium to be mobilized as manifested by diuresis and loss of weight.[44]

Although restoration of intravascular volume usually results in resolution of metabolic acidosis, patients with severe acidosis may require the administration of sodium bicarbonate especially if arterial blood pH is less than 7.20.[44] Persistent acidosis may adversely affect the action of medications as well as depress myocardial function and cause dysrhythmias. Sodium bicarbonate is used at the dosage of 1–2 mEq per kilogram with subsequent doses based on body weight and base deficit. Once arterial pH is greater than 7.25 to 7.30, bicarbonate infusions are usually no longer necessary.[44] It may also be necessary to replace calcium, magnesium or phosphorus ions if deficiencies are identified. Hypocalcemia can result in depressed myocardial function, tachycardia, hypotension, acidosis, and alterations in mental status.[44] Phosphate deficiency can cause respiratory failure, myocardial damage, diminished phagocytosis, platelet dysfunction, hepatocellular damage and neurologic abnormalities.[44] Restoration of calcium, phosphorus or magnesium deficiencies should be done with care as rapid administration or excess can be harmful.

Patients with mild degrees of hypoxemia will benefit from oxygen administration. Patients with hypoxemia, hypercarbia, or respiratory failure may require ventilatory support. On occasion, neuromuscular blocking agents are necessary for agitated patients needing assisted ventilation. Respiratory therapy may range from continuous positive airway pressure to full ventilatory support. Positive end expiratory pressure may be useful in patients with pulmonary edema, but excessive pressures can result in pulmonary damage.[44] Monitoring of blood gases and continual adjustment of the ventilator are often necessary to maintain optimal oxygenation and carbon dioxide levels. Excessive pressures and oxygen can damage lungs, further contributing to respiratory difficulties.

Judicious use of diuretics such as furosemide and mannitol may be useful in patients with pre-renal azotemia, pulmonary edema, cerebral edema or cardiac failure. Diuretic agents and osmotic diuretics should not be used in the presence of renal failure. If renal failure is present, dialysis may be necessary, usually by the peritoneal route. Dosages of antibiotics and other medications may need to be adjusted depending upon the degree of renal impairment.

The presence of disseminated intravascular coagulation indicates the need for replacement of circulating clotting factors. Vitamin K may be useful with intact hepatic function. Platelet transfusions and fresh frozen plasma supply needed clotting components. Therapy is determined by following clotting function tests. In general, heparin therapy for disseminated intravascular coagulation has little beneficial effect and is potentially dangerous.[48,49] However, some experts recommend its use in the face of extensive purpuric lesions.[48] It is probably safer to use heparin as a continuous infusion. Clotting time should not exceed 20 minutes when heparin is used.

If blood pressure cannot be restored by crystalloid or colloid infusions, or cardiac failure ensues, or there is an unacceptable rise in the central venous pressure, drugs which increase myocardial contractility or peripheral vascular tone are indicated. Medications usually used in this situation include isuprel and dopamine. Isuprel may divert cardiac output to noncritical tissues such as skeletal muscle and contribute to dysrhythmias, although it does have inotropic and chronotropic effects.[44] Dopamine is usually the drug of choice. At lower doses, (5 to 10 micrograms/kg/min) it stimulates cardiac beta receptors and causes a selective dilation of renal and mesenteric beds allowing blood flow to vital organs while constricting vasculature elsewhere.[44] Higher doses may be harmful as renal blood flow may be compromised and pulmonary vascular resistance increased. Digitalis glycosides have a rather delayed onset of activity and although they may augment myocardial contractility, there may be a reflex peripheral vaso-constriction which negates the effect of the medication.[44] The myocardium in septic shock may be particularly sensitive to digitalis resulting in dysrhythmias at, ordinarily, therapeutic dosages. Choice of medications to affect cardiac functioning and peripheral vascular tone will depend upon knowledge of their pharmacological actions and the patient's cardiovascular status.[44]

Although somewhat controversial, the use of corticosteroids is probably indicated in the septic shock syndrome.[50] The earlier steroids are used, the more likely they will have a beneficial effect. Steroids stabilize the polymorphonuclear cell membrane preventing the release of lysosomal contents into the environment and also block the effect of complement fraction 5a which activates neutrophils.[51] Corticosteroids may also, to a certain extent, stabilize the microvasculature preventing bleeding and capillary leak.[34] Steroids such as hydrocortisone or decadron should be used in very high doses for no longer than 72 hours.[44,50]

Animal experimentation suggests that endorphins may have a role in septic shock that can be reversed with opiate antagonists.[52] In one study, Naloxone, a narcotic antagonist was shown to have a beneficial effect on hypotension in patients with septic shock.[53] This observation requires substantiation before Naloxone can be accepted as routine therapy in the treatment of septic shock. A human antiserum has been developed by immunizing volunteers with heat killed *E. Coli* J5, a mutant organism with an exposed core. This antiserum also holds promise in the treatment of septic shock syndrome.[54]

Patients with septic shock syndrome require many days of intensive care and often weeks of hospitalization. In the rush to provide intensive medical and supportive care, the patient's nutritional requirements may be overlooked. Without adequate nutritional support repair of damaged organs cannot take place. Parenteral nutrition should be administered when the patient cannot take food orally.

Prevention

There is probably no way to prevent the septic shock syndrome which occurs in patients who are at home or those who develop meningococcemia. Parents of children who are at high risk should be warned of the early signs of the septic shock syndrome so that they may rapidly seek medical care in the hopes of preventing progression to the later stages of the process. Patients in the hospital who are at risk for septic shock syndrome should be identified. Careful attention should be paid to medical devices which are used to support life and yet may provide a source for access of endogenous and exogenous bacteria. Aseptic techniques should be used for management of urinary and intravascular catheters. Catheters should be replaced at regular intervals and cultured should the patient develop fever. The physician should be aware of the resistance patterns of bacteria isolated in the hospital. Careful attention should be paid to proper care and sterilization of equipment. It may be necessary to periodically culture high-risk patients and equipment used to care for them.[34] The physician should be aware of the premonitory signs of septic shock syndrome, as the more rapidly the process is identified and therapy initiated the better the prognosis.

Pneumonia

Introduction

Pneumonia in childhood has a multitude of causes, infectious and noninfectious. Most pneumonia in children is caused by viruses and can be managed in an ambulatory setting.[55] Only a small fraction of children with pneumonia require intensive care. Intensive care is more likely to be necessary for pneumonia occurring in infants and immunosuppressed children. Because of the wide variety of causes and the likelihood that respiratory culture will be contaminated by oropharyngeal flora, it is often difficult to establish an etiology in childhood pneumonia. Clinical features such as geographic history, underlying illnesses, presenting signs and symptoms and chest roentgenogram findings[55,66] may help to differentiate pneumonias with varying causes. Since treatment varies significantly with the etiology of pneumonia, and unnecessary antibiotic therapy may result in secondary opportunistic infections by hospital pathogens, an attempt should be made to identify the cause of pneumonia in hospitalized children in advance of initiating therapy. Intensive care for infants and children with pneumonia is required when respiratory function is severely compromised irrespective of the cause. Pneumonia may occur in patients hospitalized for other reasons. Patients with communicable pneumonias are appropriately isolated from other patients in the intensive care unit.

Pathophysiology

The lung and tracheobronchial tree are usually sterile. Pneumonia or inflammation of the lung occurs when infectious or toxic agents gain access to the lung by inhalation, aspiration, or hematogenous dissemination. In the event that local defenses are unable to clear the lung, infection and an inflammatory response ensues.[56] The type and rapidity of inflammatory changes, edema or purulent exudate are pathogen and host dependent. There may be predominant involvement of the interalveolar spaces, the interstitium or the bronchioli. The pneumonia may be confined to a specific area of the lung, contiguous areas or may involve all lobes. Edema fluid or pus obstructs respiratory passages or aveoli, reducing air exchange and surface area for gas transport. Lung necrosis may occur. Noninfectious pneumonias include but are not limited to those resulting from aspiration of gastric content, aspiration of toxic agents such as hydrocarbons, inhalation of noxious fumes, aspiration of a foreign body,[55] or hypersensitivity pneumonia.[57] Children with underlying lung disease such as cystic fibrosis or asthma are susceptible to pneumonias and have less pulmonary reserve function.

Once infection is established, it may spread to adjacent portions of the lung secondarily, via the pores of Kohn or by destruction of tissue with local extension.[56] Infectious agents may enter the blood stream or lymphatic system and spread to other areas of the lungs or to distant foci. Bacterial infections may extend to the pleural space with concomitant pleural exudation or empyema. Tuberculosis and malignancies may cause a pleural exudate without empyema formation. Aspiration of oral anaerobic bacteria or a foreign body may lead to a pulmonary abscess. Certain pyogenic bacteria such as staphylococci and klebsiella can also cause pulmonary abscesses.[55,58]

If the infectious process causes bronchiolar wall edema, the resultant inhibition of air flow may lead to severe respiratory distress. Inspiratory and expiratory wheezing as well as air trapping are found. This process (bronchiolitis) is almost always viral and occurs in infants.[55] Infectious processes within the lung may result in ventilation perfusion defects and pulmonary vascular shunting leading to hypoxemia and hypercarbia. Tachypnea and increased respiratory effort may cause fatigue. In viral pneumonias there may be air trapping with hyperexpansion whereas in bacterial pneumonias the alveoli are filled with purulent exudate and there is often loss of volume.[55] Inappropriate secretion of antidiuretic hormone has been reported in infants with respiratory infections.[59]

Clinical Presentation

The clinical characteristics of childhood pneumonia vary depending upon the age of the child and the cause for the pneumonia. In older children tachypnea is usually present; fever and cough may or may not be present. Chills, malaise, headache, chest pain, and abdominal pain may also be noted.[56] The child may complain of breathlessness or pain on inspiration. Occasionally, infants with pneumonia may not manifest tachypnea; however, they will usually demonstrate nonspecific signs of infection such as fever, hypothermia, decreased activity, poor feeding, abdominal distension, or apnea-bradycardia spells. Sputum production will not be seen in infants and is quite variable in older children.

Depending upon the type and extent of pneumonia, physical findings may differ; however, in most older children, rales will be present on auscultation. Bronchial breath sounds, dullness to percussion, splinting of the chest, and increased vocal fremitus may also be present.[56] Small infants with pneumonia may not have characteristic auscultatory findings. In young infants who have bronchiolitis or who have aspirated a foreign body, inspiratory and expiratory wheezing may be associated with respiratory distress and cough. In severe pneumonias, the child demonstrates air hunger, use of accessory respiratory muscles, retractions, nasal flaring and cyanosis.

Diagnosis

The diagnosis of pneumonia is usually established by the identification of pulmonary infiltrates on a chest roentgenogram. Pulmonary infiltrates may be delayed 12 to 24 hours in patients with pneumonia who are severely dehydrated or who have aspirated hydrocarbons.[55] The pattern of infiltration may aid in the differentiation of the type of pneumonia.[55] The chest roentgenogram should also be examined for pleural effusion, pneumatocoeles, abscesses, cavities and hyperinflation. In patients that are to be hospitalized for pneumonia, the initial laboratory investigation should include a chest roentgenogram, a blood culture, a complete blood count with differential, and an attempt at a respiratory culture. Most initial pediatric sputum cultures will be obtained in such a way as to be contaminated by oropharyngeal flora. The degree to which contamination occurs will determine the usefulness of the culture with respect to establishing an infectious etiologic agent or agents.[60,61] Depending upon the situation, other laboratory tests which may be obtained include skin tests for tuberculosis and fungi, acute serological tests for fungi and viruses, and testing of sputum or urine by counterimmunoelectrophoresis or other means of identifying specific bacterial antigens.[62]

Respiratory cultures are often difficult to obtain in infants and children. There is little likelihood of obtaining sputum on command, and cultures are obtained through the oropharynx. Sputum obtained by expectoration or through a Leukens trap aspirate may provide useful information depending upon the degree of contamination by upper respiratory flora. A system for classifying sputum specimens based upon the number of polymorphonuclear cells they contain per high power field as compared to the number of epithelial cells is used.[60,61] Epithelial cells are indicative of upper respiratory contamination. Most laboratories will not culture specimens which contain an untoward number of epithelial cells. However, if there is a predominance of polymorphonuclear cells, alveolar macrophages and a prominent organism on gram stain the culture may reveal a bacterial pathogen.[56,60] Sputum specimens may also be cultured for mycobacteria and fungi as well as chlamydia and viruses. Sputum or upper respiratory cultures for viruses may be indicated in pneumonia if there is the possibility of response to antiviral chemotherapy or where useful epidemiological information may be gained, as in hospital outbreaks.

In hospitalized infants and children with pneumonia, it may not be possible to identify the cause by either blood or sputum cultures. The physician must then make a decision as to the necessity of using more invasive diagnostic procedures. This decision will depend upon the type of pneumonia, the clinical course, and the age of the child. Bronchoscopy, using a fiber-optic bronchoscope, is a useful technique for acquiring respiratory cultures in children although pharyngeal contamination of the specimen may occur.[63]

Cultures can be obtained by instillation and aspiration of sterile nonbacteriostatic saline, collection of purulent drainage in the bronchi, bronchial brushings or a bronchial culture with a protected catheter. The latter method appears to incur the least oropharyngeal contamination.[64] Transtracheal aspiration has limited usefulness in children; however, in older children it may be attempted by a person expert in the procedure if it is deemed necessary to establish a diagnosis. This procedure avoids oral contamination and allows for anaerobic cultures. Transthoracic aspiration of the lung using a syringe with nonbacteriostatic saline and a 21 or 22 gauge needle may be useful in children who have pneumonias which can be reached with a needle.[55] The procedure may be done under fluoroscopic control. In one large series, there were minimal side effects, and the procedure was more useful than sputum analysis for establishing the diagnosis of cryptic pneumonias.[65] Bleeding and pneumothorax are occasional complications of percutaneous lung puncture. Lung biopsy, drainage of an abscess or removal of a foreign body can be performed through a bronchoscope. Percutaneous lung biopsies have a high incidence of complications and probably should not be obtained in children. If the etiology of pneumonia cannot be established by other means and the patient's condition is deteriorating, an open lung biopsy will provide sufficient material for diagnosis, in most cases, and allow for pathological examination from an area which can be ascertained to be involved visually at the time of biopsy.[56] This procedure does incur the risk of anesthesia and an open surgical procedure in a severely ill child.

In pneumococcal pneumonia, which is the most common bacterial pneumonia seen in children, there is often a consolidated lobe, high temperature, high white count with left shift and a toxic appearing patient. Pneumonia due to klebsiella also causes a consolidated process usually of an upper lobe. The upper lobe fissure may bulge into the middle lobe and there may be abscess formation. Pneumonia due to *Staphylococcus aureus* usually progresses rapidly with consolidation and the formation of pneumatocoeles and pleural empyema.[55] Pneumonia due to group A streptococci is rare in children. This is also a rapidly progressive pneumonia, usually with pleural effusion present.[67] Pneumonia due to Gram-negative enteric bacteria usually occurs in immunosuppressed children. There is usually consolidation and pleural empyema. In pneumonia due to *Hemophilus influenzae* type b, the accumulation of pleural empyema, if it occurs, is usually slower.[66] The presence of pleural effusion gives the physician the opportunity to aspirate the pleural space to improve respiratory function and culture the causative agent.[55] Tuberculosis may also cause a consolidated pneumonia in young children. There may or may not be a pleural exudate. Ipsilateral hilar adenopathy may provide a clue to a tuberculous or fungal etiology. Children who have aspirated foreign bodies may also have consolidated pneumonia usually behind the obstructed bronchus and there may be abscess formation. The presence of a foreign body may be ascertained by mediastinal shift when comparing inspiratory and expiratory chest roentgenograms, but this is often difficult in children. Bronchopneumonia (diffuse) may be caused by a wide variety of organisms and noninfectious causes, and if necessary, the diagnosis may have to be established by sophisticated cultures serological techniques and invasive procedures as outlined above. Peribronchial infiltrates and pulmonary hyperexpansion suggest bronchiolitis.[55]

Severe nonbacterial pneumonias may occur in children, primarily infants, and those who are immunosuppressed. Viral agents which may cause such pneumonias include, but are not limited to, respiratory syncytial virus,[68] adenovirus,[55] cytomegalovirus,[69] and herpes virus.[70] *Chlamydia trachomatis* has recently been described as causing a pneumonitis syndrome in young infants. There is a bronchopneumonia pattern on chest roentgenogram associated with a staccato, paroxysmal cough and peripheral eosinophilia.[71] Fifty percent of such infants will have had inclusion conjunctivitis. Immunosuppressed patients may have fatal pneumonias as a consequence of dissemination of common childhood viruses such as varicella or rubeola. Other nonbacterial agents which can cause pneumonia in this group of patients include *Pneumocystis carinii.* The diagnosis of this pneumonia is established by bronchial brushings or biopsy via bronchoscope or lung biopsy. Rarely, pneumonia in children will be caused by tuberculosis or deep mycoses such as coccidioidomycosis or histoplasmosis. *Candida albicans* may cause an opportunistic pneumonia in children on broad-spectrum antibiotics. Hospitalized children may also suffer pneumonia from opportunistic antibiotic-resistant Gram-negative enteric organisms such pseudomonas and serratia. Very rarely, pneumonia due to brucellosis, tularemia, plague and legionnaire's disease will be seen in children.[56,77]

Treatment

An infant or child with pneumonia requires intensive care because a respiratory function is compromised to the point that supportive measures are needed. Depending upon the degree of fatigue and derangement of blood gas measurements, the patient may require only supplemental oxygen. Ventilatory support may be necessary when hypoxemia, hypercarbia or fatigue are present. In infants with bronchiolitis, cold mist and oxygen are often all that is necessary. Vital signs, blood gas determinations and serum electrolytes should be monitored at intervals commensurate with the severity of the illness. Patients with pneumonia and tachypnea have a greater than usual insensible water loss which should be taken into account when calculating fluid replacement therapy. Pleural empyema may require chest tube placement. Rarely, infants with severe pneumonia may have inappropriate antidiuretic hormone secretion in which case fluid restriction is necessary.[59]

Specific anti-infective treatment will depend upon the etiology of the pneumonia. Prior to the availability of cultures the choice of antibiotics depends on clinical features. Pneumococcal pneumonia is most appropriately treated with penicillin or ampicillin. Penicillin-resistant strains of pneumococcus have rarely been encountered in the United States. Staphylococcal pneumonia requires an antistaphylococcal penicillin such as nafcillin or methicillin. It may be necessary to treat the patient intravenously for four to six weeks as this pneumonia is usually slow to resolve. In *Hemophilus influenzae* pneumonia, ampicillin is usually used unless the organism is found to produce beta-lactamase in which case chloramphenicol is appropriate. For opportunistic Gram-negative bacterial infections, an aminoglycoside should be part of the antibiotic regimen which can then be modified as the organism is identified and antibiotic susceptibilities become available.

Trimethoprim-sulfamethoxazole is the drug of choice in *Pneumocystis carinii* infections. Chlamydial pneumonia or rarely legionnaire's agent pneumonia will require erythromycin therapy. Specific antiviral chemotherapy such as acyclovir or adenosine arabinoside may be considered in opportunistic and neonatal viral pneumonias due to herpes and possibly varicella or cytomegalovirus. Tuberculous pneumonia is treated with antimycobacterial agents, and fungal pneumonia with amphotericin B. Often in severe viral pneumonias only supportive care is available and antibiotics may lead to opportunistic superinfection.

Prevention

Pneumonia, in otherwise healthy children, acquired in the community is difficult to prevent. However, pneumonia in neonates and other hospitalized children may, to a certain extent, be prevented by proper sterilization of respiratory devices and attention to hand-washing and aseptic technique.

Conclusion

Infections in children may, on occasion, be severe enough to require intensive care. Those infections discussed in this chapter may be illustrative of principles common to the intensive care of all children with infections. Infections in children whom require intensive care may be communicable and in an effort to provide comprehensive expert management, the physician must not overlook the necessity for isolation. Often, many physician specialists and paramedical personnel will be involved in the care of such children. It is usually appropriate that the patient's pediatrician or an intensivist assume primary responsibility for the management of the patient and coordinate the recommendations of consultants in light of his perceptions of the patient's condition and clinical progress. Examples of specialists who may help in the intensive care management of children with infections include pediatric intensivists, pulmonologists, infectious disease specialists, surgeons, nephrologists, hematologists, pharmacologists, respiratory therapists, and skilled intensive care nurses. The responsible physician should coordinate the efforts of all these individuals for a coherent unified approach to patient management.

It may be appropriate to transfer certain types of infectious patients to more sophisticated medical facilities for more skilled intensive care. In some patients whose infections cannot be treated primarily, supportive care is all that can be offered. A physician caring for an intensively ill child with infection should be aware of the potential effects on organ systems and body functions not primarily involved in the infectious process. Antibiotics are certainly necessary for some infections. Antimicrobial therapy should be based upon the likely infectious agents and therapy should be modified as new information as to etiologic agent and drug susceptibilities become available. Broad-spectrum antibiotics used in the intensive care unit may lead to invasion and secondary infection by opportunistic resistant hospital organisms.

References

1. Greene GR: Management of the child with fever and infection. *Top Emerg Med* 3:19–42, 1981.
2. McCarthy PL, Jekel JF, Stashwick CA, et al: History and observation variables in assessing febrile children. *Pediatrics* 65:1090–1095, 1980.
3. Naiman HL, Albritton WL: Counterimmunoelectrophoresis in the diagnosis of acute infection. *J Infect Dis* 142:524–531, 1980.
4. Daum RS, Siber GR, Kamon JS, et al: Evaluation of a commercial Latex particle agglutination test for rapid diagnosis of Haemophilus influenzae type B infection. *Pediatrics* 69:466–471, 1982.
5. Kaplan SL, Feigin RD: Rapid identification of the invading microorganism. *Pediatr Clin North Am* 27:783–803, 1980.
6. Maguire GC, Nordin J, Myers MG, et al: Infections acquired by young infants. *Am J Dis Child* 135:693–698, 1981.
7. Hemming VG, Overall JC, Britt MR: Nosocomial infections in a newborn intensive care unit. *N Engl J Med* 294:1310–1316, 1976.
8. Hall CB: Nosocomial viral respiratory infections: Perennial weeds on pediatric wards. *Am J Med* 70:670–676, 1981.
9. Young LS: Infection in the compromised host. *Hosp Pract* 16:73–84, 1981.
10. Konerding K, Moffet HL: New episodes of fever in hospitalized children. *Am J Dis Child* 120:515–519, 1970.
11. Bornstein DL: Fevers of nosocomial origin. *J of Med* 11:275–292, 1980.
12. Valenti WM, Clarke TA, Hall CB, et al: Concurrent outbreaks of rhinovirus and respiratory syncytial virus in an intensive care nursery: Epidemiology and associated risk factors. *J Pediatr* 100:722–726, 1982.
13. Baker CJ: Nosocomial septicemia and meningitis in neonates. *Am J Med* 70:698–701, 1981.
14. Siegel JD, McCracken GH Jr: Sepsis neonatorum. *N Engl J Med* 304:642–647, 1981.
15. Wasserman RL: Neonatal sepsis: The potential of granulocyte transfusion. *Hosp Pract* 17:95–104, 1982.

16. Yaffe SJ: Antimicrobial therapy and the neonate. *Obstet Gynecol* 58:85–93 (Suppl), 1981.
17. Gotoff SP: Neonatal immunity. *J Pediatr* 85:149–154, 1974.
18. Ogra PL: Ontogeny of the local immune system. *Pediatrics* 64:765–774, 1979.
19. Johnston Jr RB, Altenburger KM, Atkinson Jr AW, et al: Complement in the newborn infant. *Pediatrics* 64:781–786, 1979.
20. Stites DP, Pavia CS: Ontogeny of human T cells. *Pediatrics* 64:795–802, 1979.
21. Mills EL, Thompson T, Bjorksten B, et al: The chemiluminescence response and bactericidal activity of polymorphonuclear neutrophils from newborns and their mothers. *Pediatrics.* 63:429–434, 1979.
22. Miller ME: Phagocyte function in the neonate: Selected aspects. *Pediatrics* 64:709–712, 1979.
23. Christensen RD, Rothstein G: Exhaustion of mature marrow neutrophils in neonates with sepsis. *J Pediatr* 96:316–318, 1980.
24. Ablow RC, Driscoll SG, Effman EL, et al: A comparison of early-onset group B streptococcal neonatal infection and the respiratory-distress syndrome of the newborn. *N Engl J Med* 294:65–70, 1976.
25. Freedman RM, Ingram DL, Gross I, et al: A half century of neonatal sepsis at Yale. *Am J Dis Child* 135:140–144, 1981.
26. McCracken Jr GH, Glode MP, Sarff LD, et al: Between escherichia coli k1 capsular polysaccharide antigen and clinical outcome in neonatal meningitis. *Lancet* 2:246–250, 1974.
27. Halliday HL, Hirata T: Perinatal listeriosis: A review of twelve patients. *Am J Obstet Gynecol* 133:405–410, 1979.
28. Boyle RJ, Chandler BD, Stonestreet BS, et al: Early identification of sepsis in infants with respiratory distress. *Pediatrics* 62:744–750, 1978.
29. Squire E, Favara B, Todd J: Diagnosis of neonatal bacterial infection: Hematologic and pathologic findings in fatal and nonfatal cases. *Pediatrics* 64:60–64, 1979.
30. Baker CJ, Webb BJ, Jackson CV, et al: Countercurrent immunoelectrophoresis in the evaluation of infants with group B streptococcal disease. *Pediatrics* 65:1110–1114, 1980.
31. Kafetzis DA, Brater DC, Kapiki AN, et al: Treatment of severe neonatal infections with cefotaxime. Efficacy and pharmacokinetics. *J Pediatr* 100:483–489, 1982.
32. Perkin RM, Levin DL: Shock in the pediatric patient. Part I. *J Pediatr* 101:163–169, 1982.
33. Hodes HL: Care of the critically ill child: Endotoxin shock. *Pediatrics* 44:248–260, 1969.
34. *Septic Shock.* The Upjohn Company, Kalamazoo, Michigan, 1977.
35. Weissmann G, Smolen JE, Korchak HM: Release of inflammatory mediators from stimulated neutrophils. *N Engl J Med* 303:27–34, 1980.
36. Mathies Jr AW: Meningococcal infections. *Brennemann's Practice of Pediatrics.* Vol. II, Harper & Row, Publishers, Inc., Hagerstown, Maryland, 1970.

37. Edwards MS, Baker CJ: Complications and sequelae of meningococcal infections in children. *J Pediatr* 99:540–545, 1981.
38. Todd J, Fishaut M, Kapral F, et al: Toxic-shock syndrome associated with phage-group-I staphylococci. *Lancet* 2:1116–1118, 1978.
39. Dan BB, Shands KN: Toxic-shock syndrome. *Pediatr Ann* 10:29–34, 1981.
40. Merskey C: DIC: Identification and management. *Hosp Pract* 17: 83–94, 1982.
41. Jacob HS, Craddock PR, Hammerschmidt DE, et al: Complement-induced granulocyte aggregation. *N Engl J Med* 302:789–794, 1980.
42. Weil MH, Nishijima H: Cardiac output in bacterial shock. *Am J Med* 64:920–922, 1978.
43. Divertie MB: The adult respiratory distress syndrome. *Mayo Clin Proc* 57:371–378, 1982.
44. Perkin RM, Levin DL: Shock in the pediatric patient. Part II. Therapy. *J Pediatr* 101:319–332, 1982.
45. Schlievert PM, Shands KN, Dan BB, et al: Identification and characterization of an exotoxin from *Staphylococcus aureus* associated with toxic-shock syndrome. *J Infect Dis* 143:509–516, 1981.
46. Bergdoll MS, Crass BA, Reiser RF, et al: A new staphylococcal enterotoxin, enterotoxin f, associated with toxic-shock-syndrome *staphylococcus aureus* isolates. *Lancet* 1:1017–1021, 1981.
47. Reingold AL, Dan BB, Shands KN, et al: Toxic-shock syndrome not associated with menstruation. *Lancet* 1:1–4, 1982.
48. Corrigan JJ: Heparin therapy in bacterial septicemia. *J Pediatr* 91:695–700, 1977.
49. Sheagren JN: Septic shock and corticosteroids. *N Engl J Med* 305:456–458, 1981.
50. Schumer W: Steroids in the treatment of clinical septic shock. *Ann Surg* 184:333–341, 1976.
51. Skubitz KM, Craddock PR, Hammerschmidt DE, et al: Corticosteroids block binding of chemotactic peptide to its receptor on granulocytes and cause disaggregation of granulocyte aggregates *in vitro*. *J Clin Invest* 68:13–20, 1981.
52. Faden AI, Holaday JW: Experimental endotoxin shock: The pathophysiologic function of endorphins and treatment with opiate antagonists. *J Infect Dis* 142:229–238, 1980.
53. Peters WP, Johnson MW, Friedman PA, et al: Pressor effect of naloxone in septic shock. *Lancet* 1:529–532, 1981.
54. Ziegler EJ, McCutchan JA, Fierer J, et al: Treatment of Gram-negative bacteremia and shock with human antiserum to a mutant *escherichia Coli*. *N Engl J Med* 307:1225–1230, 1982.
55. Eichenwald HF: Pneumonia syndromes in children. *Hosp Pract* 11:89–96, 1976.
56. Leedom JM, Brown JD: Pneumonias, bacterial. *In* Wehrle PF, Top FH (eds): *Communicable and Infectious Diseases*. Chapter 53, St. Louis, The C.V. Mosby Company, 1981, pp. 429–503.

57. Schatz M, Patterson R, Fink J: Immunologic lung disease. *N Engl J Med* 300:1310–1320, 1979.
58. Asher MI, Spier S, Beland M, et al: Primary lung abscess in childhood. *Am J Dis Child* 136:491–494, 1982.
59. Rivers RPA, Forsling ML, Olver RP: Inappropriate secretion of antidiuretic hormone in infants with respiratory infections. *Arch Dis Child* 56:358–363, 1981.
60. Bartlett JG, Brewer NS, Ryan KJ: Laboratory diagnosis of lower respiratory tract infections. *Cumitech* 7, pp. 1–15, American Society for Microbiology, Septermber, 1978.
61. Murray PR, Washington II JA: Microscopic and bacteriologic analysis of expectorated sputum. *Mayo Clin Proc* 50:339–344, 1975.
62. Congeni BL, Nankervis GA: Diagnosis of pneumonia by counter immunoelectrophoresis of respiratory secretion. *Am J Dis Child* 132: 684–687, 1978.
63. Dudley JP, Martin WJ: Bronchoscopy as an aid in the diagnosis of pneumonia in pediatric immunosuppressed patients. What to order. *Laryngoscope* 91:1379–1383, 1981.
64. Wimberley, NW, Bass JB, Boyd BW, et al: Use of a bronchoscopic protected catheter brush for the diagnosis of pulmonary infections. *Chest* 81:556–561, 1982.
65. Mimica I, Donoso E, Howard JE, et al: Lung puncture in the etiological diagnosis of pneumonia. *Am J Dis Child* 122:278–282, 1971.
66. Zornoza J, Goldman AM, Wallace S, et al: Radiologic features of Gram-negative pneumonias in the neutropenic patient. *Am J Roentgenol* 127:989–996, 1976.
67. Molteni RA: Group a B-hemolytic streptococcal pneumonia. *Am J Dis Child* 131:1366–1371, 1977.
68. Bruhn FW, Mokrohisky ST, McIntosh K: Apnea associated with respiratory syncytial virus infection in young infants. *J Pediatr* 90:382–386, 1977.
69. Stagno S, Brasfield DM, Brown MB, et al: Infant pneumonitis associated with cytomegalovirus, chlamydia, pneumocystis, and ureaplasma: A prospective study. *Pediatrics* 68:322–329, 1981.
70. Greene GR King D, Romansky, G, et al: Primary herpes simplex pneumonia in a neonate. *Am J Dis Child* 137:464–466, 1983.
71. Beem MO, Saxon EM: Respiratory-tract colonization and a distinctive pneumonia syndrome in infants infected with chlamydia trachomatis. *N Engl J Med* 296:306–310, 1977.
72. Orenstein WA, Overturf GD, Leedom JM, et al: The frequency of legionella infection prospectively determined in children hospitalized with pneumonia. *J Pediatr* 99:403–406, 1981.

Part VI

Foreign Bodies in Children

The topic of foreign bodies in children has, thus far, been separated from the entire text. Foreign bodies can be found in any organ or system in the pediatric age group, with the most common sites including the respiratory and the gastrointestinal tracts. This part emphasizes the invasive approach to the child with suspected foreign body aspiration.

24

Foreign Bodies in Children

Seymour R. Cohen, M.D., M.S., F.A.A.P.

Introduction

Ubiquitous and in many forms (Fig. 1) foreign bodies may be found in every orifice of the child's body. None produce more dramatic, alarming symptoms or potential hazards than when they enter the airway and food passages of the child.

Choking on foods has been estimated to cause approximately 2500 to 3900 deaths yearly.[1] It is the sixth most common cause of accidental death. The respiratory tract is involved in 55% of cases of ingested foreign bodies in children six months to four years of age.[2] In over one-third of these children, the accident or incident has not been suspected or observed. This fact, together with the tendency on the part of physicians to exclude inhaled or ingested foreign material from the differential diagnosis, contributes to the many complications and high incidence of morbidity.

It is hopeful that physicians will be alerted to the fairly common occurrence of this problem and will include foreign body aspiration and ingestion in the differential diagnosis of dysphagia, symptoms of airway obstruction and pulmonary disorders.

The young infant who first learns to crawl and who is in the oral phase of his development must be protected from the hazards of his explorations. The child must not be allowed foods requiring thorough mastication until his molar teeth have erupted. Nut-

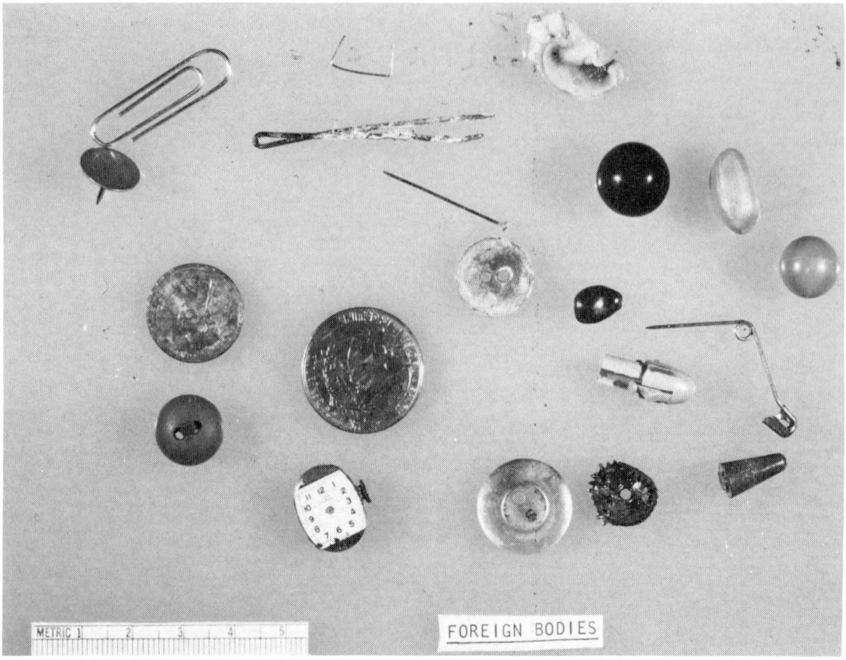

Figure 1. Numerous foreign bodies removed from the larynx, tracheobronchial tree, and esophagus of children.

meat, the most common inhaled foreign body, must not be given to children until they are at least three years of age. Parents must be careful to avoid using the lips and mouth as "storage bins," since the child will copy this dangerous and universally bad habit.

When a positive history of choking on a foreign object is obtained, the diagnosis and management should pose few, if any, problems for the physician in the care of the child.

Pathophysiology

A foreign body is defined as anything abnormal in the place in which it is found. The pathology produced by foreign bodies and the potential for damage is dependent upon whether they remain lodged in the oropharynx, larynx, tracheobronchial tree or esophagus. In general, the initial effect of foreign body intrusion is to create a violent reaction to its presence and there will be reflex attempts to expel the intruder. When the foreign body is too large to be spontaneously evacuated, removed manually, or travel distally, progressive occlusion of the airway will occur with hypoxia, cardiac arrest and death.

If the foreign body is extruded, only mild inflammatory changes will occur in the organ from which it was expelled. These changes will usually subside spontaneously. However, if the foreign body does not cause serious obstruction which leads to death, the reflex response subsides presumably from fatigue of nerve endings and the silent period ensues.[3,4] The small caliber of the trachea and bronchi, together with the ineffectual cough of the infant, is a cause for extensive disease and illness when foreign bodies are aspirated, which in older children and the adult would be relatively insignificant.[3]

The foreign body lodged in the larynx may produce a bypass type of obstruction and will cause inflammatory changes. The type of reaction will be determined by the composition of the foreign body, whether it is organic or nonorganic, its texture and size and its position within the larynx. Early inflammatory changes occur within the laryngeal structures, and edema becomes intense, producing increasing airway obstruction. Superficial ulceration with bacterial invasion produces pyogenic granulations. Subglottic stenosis develops, a problem much more prominent in the younger child, and symptoms simulating "croup" develop. These changes create dysfunction of the larynx with associated dysphonia and dysphagia. If blood vessels are eroded, hemoptysis will occur.

If the foreign body bypasses the larynx and is large, it may become wedged in the lumen of the trachea. Total obstruction and death may occur. The reaction within the trachea, as in the larynx, will again be determined by the type of foreign body. Organic material, particularly nuts, produces a severe response. Fortunately, tracheal foreign bodies will be easily detected by the alarming symptoms of airway obstruction which they produce. If not recognized, total obstruction may result. Fortunately, most tracheal foreign bodies retreat into the bronchial tree.

Inflammatory changes in the bronchi are dependent upon the type of foreign body, and changes similar to those in the larynx occur. Here also, organic material such as meat, bone, vegetable substances especially nuts, produces serious reactions. Metallic foreign bodies produce little, if any, reaction. Dried encapsulated fruits or vegetables moistened by secretions gradually swell and produce total obstruction of the lumen. Two factors which cause reactions are: (1) infection due to the introduction of bacteria with the inhalation of the foreign body, and (2) the irritation of the material which was aspirated. Trauma to the mucosa by sharp or rough surfaces leads to inflammation, edema, ulceration, bacterial infection and granulation tissue. These reactions, together with the space occupied by the foreign object, produce increasing obstruction with impairment of mucociliary function. This results in lower tract and parenchymal disease. Suppurative bronchitis with atelectasis, pneumonia, lung abscess and bronchiectasis may develop.

Foreign bodies in the airway once having passed the larynx, gradually ratchet downward into the trachea, the mainstem bronchi and finally into the peripheral bronchi.

Normally, the bronchi are not absolutely sterile at all times. The bronchi are less contaminated at the peripheral extent aided by mucociliary clearance, local immunity and the cough reflex. The latter is a major factor in the vulnerability of this age group to foreign body intrusion and the difficulties in expelling the foreign body.[3]

The normal tracheobronchial tree is a dynamic organ during normal respirations. The tree lengthens and widens during inspiration, and shortens and narrows during expiration. These changes produce peripheral wandering of the foreign body until it arrives at a lumen which no longer permits its more distal movement. These dynamic changes of the lumen allow the creation of either a ball valve or flapping valve type of obstruction. The ball valve type of obstruction produces obstructive emphysema which, if permitted to progress, will cause a pneumomediastinum, subcutaneous emphysema and eventually a tension pneumothorax. The flapping type of obstruction results in atelectasis.

Foreign objects or excessively large pieces of food may become impacted in the esophagus. There are three normally narrowed areas in the esophagus: the thoracic inlet; the aortic arch level; and the hiatus of the diaphragm. If the foreign body cannot be evacuated by voluntary or reflex efforts, the very powerful inferior constricture muscle will push the intruder into the esophagus through the cricopharyngeus sphincter. Foreign body impaction occurs in the normal as well as the abnormal esophagus. Strictures, sphincteric dysfunction and abnormal esophageal motility cause a higher incidence of foreign body impaction. Most foreign bodies too large to pass through the lumen will arrest at the level of the thoracic inlet. The relative weakness of the propulsive mechanism in the esophagus causes stagnation at the level of the thoracic inlet. In the strictured esophagus, the foreign body will become impacted above the level of the narrowed area. Once having passed the superior aperture, foreign bodies will usually pass through the esophagus into the stomach. However, they may become lodged at the cardioesophageal junction.

Should the foreign body remain in the esophagus because of its size, contour, transverse presentation or impaction, the pressure or point penetration will produce ulceration, infection, granulations, periesophagitis, retropharyngeal or peripharyngeal infection and abscesses. When in the hypopharynx or oropharynx, perforation of these organs may result in a retropharyngeal abscess, mediastinitis and cervical abscess.

Ultimately, a foreign body in the esophagus which remains for a prolonged time will produce a stricture or tracheo-esophageal fistula. Small alkaline batteries used in computers and hearing aids impacted in the esophagus may leak and produce alkaline corrosion of the esophagus with septic mediastinitis, hemorrhage and death.

Symptoms and Clinical Presentations

If the foreign object is excessively large and cannot be removed, asphyxia and death may occur. Frequently, the initial inhalation or ingestion of a foreign body has not been observed by an adult. When the episode is observed, violent wretching and choking are seen as the foreign body contacts or enters the larynx or upper esophagus. Gagging, coughing, dyspnea and cyanosis may occur. The foreign body may be evacuated by the strong reflex activity or may be dislodged from the larynx and then swallowed. It may then pass into the stomach or become lodged in the esophagus.

Should efforts to expel the object fail, attempts to fill the now practically empty lungs draw the object inward and if too large to pass into the trachea or swallowed into the esophagus, it may become impacted more tightly into the glottis. Fortunately, the intruder is usually of such a size and consistency that if it cannot be expelled, it will pass into the tracheobronchial tree. Repeated coughing paroxysms occur until the laryngeal sensations are fatigued and the silent period ensues. This is the interval in which the larynx has become accustomed to the foreign object and accepts its occupancy.

After the initial phase, symptoms will be determined by the site of impaction of the foreign body. In the larynx, the symptoms are inspiratory stridor, croupy cough, paroxysms of coughing, dysphonia, progressive airway obstruction and retractions of the chest wall. The symptoms may simulate croup and epiglottitis. Dyspnea and cyanosis, with drooling and dysphagia, may be concomitant symptoms.

The symptomatology in the tracheobronchial tree will depend on whether the foreign body has produced a bypass or check valve type of obstruction. Clinically, the child presents with a brassy cough, either dry or productive; asthmatoid wheezing during the expiratory phase of respirations heard at the mouth or over the chest; occasionally hemoptysis with dyspnea and chest pain. Cyanosis may occur when obstruction is severe and retractions of the suprasternal notch, xiphoid and intercostal areas may be seen.

When the foreign body is in the oropharynx or esophagus, the child may dig at his mouth with his fingers, drool, gag and cough and choke when feeding is attempted. Vomiting will occur if the foreign body occludes the esophageal lumen.

Physical Findings

If the child is not seen during the initial phase of the foreign body ingestion or inhalation, he may appear perfectly normal and have no positive physical findings. In many instances, examination will show typical signs of obstruction to the airway. If the foreign body is within view of an oral examination it will usually be seen at the base of the tongue or lying within the tonsil or hypopharyngeal area. A mirror examination may reveal the foreign object in the hypopharynx or larynx. If complications of an oropharyngeal or upper esophageal foreign body occur, redness, tenderness, and swelling in the neck will be noted. The oropharynx may be filled with saliva and the child may drool. The neck may be held stiffly if a retropharyngeal inflammatory process develops.

If the foreign body is in the trachea and lies loosely in the lumen, an audible slap may be heard or a thud may be palpated over the larynx and trachea. Wheezing can be heard at the mouth (asthmatoid) or may be heard on auscultation of the chest.

There may be no positive findings in patients with endobronchial foreign bodies. This is particularly true early in the course of the disease, and if there is a bypass type of obstruction. Examination of the chest may show differential aeration of the chest cage with hyperexpansion on one side or flattening on the other. This is particularly true where there is a ball valve obstruction causing hyperexpansion of the lung or a flap valve obstruction causing atelectasis. Wheezing and rhonchi and rales may be heard over the entire chest, but will be more prominent over the site of the foreign body.

If the lung becomes excessively hyperaerated, the breath sounds will be diminished and percussion will detect hyperresonance. On the atelectatic side, breath sounds will be absent or the chest will be dull or flat to percussion. When pneumonia is present bronchophony or rales may be heard. If the foreign body is at the carinal level, it may flop from side to side producing emphysema of one lung and atelectasis of the other. (See Table I.)

Radiographic Findings

The radiographic findings will depend upon the type and composition of the foreign object. If the foreign object is opaque and adequate studies are obtained, it will be nicely demonstrated on an X-ray film (Fig. 2).

With the development of plastic materials, increasing numbers of nonopaque foreign bodies are ingested and inhaled. The nonopaque foreign body presents problems in radiographic diagnosis. When complications develop, however, these will be readily seen within the roentgen study. A single X-ray film may be perfectly normal.

In all cases of suspected foreign bodies, a lateral film of the

Table I
Physical Findings

Symptoms	*Larynx*	*Trachea*	*Bronchi*	*Esophagus*
Voice	hoarse or aphonic	normal	normal	normal
Cough	croupy	brassy	dry or productive	with aspiration
Stridor	inspiratory early, to & fro later	expiratory early, to & fro later	expiratory, asthmatoid wheeze	to & fro if trachea is compressed
Dyspnea	moderate	severe	little unless bilateral	if trachea is compressed
Cyanosis	with severe obstruction only	moderate to severe	with bilateral obstruction only	rare unless total obstruction
Hemoptysis	with sharp objects	with sharp objects	sharp objects or with prolonged sojourn	hematemesis
Airway Obstruction	little to severe	severe	severe only with bilateral obstruction	only with large foreign body
Chest Examination	clear	clear with rhonchi	emphysema = depr. B.S., atelectasis = depr. B.S.	clear or wheezing if large foreign body
Pooling Saliva	none	none	none	may pool saliva
Dysphagia	rare	rare	rare	common
Vomiting	none	none	with severe coughing spasms	moderate to severe

depr. B.S. = depressed breath sounds

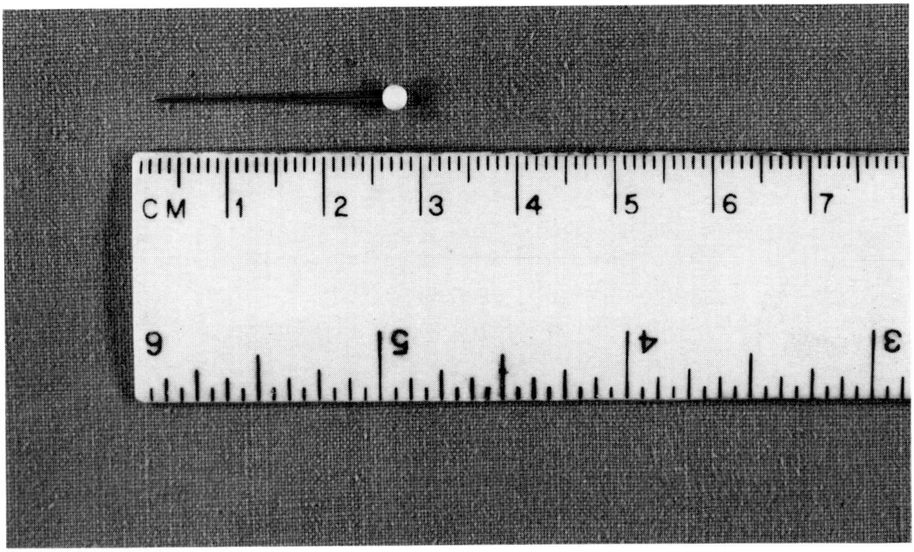

Figure 2A.

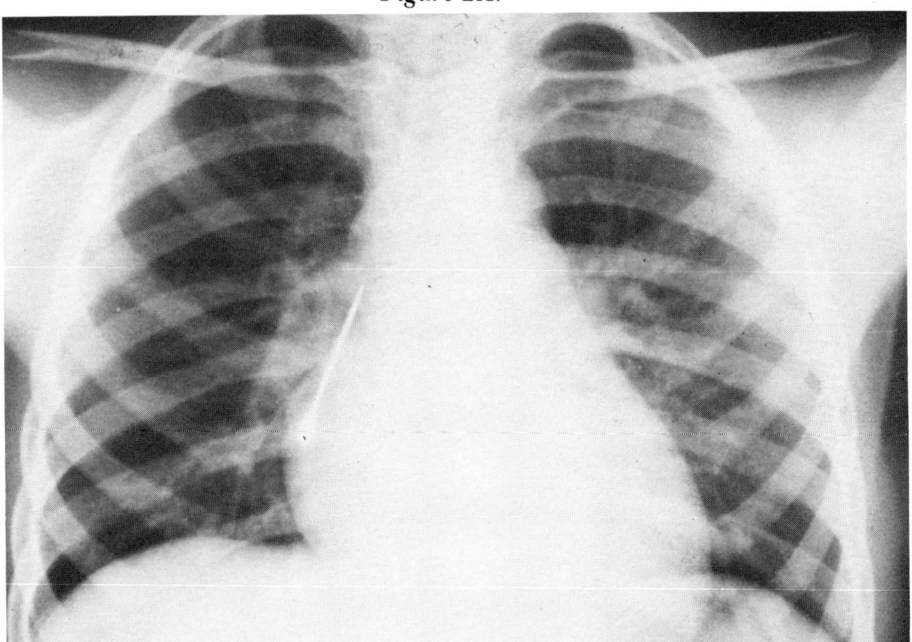

Figure 2A and B. A hatpin in the right lower lobe bronchus demonstrates easy visualization of an opaque foreign body.

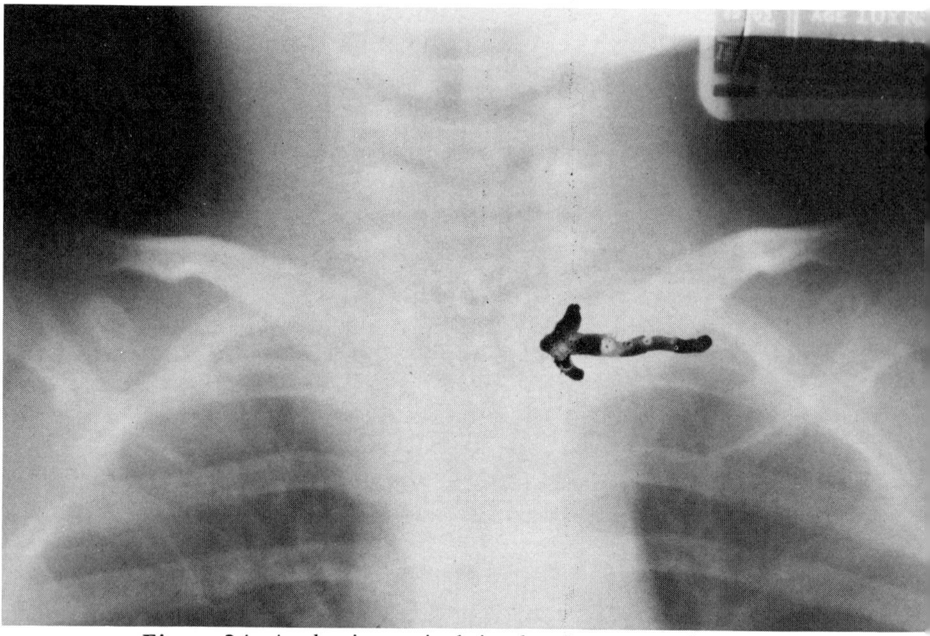

Figure 3A. A plastic toy jack in the upper esophagus.

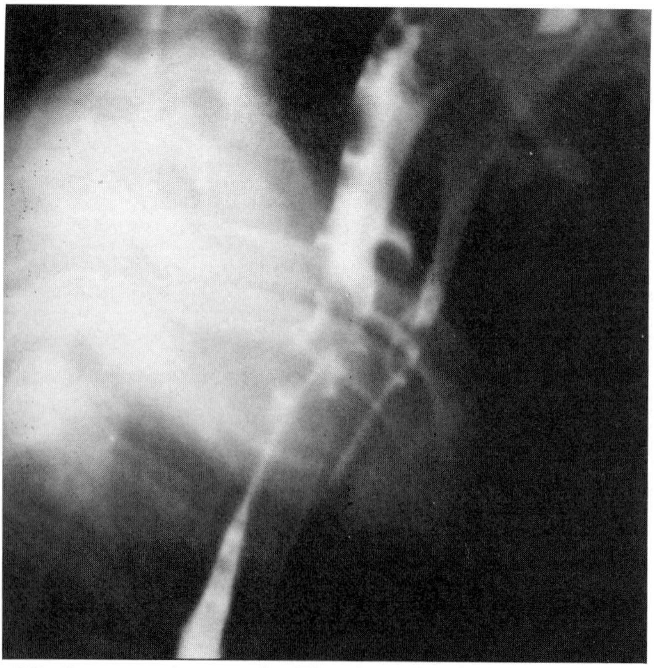

Figure 3B. Same patient as in Fig. 3A with barium esophagram showing a tracheoesophageal fistula.

entire airway, from the nasopharynx to the carina, is essential. Inspiratory and expiratory chest x-rays should be obtained. The abdomen should be included in the x-ray study. A barium esophagram is essential if a nonopaque esophageal foreign body is suspected (Figs. 3A, 3B). Multiple studies such as decubitus x-rays, fluoroscopic examinations and xeroradiograms should be discouraged. When the x-ray studies are completely normal and a foreign body is suspected, endoscopic examination is necessary.

When a nonopaque foreign body is lodged in the larynx, a lateral x-ray film of the neck and upper airway may show evidence of edema, obliteration of the laryngeal ventricle and narrowing of the subglottic space. If the nonopaque foreign body is in the trachea, the lumen may be narrowed or the lateral x-ray film may be completely normal. If the nonopaque foreign body is in the bronchial tree, the roentgenogram of the chest may be normal early in the course of the disease. If, however, obstruction occurs, emphysema, atelectasis, pneumonia and shift of the mediastinum may be seen. Where ball valve obstruction is severe, the foreign object may produce mediastinal emphysema, pneumomediastinum, pneumothorax and subcutaneous emphysema (Figs. 4A, 4B).

Fluoroscopic examination, if performed, may show the shift of the mediastinum with inspiration and expiration, and also reveal the restricted movements of the diaphragm. Inspiratory and expiratory studies are essential when nonopaque foreign bodies are suspected. A single x-ray study of the chest is inadequate to diagnose the presence of a nonopaque foreign object.

When inspiratory and expiratory x-ray studies of the chest are obtained and a ball valve obstruction is present, the following findings will be seen. The diaphragm will be depressed on the affected side. During expiration, the mediastinal structures will shift towards the uninvolved side. During deep inspiration both lungs are completely inflated and the mediastinum may be in the almost normal position. Only during expiration is the air trapped lung usually demonstrated (Fig. 5).

When a bronchus is completely obstructed, shift of the mediastinum to the involved side is seen during both phases of respiration. The diaphragm will either be fixed or elevated on the side of the atelectatic lung. Compensatory emphysema of the normal lung can usually be seen (Figs. 6A, 6B).

It should be emphasized that when there is a bypass obstruc-

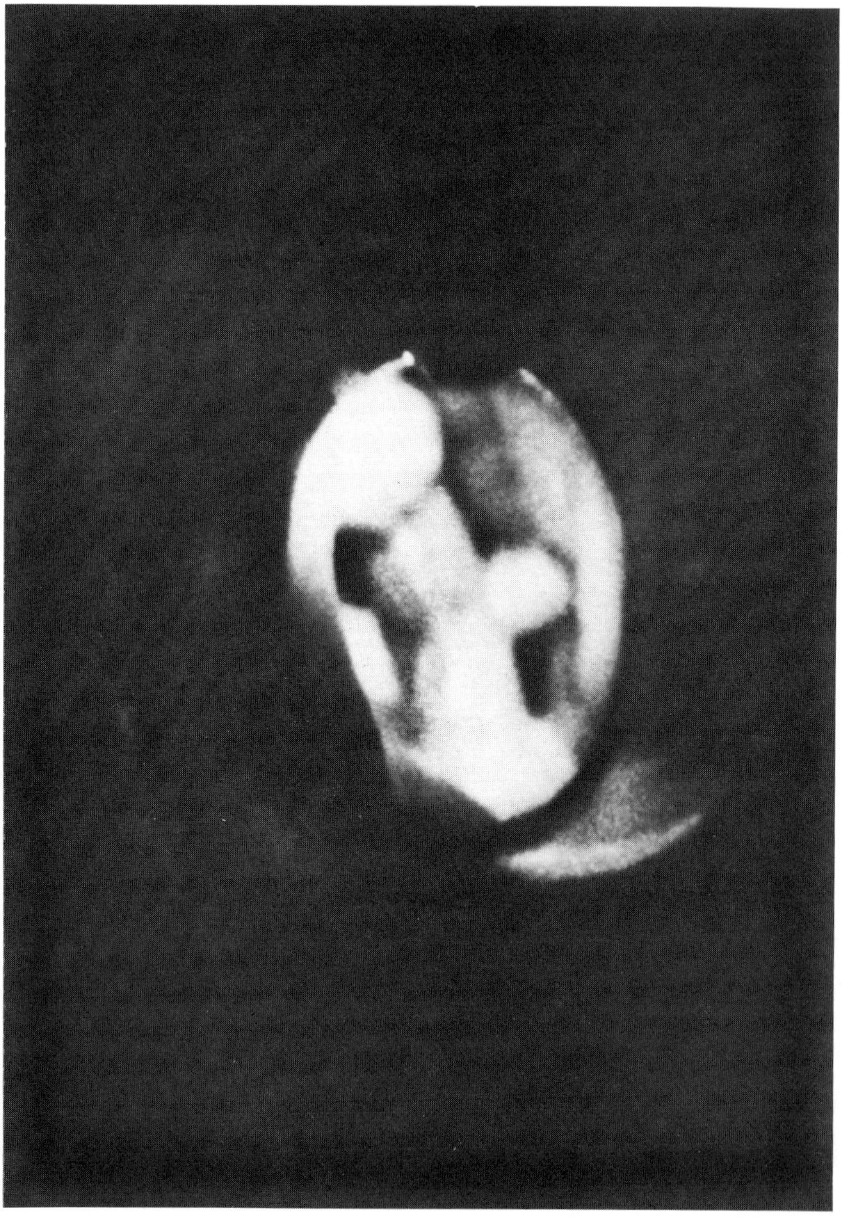

Figure 3C. The foreign body is seen within the esophageal lumen penetrating the anterior party wall.

tion and the lung ventilates normally, the chest roentgenogram will be normal except when there are associated complications.

Since the coin is the most common foreign body in the esophagus, a lateral film and posteroanterior x-ray of the chest will be adequate to demonstrate its presence (Figs. 7A, 7B, 7C). It is essential that the neck be included in the x-ray study of the chest or that a film of the neck be obtained to rule out a hypopharyngeal or cervical esophageal foreign body.

Roentgen studies are necessary to determine the position and type of foreign body in preparation for its removal. With small opaque objects, x-ray studies prior to endoscopy are necessary to insure that the object has not passed spontaneously into the gastrointestinal tract.

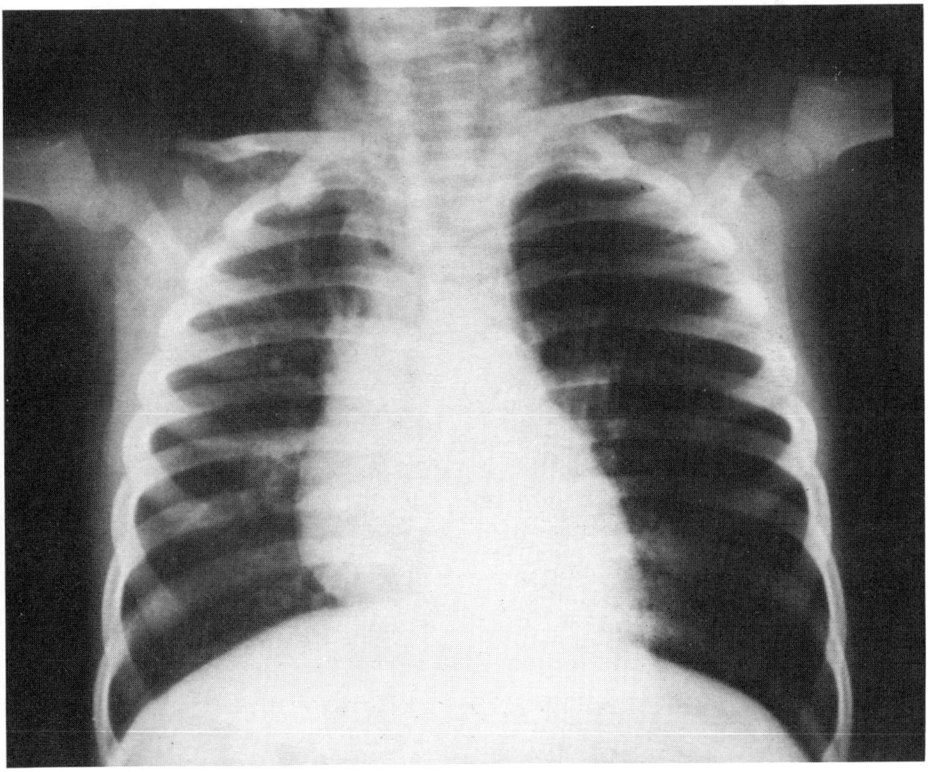

Figure 4A. Postero-anterior roentgenogram showing obstructive emphysema of the left lung and shift of the mediastinum to the right. There is a pneumomediastinum and subcutaneous emphysema.

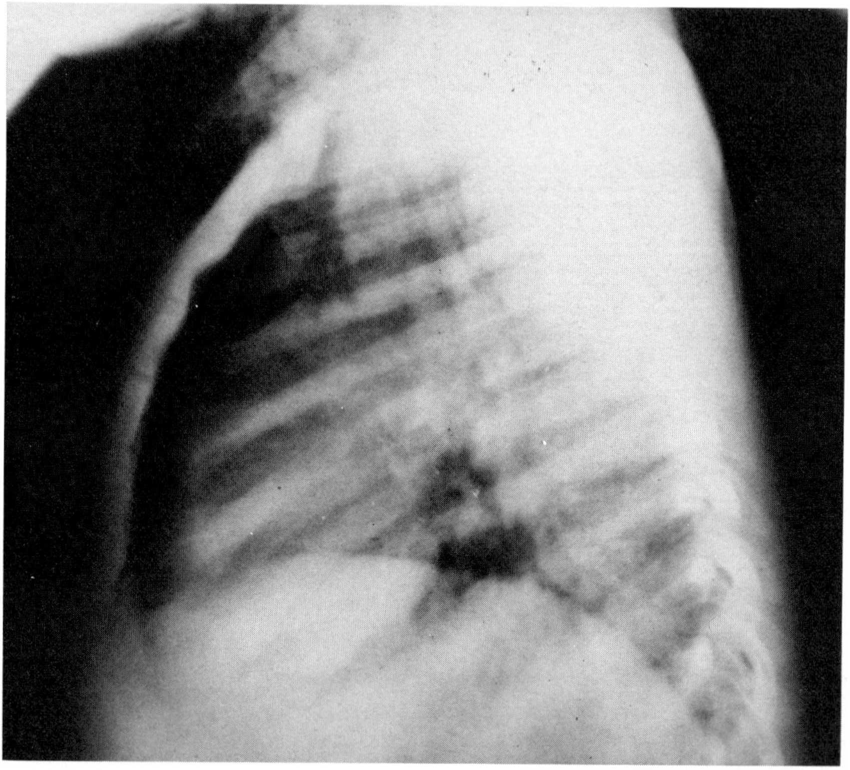

Figure 4B. A lateral x-ray film showing pneumomediastinum and subcutaneous emphysema due to extensive air trapping of the left lung.

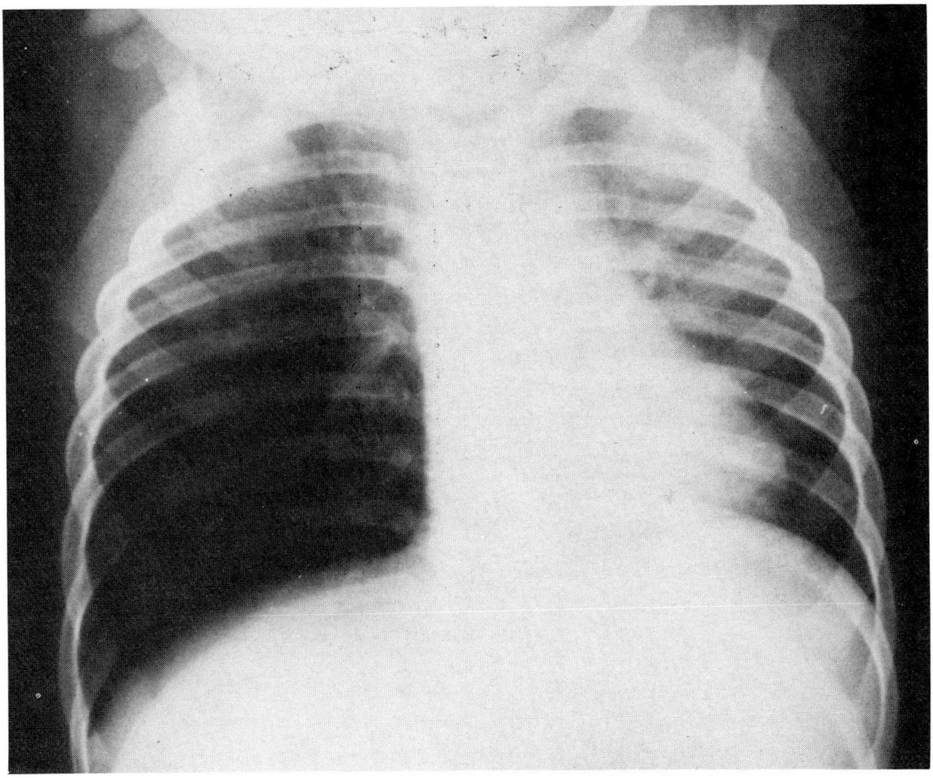

Figure 5. A postero-anterior X-ray in expiratory phase of respiration showing obstructive emphysema due to obstruction of the right mainstem bronchus with shift of the mediastinum to the left. Note depressed diaphragm on the right side.

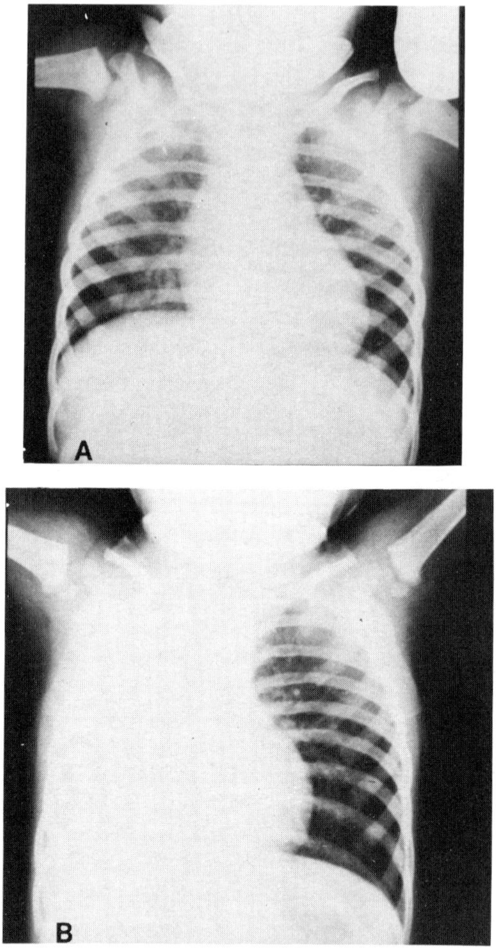

Figure 6A. Postero-anterior X-ray film shows complete atelectasis of the right lung with shift of the mediastinum to the right and elevation of the diaphragm on the right. There is compensatory emphysema on the normal left side. ***(6B.)*** A post-operative X-ray study after removal of the bean from the right mainstem bronchus. The lungs are equally ventilated and the mediastinum has returned to normal.

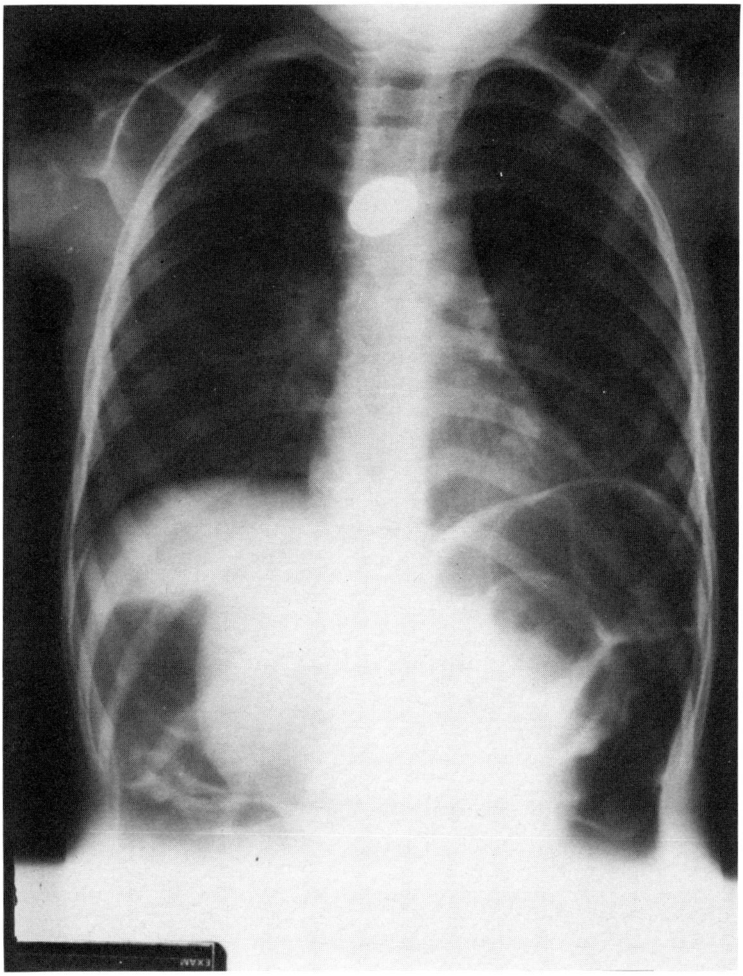

Figure 7A. A postero-anterior x-ray film of a coin in the esophagus.

Illustration continued on the following page

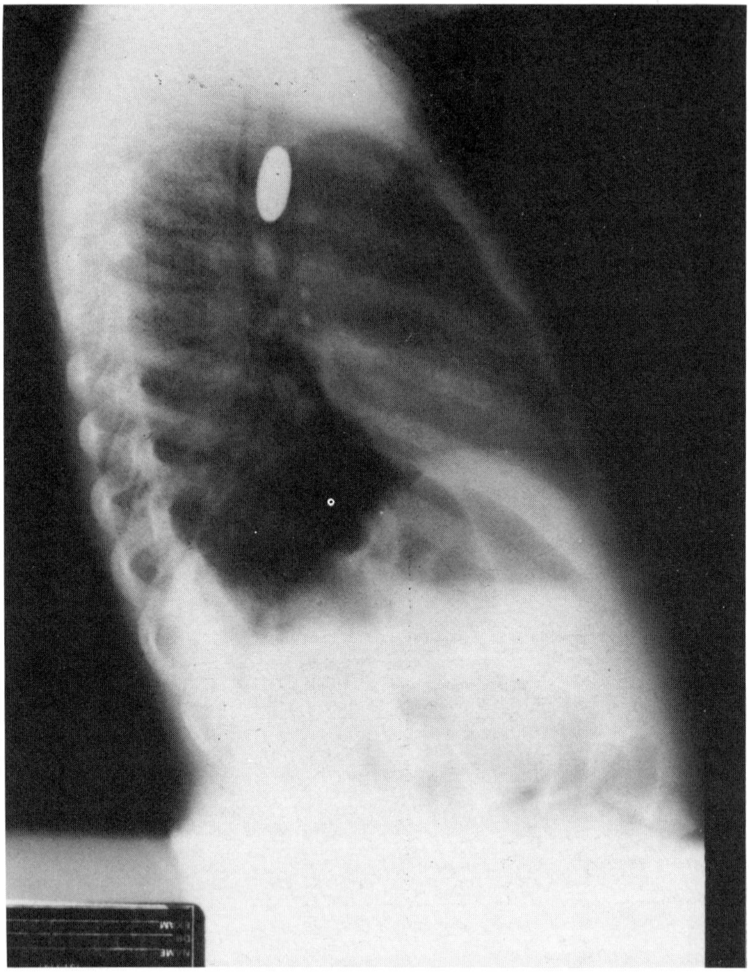

Figure 7B. Lateral x-ray film shows that the coin is not within the esophageal lumen. It lies between the esophagus and into the tracheal airway.

Illustration continued on the opposite page

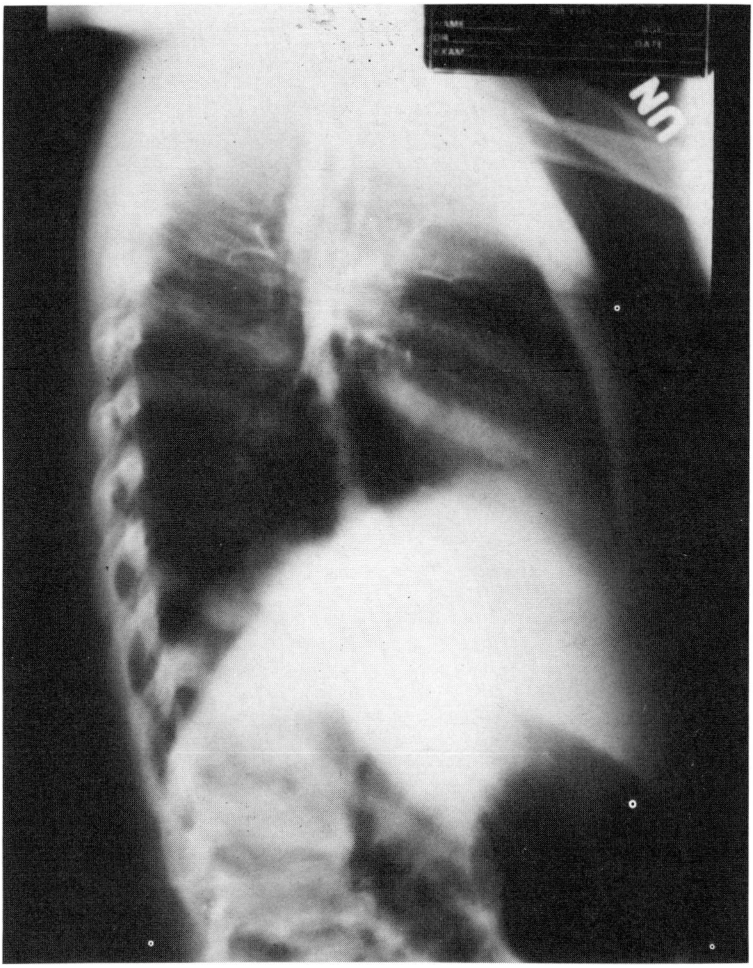

Figure 7C. Same patient as in Fig. 7B with barium esophagram. A tracheoesophageal fistula is demonstrated.

When the foreign body in the esophagus is nonopaque, the addition of a contrast material such as hypaque or barium will outline the foreign object and demonstrate any type of complication which may have developed. (See Figs. 3A, 3B.) The contrast material will demonstrate whether the foreign body is still within the lumen of the esophagus or if a tracheoesophageal fistula has developed.

Diagnosis

The diagnosis is simplified when a positive history is obtained. The child may have been observed choking after placing something within the mouth or during feeding.

A positive history, even in the absence of positive physical or roentgen findings, should alert the physician to the presence of a foreign object in the air or food passages until proven otherwise. One must remember the silent asymptomatic period. A complete examination of the child is essential. This should include examination of the oral cavity, the oropharynx, the neck and the chest. The child should be stressed so as to be able to hear the voice and determine the presence of stridor. Complete roentgen studies, which include the nasopharynx, oropharynx, cervical esophagus, larynx, chest and abdomen should be obtained.

When a child presents with persistent dysphagia, sudden onset of wheezing, vomiting which persists, chronic cough, airway obstruction, persistent "croup", recurrent pneumonias or failure of a lung disorder to respond to adequate therapy, a foreign body should be suspected. This is particularly true when any symptoms related to the airway and esophagus persist in spite of what is considered adequate therapy for the diagnosis (Fig. 8).

Differential Diagnosis

The differential diagnosis of foreign bodies in the airway and food passages is related to the presenting symptomatology, the physical findings and roentgen studies. (See Table II.) The symp-

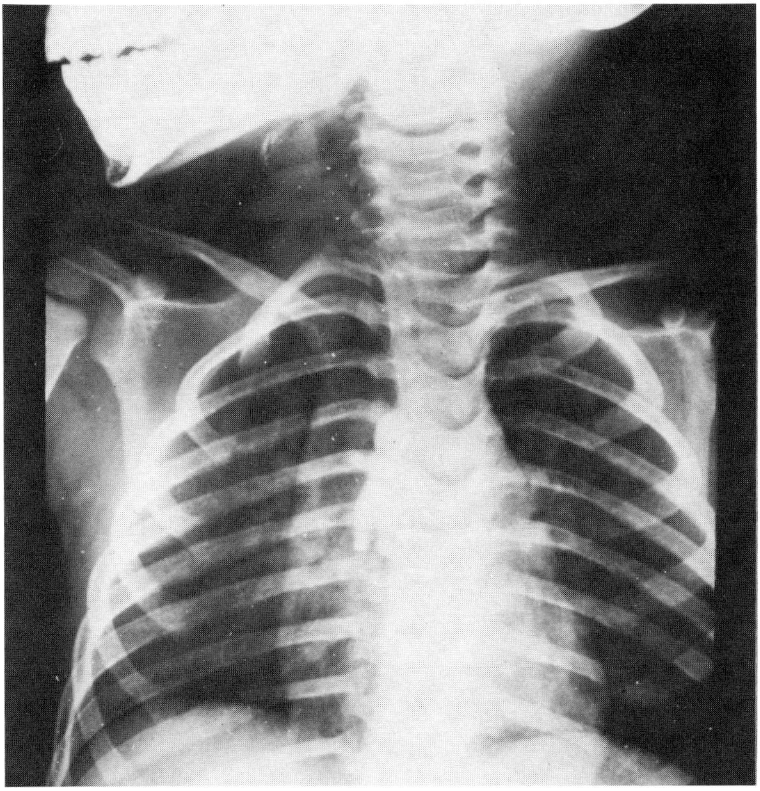

Figure 8. Postero-anterior x-ray film of the chest which shows a doll in the esophagus. The large foreign body compressed the tracheoesophageal wall causing obstruction and a clinical picture of asthma. Unsuccessful treatment for asthma resulted in this x-ray which showed the true pathology.

toms and physical findings will be dependent upon the site of impaction of the foreign object.

A foreign body in the larynx can mimic any disease. Anomalies of the larynx such as webs, cysts, laryngomalacia and clefts must be ruled out. Neurological lesions with laryngeal paralysis should be considered. Infections such as laryngotracheitis and epiglottitis produce symptoms similar to foreign bodies within the larynx.

Table II
Differential Diagnosis

Oropharyngeal	*Laryngeal*	*Tracheobronchial*	*Esophagus*
peritonsillar abscess	croup	tracheobronchitis	strictures
retropharyngeal abscess	epiglottitis	defects of trachea	corrosive ingestion
parapharyngeal infection	congenital defects	vascular rings	diverticuli
peritonsillitis	tumors of the larynx	vascular slings	tumors
tumors	trauma to the larynx	mediastinal tumors	chalasia
	granulomatous disease	cardiovascular defects	achalasia
		asthma	nonsphincteric spasm
		tumors	tracheoesophageal fistulae
		granulomatous disease	collagen disease
			granulomatous disease

Tumors and trauma, external or from intubation, may produce laryngeal symptoms simulating foreign bodies.

At the tracheobronchial tree level, the following are to be considered. Tracheobronchial abnormalities with intrinsic stenosis, fibrous or cartilaginous defects, webs, vascular compression by rings and slings, mediastinal tumors and progressive autoimmune diseases such as Wegener's and lupus erythematosus. Other considerations are tracheo-esophageal fistulae, dysphagia with aspiration from central nervous system and neuromuscular disorders.

The differential diagnosis of foreign bodies in the esophagus are strictures, corrosive ingestions, diverticuli, benign and malignant tumors, chalasia and achalasia and nonsphincteric diffuse spasm of the esophagus.

Therapy

The treatment of foreign bodies, either aspirated or ingested, is removal. Therapy should be directed to the immediate or the delayed aspects of the inhalation or ingestion episode.

The immediate treatment of the acute phase of foreign body aspiration or ingestion is to allow the patient's normal reflex to extrude the object without outside interference. If, however, after a short period of time expulsion or improvement of the obstruction does not occur, the child's mouth should be opened and examined. If a foreign object is seen or palpated, it should be digitally removed. The danger of this maneuver is that digital manipulation, if not carefully performed, may force the foreign body downward and cause its impaction. The manipulation should be carefully performed with a sweeping motion of the index finger. If, after opening the mouth and palpation of the oropharynx reveal no foreign body, a firm slap on the back between the shoulder blades with the patient in the knee-chest position may aid in expelling the foreign body.[5–6] There is controversy regarding back blows which have been recommended by the conference on CPR and ECC. It is possible and there have been studies which show that back blows may produce further impaction of the foreign body. It, therefore, may be more harmful than good. The Heimlich procedure should be performed when obstruction is noted, is severe and there is no voice.[7] While these efforts are being performed, a call for expert help should be made. If necessary, cardiopulmonary resuscitation should be applied when indicated.

After the acute symptoms resolve, the child should immediately be taken to his physician or an emergency room for a complete physical examination and X-ray studies.

Endoscopic removal is the method of choice and will in almost all cases of ingestion or aspiration be essential. All techniques such as awaiting spontaneous expulsion, the use of bronchodilators, steroids and racemic epinephrine followed by postural drainage and percussion are to be discouraged and may be dangerous. At no time should the child be tilted upside down to attempt evacuation of the foreign body by gravity. This maneuver may cause the foreign object in the trachea or bronchi to become impacted in the larynx producing spasm and complete obstruction and death.

Should mouth-to-mouth breathing fail to ventilate the child, emergency intubation, if possible, or a tracheotomy or cricothyroidotomy may be necessary. In rare instances when there is no other available methodology, the use of a needle to institute an airway may be used as a heroic and desperate measure.

Controversy exists regarding the type of instrumentation and preferable method of removing foreign objects. It is the consensus of opinion of those with years of experience that open rigid tube endoscopy with complete control of the airway is the safest method of treating foreign bodies in the air and food passages. This technique, performed under general anesthesia and in an operating room, is the best guarantee of the child's safety and successful care. The use of fiberoptic bronchoscopes to remove foreign bodies from the airway of children by individuals not expert with the use of rigid endoscopes is extremely risky.

The treatment of esophageal foreign bodies should be by direct endoscopic techniques.[8] Blind probing or nasogastric tube manipulation, the use of emetics, the use of papain and caroid to enzymatically reduce food boluses in an attempt to allow spontaneous passage are all contraindicated. Severe complications such as perforation of the esophagus have occurred using these techniques.

The recent addition of the use of a Foley catheter to remove foreign bodies under fluoroscopic guidance in the radiological amphitheatre has further added to the hazards of foreign body removal. This method purported to reduce psychic trauma and cost of medical care has been reported to have been associated with severe airway obstruction and death.

The removal of a foreign body should not be attempted at the site of its ingestion or inhalation except in the most desperate of situations. This principle should be expanded to the bedside, emergency room and even the radiological treatment room.

Once the foreign body has passed into the stomach or intestine, one needs only to await the arrival at its final destination. However, while most objects reaching the stomach will pass through the gastrointestinal tract, long-pointed foreign objects such as hatpins, bobbypins, long needles or toothpicks should be removed surgically prior to passing out of the stomach. These long foreign objects will not make the turns of the duodenum and may cause intestinal perforation.

Prevention

There would be a remarkable reduction in the occurrence of foreign body aspiration and ingestion if parents were alerted to methods of prevention. Children copy the actions of parents, and, therefore, nothing except food should be placed in the mouth. The infant without molar teeth, and children prior to three or four years of age, should not be given peanuts or nut meat. These are the most common foreign bodies in the tracheobronchial tree. Young children should not be given coins until old enough to use them appropriately.

Feeding time should be quiet and not associated with comedy. Only foods appropriate for age in texture, size and preparation should be permitted. The crawling infant and toddler should be protected during his adventures by thorough removal of all possible objects which could be placed into the mouth. Only toys, approved by governmental agencies as to safety, which have no removable parts should be permitted.

Conclusions

To prevent complications and increased morbidity from foreign body ingestions and inhalations, it is essential for the physician to include foriegn bodies as a not uncommon possibility in the differential diagnosis of airway and esophageal diseases.[9] By early diagnosis and institution of appropriate therapy, complications such as periesophageal perforation with abscess, mediastinitis, bronchiectasis, tracheoesophageal fistulae, recurrent pneumonias and pulmonary hemorrhage may be prevented. The reduction in cost to society and morbidity would indeed be remarkable.

It is incumbent upon the physician never to assume that a negative history excludes the possibility of a foreign body. The physician should be alert to symptoms reported by the parents which may indicate possible aspiration or ingestion of something abnormal. Negative or inadequate roentgen studies must not be accepted as conclusive evidence that a foreign body is not present.

Skillful open tube endoscopy, together with skillful expert anesthesia remains the sole proven safe technique for removal of foreign bodies in the airway and in the esophagus.

References

1. Eller WC, Haugen RK: Food asphyxiation. *N Engl J Med* 289:81, 1973.
2. Anderson DL: Death from improper mastication. *Int Dent J* 27: 349–354, 1977.
3. Jackson C, Jackson CL: *Bronchoesophagology*. Philadelphia and London. W.B. Saunders Co, 1950, Section 3:13.
4. Lederer FL: *Diseases of the Ear, Nose and Throat*. Philadelphia. FA Davis Company, 1952. Chapter 75:990.
5. Greensher J, Mofenson HC: Emergency treatment of the choking child. *Pediatrics* 70:110–112, 1982.
6. Day RL, Crelin ES, Du Bois AB: Choking: The Heimlich abdominal thrust vs back blows: An approach to measurement of inertial and aerodynamic forces. *Pediatrics* 70:113–119, 1982.
7. Heimlich HJ: Special Commentary: First aid for choking children: Back blows and chest thrusts cause complications and death. *Pediatrics* 70:120–126, 1982.
8. Cohen SR, Herbert WI, Lewis GB, et al: Foreign bodies in the airway. Five-year retrospective study with special reference to management. *Ann Otol Rhinol Laryngol* 89:437–442, 1980.
9. Cohen SR: Unusual presentations and problems created by mismanagement of foreign bodies in the aerodigestive tract of the pediatric patient. *Ann Otol Rhinol Laryngol* 90:316–322, 1981.

Part VII

Near Miss Sudden Infant Death Syndrome and Physiology/Methodology of Sleep Apnea

This final section on the sudden infant death syndrome introduces up-to-date concepts in physiology and methodology of sleep apnea. It is a newly emerging entity within pediatrics. This chapter concludes the book in an attempt to open new horizons for those readers interested in the field. However, it should be stressed that this chapter serves only as a basic introduction to this yet unknown disease entity.

25

Near-Miss Sudden Infant Death Syndrome and Physiology/ Methodology of Sleep Apnea

Barry J. Fisher, M.D.
Kathleen Tripp, R.N., M.S.

Since the First International Sudden Infant Death Syndrome (SIDS) Conference in 1963, there has been a progressive worldwide increase in interest concerning the etiology of this puzzling disorder. In the United States, SIDS kills 1 in 500 live-born infants during the first year of life, making it the most common cause of infant mortality after the first month of life. The sudden and unexpected death of an apparently healthy infant is disheartening, but it is even more distressing when no obvious cause can be found on routine autopsy examination. The purpose of this chapter is to present our approach to the identification, evaluation, and treatment of potentially high-risk infants.

History of Program

We initiated our program in April 1980 and it has continued to grow in size and scope so that we now evaluate over 300 infants annually. Various factors which have contributed to the design and continued refinement of our program include: literature review, analysis of comparable programs elsewhere in the country, identification of problems unique to our geography and population, and trial and error. We attempt to maintain flexibility so that modification can be made easily as new scientific data emerge.

Since it is beyond the scope of this chapter to summarize the world's literature, the reader is referred to several excellent reviews.[1–5] The apnea and/or bradycardia hypothesis as well as aberrations in the neurological control of autonomic function are leading etiologic considerations and serve as the foundation for our assessment of these infants.

Guntheroth[6] initially suggested the apnea hypothesis, basing his observations on infants seen during cardiopulmonary emergencies. The infants were found not breathing, but often still having a heart beat. This observation led to the concept known as the near-miss SIDS episode. In 1972, Steinschneider[7] studied five infants in the sleep laboratory who had been referred for evaluation of apnea and/or cyanotic episodes. All five infants demonstrated apnea greater than 15 seconds in duration (considered prolonged apnea) as well as periodic breathing. He defined periodic breathing as recurring apneic episodes of at least two seconds in duration occurring mostly during REM sleep. Curiously, both prolonged apneic episodes and periodic breathing increased when the infants had nasal pharyngitis. This work has served as stimulus for countless studies during the past decade.

Types of Apnea

There are three different types of apnea. *Central apnea* is defined as a lack of air flow at the nares or mouth associated with the lack of chest wall and/or diaphragmatic movement (Fig. 1), apparently due to a lack of central neurological stimulation to the chest wall and diaphragm. *Obstructive apnea* is the absence of nasal and/or oral air flow associated with continuation of chest wall and diaphragmatic movements. When these apneic episodes are observed, the chest wall movements often appear more vigorous than usual. *Mixed apneic episodes* are a combination of the above with the majority of these episodes beginning as central episodes and terminating as obstructive episodes. At any given apneic length, ob-

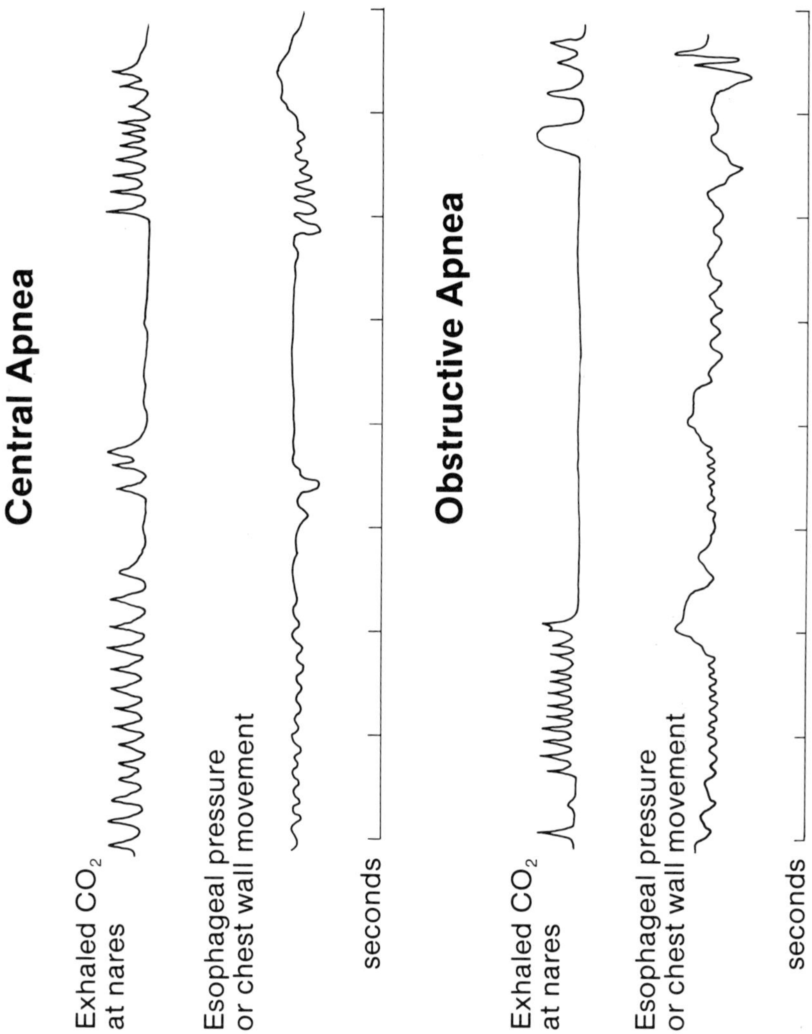

Figure 1. Types of apnea.

structive apneic episodes tend to result in more significant bradycardia and/or hypoxemia than central apneic episodes. A probable explanation for this observation is that oxygen debt increases more readily in obstructive apnea because of the continued vigorous chest wall movements.

Since anatomical upper airway obstruction is rarely observed, several investigative groups[8–10] have suggested that there is functional upper airway obstruction produced by relaxation of muscles maintaining patency of the upper airway, most notably the genioglossus. When relaxation occurs, the tongue falls back into the airway and upper airway obstruction results. In general, the harder the infant struggles to breathe, the less effective ventilation becomes. Often, these infants must experience at least a partial arousal and/or change position to break the obstruction. The most frightening episodes occur when there is a lack of arousal and/or a lack of movement on the infant's part (Fig. 2). These infants rapidly develop significant bradycardia and/or hypoxemia and may require vigorous stimulation or resuscitation, even in the sleep lab.

In our experience, obstructive apnea is more common among premature infants than full-term infants. Obstructive apnea decreases with increasing maturity, being infrequently observed beyond 56 weeks post-conceptional age, except when significant gastroesophageal reflux (GER) is present. Since impedance pneumography does not identify obstructive apnea, we study premature infants who have had a history of significant apnea and/or bradycardia prior to their discharge from the NICU in the sleep lab where nasal air flow can be measured. We prefer to study these infants when they are not on a theophylline preparation so that potential abnormalities are not masked by this drug.

Between April 1980 and October 1982, 138 different premature infants were studied in our sleep laboratory. Premature infants (less than 37 weeks gestational age) with a history of repeated or persistent apnea and/or bradycardia and/or a family history of SIDS comprised the study group. Obstructive apnea above 15 seconds in duration was present in 43 of 138 or 31.2% of these infants (Fig. 3) with the duration of apnea ranging between 15 and 62.5 seconds. In addition, 27.9% of these infants (12 of 43) had periodic breathing above 10% of total sleep time ranging between 10 and 83.3%. In our laboratory, periodic breathing is defined as a minimum of three successive apneic pauses above three seconds

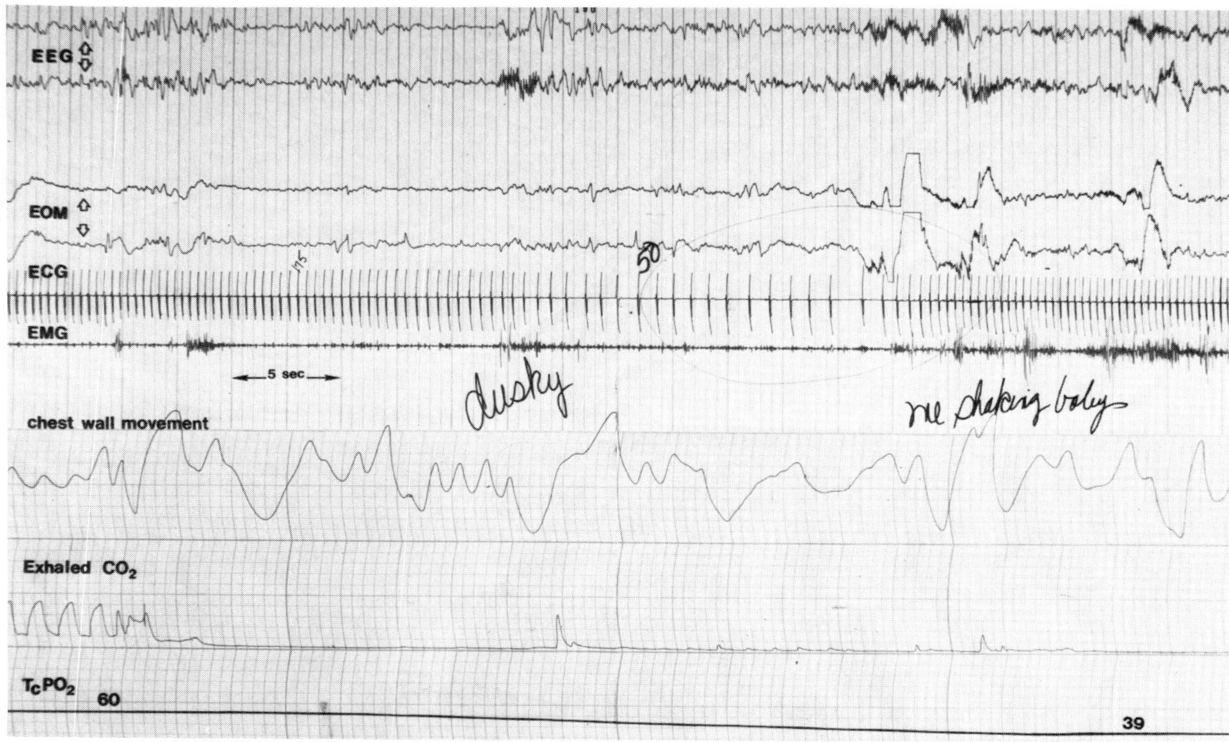

Figure 2. One-minute epic from sleep study of premature infant with obstructive apnea above 50 seconds in duration associated with bradycardia and hypoxemia unassociated with arousal. *(For abbreviations, see text.)*

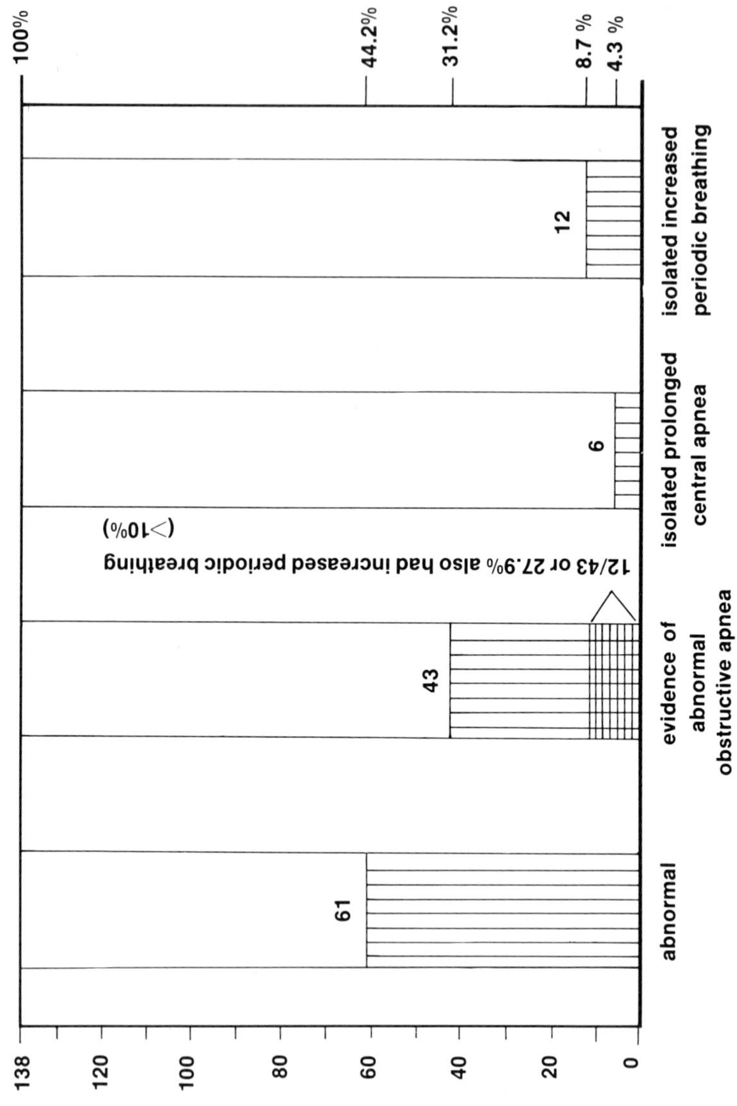

Figure 3. Summary of premature polygraphic sleep studies between 4/80 and 10/82. *(For complete details, see text.)*

in duration but under 15 seconds in duration interrupted by no greater than 20 seconds of normal breathing between each apneic pause (Fig. 4).[13] Prolonged central apneic episodes above 15 seconds in duration were present in only 6 of 138 or 4.3% of these infants. Isolated periodic breathing above 10% of total sleep time was present in 12 of 138 or 8.7% of the infants with the range of 11–93% of total sleep time.

This preliminary analysis of our data suggests that pneumocardiograms (impedance pneumography + 1 ECG channel) are not sufficient to evaluate premature infants because they failed to identify significant obstructive apnea in one-third of our premature patients. We believe it is necessary to measure nasal air flow to determine if obstructive apnea is present if premature infants are to be comprehensively evaluated. In our experience significant obstructive apnea is uncommon in full-term infants unless there is associated severe gastroesophageal reflux. Therefore, we believe "home" pneumocardiograms can be used either as a screening study in full-term infants or as a follow-up study in patients with either prolonged central apnea or inceased periodic breathing or both. Since bradycardia frequently accompanies obstructive apnea, we perform a polygraphic sleep study where nasal air flow can be measured if unexplained bradycardia is found on the pneumocardiogram.

Sleep Study Methodology

As previously alluded to, we utilize two types of sleep studies at our Pediatric Sleep Disorders Center. In addition to "home" pneumocardiograms, "in laboratory" polygraphic sleep studies are performed. These latter studies include two to six channels for EEG along with two channels for external ocular movements (EOM), one channel for ECG, one channel for electromyogram (EMG), one channel for chest wall impedance or diaphragmatic movements using a mercury strain gauge, one channel for exhaled carbon dioxide at the nares and/or mouth using a capnograph, and one channel for transcutaneous Po_2 ($TcPo_2$). When indicated, an additional channel is added for continuous esophageal pH monitoring.

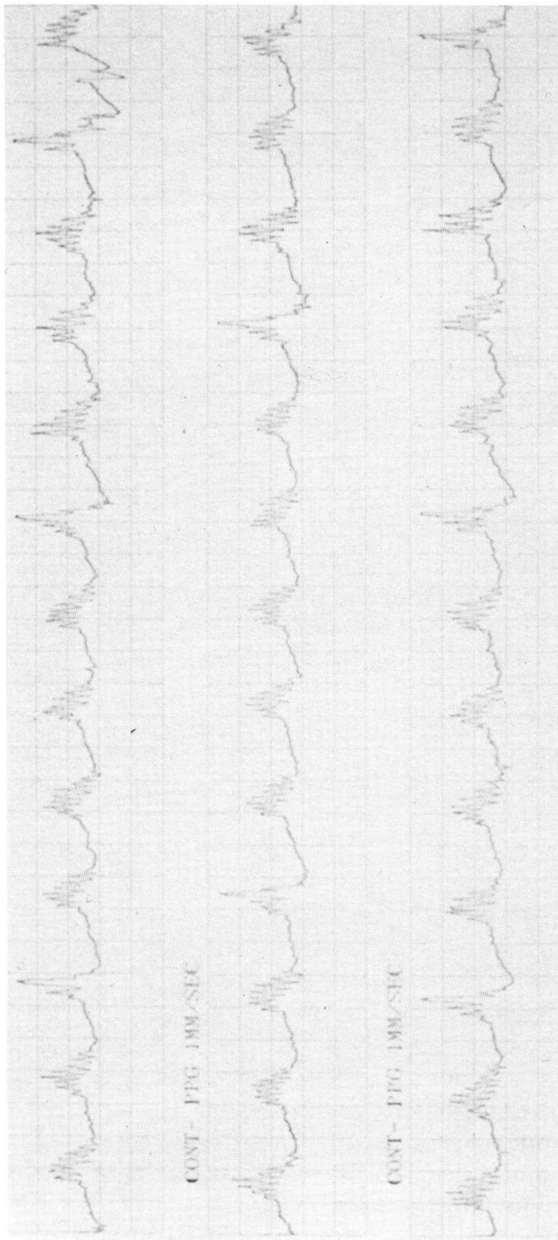

Figure 4. Continuous periodic breathing for 9 minutes and 30 seconds.

Figure 5 demonstrates a 30-second epic from a normal sleep study while Figure 2 illustrates an epic from a premature infant with a prolonged obstructive apneic episode associated with bradycardia and hypoxemia. We define significant bradycardia in an infant under one month of age as a decrease in heart rate to under 80 bpm for at least five seconds. After one month of age, bradycardia is defined as a decrease in heart rate to under 70 bpm for at least 5 seconds. Comparable normative data for older infants is not available. Suggestive bradycardia is defined as a decrease in heart rate from baseline of at least 40 bpm, but not down to the absolute values described above. Significant hypoxemia is defined as a decrease in $TcPo_2$ of at least 10% from baseline.

Studies can be performed during the day, evening, or night. The age of the patient dictates when a study should be performed. All patients above four months of age are studied overnight. Infants between three to four months of age are studied during the evening or overnight depending upon their sleeping habits. Chloral hydrate (50–60 mg/kg/po) is rarely utilized to induce sleep. We prefer to restudy any patient who does not sleep during a scheduled study. For infant studies, we strive for a minimum of four hours of sleep time. The average study lasts five to six hours after electrodes have been placed. We recommend two successive, uninterrupted sleep cycles before we consider the data valid.

In the sleep lab, we try to recreate a home bedroom atmosphere. Regular bedroom furniture is used and the patient studied in a dark, quiet room visually observed using low light TV cameras. All patient cables enter the central recording area via a pass through in the wall. The recording equipment is outside the patient's room where the technical staff can monitor the study in progress.

Sleep Study Scoring

All studies are manually scored with each successive 30-second period or epic evaluated for sleep state, heart rate, presence of and type of apnea, and periodic breathing. Results are recorded for each epic and a detailed summary of each study can then be consolidated onto one or two pages. This permits a rapid overview of each study. Areas where abnormalities are present can then be reviewed in great detail.

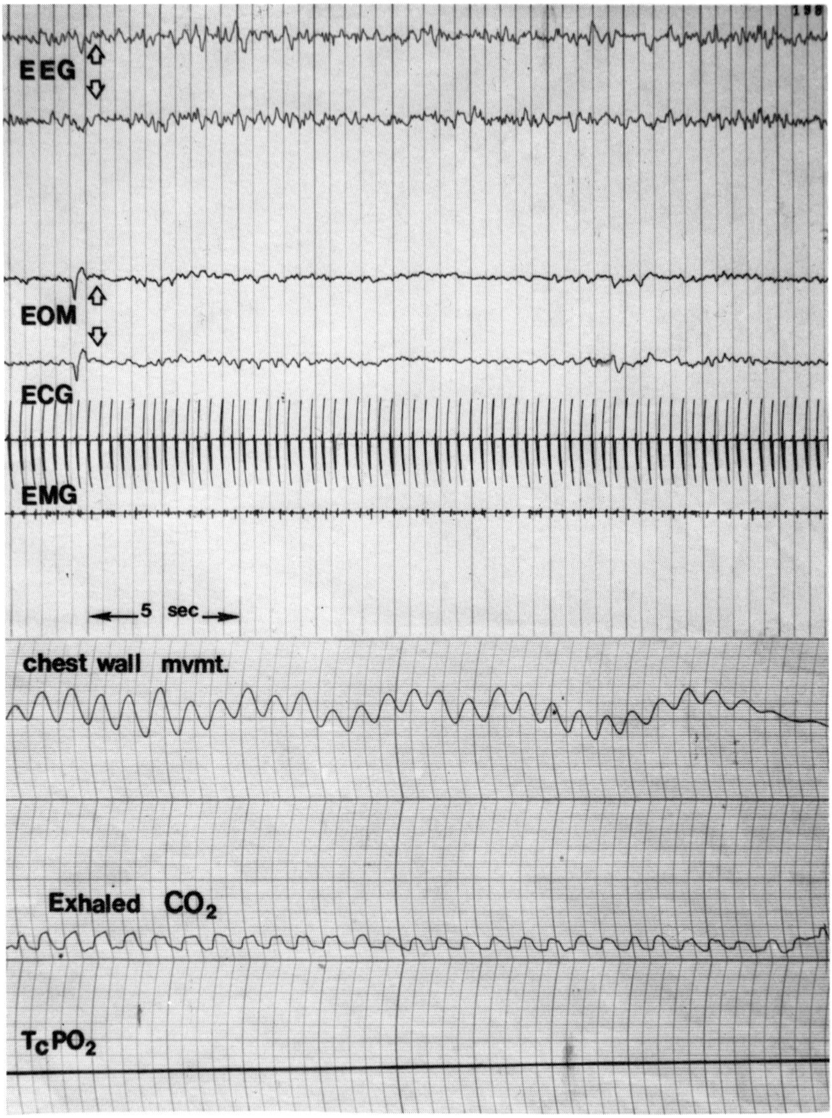

Figure 5. 30-second epic from a normal polygraphic sleep study. *(For abbreviations, see text.)*

Staging of sleep during infancy is difficult, particularly in premature infants. The differentiation between REM and NREM sleep is generally quite apparent. EEG criteria, eye movements, and muscle tone are all used to make this differentiation. Detailed criteria for identification of infant sleep stages are available.[11] The staging of the various NREM sleep stages are more difficult, particularly in premature and young full-term infants. Sleep spindle formation (used to identify stage two NREM sleep) is poorly developed in newly born infants. Trace alternants is a common normal immature NREM sleep pattern observed in premature and very young full-term infants. It is associated with rhythmic alternating cycles of high voltage brain wave activity and minimal or very low voltage activity (Fig. 6). REM sleep is characterized by an irregular heart rate and respiration along with random frequency, variable voltage EEG waves associated with asynchronous rapid eye movements. In addition, there is either an absence of muscular activity or a random burst of muscular activity on an electromyogram. There is generally a progression from faster to slower and from smaller to larger amplitude EEG waves as the infant advances from the awake state to progressively deeper sleep.

Summary data (Fig. 7) include total recording time (TRT), total sleep time (TST), total number of apneic episodes exclusive of periodic breathing, and total apnea time including periodic breathing/TST. The next section of the sleep scoring summary subdivides the total number of both REM and NREM apneic episodes into central, obstructive, and mixed. The longest apneic episode is identified as well as sleep stage, type, duration of apnea, and associated bradycardia and/or hypoxemia. This is followed by the mean duration of apneic episodes during both REM and NREM sleep. Similarly, mean transcutaneous Po_2 during these two stages of sleep is also reported, as is the lowest recorded $TcPo_2$, permitting correlation with an individual epic and/or apneic episode. We are now recording during feedings, observing for apnea, bradycardia and/or hypoxemia to assess the infant's ability to coordinate swallowing and breathing.[12]

Kelly and co-workers[13–15] have suggested normal values for periodic breathing. Table I summarizes these values. There are suggestive data that acceptable upper limits of periodic breathing are inversely related to gestational age. This observation may explain why higher levels of periodic breathing appear to be accept-

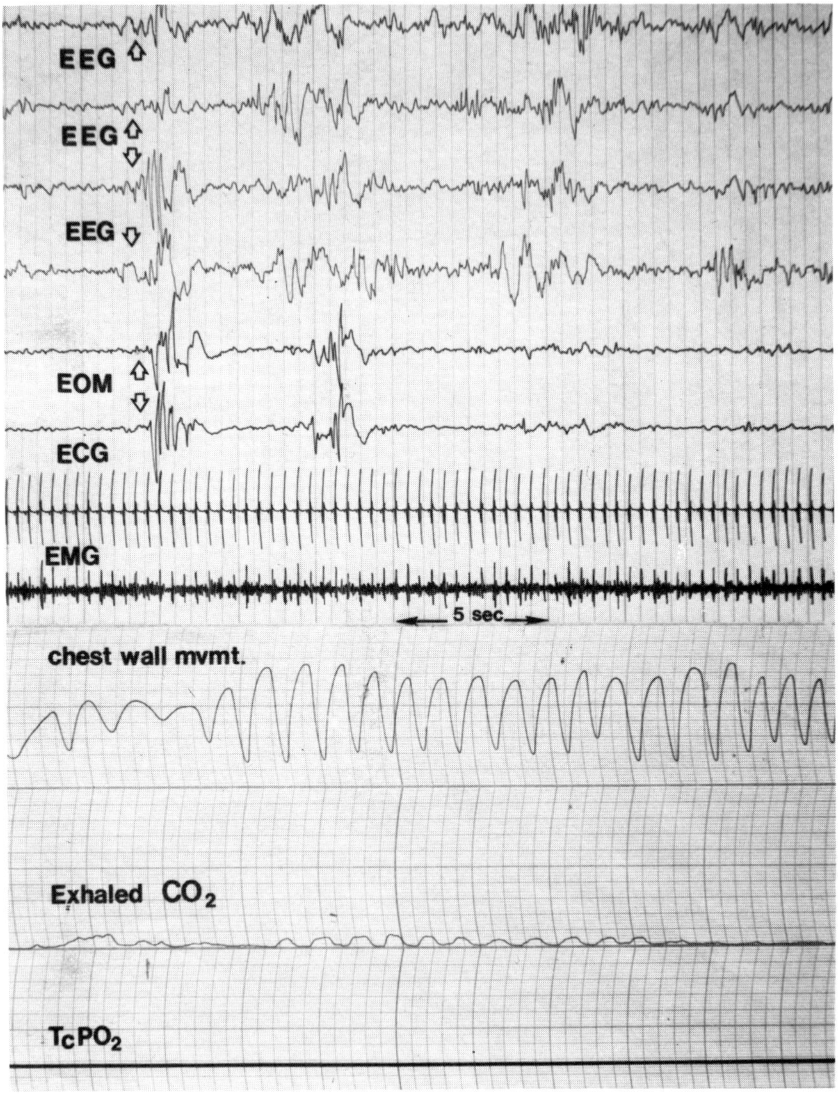

Figure 6. Tracé alternants. *(For description and abbreviations, see text.)*

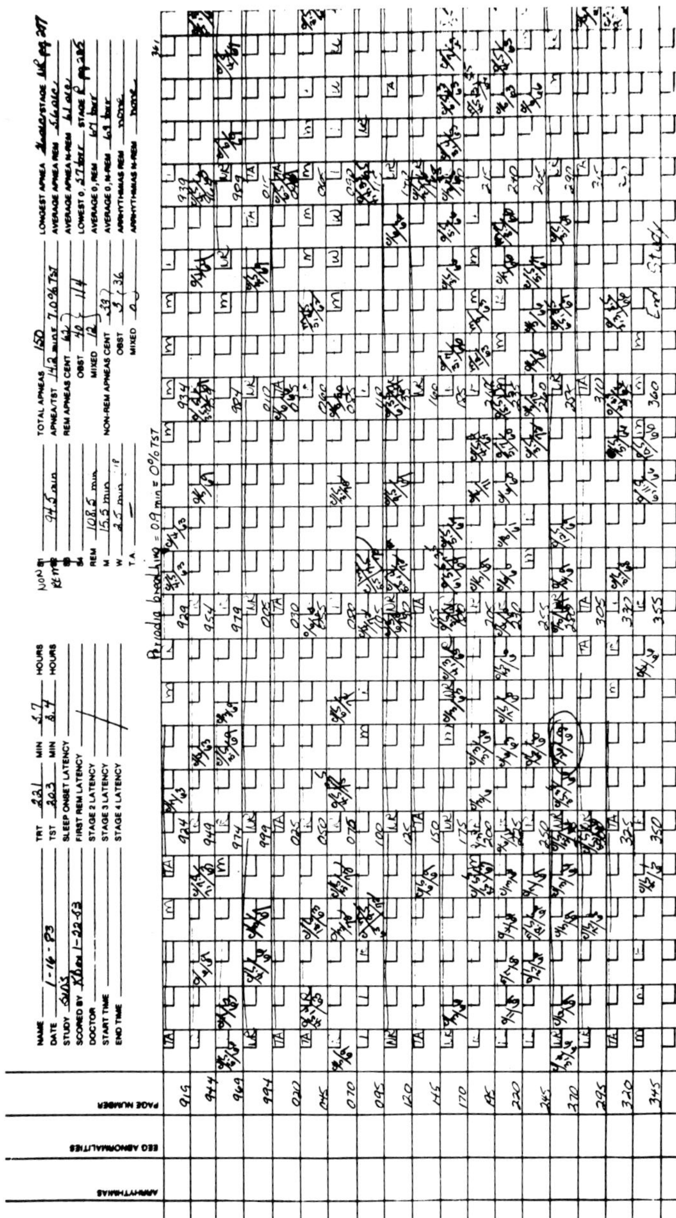

Figure 7. Scoring sheet for polygraphic sleep studies. Small square at upper right hand corner of each square is for sleep staging. TA = trace alternants, R = REM sleep, NR = non-REM sleep. In large square, apneic episodes are described by type above top line with C = central apnea, O = obstructive apnea, and M = mixed apnea. The number below the top line describes the duration of the apneic episode in seconds, while the bottom number is the transcutaneous pO_2. Each large square represents a 30-second epic. *(This figure is shown for illustrative purposes only to present a representative overview of our method of scoring.)*

Table I
Periodic Breathing Criteria

Under 30 days of age	<3.5%
Over 30 days, but under 60 days	<2.5%
Over 60 days, but less than 90 days	<1.5%
Over 90 days of age	<1.0%
Prematures	<10.0%

able for the premature infant when compared to the full-term infant. Once an infant reaches 40 weeks post-conceptual age, the criteria for periodic breathing recommended for full-term infants are used.

For full-term infants, a sleep study is considered positive if there is apnea beyond 15 seconds in duration, if there is periodic breathing above 3.5% of total sleep time, or if an apneic episode of any duration is associated with either significant hypoxemia and/or bradycardia (as described above). The criteria for premature infants (less than 37 weeks gestational age) are that any apneic episode above 20 seconds in duration is abnormal, but an apneic episode of any duration is abnormal if associated with significant bradycardia and/or hypoxemia. The upper acceptable limit for periodic breathing for premature infants is less than 10% of total sleep time.

We are just beginning to adjust ambient oxygen environments to simulate the hypoxic environment of high altitude as well as performing evaluations of arousal responses to hypercarbic and hypoxic stimulation.[16] Patients from Northern Arizona may live as high as 8000 feet above sea level and a recording performed at 1100 feet does not accurately reflect what happens at high altitude since apnea and periodic breathing increase at high altitude. The performance of pneumocardiograms at high altitude affords another mechanism for assessing the effects of altitude.

Study Groups

Currently we are evaluating four groups of infants whom we consider to be at increased risk for SIDS. The groups that we study include premature infants[1] (less than 37-weeks gestation by neurological dating) who have a history of recurrent or persistent apnea and/or bradycardia. We also study premature infants who are siblings of infants who have died of SIDS or who have had a so-called "near-miss" episode. We make an attempt to study these infants when they have been off a theophylline preparation for at least five days.

The next study group includes siblings of a previous child who either died of SIDS or who had a "near-miss" episode. We receive numerous requests to study infants when there has been a history of SIDS in the family (uncles, aunts, cousins, etc.). We generally screen these infants with pneumocardiograms although there are no data concerning the risk of SIDS in these infants. In our experience, the risk appears greater than 1 in 500, but less than the risk of subsequent siblings. However, our study group is not yet large enough to permit statistical evaluation.

The third group includes infants who experience an apparent apneic episode associated with cyanosis and/or pallor, often requiring resuscitation (apparent near-miss SIDS episode). These infants frequently look "perfectly well" when seen by medical or paramedical personnel, but this observation should not preclude their evaluation. From a historical perspective, it is impossible to determine if any particular episode is significant without a detailed evaluation (see later discussion).

The fourth group of infants whom we believe should be evaluated include other infants who have statistically been shown to be at high risk. Many of these infants will already have been identified as high risk patients, because they fall in one of the above categories. For example, infants born to unwed mothers under 15 years of age[17–18] have been shown to be at increased risk. However, the rate of prematurity is greater among these women as well and these infants may already be identified. Another group at very high risk are infants born to drug-addicted mothers, where the incidence of SIDS is reported to be as high as ten times the general population.[19] Therefore, we believe that all infants born to drug-addicted mothers should be evaluated. Another group of infants who will probably receive more attention in the future are infants born to mothers with gestational infection, most notably, amnionitis. Naeye[20] believes that the risk for SIDS is dramatically increased in this population.

Operations and Protocol

The following is a discussion of our operations and protocols. Infants who are siblings of SIDS or "near-miss" infants are screened with a pneumocardiogram at 5–7 days of age. If this pneumocardiogram is normal, no further intervention is taken at that time, but a repeat pneumocardiogram is performed at one month of age. If the second pneumocardiogram is also normal, we feel reasonably comfortable telling the family that the infant does not appear to be at increased risk for SIDS. We believe no further studies or therapy are needed unless the infant has a severe apneic episode associated with cyanosis and/or pallor. To date, this has occurred in only one patient from a total studied population called normal in excess of 600. That child was found to have a seizure disorder and apneic symptoms were controlled with anticonvulsant therapy. There have been no deaths to date in any way attributable to SIDS in any infant studied whom we considered to be at no increased risk for SIDS. Some of the families who had previously lost a child to SIDS have insisted upon having a monitor for their newly born infant but almost all of them were willing to give up the monitor after two normal pneumocardiograms. If either pneumocardiogram is abnormal, a more extensive workup is then carried out and the child is followed by protocol. The criteria for premature infants have already been described and no further "SIDS" evaluation is performed unless the sleep study is abnormal.

The near-miss infants who have had a severe apneic episode associated with either cyanosis or pallor are admitted for a workup. Their work-up is more extensive and includes:

- Complete history and physical examination
- CBC and WBC differential
- Electrolytes, BUN, glucose, and calcium determinations
- Barium swallow or radionucleotide study looking for gastroesophageal reflux
- EEG
- In-laboratory polygraphic sleep study
- Heart rate and respiratory monitoring in the hospital
- Parental instruction in CPR
- Referral to the pediatric sleep disorders nurse specialist

In our setting, this work-up can generally be accomplished

within a 48-hour period of time. The results of all the studies are then reviewed with the family and recommendations are made.

If seizure activity is noted on the EEG, the infant is begun on anticonvulsant therapy. Additional studies are ordered as deemed appropriate. CT scans and lumbar punctures are not routinely performed. In infants with EEG evidence of seizure activity the sleep study may also be abnormal, demonstrating either increased periodic breathing or abnormal apnea or both. In this case, the family receives full instruction (see later discussion) and the baby is discharged home on the monitor. A theophylline preparation is generally not prescribed along with anticonvulsant medication. One month after anticonvulsant therapy has been initiated, a repeat pneumocardiogram or in-laboratory sleep study (if indicated) is performed. If no abnormalities are found, home monitoring may be discontinued, but anticonvulsant therapy is continued for six months. However, if the follow-up sleep study is again abnormal, home monitoring is continued and the patient is followed according to our protocol.

If the patient has radiographic or radionucleotide evidence of significant GE reflux, an esophageal pH study is performed.[21] This study may be performed as an independent study or as a part of the multichannel sleep study where correlations can be made with the apneic events. Reflux precautions are instituted if significant GER is identified. These precautions include upright positioning in an infant seat, thickened feedings, and the possible use of urecholine. The families are instructed in proper feeding techniques. We believe that gastrostomy or jejunostomy feedings are not helpful, since we find that reflux often persists in patients with GE reflux after these procedures. Surgical plication of the gastroesophageal sphincter is reserved for children who fail to respond to aggressive medical management. Several patients have been treated with intravenous hyperalimentation while waiting for GER to abate. This technique has been helpful in about one-half the cases and we consider its use before recommending surgical intervention.

The syndrome of severe GE reflux, chronic repeated pulmonary aspiration, and significant obstructive apnea associated with severe bradycardia and/or hypoxemia presents a major management challenge. These infants, often premature nursery graduates, are difficult to care for, often fail to thrive, and frequently have prolonged hospitalizations. Randomly occurring severe apneic episodes requiring resuscitation and prolonged hospitalizations stimulate high levels of parental anxieties and tension. These families require a great deal of psycho-social support, and they express appropriate anxiety about caring for these children. Extreme patience and diligence is necessary for their successful care.

Figure 8 is a graphic representation of the various protocols and interventions currently in operation. If a sleep study or pneumocardiogram abnormality consists only of increased periodic breathing, the infants are begun on theophylline at 2 mg/kg/24 hrs divided every 8 hours orally. This dose is lower than the dose used at various other centers, but Milsap and co-workers[22] have reported that low dose theophylline was equally as effective as higher dose theophylline (8–10 mg/kg/24 hrs) in decreasing apnea of prematurity. Toxic side-effects were reduced at this lower level.

We elected to try this lower dosage of theophylline to evaluate its efficacy in shortening the duration and lowering the frequency of occurrence of long central apneas (greater than 15 seconds in duration) and reducing the amount of periodic breathing. We attempt to maintain serum theophylline levels between 3 and 6 μg/ml[22] and find that this dosage usually gives these levels. Our preliminary results to date indicate that low dosage theophylline is equally as effective as the higher dosage in suppressing periodic breathing or decreasing the duration and lowering the frequency of central apnea. Idiosyncratic hyperactivity reactions persist at a rate comparable to that seen at higher dosages. We believe that this reaction is independent of the dosage or preparation of theophylline employed. Gastrointestinal side-effects are rarely seen with low dose theophylline therapy. No hypertension or seizure activity has been observed. The administered dosage is increased as the child grows so as to maintain a steady mg/kg/day schedule.

The infants with increased periodic breathing and/or prolonged central apnea, are discharged on a home monitor along with theophylline. After serum theophylline levels between 3 and 6 μg/ml are achieved on an ambulatory basis, a repeat home pneumocardiogram is performed. If this follow-up study demonstrates normal levels of periodic breathing and/or no prolonged central apneic episodes, then home monitoring is discontinued and the infant is maintained on theophylline for the next three months.

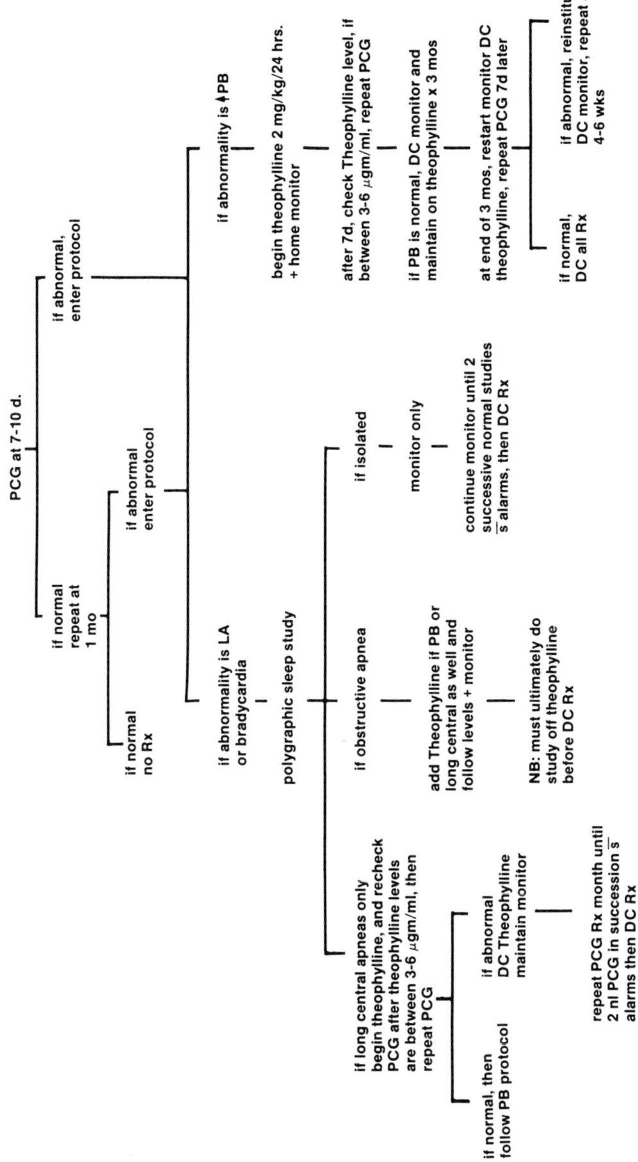

Figure 8. SIDS protocol. *(For details, see text.)*

At that time the monitor is reinstituted, the theophylline preparation is discontinued, and a home pneumocardiogram performed 5–7 days later. If this study is normal, then all therapy is discontinued. If increased periodic breathing or prolonged central apnea is still found, theophylline is resumed, the monitor discontinued, and the entire process described above repeated in 4–6 weeks.

The home-care company we utilize provides the monitors on a 2-week rental basis. The average infant with periodic breathing uses the monitor for only 4–6 weeks. Several families have preferred to use the home monitor exclusively and not use theophylline at all. In this case, repeat home pneumocardiogram is performed after three months and, if normal, the home monitor is discontinued. In addition to a normal study, it is imperative that there be no monitor alarms other than loose lead or disconnect alarms for the preceding month.

If there is prolonged obstructive apnea or obstructive apnea associated with hypoxemia and/or bradycardia, home monitoring alone is instituted. Follow-up laboratory multichannel sleep studies are performed at 4–6 week intervals until there are 2 successive normal studies with no intervening significant alarms (as described above). In infants who have increased periodic breathing in addition to significant or prolonged obstructive apnea, theophylline is added in addition to monitor usage. However, after one normal in-laboratory study, theophylline is discontinued while home monitoring is continued, so that a representative study can be obtained with the next study and a valid therapeutic decision made. Our experience with babies who have had increased periodic breathing and/or significant central or obstructive apnea is that home monitoring and/or treatment with theophylline is generally completed by 5–6 months of age. Occasionally families insist on continuing the monitor beyond the age of the previous sibling's death from SIDS or until 6 months of age. We have emphasized to them that over 90% of infants who die of SIDS die before 6 months of age.

We have increased ambient inspired oxygen to 30% on six occasions and observed a minimum 50% decrease in periodic breathing. Because approximately one-third of Arizona residents live above 5000 feet, an evaluation at 1000 feet does not give representative data. If evaluation at 1000 feet is abnormal, monitoring is obviously instituted. We attempt to perform follow-up pneumocardiograms at high altitude, where apnea and periodic breathing are increased, probably on a hypoxic basis. However, if our studies are normal, but the history is suggestive, monitoring will be instituted and a pneumocardiogram performed at high altitude. We recommend that the patients be at high altitude at least 24 hours before the study is performed. During a 30-month period, we have cared for 20 infants who had normal evaluations at 1000 feet, but marked increases in periodic breathing (highest value = 35%) and/or prolonged central apnea at high altitude.

Educational and Psycho-social Aspects of Home Monitoring

The preceding discussion has described the evaluation and identification of infants at high risk for SIDS. The following section discusses the concepts, methodology, and psycho-social impact of home monitoring.

The initial use of home apnea monitoring elicited well-founded skepticism because of its potential impact on family life. Authors of an early commentary[28] cautioned that "there is reason to be seriously concerned about adverse effects of monitors on parental behavior and familial emotional health." Subsequent practitioners alluded to both the potential positive and negative effects of monitoring in the home[23,30–32] and to more specific aspects of familial adaptation.[29] Only recently has any systematic attempt been made to investigate these potential impacts. In fact, only one such study is reported in the literature.[27] During the past year, however, authors are beginning to share specific suggestions for enabling families to cope better with the potential impact of home monitoring.[5,25,26] The following discussion will suggest guidelines that we have found useful in working with monitored families. This approach will vary given the nature of each particular circumstance, each individual family system, and each practitioner's style and personal strengths.

In our experience, there are three distinct groups of families whose needs differ due to circumstance: families of a prematurely born infant; families who have previously lost a child to SIDS; and families whose infant experienced a potentially life-threatening apneic episode with cyanosis or pallor "near-miss". Although all families should receive the core educational material, their support needs will vary. Typically, families who have spent time in the premature nursery are less frightened by the prospect of home monitoring. They have become accustomed to complex machinery and monitors in the nursery, have seen their baby survive severe threats, and have observed marked improvements. They are eager to have the baby home and tend to view monitoring with ambivalent acceptance. Unless there are other complications or unless they have observed recent apneic episodes, they tend to be more casual, report less compulsive use of the monitor, and relegate it more quickly to bedtime use only.

In contrast, parents who have previously lost a child to SIDS tend to be very anxious and extremely faithful in their use of the monitor. Subsequent births often elicit unresolved grief complicating the emotional environment. These families frequently request a monitor in spite of normal sleep studies and tend to use the monitor beyond the point of pure "medical" indication, often preferring to use the monitor beyond the age at which the previous sibling died.

The response of parents whose baby had an apparently life-threatening apneic episode tends to vary with parental perception of the event's severity. If parents, in retrospect, question the validity of their observations, they may have difficulty accepting the necessity of home monitoring. Conversely, parents who experienced a severe event and perceive this episode to be a life-threatening "near-miss" tend to welcome home monitor as the only alternative to 24-hour visual surveillance of the infant. If the initial event occurs during the immediate post-partum hospital stay or if the event was not witnessed by the parents, monitoring may be perceived negatively. Such parents may consider monitoring an unnecessary nuisance for their "perfectly healthy" baby.

The parent's emotional environment can be further affected by their anxiety level; by complex post-partum transitions;[24] by accessibility or lack of accessibility of strong support systems; by their coping ability and personal strengths; and by other life stresses impacting upon the family unit. Thus, the reader can see that each family must be assessed individually to identify the most appropriate approach to meet each family's unique support needs. By understanding each family's needs, the health care provider can facilitate the learning of essential content related to home apnea monitoring and identify psycho-social support mechanisms.

It is essential to provide families with information that will enable them to understand the nature of their child's problem, to comply with the treatment regimen, to appropriately use and respond to monitor alarms, and to maintain healthy family dynamics. This information, though fairly standardized, must be individually tailored to each family depending upon their intellectual capacity, emotional stability, and value orientation as previously discussed. If managed well, each encounter between family and health care provider can build on previously learned information; thus providing a sense of coherency, continuity, and reinforcement of previous learning.

The initial familial contact with caretakers is crucial to the development of mutual respect and to the facilitation of understanding the diagnostic process. This contact often occurs over the telephone or upon hospital admission. In the case of a SIDS sibling, the contact may even be prior to birth of the subsequent child. In most cases this contact is made prior to final determination of need for home apnea monitoring. Thus, the health care provider has the opportunity to provide anticipatory guidance and conduct an informal family assessment.

It has been our experience that if parents understand the nature of and rationale for the various diagnostic tests they will more readily tolerate any inconveniences to themselves or their infant. Parents need to have a realistic concept of the time element involved with the diagnostic tests and the family teaching, so that they can make decisions about their work schedule, childcare arrangements and involvement of other family or friends. Definitions of terms and concepts that parents are likely to hear is helpful for allaying unnecessary anxiety and for establishing the foundation for future teaching.

Perhaps the most effective means of providing the initial information is by assessing the parents' perceptions of each area. The health care provider can then immediately identify areas of misunderstanding or unrealistic expectation and clarify those issues. This method may be initially more time consuming but can prevent later dissatisfaction. Table II outlines suggested content for the initial encounter between caretakers and families and a member of the health care provider team.

We urge that parents of all infants who are hospitalized for an apnea workup learn CPR prior to discharge. Though this may be initially traumatic for parents, we have found that once they

Table II
Suggested Guidelines for Initial Encounter with Caretakers

Introduce self and explain position in the program hierarchy

Conduct family assessment
- Presenting problem
- Parents' perceptions and expectations
- Family support network
- Financial status

Provide anticipatory guidance
- Define commonly used terms: eg. apnea, bradycardia
- Clarify evaluation, testing and duration of hospitalization
- Describe scope of caretaker teaching
  - CPR teaching (1-2 hours)
  - monitor demonstrations (2 hours)
  - family instruction by nurse specialist (1-2 hours)
  - schedule meeting times

have received the training and have practiced their technique, they generally feel more confident of their ability to respond in an emergency. We encourage not only parents, but any potential caretaker (grandparents, friends, older siblings) to attend this session. The session may be conducted for one or more families.

The session should open with introduction of people to one another to promote a sense of group cohesion. To allay anxiety, the teacher should reassure people that a doll will be used for practice and that repetition will be provided. We have found the use of a slide-tape presentation (Trainex, 1968) an effective way of introducing CPR technique for infants. The presentation we use is straight-forward and factual. It demonstrates each step with the use of a resuscibaby so as not to arouse undue emotion.

After the slide presentation, the teacher reviews the steps and demonstrates CPR on a resuscibaby. If it is already known that the family(s) present will be using a monitor, then it is helpful to demonstrate each of the steps from the first sound of a monitor alarm (i.e., the graded responses). Questions are encouraged.

The final step in CPR teaching permits each member of the group to practice their technique. Starting with the most confident member allows more reticent ones to gain courage and learn by role-model and repetition. The teacher emphasizes strong points in technique, but also makes constructive suggestions for improving weak points. If the group seem inhibited by the presence of an "expert" they are left alone with written instructions and the doll and encouraged to practice at their own pace. However, at some point each caretaker should give a return demonstration so that their technique can be evaluated. The doll and slide tape is made available to families for review and practice upon request throughout the infant's hospitalization.

Once it is determined that a monitor is indeed indicated, then teaching can proceed to more specific aspects of home monitoring. Parents need specific information about monitoring, medications, and follow-up plans. They also need anticipatory guidance about adaptation to life with a monitor. Often this information can be provided in response to caretaker's questions. Information not elicited by parent questions can then be presented by the health care provider and discussed.

Initial concerns generally focus on the monitor, when to use it, and what to do when it alarms. Parents are exhorted to use the monitor whenever they are not closely observing the baby and during all sleep periods, both day and night. If they are going to a friend's home for an evening, they are encouraged to take the monitor along. If the monitor is not portable, parents are advised to visually monitor the baby. We do not encourage them to drive alone in a car with the baby, since it is impossible to drive and monitor and/or resuscitate at the same time. In the event the baby is taken out with only one person in the car, we advise that one hand be kept on the baby to monitor breathing movements.

When the baby is on the monitor, we counsel parents to be within a 10-second run. We further suggest that they experiment with the monitor-intercom system to delineate limits of sound and distance. We caution parents about activities that could prevent them from hearing alarms: showers, vacuuming, washing machines, hanging-out clothes, blenders, loud music, etc. If an activity potentially prevents hearing the monitor alarm, we counsel parents to arrange their schedules so that such actions are conducted when another person is present to answer alarms. Such counsel often necessitates a major reorganization of the family schedule and division of labor.

Caretakers are taught a graded response to alarms. When the

monitor alarms, they are instructed to go to baby and "stop, look and listen." They specifically observe for color and respiratory activity. Most often, the infant will have self-corrected spontaneously and nothing more than verification of normal respiration and heart rate is needed. However, if the baby is still apneic, but color is good when they arrive, we recommend they observe the baby for up to 10 seconds (counting one-thousand one, one-thousand two . . . one-thousand ten) to allow him or her to self correct. If, after ten seconds, no respirations are detected or if circumoral pallor or duskiness develops, the caretaker is advised to mildly stimulate the infant (a gentle shake). Obviously, if gentle stimulation does not arouse the infant, stimulation should become progressively more vigorous. If the baby still does not arouse after being picked up, called, and vigorously shaken, CPR should be initiated and help summoned.

We recommend that an apnea and bradycardia log be kept of all alarms that cannot be proven false. A variety of formats exists for logging. We observed that parents seemed intimidated if the log is complex. We provide families with a representative logging form and encourage them to develop their own system for recording, if they wish. If an infant's primary problem is pure obstructive apnea, we request that the parents document persistent bradycardia alarms (greater than five beeps) that occur during sleep and record any bradycardia associated with circumoral pallor or duskiness.

We provide caretakers with 24 hour per day telephone numbers to contact members of the hospital based health care provider team in an emergency or for any other reason (test results, concerns, support). They are exhorted to contact either their pediatrician or the program physician if: (1) there is a sudden increase in the frequency or severity of apnea within a 24-hour period (i.e., three more episodes than their child's normal rate); (2) the infant suddenly requires vigorous stimulation; and (3) and if CPR was necessary.

Parents can often account for unusual events that might have fatigued the infant, resulting in deeper sleep (i.e. circumcision, immunizations, disrupted sleep schedule, over-warm or cold). Caretakers are warned that these events might precipitate apnea[33] and are encouraged not to overprotect their infant, they are advised that these "unusual" events may produce more apnea and that they should respond appropriately. If no precipitating event for the worsening apnea is obvious, then other stimuli such as an early otitis or other infections should be searched for.

If CPR is initiated, paramedics should be summoned to the scene and the baby transported to the nearest emergency center until stable. The program physician should then be notified and, most likely, the baby will be transferred back to the program center for further observation and possible testing.

Parents are instructed to identify the appropriate emergency services in their area, such as ambulance, paramedic, fire department, or police. They are encouraged to call the number to ensure its accuracy and to inform them that their baby is being monitored. Although this practice may not be useful to the rescue squads in large metropolitan areas, it does ensure that the parents have the correct number. In outlying regions, it alerts the potential rescuers of the family's location so they can respond appropriately in an emergency. Families are encouraged to write all emergency numbers in one place and keep them by every phone in the home. This information should also include their address and directions to their home so that anyone could, in a state of panic, read the information over the telephone in case of emergency.

Families are particularly concerned about the anticipated duration of home monitoring. It is generally possible to give them a minimum amount of time and an anticipated maximum, though this is always conditional on the infant's progress. The protocol criteria and follow-up plans for the infant should also be described to the caretakers, for example when the next test will be done and which test will be performed.

A letter is sent by the program to the family's utility company upon initiation of monitoring. With this letter the residence is placed on a medical priority list so that electricity would not be terminated without prior notification and so that power may be restored on a priority basis, if possible. Parents are directed to visually monitor the infant in the case of a power outage unless their monitor is battery operated. Power failure alarms are provided to families using electrical monitors. When monitoring is discontinued, the utility company is so notified by the program.

If medication is prescribed, caretakers need to be taught how to measure the dose, administer the drug, and how to increase the dose per pound of weight gain. Parents are alerted to potential side effects and what action to take if side effects are observed. Better compliance is generally achieved if parents understand the rationale for drug usage.

Finally, the health care provider can help parents anticipate potential problems and identify strategies for coping. The family should identify their local support systems (significant others), such as family, friends, clergy, etc. and if possible invite at least one of these individuals to attend all teaching sessions.

Parents are warned of the potential for social isolation due to the fear of others about the monitoring situation. Primary caretakers are further cautioned about possible "cabin fever". Parents are encouraged to identify a babysitter, so as to enjoy time out alone together. We suggest that they invite their friends in and explain to them about the monitor. If friends remain reluctant to visit, then parents are encouraged to take the baby and monitor out for a visit.

Respite care can be a severe problem, especially for families with little local support and for working mothers. A few insurance companies will pay for a small amount of regular respite care. Sometimes pediatric nurses or other monitor parents will babysit. Some home care agencies have staff who are trained to care for monitored infants. The major requirement is that any caretaker be trained in CPR, know how to use the monitor, and know how to respond appropriately to alarms.

Older siblings can present special problems as well. Parents should be helped to identify a strategy for explaining the monitor to the other family children in terms they can understand. Older siblings above 10–12 years of age can be a valuable resource and can effectively participate in the care of the infant.

In addition to this specific discussion about life with a monitor, families need an understanding of basic monitor mechanics. The monitor demonstration should focus on mechanics (i.e. how to identify lead problems, how to correct the causes of false alarms etc.) and can reinforce or be reinforced by the previously discussed information depending upon the sequence of the sessions. Home set-up and review of monitoring techniques by monitoring company personnel generally occurs within 24 hours of discharge. If the new monitoring family lives in an outlying or distant area, the above follow-up visit may not be feasible. In that case, the assistance of the primary physician, local social agencies, and the VNA are sought. Theoretically, a home-visit by a member of the health care provider team would be ideal for assessment of the home environment and initial adaptation to the monitor. Our team is not large enough to provide that service on a regular basis. Coordination between team members and public health agencies can prevent duplication of services. Follow-up by our health care provider team is generally conducted by telephone.

Content and frequency of follow-up calls varies with the particular support needs of individual families. We find that families who have previously lost an infant tend to require the most support initially. Emotional support requirements appear greatest for most families during the first weeks of monitoring and when monitoring is discontinued. Table III suggests a list of subjects for follow-up and assessment. If good rapport has been established during the initial contact and teaching session(s), then caretakers are more likely to express other concerns and respond honestly to questions.

As previously alluded to, parents who accept monitoring appear to go through a series of stages. First they try to understand the nature of the problem and the rationale for monitoring. Then they work to develop technical expertise so that they can use the monitor confidently. As they gain experience at home they begin to trust their ability to respond to alarms while learning to trust the monitor to alarm at the appropriate time.

Families who experience no alarms tend to find the monitor reassuring, but develop confidence in their infant's ability to self-arouse. Families who experience frequent false alarms may become disgusted, and, unless the situation is quickly remedied, begin to lose confidence in the monitor. Families who experience "true" alarms and observe apneic episodes tend to trust the monitor and can develop dependently on it for the relative security it affords.

Families who have found the monitor reassuring often find its discontinuation as traumatic as its initiation. They are now confronted with the task of transferring their dependence from the monitor back to themselves and the baby. Thus, our support efforts extend to the point where the caretakers feel comfortable living without the monitor.

We try to help parents anticipate discontinuation of the monitor by discussing the probable event in advance of its final occurence. We encourage parents to develop their own mutually agreed-upon plan. They may choose to go "cold turkey" or "wean" them-

Table III
Suggested Follow-Up Assessment Guide

Assess family's coping with monitor and baby
Baby's sleeping location
Location and use
Monitor problems
Sibling and significant other reactions
Changes in lifestyle and family relationships
Assess caretaker's response to monitor alarms
CPR review
Apnea log
Plan of response to life threatening episode
Assess family understanding of hospital test results and follow-up program
Assess family understanding of other medical problems and treatment regimes
Gastroesophageal reflux
Seizures
Aminophylline

selves more gradually. In either case *they* set the target date for actual return of the monitor and *they* make the phone call to ask for monitor pick-up. This allows the parents to be in total control of their monitor return. In our experience with this system, most parents have returned the monitor within one to three weeks of medical discontinuation.

Some parents find contact with other "monitor-families" to be an aid in coping. Families can be a valuable resource to guide, encourage, and support one another during and after the monitor experience. A caretaker's group can provide families with a sense of cohesiveness. Furthermore, such a group can work together to increase community awareness of infantile apnea and home monitoring and to raise money for medically indigent families, research, and parent education aids. In our experience, it is the post-monitor families who have the time, energy, and desire to be involved in such a group. During the course of monitoring phone contact between monitor-families is most helpful. Such family support networks should be enthusiastically supported.

We provide the name and telephone number of our home monitoring "parent's group" to all new monitoring families. If agreeable to the new monitoring family, their name, address, and phone number is also given to the parent's organization. This permits the parent's organization to contact them and help them through the difficult adaptation period. The parent's support group holds monthly meetings at the hospital and invitations are extended to all current monitoring families. The first part of each meeting is devoted to a review of CPR by a member of the health care provider team and families are encouraged to obtain additional supervised experience if they feel it would be helpful. The remainder of the program is totally arranged by the parents. It may include an open discussion of life with the monitor, invited lectures, or a question and answer session. A 24-hour a day parent's group telephone hotline is now in operation.

Another significant role of the hospital based health care provider team is to educate the medical and lay community about SIDS, its possible prevention, and provide information about the identification and referral of high risk infants. To that end, presentations to community nursing groups, ER staffs, medical societies, and community organizations such as the Kiwanis Club, the fire department, and ladies clubs is imperative.

We have alluded to the vague concept of "program". We have shared what "we" do with our families. However, the type of program developed will vary depending upon local needs and resources. The essential staff should include a physician with expertise in sleep testing, an experienced nurse to provide parent-education and psycho-social support and technicians able to conduct the sleep testing and demonstrate monitor mechanics. If the program is to extend beyond families to the community, then a masters-prepared nurse with expertise in program planning, community health, and public speaking can be an asset.

We would concur with Cain, Kelly, and Shannon[27] that "with availability of a psycho-social support system, electronic home monitoring of infants can be conducted by parents without constant and extreme anxiety and . . . can even be a satisfying experience."

References

1. Shannon DC, Kelly DH: SIDS and near-SIDS. *N Engl J Med* 306:959, 1982.

2. Shannon DC, Kelly DH: SIDS and near-SIDS. *N Engl J Med* 306:1022, 1982.
3. Valdes-Dapena MA: Sudden infant death syndrome: A review of the medical literature 1974–1979. *Pediatrics* 66:597, 1980.
4. Valdes-Dapena MA: Sudden and unexpected death in infancy: A review of the world literature 1954–1966. *Pediatrics* 39:123, 1967.
5. Guntheroth WG: *Crib Death: The Sudden Infant Death Syndrome,* Mount Kisco, New York, Futura Publishing Company, 1982.
6. Guntheroth WG: *In* Wedgewood RJ, Banditt EP, (eds): *Sudden Death in Infants.* USPHS publication No. 1412, p. 6.
7. Steinschneider A: Prolonged apnea and the sudden infant death syndrome: Clinical and laboratory observations. *Pediatrics* 50:646, 1972.
8. Tonkin S: Sudden infant death syndrome: Hypothesis of causation. *Pediatrics* 55:650, 1975.
9. Stark AR, Thach BT: Mechanisms of airway obstruction leading to apnea in newborn infants. *J Pediat* 89:982, 1976.
10. Brouilette RT, Thach BT: A neuromuscular mechanism maintaining extrathoracic airway patency. *J Appl Physiol* 46:772, 1979.
11. Anders T, Ende R, Parmalee A: *A manual of standardized terminology and criteria for scoring of states of sleep and wakefulness in newborn infants.* UCLA Brain Information Service/BRI Publications Office, Los Angeles, California, Ninds Neurological Information Network, 1971.
12. Steinschneider A, Weinstein SL, Diamond E: The sudden infant death syndrome and apnea/obstruction during neonatal sleep and feeding. *Pediatrics* 70:858, 1982.
13. Kelly DH, Shannon DC: Periodic breathing in infants with near miss sudden infant death syndrome. *Pediatrics* 63:355, 1979.
14. Kelly DH, Walker AM, Cahen L, et al: Periodic breathing in siblings of sudden infant death syndrome victims. *Pediatrics* 66:515, 1980.
15. Kelly DH, Shannon DC: personal communication.
16. McCulloch K, Brouilette RT, Guzzetta AJ, et al: Arousal responses in near-miss sudden infant death syndrome and in normal infants. *J Pediat* 101:911, 1982.
17. Kraus JF, Borhani NO: Post neonatal sudden unexplained death in California: A cohort study. *Am J Epidemiol* 95:497, 1972.
18. Naeye RL, Ladis B, Drage JS: Sudden infant death syndrome: a prospective study. *Am J Dis Child* 130:1207, 1976.
19. Finnegan LP: In utero opiate dependence and sudden infant death syndrome. *Clin Perinat* 6:163, 1979.
20. Naeye RL: Placental abnormalities in victims of the sudden infant death syndrome. *Biol Neonate* 32:189, 1977.
21. Jolley SG, Herbst JJ, Johnson DG, et al: Esophageal pH monitoring during sleep identifies children with respiratory symptoms from gastroesophageal reflux. *Gastroenterology* 80:1501, 1981.
22. Milsap RL, Krauss AN, Auld PAM: Efficacy of low dose theophylline. *Sem Perinat* 5:321, 1981.
23. Steinschneider A: A re-examination of the "apnea monitor business". *Pediatrics* 58:4, 1976.

24. Mercer RT: The nurse and maternal tasks of early postpartum. *Maternal Child Nursing* 6, 341. Sept/Oct., 1981.
25. Lundeen KW: When baby makes three . . . Challenges. *Nursing* 74, 1982.
26. Rodenberger DJ: Apnea monitoring. *Nursing* 9, 1982.
27. Cain LP, Kelly DH, Shannon DC: Parents' perception of the psychological and social impact of home monitoring. *Pediatrics* 66:37, 1980.
28. Bergman AB, Beckwith JB, Ray CG: The apnea monitor business. *Pediatrics* 56:1, 1975.
29. Task Force on Prolonged Apnea. Prolonged apnea. *Pediatrics* 61:561, 1978.
30. Nelson NM: But who shall monitor the monitor? *Pediatrics* 61:663, 1978.
31. Committee on infant of preschool child. Home monitoring for sudden infant death. *Pediatrics* 55:144, 1975.
32. Shannon DC: Monitoring for SIDS. *J Res Dis* 2:104, 1981.
33. McGinty DJ, Harper RM: Sleep physiology and SIDS: Animal and human studies. *In* Robinson RR, (ed): *SIDS*. Canada, Canadian Foundation for the study of infant deaths, 1974. p. 201.

Index

Abdominal examination
coma, 46
intestinal injury, 385
shock, 141
Abdominal injury, 373, 376–378
Absorption, of poisons, 438–444
Accidental poisonings, 427
Accidents, 55
Acetazolamide, 49
Acidosis, 300–301
Activated charcoal powder, 440–441, 442–443
Activated partial thromboplastin time (APTT), 469–470
Acute bacterial meningitis, 96–109
Enterobacteriaceae, 103–105
group B streptococcus, 102–103
Hemophilus influenzae, 96–99
initial antimicrobial therapy for, 107–109
Listeria monocytogenes, 105–106
Mycobacterium tuberculosis, 106–107
Neisseria meningitidis, 99–101
Streptococcus pneumoniae, 101–102
See also Meningitis
Acute epiglottitis. *See* Epiglottitis
Acute hemorrhagic leukoencephalopathy, 38–39
Acute infections. *See* Infections
Acute laryngotracheobronchitis, 281, 282
Acute streptococcal pneumonia, 241
Addison's disease, 48
Adenoid tissue, 182
Adenosine arabinoside, 110
Adenosine-triphosphate (ATP), 27
Adult respiratory distress syndrome (ARDS), 140, 228, 232–233, 309–324
clinical course and complications in, 313–314
clinical features of, 312–313
differential diagnosis of, 316–317
historical aspects of, 309–310
laboratory findings of, 316
mortality and morbidity in, 311
pathology of, 315–316
proposed etiology, 311–312
radiology and, 228, 232–233, 314–315
treatment of, 317–321
Aerosolized medication, 344–345
Aerosol masks, 342
Aerosol units, 340
Airway
angioneurotic edema, 284
cardiopulmonary resuscitation, 152–153
coma, 44, 50
croup, 281–282, 289
epiglottitis, 280
foreign bodies, 517
inhalation injury, 412
obstruction causes, 283
status asthmaticus, 300
sudden infant death syndrome, 548
traumatic injury, 372
See also Obstructive airway lesions; Respiration
Airway (artificial), 292–293, 295
Albumin
pleural effusion and, 326–327
septic shock syndrome, 499
shock, 143
Alcohol abuse
coma, 39–40, 46, 52
head injury, 62
Alpha-2-antiplasmin, 458
Alveolar edema, 228
American Burn Association, 409
American Heart Association, 149
American Thoracic Society, 299
Aminoglycosides, 104
Amphotericin B, 111–112
Ampicillin, 96, 102, 103, 104, 105, 106
adult respiratory distress syndrome, 319
epiglottitis, 295
Angiofibroma, 185, 187
Angioneurotic edema, 284
Anomalous pulmonary artery, 203, 209
Antibiotics
adult respiratory distress syndrome, 319
central nervous system infection, 95
croup, 291
epiglottitis, 294–295
infection and, 483–484
neonatal sepsis syndrome, 488, 492–493
nosocomial infection, 487
pneumonia, 509
septic shock syndrome, 498–499
skull injury, 63
status asthmaticus, 305
Anticonvulsants
central nervous system infections, 112
poisonings, 437–438
status epilepticus, 88–92
Antidiuretic hormone (ADH), 112–113
Antidotes, 447–448, 450–453
Anxiety
croup, 288–289
ventilators and, 349–350
Aortic tear, 263–264
Apnea
sudden infant death syndrome and, 546, 564
types of, 546–551
See also Sudden infant death syndrome
Apomorphine, 438, 439
Aqueduct of Sylvius, 6
Arachnoid villi, 7
ARDS. *See* Adult respiratory distress syndrome
Arnold-Chiari malformations, 43, 44
Arterial blood gases, 126–127
See also Blood gases
Arterial carbon dioxide tension, 10, 11
Arterial pressure, 126, 127–128
See also Blood pressure
Artificial airway, 292–293, 295
Aryepiglottic cysts, 189, 194
Aseptic meningitis, 110
See also Meningitis
Aspergillosis, 243
Asthma. *See* Status asthmaticus
Astrogliao cells, 6
Ataxia, 432
Atelectasis, 248
Atropine, 154
Automobile accidents, 371, 394

Back blows, 539
Bacterial meningitis. *See* Acute bacterial meningitis; Meningitis
Barbiturate coma, 29–30
Barbiturate therapy, 32
Barometric pressure, 269, 271
Basal ganglia, 6
Basilar skull fracture, 63

Beckwith-Wiedemann syndrome, 188
Benzathine penicillin G, 102
Bleeding and clotting disorders, 457–478
  clinical presentation of, 459–467
  cyanotic congenital heart disease, 465–466
  diagnosis, 461
  differential diagnosis, 461, 471–474
  disseminated intravascular coagulation, 462–463, 464
  immune thrombocytopenic purpura (ITP), 466
  kidney, 465
  laboratory and, 468–471
  liver, 463–464
  massive blood loss, 467
  pathophysiology of, 458
  prognosis, 477
  septic shock syndrome, 494–495, 501
  surgery and, 461–462
  therapeutic considerations in, 474–477
  von Willebrand's disease, 466–467
Bleeding time, 471
Blood-brain barrier, 8, 72, 82
Blood gases
  adult respiratory distress syndrome, 316, 317
  burns, 412, 419
  cardiovascular monitoring, 126–127
  cor pulmonale, 164
  croup, 285
  monitoring devices for, 133
  oxygen therapy, 344
  respiratory care, 357–358, 361–362, 364
  respiratory failure, 271, 272–273
  shock, 142
  status asthmaticus, 302
  thoracic injury, 375
  traumatic injury, 373
Blood loss (massive), 467
Blood pressure
  brain injury, 71
  cardiovascular monitoring, 126–130
  cerebral blood flow and, 9
  coma, 42
  near-drowning, 30
  septic shock syndrome, 501
  shock, 142, 144–145
  See also Arterial blood pressure
Blood tests
  bleeding disorders, 468
  coma, 47
  epiglottitis, 295
  shock, 143
  sites for obtaining, 357
  status epilepticus, 87
Blood transfusion
  bleeding disorders, 462, 467, 476
  neonatal sepsis syndrome, 492
Blood volume, 8
Body temperature
  cardiovascular monitoring, 125
  hemoperfusion, 447
  infections and, 482
  near-drowning, 29
  shock, 141, 143
  skull injury, 63
  spinal cord injury, 404
  See also Fever; Hypothermia
Body weight, 126
Bone marrow production, 457, 458
Bradycardia, 546, 548
Brain
  anatomy of, 6–7
  cardiopulmonary resuscitation and, 156, 157
  coma, 42–43, 45–46
  intracranial hemorrhage, 466
  near-drowning, 26, 27
  pathology of, 17–19
  physiology of, 7–12
Brain (*Continued*)
  physiopathology and clinical considerations, 19–20
  shock, 140
  volume-pressure relationships, 12–15
  See also Head injury; Skull injury
Brain abscesses, 37, 49
Brain death, 19, 51–52
Brain metabolism, 8, 27
Brain parenchyma, 6
Brain tumors, 49
Breath odor, 433
Breech delivery, 394
Bronchi, foreign bodies in, 520
Bronchial fracture, 263
Bronchial injury, 375
Bronchopulmonary dysplasia, 166
Brooke formula, 416, 417
Burn evaluation charts, 414
Burns, 409–426
  early management, 412–420
  frequency of, 409
  initial evaluation, 410–412
  management concerns in, 420–424
  prevention of, 409

Caesarean section, 394
Calcium, 143, 500
Calcium chloride, 154–155
Cancer, 331, 335–336
Candida albicans, 508
Candida spp., 111
Cannulation, 364–366
Capillaries, 8
Capnography, 360–361
Carbon dioxide, 8, 161–162
Carbon monoxide poisoning, 410, 412
Cardiac arrest, 150, 152–156
Cardiac catheterization, 156–166
Cardiac injury, 264
Cardiac output, 152, 413, 416
Cardiac tamponade, 239–240
Cardiogenic shock, 137, 138
  catheterization, 142
  pathophysiology of, 138
Cardiopulmonary by-pass, 138
Cardiopulmonary resuscitation (CPR), 28, 149–158
  blood flow during, 151–152
  complications in, 157
  development of, 149
  foreign bodies, 540
  sudden infant death syndrome and, 567–568, 571, 572
  termination of, 156
  See also Cerebral-cardiopulmonary resuscitation
Cardiovascular monitoring, 123–135
  ancillary devices for, 132–134
  arterial blood gases, 126–127
  arterial pressure, 126, 127–128
  body temperature, 125
  body weight, 126
  cardiac output, 130–131
  central venous pressure, 129–130
  echocardiography, 131–132
  electrocardiograph, 124
  equipment for, 124–134
  fluoroscopy, 131
  goals of, 123
  pulmonary wedge pressures, 128–129
  urine output, 125–126
Cathartics, 441, 443–444
Catheterization
  abdominal injury, 377–378
  adult respiratory distress syndrome, 320–321
  arterial pressure monitoring, 128–129
  brain injury, 69–70

Catheterization (*Continued*)
burns, 418, 419
cor pulmonale, 165–166
kidney injury, 382
nasal catheters, 341
respiratory failure, 273–274
septic shock syndrome, 498
shock, 141–142
status asthmaticus, 302
traumatic injury, 373
urethral injury, 390
urine output measurement, 125–126
CBF. *See* Cerebral blood flow
Cefamandole, 295
Centilators, 352–354
Central apnea, 546, 547
Central nervous system infection, 95–115
acute bacterial meningitis, 96–109
supportive therapy, 112–113
viral, 109–110
Central venous pressure, 129–130
Cephalosporins, 100, 105
Cerebral blood flow (CBF), 8–12, 81, 82
Cerebral-cardiopulmonary resuscitation, 25, 31–34
See also Cardiopulmonary resuscitation (CPR)
Cerebral concussion, 61
Cerebral death. *See* Brain death
Cerebral edema, 19, 33
Cerebral metabolic rate (CMR), 81
Cerebral perfusion pressure (CPP)
brain injury, 69
cerebral blood flow and, 9–10
near-drowning, 25–26, 27, 29, 30, 32–33
Cerebral swelling, edema contrasted, 19
Cerebrospinal fluid (CSF)
brain injury, 70
brain physiology and, 7
coma and, 48, 49
head injury, 58
raised intracranial pressure, 16–17
Reye's syndrome, A–2
skull injury, 60, 63
volume-pressure relationships, 12–15
Cerebrospinal fluid fistula, 57
Cervical spine. *See* Spinal cord injury
Charcoal. *See* Activated charcoal powder
Chemical burns, 410
Chest physiotherapy (CPT), 345–346
Chest tube drainage, 335–336
Child abuse
brain injury, 65
burns, 410–411
coma, 45
head injury and, 74
skull injury and, 60
Chlamydial pneumonia, 241
Chlamydia tracomatis, 508
Chloramphenicol, 96–97, 98–99, 101–102, 104, 106, 295, 493
Chloramphenicol succinate, 100
Choanal atresia, 175, 180–185
Choking, 517
Chronic lung disease, 161
Chylothorax, 331, 334
Cine-angiography, 151
Cingulate herniation, 18
Circulatory insufficiency. *See* Shock
Clotting disorders. *See* Bleeding and clotting disorders
Clotting factor, 460
Coagulation, 140
Coagulation laboratory, 471
Colic, 433
Colonic injuries, 388–389
Coma, 35–53
cardiopulmonary resuscitation, 157
definitions, 35–36
Coma (*Continued*)
definitive diagnosis, 47–49
diagnosis, 44–49
Glasgow Coma Scale, 62, 63
head injury, 61–62
irreversible, 51–52
near-drowning, 25–26, 28–30
physiopathology of, 36–44
poisonings, 432, 435, 437, 445, 447
prevention, 52–53
prognosis, 50–52
spinal cord injury, 401
therapy, 49–50
therapy directed diagnosis, 44–47
traumatic injury, 373
Comminuted depressed skull fracture, 60
Compliance, 14, 15
Compliance studies, 358–359
Computed tomography
brain injury, 67
coma, 45, 46, 47
head injury, 57–58
intestinal injury, 385
nasopharynx, 185
obstructive airway disease, 174–175
pleural effusion, 328
seizures, 48
See also Radiology
Concussion. *See* Cerebral concussion
Congenital diseases and anomalies
bleeding disorders, 457
coma, 43–44
heart disease, 457
lobar emphysema, 235
Congestive heart failure, 334
Contact phase, 458
Continuous partial status epilepticus, 79
Continuous Positive Airway Pressure (CPAP), 353–354
Convulsions, 432, 437–438
Convulsive status epilepticus, 79
Cor pulmonale, 159–169
clinical presentation and evaluation, 163–166
defined, 159
differential diagnosis, 166
etiology, 160
incidence, 160
pathophysiology, 159–163
prognosis, 167–168
therapy, 166–167
Corticosteroids, 107
adult respiratory distress syndrome, 232–233, 318–319
inhalation injury, 412
septic shock syndrome, 501–502
shock, 147
status asthmaticus, 305
See also Steroids
Coughing, 346
CPP. *See* Cerebral perfusion pressure
CPR. *See* Cardiopulmonary resuscitation
Croup (laryngotracheobronchitis), 281–282
clinical features, 279
foreign bodies and, 519
incidence, 278
pathophysiology, 284–287
radiology, 194
therapy, 288–293
Cryptococcus neoformans, 111
CT scan. *See* Computed tomography
Cushing's disease, 48
Cyanotic congenital heart disease, 465–466, 468
Cystic fibrosis, 166, 167, 168
hypercapnia and, 48
Cystic hygroma, 188

Dandy-Walker syndrome, 43, 44

Decannulation, 364–366
Decompressive laminectomy, 404
Defibrillation, 155–156
Dehydration, 137, 301
Depressed skull fracture, 63
Developmental anomalies, 43–44
Dexamathasone sodium phosphate, 30
Dialysis, 445, 446
Diaphragmatic hernia, 252–253
Diaphragmatic injury, 264
Diastolic blood pressure, 127
  See also Blood pressure
Diazepam, 88–89, 91
Digitalis, 166
Disseminated intravascular coagulation (DIC), 460, 462–463, 464, 477
Diuresis, 444–445
Diuretics, 500
Dobutamine, 145, 146
Dopamine, 30, 145–146
Doppler echocardiography, 132
  See also Echocardiography
Drowning
  cerebral-cardiopulmonary resuscitation, 25
  defined, 26
  incidence, 26
  types of, 26
  See also Near-drowning
Drug abuse
  coma, 39–40, 52
  head injury, 62
  poisonings by, 429, 430, 435
Duodenal injury, 385–386

Ear, 60–61
Ear oximetry, 362
Echocardiography, 131–132, 142, 151, 164–165
EEG. *See* Electroencephalograph
Ehlers-Danlos syndrome, 460, 473
Elastance, 14, 15
Electrocardiograph
  cardiovascular monitoring, 124
  cor pulmonale, 164
  poisonings, 437
  shock, 142
Electroencephalograph (EEG)
  brain injury, 71
  cerebral blood flow, 10
  near-drowning, 30
  seizures, 48
  status epilepticus, 85, 86
  sudden infant death syndrome, 561
Electrolytes, 301, 437
Emesis
  activated charcoal, 441
  brain injury, 65
  contraindications, 440
  poisons, 433, 438–439
Emphysema (congenital lobar), 235
Empyema, 331
Encephalitis
  coma, 37, 48
  herpes simplex virus, 110
  intoxications, 39
Encephalopathy, 49
Endobronchial foreign bodies, 212–213, 216
Endorphins, 502
Endotoxic shock, 137, 138
Endotracheal tube
  cardiopulmonary resuscitation, 153
  care and monitoring, 355
  croup and epiglottitis, 292, 293
  intubation, 347
Enterobacteriaceae, 103–105
Enterococcus, 314
Epidural hematoma, 67
Epiglottitis (supraglottitis), 278–280
Epiglottitis (supraglottitis) (*Continued*)
  acute, 194, 200–201
  clinical features, 279–280
  diagnosis, 283–284
  incidence, 277
  pathophysiology, 284–287
  radiology, 194, 200–201
  therapy, 293–295
Epilepsy. *See* Status epilepticus
Epinephrine, 145, 154, 290–291, 294
Epistaxis, 460
Eschar separation, 423
Escharotomy, 420
Escherichia coli, 490, 502
Esophageal foreign bodies, 221–225, 520–521
Esophageal injury, 375–376
Ethambutol, 107
Evans formula, 417
Extrahepatic biliary tree, 384
Extubation, 364–366
Eye
  poisonings, 432
  skull injury, 60, 61–62, 63
  See also Pupillary response

Facial fracture, 209
Falx cerebri, 6
Family history. *See* Patient history
Fasciotomy, 420
Fever, 472, 484–485
  See also Body temperature
Fibrinogen, 458, 459, 470
Fibrothorax, 331
Fick principle, 130
First degree burns, 411
Flucytosine, 111–112
Fluids
  burns, 413, 416–419, 421–422
  poisonings, 437
  shock, 144–145
Fluoroscopy, 131
Foley catheter. *See* Catheterization
Foramen magnum herniation, 18
Foreign bodies, 517–542
  croup and epiglottitis differentiated, 283
  diagnosis, 536
  differential diagnosis, 517, 536–539
  endobronchial, 212–213, 216
  hypopharyngeal, 210
  laryngo-tracheal, 210, 212
  pathophysiology, 518–521
  physical findings, 522–523, 524
  prevention, 541
  radiology, 209–225, 523–536, 537
  symptoms and clinical presentation, 521–522
  therapy, 539–541
Fresh water drowning, 27, 31
Fungal meningitis, 38, 111–112
Furosemide, 49

Gall bladder, 384
Gastric injury, 385
Gastric lavage, 438, 440
Gastroesophageal reflux (GER), 248–249, 548, 561
Gastrointestinal bleeding, 460
Gastrointestinal tract, 405
Genitourinary injury, 390
Glasgow Coma Scale, 62, 63, 64, 65, 66, 68, 72, 74
Gluconate, 154
Glucose, 143–144, 333–334
Gregory hood, 354
Grey matter, 6, 8
Group B streptococcus, 102–103, 490
Growing skull fracture (leptomeningeal cyst), 60

Hageman factor, 494, 495
Head injury, 55–77
  clinical presentation and diagnosis, 59–62
  frequency, 55
  mortality, 55
  pathology, 56–58
  physiopathology, 59
  prevention, 74
  prognosis, 56, 59, 61–62, 72–74
  seizures, 48
  therapy, 62–72
  traumatic injury, 373
  See also Brain; Skull injury
Heart
  cardiac output, 130
  cardiopulmonary resuscitation, 151–152, 153, 156, 157
  cyanotic congenital heart disease, 465–466
  poisonings, 437
  septic shock syndrome, 501
  shock, 139, 141, 145
  spinal cord injury, 403–404
  status epilepticus, 82
  thoracic injury, 375
  See also entries under Cardiac; Cardio-
Heart surgery, 462
Heimlich procedure, 539
Helium-oxygen therapy, 292
Hemangioma, 189
Hemarthrosis, 460
Hematoma
  bleeding and clotting disorders, 460
  duodenal, 386
  epidural, 67
  head injury, 58, 59
  intracranial, 67
  kidney, 283
  liver, 384
  lung, 256
  subgaleal, 62–63
Hematuria
  bleeding disorders, 460
  kidney injury, 382
Hemodialysis, 445
Hemodynamic monitoring. *See* Cardiovascular monitoring
Hemoperfusion, 445, 446, 447
Hemophilus influenzae, 96–99, 200, 278, 294–295, 507, 509
Hemorrhage
  bleeding disorders, 460
  coma, 42
  intracranial, 466
  shock, 137, 143
  traumatic injury, 373
Hemostasis. *See* Bleeding and clotting disorders
Hemothorax, 331, 374–375
Hemotympanum, 60–61
Heparin, 477
Hepatic injury. *See* Liver
Hernia (diaphragmatic), 252–253
Herpes encephalitis, 37, 48, 110
High Frequency Ventilation (HFV), 354–355
Histoplasma capsulatum, 111
Hoods (oxygen), 342–343
Humidification
  croup, 288, 289–290
  epiglottitis, 294
  respiratory care, 340, 356
Hydration
  croup, 290
  near-drowning, 29
  status asthmaticus, 304
Hyperbaric oxygenation
  cerebral edema, 33
  See also Oxygen therapy
Hypercapnia, 300
Hypertension
  cor pulmonale, 161, 162–163
  See also Blood pressure; Intracranial hypertension
Hyperthermia
  spinal cord injury, 404
  See also Body temperature; Fever
Hypoglycemia, 46, 48
Hyponatremia, 112
Hypopharyngeal foreign bodies, 210
Hypotension
  coma, 44–45
  poisonings, 437
  shock, 139, 141
  See also Blood pressure
Hypothermia
  burns, 410
  intoxications, 40
  near-drowning, 31, 33
  See also Body temperature
Hypothyroidism, 188
Hypovolemic shock, 137–138, 141
  catheterization, 142
  central venous pressure, 130
  pathophysiology, 138
  See also Shock
Hypoxemia
  adult respiratory distress syndrome, 313
  croup, 285, 289
  status asthmaticus, 300
Hypoxia, 271, 272, 273

Iatrogenic coma, 40
ICP. *See* Intracranial pressure
Idoxuridine, 110
Ileus, 419
Immune thrombocytopenia purpura (ITP), 466
Immunology
  adenoid tissue, 182
  bleeding disorders, 457
  burns, 420
  croup and epiglottitis, 283–284
  neonates, 489
Immunosuppressive therapy, 138
Immunotherapy, 449
Impairment of consciousness, 35–36
Incubators, 343
Infants and infancy
  coma, 36–37
  herpes simplex encephalitis, 110
  meningitis, 102, 104, 108
  shock, 138
  status epilepticus, 82, 85–86
  See also entries under Neonatal
Infection
  burns, 422–424
  central nervous system, 95–115 *See also* Central nervous system infection
  coma and, 36–39, 48–49
  cor pulmonale and, 167
  croup, 282
  empyema, 331
  epiglottitis, 278
  foreign bodies and, 520
  general considerations in, 481–484
  hospital acquired, 484–488 *See also* Nosocomial infection
  lung, 241–243
  neonatal sepsis syndrome, 488–493 *See also* Neonatal sepsis syndrome
  pneumonia, 503–510 *See also* Pneumonia
  septic shock syndrome, 138, 493–503 *See also* Septic shock syndrome
  shock, 143
  viral, 109–110
Inhalation injury, 410, 412

Interhemispheric cisterns, 6
Intermittent Mandatory Ventilation (IMV), 351
Intermittent Positive Pressure Breathing (IPPB), 344
Internal bleeding, 460
Interstitial edema, 228
Intestinal injuries, 385–389
Intoxications
 coma, 39–40, 46, 49, 50, 52
 pupillary response and, 46–47
Intracranial hematoma, 67
Intracranial hypertension, 8
Intracranial pressure (ICP), 15–17
 brain injury, 69, 70–71
 cerebral blood flow and, 9
 cerebrospinal fluid, 7
 clinical considerations, 19–20
 coma, 49
 drowning, 25–26
 factors in, 20
 head injury, 59
 intracranial hypertension and, 8
 monitoring of, 5
 near-drowning, 27, 29, 30–31, 32, 33–34
 normal, 15–16
 pathology, 17–19
 raised, 16–17
 tumors, 39
 volume-pressure relationships, 12–15
Intracranial tumors, 39
Intravascular coagulation, 140
Intubation
 extubation, 364–366
 radiology, 355
 respiratory care, 346–348
Ipecac, 438–439, 440, 441
Irreversible coma, 51–52
Isolettes, 343
Isoniazid, 106, 107
Isoproterenol, 145, 275, 304–305, 306–307

Jejunoileal injuries, 388

Ketoconazole, 112
Kidney
 bleeding disorders, 465
 disease of, 457
 injury, 376, 377, 382–383
 poisonings, 444–445
 septic shock syndrome, 500–501
 shock, 142–143

Lactic acidosis, 141
Laparotomy, 384, 385, 386
Laryngomalacia, 189
Laryngo-tracheal foreign bodies, 210, 212
Laryngotracheobronchitis. *See* Croup
Larynx
 foreign bodies, 519, 537
 fracture, 209
 radiology, 189, 194
Law, brain death and, 52
Lennox-Gastaut syndrome, 84
Leptomeningeal cyst, 60
Lesion. *See* Obstructive airway lesions
Lethargy, 35
Leukemia, 39, 457
Leukoencephalopathy (acute hemorrhagic), 38–39
Lidocaine, 154, 155
Linear skull fracture, 60
Listeria monocytogenes, 105–106, 490
Liver
 cardiopulmonary resuscitation, 157
 cor pulmonale, 164
Liver (*Continued*)
 disease of, 457, 463–464
 injury to, 376, 377, 383–384
 septic shock syndrome, 496, 501
 shock, 143
Lobar collapse, 249, 252
Lumbar puncture, 46, 48
Lung
 contusion, 254, 256
 cor pulmonale, 159
 drowning, 27
 foreign bodies, 523
 lobar collapse, 249, 252
 pleural effusion, 325–337 *See also* Pleural effusion
 pulmonary laceration, 256, 260
 shock lung, 140, 141, 142
 trauma to, 253–254
 See also Thorax
Lung disease
 cor pulmonale and, 161
 hypercapnia, 48
Lung hematoma, 256
Lung infection, 241–243
Lupus erythematosis, 460
Lupus inhibitor, 460
Lymphoma, 185, 186

Macroglossia, 188
Mafenide, 422–423
Magnesium, 500
Malnutrition, 41
Mannitol, 30
Masks (oxygen), 341–343
Measles, 284
Meningitis
 aseptic, 110
 coma, 36–37, 46, 48, 49, 50
 fungal, 111–112
 septic shock syndrome, 496
Meningococcemia, 496, 497
Metabolic measurement system, 133–134
Metabolism
 brain, 8, 27
 burns, 421–422
 coma, 40–41, 42, 50
Metaproterenol, 304–305
Minocycline, 100
Mixed apneic episodes, 546, 548
M-mode echocardiography, 131–132, 142, 165 *See also* Echocardiography
Monro-Kellie hypothesis, 5, 12, 13
Mouth
 poisonings, 433
 radiology, 188
Moxalactam, 99
Muscular paralysis, 29
Mycobacterium tuberculosis, 106–107
Myelosuppression, 112

Naloxone, 437
Nasal cannulae, 341
Nasal prongs, 354
Nasopharyngeal angiofibroma, 185, 187
Nasopharynx, 175, 180–185
National Clearinghouse for Poison Control Centers, 449
Near-drowning
 adult respiratory distress syndrome, 314
 cerebral-cardiopulmonary resuscitation, 31–34
 coma, 49
 defined, 26
 neurological classification, 28–30
 pathophysiology, 27
 therapy, 27, 28–30

Near-drowning (*Continued*)
types of, 26
Neisseria meningitidis, 99–101
Neonatal sepsis syndrome, 488–493
clinical presentation, 491–492
pathophysiology, 489–490
prevention, 493
prognosis, 493
therapy, 492–493
Neonates. *See* Infants and infancy
Neurogenic bladder, 405
Nonconvulsive status epilepticus, 79
Nontoxic agents, 431
Nosocomial infection, 484–488
clinical presentation, 485–486
diagnosis, 486
pathophysiology, 485
prevention, 487–488
prognosis, 487
risk of, 484
therapy for, 487
Nuchal rigidity, 46
Nuclear camera, 133
Nutrition, 421–422
See also entries under Vitamin deficiency

Obesity, 48
Obstetrics, 394
Obstructive airway lesions, 173–175
See also Airway
Obstructive apnea, 546, 547, 548, 564
Obtundation, 35
Oral cavity
poisonings, 433
radiology, 188
Orotracheal tubes, 348
Oxygen hoods, 342–343
Oxygen tents, 342
Oxygen therapy
adult respiratory distress syndrome, 318, 319
aerosolized medication administration, 344–345
aerosol units, 340
blood gases, 357
burns, 412
cor pulmonale, 166–167
croup, 289, 292
epiglottitis, 294
hazards and complications in, 344
humidifiers, 340
masks, 341–343
nasal cannulae, 341
near-drowning, 28, 29, 30–31, 33
respiratory care, 340–355
respiratory failure, 273
status asthmaticus, 303
status epilepticus, 87

Pancreas
injury to 386–388
shock, 143
Pancuronium (Pavulon), 29
Papillomas, 189
Para-amino salicyclic acid, 107
Parainfectious encephalomyelitis, 38
Para-influenza virus type 1, 282
Paraldehyde, 91
Paralysis, 432
Parkland formula, 416, 417, 418
Patient history
bleeding disorders, 459–460, 461
burns, 415
coma, 45
infections, 482
poisonings, 428
status asthmaticus, 301
Pavulon (Pancuronium), 29
Pelvic injury, 389–390
Penicillin, 99, 100, 101–102, 103, 106, 423
Pentobarbital coma, 29–30
Percussion, 346
Percutaneous liver needle biopsy, 47
Perfusion pressure, 11, 12
Periorbital ecchymosis, 60
Peritoneal dialysis, 445
Peritoneal lavage, 377, 378
Pharynx, 188
Phenobarbital, 89–91
Phenytoin, 67, 89–91
Pheochromocytoma, 48
Phosphorus, 500
Phosphorylase, 82
Pickwick syndrome, 48
Pierre-Robin syndrome, 188
Plasma, 475, 476
Plasmin, 458
Platelet count, 470
Platelet disorders, 457, 460, 473
Platelets
bleeding disorders, 474–475
factors of, 458
Pleural effusion, 325–337
clinical presentation, 327
diagnosis, 327–328
differential diagnosis, 331–334
pathophysiology, 326–327
prevention, 336
prognosis, 336
therapy, 334–336
Pleural fluid, 238–239
Pneumatocele, 260
Pneumoccocal meningitis, 37
Pneumocystic carinii, 508, 509
Pneumomediastinum, 235, 237–238, 248
Pneumonia
clinical presentation, 505
diagnosis, 505–508
pathophysiology, 503–504
pleural effusion, 334, 336
prevention, 510
radiology, 241
treatment, 509–510
Pneumopericardium, 239–240
Pneumothorax
asthma, 248
radiology, 233–235, 236
traumatic injury, 374–375
Poiseuille law, 8
Poison Prevention Packaging Act (1970), 427
Poisonings, 427–456
absorption prevention, 438–444
accidental versus self-induced, 427
agents in, 428
antidotes, 447–448, 450–453
coma, 41, 52
diagnosis, 428–436
dialysis, 445, 446
forced diuresis, 444–445
future trends in treatment of, 449
hemoperfusion, 445, 446, 447
incidence, 427–428
information centers, 448–449
symptoms and signs, 432–433
treatment, 437–449
Porphyria, 48
Portable nuclear camera, 133
Positive End Expiratory Pressure (PEEP), 351–354, 359–360
Postinfectious encephalomyelitis, 38
Postural drainage, 345
Potassium, 111, 143, 421
Premature infants
fungal meningitis, 111
neonatal sepsis syndrome, 488
sudden infant death syndrome, 548

Pressure-volume index, 15
Prothrombin time (PT), 468–469
Pseudocysts, 387–388
Pulmonary arterial and capillary wedge pressure (PCWP), 128–129
Pulmonary artery, 203, 209
Pulmonary artery wedge pressure, 142
Pulmonary contusion, 375
Pulmonary edema, 225–226, 286–287
Pulmonary embolism, 473–474
Pulmonary heart disease. See *Cor pulmonale*
Pulmonary hypertension, 161, 162–163
Pulmonary sling, 203, 209
Pulsed Doppler echocardiography, 132 *See also* Echocardiography
Pulse rate, 432
Pupillary response
  coma, 46–47
  head injury, 61–62, 63
  poisonings, 432
  See also Eye

Racemic epinephrine, 290–291, 294
  See also Epinephrine
Radiology
  abdominal injury, 376
  acute epiglottitis, 194, 200–201
  adult respiratory distress syndrome, 228, 232–233
  alveolar edema, 228
  anomalous pulmonary artery, 203, 209
  aortic tear, 263–264
  asthma, 243, 248–252
  brain injury, 65, 67, 69
  bronchial fracture, 263
  cardiac injury, 264
  colonic injury, 389
  cor pulmonale, 164
  croup and epiglottitis, 194, 279, 283
  diaphragmatic hernia, 252–253
  diaphragmatic injury, 264
  duodenal injury, 386
  epiglottitis and croup, 194, 279, 283
  foreign bodies, 523–536, 537
  interstitial edema, 228
  intestinal injury, 385
  jejunoileal injuries, 388
  larynx, 189, 194
  liver injury, 383–384
  lung contusion, 254, 256
  lung hematoma, 256
  lung infection, 241–243
  lung trauma, 253–254
  nasopharynx, 175, 180–185
  obstructive airway lesions, 173–175
  oral cavity, 188
  pelvic injury, 389–390
  pharynx, 188
  pleural effusion, 327–329
  pneumatocele, 260
  pneumomediastinum, 235, 237–238
  pneumonia, 505
  pneumothorax, 233–235, 236
  poisonings, 444
  pulmonary edema, 225–226
  pulmonary laceration, 256, 260
  respiratory care, 355
  retropharyngeal space, 188–189
  rib fractures, 263
  shock, 142
  skull injury, 60
  spinal injury, 396–397, 399
  splenic injury, 378–379, 380–381
  status asthmaticus, 302
  sudden infant death syndrome, 561
  thorax, 225–264, 374–375
  tonsils, 182–183
Radiology (*Continued*)
  tumors, 203
  vascular ring, 203
  See also Computed tomography
Radionuclide cardiac angiography, 166
Radionuclide scan
  liver injury, 383–384
  spleen injury, 378–379, 380–381
Raised intracranial pressure, 16–17
REM sleep, 546, 555
Renal. *See* Kidney
Respiration
  burns, 410
  cardiac arrest, 150
  cardiopulmonary resuscitation, 152–153
  coma, 46
  epiglottitis, 280
  foreign bodies, 520
  poisonings, 432–433
  septic shock syndrome, 495–496
  shock, 140, 147
  spinal cord injury, 399, 401, 403
  status epilepticus, 82
Respirator
  adult respiratory distress syndrome, 319
  respiratory failure, 274, 275
Respiratory arrest, 40
Respiratory care, 339–368
  chest physiotherapy (CPT), 345–346
  High Frequency Ventilation (HFV), 354–355
  intubation, 346–348
  mechanical ventilation, 348–349
  monitoring, 355–366
  oxygen therapy, 340–355
  ventilators, 349–355
Respiratory distress syndrome. *See* Adult respiratory distress syndrome
Respiratory failure, 269–276
  clinical course of, 272–273
  etiology of, 269–270
  pathophysiology of, 270–271
  therapy, 273–275
  types of, 271–272
Respiratory papillomas, 189
Retropharyngeal space, 188–189
Reye's syndrome, A-1–A-6
  age distribution, A-2
  coma, 39, 47, 49
  defined, A-1
  diagnosis, A-1–A-2
  therapeutic goals, A-5
  treatment, A-3–A-5
Rhabdomyosarcoma, 185, 190, 191
Rib fracture, 263
Rickettsial infection, 37–38
Rifampin, 99, 100, 102, 107

Salbutamol, 307
Salt water drowning, 27, 31
Secondary drowning, 26
Second degree burns, 411, 412
Segmental breathing, 246
Seizures
  airway, 44
  brain abscesses, 37
  brain injury, 67
  coma, 48, 50
  head injury, 59
  microvascular occlusion, 43
  Reye's syndrome, 39
  status epilepticus, 81, 83–85
  sudden infant death syndrome, 561
  viral encephalitis, 37
Semi-coma, 35
Septic shock (endotoxic shock) syndrome, 137, 138, 493–503
  catheterization, 142

Septic shock (endotoxic shock) syndrome (*Continued*)
clinical presentation, 496
defined, 493–494
diagnosis, 497
pathophysiology, 138–139, 494–496
prevention, 502–503
treatment, 497–502
Sex differences
croup, 281
drowning, 26
Shock, 137–148
burns, 416, 417
classification and etiology, 137–138
clinical presentation, 140–141
defined, 137
liver injury, 383
monitoring of, 141–144
pathophysiology, 138–140
poisonings, 437
septic shock syndrome, 495–496
therapy, 144–147
Shock lung, 140, 142
SIDS. *See* Sudden infant death syndrome
Skin
monitoring pH of, 133
poisonings, 433
Skin grafting, 423–424
Skin temperature, 125
See also Body temperature
Skull fracture, 57
Skull injury
diagnosis, 60–61
therapy, 62–64
See also Brain; Head injury
Sleep, 546, 551–558
Sodium bicarbonate, 154–155, 305
Sodium nitroprusside, 146–147
Spasmodic croup, 281
Spinal cord injury, 393–407
biochemical factors in, 397–399
bladder and gastrointestinal tract considerations in, 405
cervical spine, 397–398
clinical features, 399–401
epidemiology, 393–395
pharmacologic treatment, 405–406
radiology, 396–397
surgical intervention, 404–405
symptomatic treatment, 403–404
thoracolumbar fracture, 398–399
transportation of victims, 402
traumatic injury, 372–373
treatment, 401–403
Spleen
abdominal injury, 376, 377
bleeding disorders, 464
injury of, 378–379, 380–381
Staphylococcus aureus, 490, 496, 507
Status asthmaticus, 299–307
assessment, 301–303
defined, 299
management, 303–306
pathophysiology, 300–301
radiology, 243, 248–252
respiratory failure, 306–307
Status epilepticus
anticonvulsant therapy, 88–92
clinical presentation, 83–85
complications, 79–80
defined, 79
diagnosis and evaluation, 87
neonates, 82, 85–86
pathology, 82–83
pathophysiology, 80–82
treatment, 86–87
Steroids
brain injury, 72
Steroids (*Continued*)
croup, 291–292
tuberculosis meningitis, 107
See also Corticosteroids
Stomach
burns, 419
injury to, 385
Streptococcus pneumoniae, 101–102
Streptomycin, 106, 107
Stupor, 35
Subarachnoid blood, 58
Subarachnoid cisterns, 6
Subarachnoid hemorrhage, 46
Subarachnoid space, 6
Subfalcine herniation, 18
Subgaleal hematoma, 62–63
Subglottic hemangioma, 189
Subglottic stenosis, 519
Suctioning, 356
Sudden infant death syndrome
apnea types and, 546–551
home monitoring, 565–575
program for, 545–546
program operations and protocol, 560–565
sleep and, 551–558
study groups in, 558–559
Sulfonamides, 99, 101, 493
Sunburn, 411
Supraglottitis
radiology, 194, 200–201
See also Epiglottitis
Surgery
bleeding disorders, 460, 461–462, 473–474
nosocomial infection, 487
Swan-Ganz catheter. *See* Catheterization
Sympathomimetic amines, 145
Sympathomimetic drugs, 304–305
Synchronized Intermittent Mandatory Ventilation (SIMV), 351
Syrup of ipecac, 438–439, 440, 441
Systemic blood pressure. *See* Blood pressure
Systolic arterial pressure, 127

Tachycardia, 150
T-bars, 343
Temperature. *See* Body temperature; Hyperthermia; Hypothermia
Tentorium cerebelli, 6
Tents (oxygen), 342
Tetanus toxoid booster, 420
Tetracycline, 100, 106
Theophylline, 304
Third degree burns, 411, 412
Thoracentesis, 334, 335
Thoracic examination, 46
Thoracic injury, 374–376
Thoracolumbar fractures, 398–399
Thoractomy, 374–375
Thorax
adult respiratory distress syndrome, 228, 232–233
alveolar edema, 228
aortic tear, 263–264
asthma, 243, 248–252
bronchial fracture, 263
cardiac injury, 264
diaphragmatic hernia, 252–253
diaphragmatic injury, 264
interstitial edema, 228
lung contusion, 254, 256
lung hematoma, 256
lung infection, 241–243
lung trauma, 253–254
pleural fluid, 238–239
pneumatocele, 260
pneumomediastinum, 235, 237–238
pneumothorax, 233–235, 236

Thorax (*Continued*)
pulmonary laceration, 256, 260
radiology, 225–264
rib fractures, 263
Thrombin, 458, 459
Thrombin time, 470
Thrombocytopathy, 473
Thrombocytopenia, 457–460, 463–464, 473
Thrombosis, 473–474
Thyroglossal cysts, 188
Tonsillar herniation, 18
Tonsils, 182–183
Toxic shock syndrome, 496, 497
Trachea
foreign bodies, 519, 523
injury to, 375
Tracheostomy collars, 342
Traction, 402
Transcutaneous monitors, 133
Transcutaneous Po_2/Pco_2, 361–362
Transient mild brain injury, 61
Transtentorial herniation, 18
Traube-Hering-Mayer phenomenon, 17
Traumatic injury, 371–391
abdominal injury, 376–378
causes, 371, 372
extent of, 371
genitourinary injury, 390
intestinal injury, 385–389
kidney injury, 382-383
liver injury, 383–384
pelvic injury, 389–390
prevention of, 371
priorities in treatment, 372–374
splenic injury, 378–379
thoracic injury, 374–376
Tuberculosis
meningitis, 37, 106–107
pneumonia, 508
Tuberculosis meningitis, 37, 106–107
Tube thoracostomy, 374–375
Tumors
airway, 203
intracranial, 39
Two-dimensional echocardiography, 132
See also Echocardiography

Ultrasound, 131–132
Universal Antidote, 441
Upward tentorial herniation, 18
Uremia, 465
Urethral injury, 390
Urinary bladder, 405
Urine output
cardiovascular monitoring, 125–126
Urine output (*Continued*)
poisonings, 444–445
shock, 142–143
Uvula
enlargement, 188
rhabdomyosarcoma, 190, 191

Valproic acid, 92
Vancomycin, 102
Vascular ring, 203
Vascular system
bleeding disorders, 458–459, 473
brain, 7–12, 19–20
cardiopulmonary resuscitation, 151–152
coma, 41–43
cor pulmonale, 161–162
pelvic injury, 389–390
septic shock syndrome, 496
shock, 139–140
spinal cord injury, 403–404
traumatic injury, 373
Vectorcardiogram, 164
Ventilation. *See* Oxygen therapy; Respiration
Ventilators, 349–355
adult ventilator modification, 349
blood gases, 357
inhalation injury, 412
modes in, 349–352
pediatric, 350
weaning from, 362–364
Venturi mask, 341–342
Vibration, 346
Viral encephalitis, 37
Viral infection
central nervous system, 109–110
croup, 281, 282
epiglottitis, 200
fungal meningitis, 111–112
lung infection, 241
nosocomial, 487
Vitamin deficiency
coma, 41, 42, 50
vitamin K, 463, 464, 501
Vocal cord paralysis, 189
Volume-pressure relationships, 12–15
Volume-pressure response, 15
Vomiting. *See* Emesis
Von Willebrand's disease, 466–467, 475

Waterhouse-Friderichsen syndrome, 496
Weight. *See* Body weight
White matter, 6, 8
Wiskott-Aldrich syndrome, 473